IMPORTANT

W9-BNO-158

BEQQ–EUG4–7KFV–PAV6–3V8X

HERE IS YOUR REGISTRATION CODE TO ACCESS MCGRAW-HILL PREMIUM CONTENT AND MCGRAW-HILL ONLINE RESOURCES

For key premium online resources you need THIS CODE to gain access. Once the code is entered, you will be able to use the web resources for the length of your course.

Access is provided only if you have purchased a new book.

If the registration code is missing from this book, the registration screen on our website, and within your WebCT or Blackboard·course will tell you how to obtain your new code. Your registration code can be used only once to establish access. It is not transferable.

To gain access to these online resources

1. **USE** your web browser to go to: **http://www.mhhe.com/hahn8e**

2. **CLICK** on "First Time User"

3. **ENTER** the Registration Code printed on the tear-off bookmark on the right

4. After you have entered your registration code, click on "Register"

5. **FOLLOW** the instructions to setup your personal UserID and Password

6. **WRITE** your UserID and Password down for future reference. Keep it in a safe place.

If your course is using WebCT or Blackboard, you'll be able to use this code to access the McGraw-Hill content within your instructor's online course.

To gain access to the McGraw-Hill content in your instructor's WebCT or Blackboard course simply log into the course with the user ID and Password provided by your instructor. Enter the registration code exactly as it appears to the right when prompted by the system. You will only need to use this code the first time you click on McGraw-Hill content.

These instructions are specifically for student access. Instructors are not required to register via the above instructions.

REGISTRATION CODE

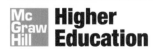

The McGraw·Hill Companies

Thank you, and welcome to your McGraw-Hill Online Resources.

13 Digit: 978-0-07-302849-1
10 Digit: 0-07-302849-5
t/a Focus on Health, 8e

Focus on Health

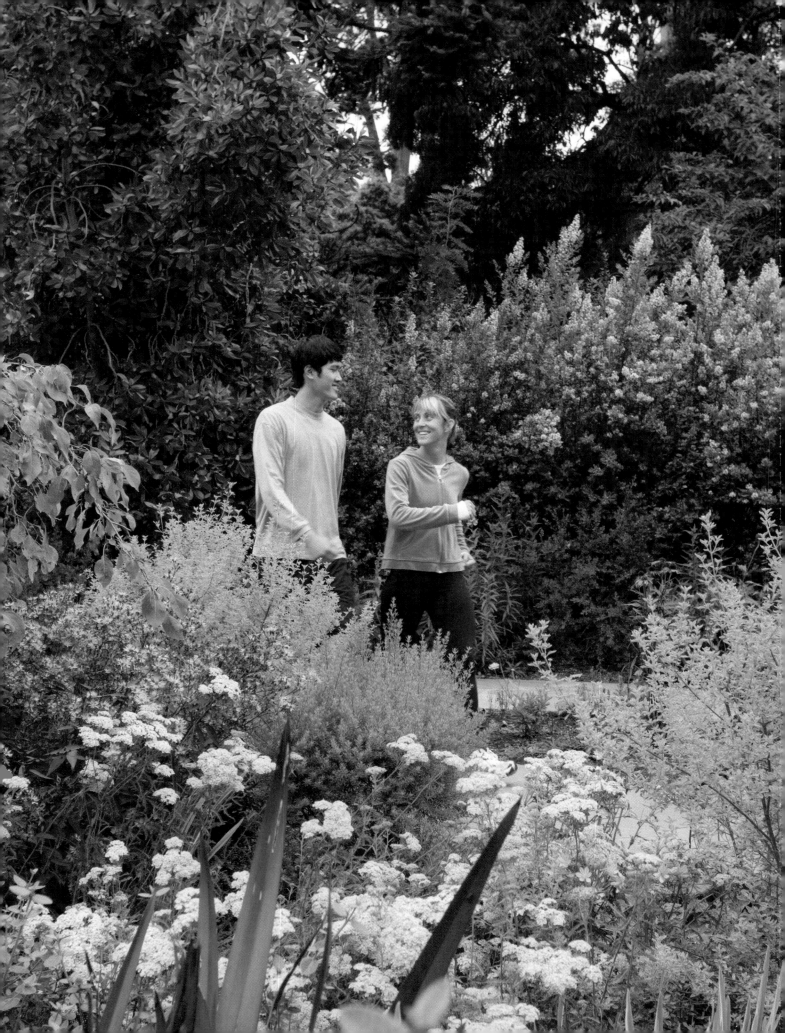

Focus on Health

Eighth Edition

Dale B. Hahn, Ph.D.

Wayne A. Payne, Ed.D.

Ellen B. Lucas, Ph.D.

All of Ball State University
Muncie, Indiana

Boston   Burr Ridge, IL   Dubuque, IA   Madison, WI   New York   San Francisco   St. Louis
Bangkok   Bogotá   Caracas   Kuala Lumpur   Lisbon   London   Madrid   Mexico City
Milan   Montreal   New Delhi   Santiago   Seoul   Singapore   Sydney   Taipei   Toronto

*To all of our students, with the hope that the
decisions they make will be healthy ones.*

The McGraw·Hill Companies

Higher Education

FOCUS ON HEALTH
Published by McGraw-Hill, a business unit of The McGraw-Hill Companies, Inc., 1221 Avenue
of the Americas, New York, NY 10020. Copyright © 2007 by The McGraw-Hill Companies,
Inc. All rights reserved. No part of this publication may be reproduced or distributed in any
form or by any means, or stored in a database or retrieval system, without the prior written
consent of The McGraw-Hill Companies, Inc., including, but not limited to, in any network
or other electronic storage or transmission, or broadcast for distance learning.
Some ancillaries, including electronic and print components, may not be available to customers
outside the United States.

This book is printed on acid-free paper.

1 2 3 4 5 6 7 8 9 0 WCK/WCK 0 9 8 7 6

ISBN-13: 978-0-07-302842-2
ISBN-10: 0-07-302842-8

Vice president and editor-in-chief: *Emily Barrosse*
Publisher: *William R. Glass*
Sponsoring editor: *Christopher Johnson*
Director of development: *Kathleen Engelberg*
Developmental editor: *Nadia Bidwell for Van Brien & Associates*
Developmental editor for technology: *Julia Ersery*
Senior marketing manager: *Pamela S. Cooper*
Media producer: *Ron Nelms*
Production editor: *Mel Valentín*
Production supervisor: *Carol Bielski*
Senior designer: *Kim Menning*
Cover design: *Yuo Riezebos*
Interior design: *Jeanne Calabrese/Glenda King*
Lead media project manager: *Marc Mattson*
Photo research coordinator: *Alexandra Ambrose*
Art editor: *Ayelet Arbel*
Art director: *Jeanne Schreiber*
Cover design: *Kim Menning*
Typeface: *10.5/12 Minion*
Compositor: *GTS—LA Campus*
Printer: *Quebecor-Versailles*
Cover image: © *The McGraw-Hill Companies, Inc./Christopher Kerrigan, photographer*

The credits section for this book begins on page C-1 and is considered an extension of the
copyright page.

Library of Congress Cataloging-in-Publication Data

Hahn, Dale B.
    Focus on health/Dale B. Hahn, Wayne A. Payne, Ellen B. Lucas—8th ed.
        p. cm.
    Includes bibliographical references and index.
    ISBN 0-07-302842-8 (alk. paper)
    1. Health. I. Payne, Wayne A. II. Lucas, Ellen B. III. Title.

RA776.H142 2006
613—dc22
                                                    2005058031

www.mhhe.com

contents in brief

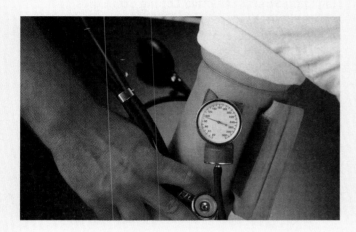

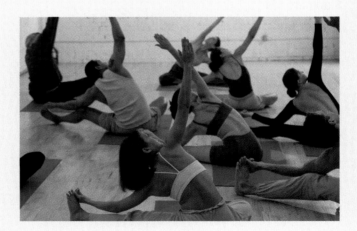

Part One: The Mind 31

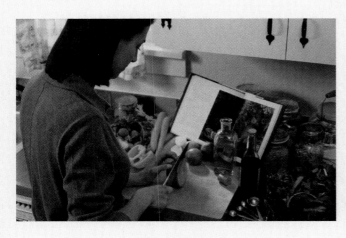

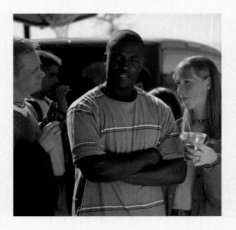

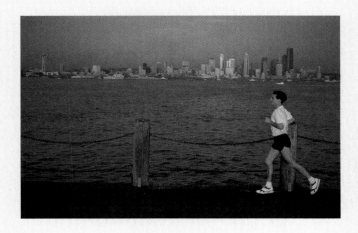

Part Four: Preventing Diseases   248

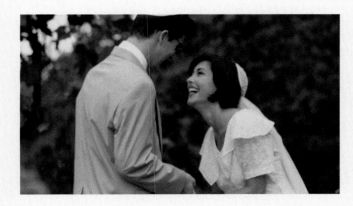

Part Five: Sexuality and Reproduction 336

Part Six: Consumer and Safety Issues   396

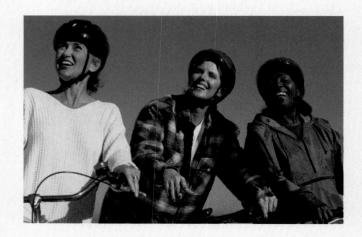

Preface

As a health educator, you already know that personal health is one of the most exciting courses a college student will take. Today's media-oriented college students are aware of the critical health issues of the new millennium. They hear about environmental issues, substance abuse, sexually transmitted diseases, fitness, and nutrition virtually every day. The value of the personal health course is its potential to expand students' knowledge of these and other health topics. Students will then be able to examine their attitudes toward health issues and modify their behavior to improve their health and perhaps even prevent or delay the onset of certain health conditions.

Focus on Health accomplishes this task with a carefully composed, well-documented text that addresses the health issues most important to both instructors and students. As health educators, we understand the teaching issues you face daily in the classroom and have written this text with your concerns in mind.

Hallmarks of the Text

Several unique themes and features set *Focus on Health* apart from other personal health texts. These successful features continue to define *Focus on Health* in its eighth edition.

A Text for All Students

This book is written for college students in a wide variety of settings, from community colleges to large four-year universities. The content is carefully constructed to be meaningful to both traditional- and nontraditional-age students. We have paid special attention to the increasing numbers of nontraditional-age students (those over age 25) who have decided to pursue a college education. The topics covered in the text often address the particular needs of these nontraditional-age students. *Focus on Health* continues to encourage students of all ages and backgrounds to achieve their goals.

Two Central Themes

Two central themes—the multiple dimensions of health and the developmental tasks—are presented in Chapter 1. Together, these two themes offer students a foundation for understanding their own health and achieving positive behavior change.

Flexible Organization

The eighth edition of *Focus on Health* has 18 chapters. The first stands alone as an introductory chapter that explains the focus of the book. The arrangement of the remaining chapters follows the recommendations of both the users of previous editions of the book and reviewers for this edition. Of course, professors can choose to cover the chapters in any sequence that suits the needs of their courses.

Wellness and Disease Prevention

Throughout this new edition, students are continually urged to be proactive in shaping their future health. Even the chapter titles invite students to take control of their health behavior.

Integrated Presentation of Aging

Topics of interest to midlife and older adults are integrated into appropriate chapters according to subject. This organization allows both traditional-age and nontraditional-age students to learn about the physical and emotional changes that take place as we age.

Timely Coverage of Cancer and Chronic Conditions

Rapid developments in cancer prevention, diagnosis, and treatment warrant a comprehensive chapter on cancer, in which we present the latest research and information. The chapter also includes information on some of the most common chronic conditions.

Technology: The Key to Teaching and Learning

Just a quick glance through the pages of *Focus on Health* shows that technology is woven throughout every chapter, both in the content and in the chapter pedagogy. Similarly, the package of supplements that accompanies the text emphasizes technology while acknowledging that printed materials also have merit. Together, the text and its supplements offer the ideal approach to teaching and learning—one that integrates the best tools that technology has to offer, challenging both instructors and students to reach higher.

Updated Coverage

As experienced health educators and authors, we know how important it is to provide students with the most current information available. The eighth edition of *Focus on Health* has been thoroughly updated with the latest information, statistics, and findings. Throughout each chapter, we have incorporated new examples and discussions, from information on newly available prescription drugs and medications (Chapters 2, 3, 11, and 15), to the latest information on dieting and supplements (Chapters 5 and 6).

Another exciting change to this edition of *Focus on Health* is the addition of a new chapter, Chapter 18, Accepting Dying and Death. Written by coauthor Ellen B. Lucas, Ph.D., this chapter presents information about the psychological stages of death; coping with grief and the loss of friends, parents, and children; hospice care; euthanasia; and physician-assisted suicide. The chapter also offers important practical advice for preparing advance health care directives.

In addition to these topics, we have once again included chapter-ending "As We Go To Press" boxes in relevant chapters. These unique boxes allow us to comment on breaking news right up to press time, ensuring that the most current issues in health are addressed. For example, in Chapter 2 we discuss the concern and controversy over prescription antidepressants for children, and in Chapter 18 we touch on the growing trend of cryogenic freezing.

New or Expanded Topics

Following is a sampling of topics that are either completely new to this edition or are covered in greater depth than in the previous edition:

Chapter 1: Shaping Your Health

- Traditional definitions of health
- Composition and role of health
- Leading causes of death for Americans under 80 years of age

Chapter 2: Achieving Psychological Health

- Advertising psychological medications
- How to say "sorry" and mean it
- Personality types
- Attention Deficit Disorder

Chapter 3: Managing Stress

- New technological stressors
- Stress is different for different populations
- Yoga
- Antidotes to anger

Chapter 4: Becoming Physically Fit

- Anterior and posterior musculature charts

Chapter 5: Understanding Nutrition and Your Diet

- Low-carb diets
- New USDA food guidelines
- Food and spirituality
- Phytochemicals
- Sample 2,000-calorie menu
- Updated fast-food choices
- Food pyramids of other cultures

Chapter 6: Maintaining a Healthy Weight

- Reality television and body image
- Religion and dieting
- Dieting myths
- Childhood obesity
- Clothing sizes around the world
- Surgical intervention

Chapter 7: Making Decisions about Drug Use

- Effects of Methamphetamine abuse
- Warning signs of a meth lab
- Ritalin and Adderall abuse on campus

Chapter 8: Taking Control of Alcohol Use

- Dangers of drinking games
- Alcohol absorption and race

Chapter 9: Rejecting Tobacco Use

- Smoking statistics by state
- Carcinogenic agents
- Sexual dysfunction and infertility
- Employment-related consequences of smoking
- International smoking bans

Chapter 10: Enhancing Your Cardiovascular Health

- Hypertension
- Cholesterol levels
- Updated statistics on cardiovascular disease

Chapter 11: Living with Cancer and Chronic Conditions

- Updated statistics on cancer
- Cancer screening guidelines
- Genetic markers
- Role of self-examination in the detection of breast cancer
- Expanded discussion of diabetes
- Changing pharmaceutical choices in treating IBDs
- Expanded discussion of multiple sclerosis
- Revised classification for Alzheimer's

Chapter 12: Preventing Infectious Diseases

- Immunization schedule
- 2004–2005 influenza vaccine shortage
- Lyme disease
- Bird influenza
- Updated HIV/AIDS statistics

Chapter 13: Understanding Sexuality

- Irregular menstrual cycles
- Changing diet to improve fibrocystic breast condition
- Same-sex marriage
- Comparison of drug treatments for erectile dysfunction

Chapter 14: Managing Your Fertility

- Contraceptive effectiveness table
- Standard Days method of periodic abstinence
- Abstinence as birth control
- New methods of contraception
- Side effects of emergency hormonal contraception

- New method of female sterilization (the Essure coil)
- Partial birth abortion
- Therapeutic cloning

Chapter 15: Becoming an Informed Health Care Consumer

- The Internet
- Alternative forms of health care
- Self-diagnosis
- Lack of health insurance
- Medicare prescription drug coverage
- The FDA's drug approval process

Chapter 16: Protecting Your Safety

- Identity theft
- Driving distractions

Chapter 17: The Environment and Your Health

- Media hype
- Religious perspectives on the Human-Environment relationship
- Non-ionizing radiation
- Polycyclic aromatic hydrocarbons
- Species extinction and the loss of natural habitats

Chapter 18: Accepting Dying and Death

- Definitions of death
- Psychological stages of death
- Advance health care directives
- Coping with specific causes of death
- Euthanasia
- Physician-assisted suicide
- Near-death experiences
- Interacting with dying people
- Discussing death with children
- Hospice care
- Death rituals

Student-Friendly Chapter Pedagogy

Each chapter of *Focus on Health* is rich with pedagogical features that offer a variety of ways to address new and emerging health issues and to pique student interest in particular topics.

Chapter Objectives

Each chapter begins with a set of clear objectives that help students distill the most important concepts in the pages that follow.

Taking Charge of Your Health

Located at the end of each chapter, these bulleted lists invite students to put the knowledge and information they've gleaned from the chapter to work in their everyday lives. Cross-referencing the text with Internet links and real-world situations allows students to see how what they've learned can be applied in their own lives.

Eye on the Media

Face it—a student's world revolves around media of all types, especially the Web. Students get most of their health information not from instructors and textbooks but from television, self-help books, popular news magazines, the Web, and the radio. To meet students on this familiar ground, we've included Eye on the Media boxes (see the inside front cover for a list of these boxes), which take a critical look at these media sources of health information.

Discovering Your Spirituality

Spirituality has become an important focus in health courses. Discovering Your Spirituality boxes (see the inside front cover for a list of these boxes) highlight the spiritual dimension of health and its effect on overall wellness. The boxes cover topics such as body image, living well with cancer or a chronic infectious disease, making decisions about sex, and having an enjoyable social life without abusing alcohol or other drugs.

Talking Points

Interspersed throughout each chapter, Talking Points offer students opportunities to explore how they might start a dialogue about specific health-related issues and situations.

Changing for the Better

These unique question-and-answer boxes show students how to put health concepts into practice. Each box begins with a real-life question, followed by helpful tips and practical advice for initiating behavior change and staying motivated to follow a healthy lifestyle.

Learning from Our Diversity

These boxes expose students to alternative viewpoints and highlight what we can learn from the differences that make us unique. Topics include the Mediterranean Food Pyramid, the male contraceptive pill, and special issues related to infectious disease among older adults.

Star Boxes

In each chapter, special material in Star boxes encourages students to delve into a particular topic or closely examine an important health issue.

Personal Assessments

Each chapter contains at least one Personal Assessment inventory. These self-assessment exercises serve three important functions: to capture students' attention, to serve as a basis for introspection and behavior change, and to provide suggestions for carrying the applications further.

Definition Boxes

Key terms are set in boldface type and defined in corresponding boxes. Pronunciation guides are provided where appropriate. Other important terms in the text are set in italics for emphasis. Both approaches facilitate student vocabulary comprehension.

Chapter Summaries

Each chapter concludes with a bulleted summary of key concepts and their significance or application. The student can then return to any topic in the chapter for clarification or study.

Review Questions

A set of questions appears at the end of each chapter to aid the student in review and analysis of chapter content.

Comprehensive Health Assessment

The Comprehensive Health Assessment at the end of Chapter 1 allows students to take a close look at their current state of health, typical health behavior, and risk factors. Using this assessment, students can pinpoint trouble spots in their own health behavior and find out what they can do to reduce their risk of disease or other health conditions. At the end of the semester, they can take a look at their previous answers to see how their behavior changed as they learned more about health and wellness issues.

Health Reference Guide

The updated Health Reference Guide at the back of the book lists many commonly used health resources. Internet addresses, phone numbers, and mailing addresses of various organizations and government agencies are provided as available. The guide is perforated and laminated, making it durable enough for students to keep for later use.

Vegetarian Food Pyramid

Many students now follow or are considering a vegetarian diet. To help them understand how such a diet meets nutrient needs, we have printed a vegetarian food pyramid along with the USDA Food Guide Pyramid in Chapter 5.

Comprehensive Glossary

At the end of the text, all terms defined in boxes, as well as pertinent italicized terms, are merged into a comprehensive glossary.

Supplements

An extensive supplements package is available to qualified adopters to enhance the teaching-learning process. We have made a concerted effort to produce supplements of extraordinary utility and quality. This package has been carefully planned and developed to help instructors derive the greatest benefit from the text. We encourage instructors to examine them carefully. Many of the products can be packaged with the text at a discounted price. Beyond the following brief descriptions, additional information about these supplements is available from your McGraw-Hill sales representative.

Integrated Instructor's Resource CD

Organized by chapter, the Instructor's Resource CD includes resources to help you teach your course. The CD will work in both Windows and Macintosh environments and includes the following elements:

- **Course Integrator Guide** This guide includes all the useful features of an instructor's manual, such as learning objectives, suggested lecture outlines, suggested activities, media resources, and Web links. It also integrates the text with all the related resources McGraw-Hill offers, such as the Online Learning Center, the HealthQuest CD-ROM, and the Health and Human Performance Discipline Page. The guide also includes references to relevant print and broadcast media.

- **Test Bank** This file includes more than 1,000 questions, including multiple-choice, true/false, and short essay. It has been rewritten to enhance clarity, and it now includes critical thinking questions and more applications questions.
- **Computerized Test Bank** McGraw-Hill's Computerized Testing is the most flexible and easy-to-use electronic testing program available in higher education. The program allows instructors to create tests from book-specific test banks and to add their own questions. It accommodates a wide range of question types, and multiple versions of the test can be created. The program is available for Windows, Macintosh, and Linux environments.
- **PowerPoint** A complete set of PowerPoint lecture slides for the course is included on the Instructor's Resource CD, as well as on the instructor's portion of the Online Learning Center. This presentation, ready to use in class, was prepared by a professional in the field of health and fitness. It corresponds to the content in each chapter of *Focus on Health*, making it easier for you to teach and ensuring that your students can follow your lectures point by point. You can modify the presentation as much as you like to meet the needs of your course.

Online Learning Center

The Online Learning Center to accompany this text offers a number of additional resources for both students and instructors. Many study tools are open to all students. Premium content such as assessments and PowerWeb require student registration using the passcode that comes free with new books. Visit this Web site to find useful materials such as the following:

For the instructor

- Downloadable PowerPoint presentations
- Course Integrator Guide

For the student

- Self-scoring chapter quizzes and online study guides
- Flash cards and crossword puzzles for learning key terms and their definitions
- Learning objectives
- Interactive activities
- Web links for study and exploration of topics in the text
- Online labs
- Wellness worksheets
- PowerWeb
- Newsfeeds
- Student success strategies

HealthQuest CD-ROM, by Bob Gold and Nancy Atkinson

The HealthQuest CD-ROM helps students explore their wellness behavior using state-of-the-art interactive technology. Students can assess their current health status, determine their risks, and explore options for positive lifestyle change. Tailored feedback gives students a meaningful and individualized learning experience without using valuable classroom time. Modules include the Wellboard (a health self-assessment); Stress Management and Mental Health; Fitness; Nutrition and Weight Control; Communicable Diseases; Cardiovascular Health; Cancer; Tobacco, Alcohol, and Other Drugs. An online Instructor's Manual presents ideas for incorporating HealthQuest into your course.

Fitness and Nutrition Log

This logbook helps students track their diet and exercise programs. It serves as a diary to help students monitor their behaviors. It can be packaged with any McGraw-Hill textbook for a small additional fee.

PowerWeb

www.dushkin.com/online

The PowerWeb Web site is a reservoir of course-specific articles and current events. Students can visit PowerWeb to take a self-scoring quiz, complete an interactive exercise, click through an interactive glossary, or check the daily news. An expert in each discipline analyzes the day's news to show students how it relates to their field of study.

PowerWeb is part of the Online Learning Center. Students are also granted full access to Dushkin/McGraw-Hill's Student Site, where they can read study tips, conduct Web research, learn about different career paths, and follow links on the Web.

Wellness Worksheets

This collection of activities and assessments helps students become more involved in their own wellness and better prepared to implement behavior change programs. It includes over 120 assessments under the topics of General Wellness and Behavior Change; Stress Management; Psychological and Spiritual Wellness; Intimate Relationships and Communication; Sexuality; Addictive Behaviors and Drug Dependence; Nutrition; Physical Activity and Exercise; Weight Management; Chronic Diseases: Cardiovascular Disease and Cancer; Infectious Diseases; Aging, Dying, and Death; Consumer Health; Personal

Safety; and Environmental Health. They are available online in the premium content or may be packaged with the text at minimal cost.

NutritionCalc Plus

http://nutritioncalc.mhhe.com

NutritionCalc Plus (ISBN 0-07-292084-X) is a dietary analysis program with an easy-to-use interface that allows users to track their nutrient and food group intakes, energy expenditures, and weight control goals. It generates a variety of reports and graphs for analysis, including comparisons with the Food Guide Pyramid and the latest Dietary Reference Intakes (DRIs). The database includes thousands of ethnic foods, supplements, fast foods, and convenience foods, and users can add their own foods to the food list. NutritionCalc Plus is available on CD-ROM or in an online version.

Video Library

The McGraw-Hill Video Library contains many quality videotapes, including selected videos from the *Films for Humanities* series and all the videos from the award-winning *Healthy Living: Road to Wellness* series. Digitized video clips are also available (see Healthy Living Video Clips CD-ROM). The library also features *Students on Health,* a unique video filmed on college campuses across the country that includes eight brief segments, 8 to 10 minutes long, featuring students involved in discussion and role play on health issues. Finally, an additional video—*McGraw-Hill Health Video*—is available. This video features brief clips on a wide range of topics of interest in personal health courses. Contact your McGraw-Hill sales representative to discuss eligibility to receive videos.

PageOut: The Course Web Site Development Center

www.pageout.net

PageOut, free to instructors who use a McGraw-Hill textbook, is an online program you can use to create your own course Web site. PageOut offers the following features:

- A course home page
- An instructor home page
- A syllabus (interactive and customizable, including quizzing, instructor notes, and links to the text's Online Learning Center)
- Web links
- Discussions (multiple discussion areas per class)
- An online gradebook
- Links to student Web pages

Contact your McGraw-Hill sales representative to obtain a password.

Course Management Systems

www.mhhe.com/solutions

Now instructors can combine their McGraw-Hill Online Learning Center with today's most popular course management systems. Our Instructor Advantage program offers customers access to a complete online teaching website called the Knowledge Gateway, prepaid, toll-free phone support, and unlimited e-mail support directly from WebCT and Blackboard. Instructors who use 500 or more copies of a McGraw-Hill textbook can enroll in our Instructor Advantage Plus program, which provides on-campus, hands-on training from a certified platform specialist. Consult your McGraw-Hill sales representative to learn what other course management systems are easily used with McGraw-Hill online materials.

Classroom Performance System

Classroom Performance System (CPS) brings interactivity into the classroom/lecture hall. It is a wireless response system that gives instructors and students immediate feedback from the entire class. The wireless response pads are essentially remotes that are easy to use and that engage students. CPS is available for both IBM and Mac computers.

The Wellness Workbook from Quia

The Wellness Workbook, developed in collaboration with Quia™, offers an electronic version of assessments and quizzes compiled from the text and its main supplements. This new online supplement offers students such benefits as interactive assessments, self-scoring quizzes, and instant feedback. Instructors benefit from a grade book that automatically scores, tracks, and records students' results and provides the opportunity to review individual and class performance. Instructors also have the ability to customize activities and features for their course by using Quia's™ activity templates. To find out more about this new online supplement and how you can package it with your textbook, contact your McGraw-Hill sales representative.

Primis Online

www.mhhe.com/primis/online

Primis Online is a database-driven publishing system that allows instructors to create content-rich textbooks, lab manuals, or readers for their courses directly from the Primis Web site. The customized text can be delivered in print or electronic (eBook) form. A Primis eBook is a digital version of the customized text (sold directly to students as a file downloadable to their computer or accessed online by a password). *Focus on Health*, eighth edition, is included in the database.

You Can Make a Difference: Be Environmentally Responsible, Second Edition, by Judith Getis

This handy text is organized around the three parts of the biosphere: land, water, and air. Each section contains descriptions of the environmental problems associated with that part of the biosphere. Immediately following the problems, or challenges, are suggested ways in which individuals and communities can help solve or alleviate them.

Annual Editions

Annual Editions is an ever-enlarging series of more than 70 volumes, each designed to provide convenient, low-cost access to a wide range of current, carefully selected articles from some of the most important magazines, newspapers, and journals published today. The articles, drawn from more than 400 periodical sources, are written by prominent scholars, researchers, and commentators. All *Annual Editions* have common organizational features, such as annotated tables of contents, topic guides, unit overviews, and indexes. In addition, a list of annotated websites is included. An Instructor's Resource Guide with testing suggestions for each volume is available to qualified instructors.

Taking Sides

www.dushkin.com/takingsides

McGraw-Hill/Dushkin's *Taking Sides* series currently consists of 22 volumes, with an instructor's guide with testing material available for each volume. The *Taking Sides* approach brings together the arguments of leading social and behavioral scientists, educators, and contemporary commentators, forming 18–20 debates, or issues, that present the pros and cons of current controversies in an area of study. An Issue Introduction that precedes the two opposing viewpoints gives students the proper context and historical background for each debate. After reading the debate, students are given other viewpoints to consider in the Issue Postscript, which also offers recommendations for further reading. *Taking Sides* fosters critical thinking in students and encourages them to develop a concern for serious social dialogue.

Acknowledgments

The publisher's reviewers made excellent comments and suggestions that were very useful to us in writing and revising this book. Their contributions are present in every chapter. We would like to express our sincere appreciation for both their critical and comparative readings.

For the Eighth Edition:

Robert Guthman, Jr.
University of Northern Colorado

Steve Hartman
Citrus College

Gary Ladd
Southwestern Illinois College

Mary Mock
University of South Dakota

Bikash Nandy
Minnesota State University

Kimberly Simpson-Kee
University of Akron

Jennifer Thomas
Emporia State University

Robert Walker
John Brown University

Bill Zuti
Radford University

For the Seventh Edition

Kari Barnumon
Moorpark College

Carol Biddington
California University of Pennsylvania

Susie Cousar
Lane Community College

William Ebomoyi
University of Northern Colorado

Caroline Crowther Fuller
Clemson University

Holly Henry
Chemeketa Community College

Marshall J. Meyer
Portland Community College–Sylvania

Lorette Oden
Western Illinois University

Todd Russell
University of Great Falls

Scott Wolf
Southeastern Illinois College

For the Sixth Edition

M. Betsy Bergen
Kansas State University

Sandra Bonneau
Golden West College

Sandra DiNatale
Keene State College

Lisa Everett
Las Positas College

Albert J. Figone
Humboldt State University

Neil E. Gallagher
Towson University

Amy Goff
Scottsdale Community College

Sharrie A. Herbold-Sheley
Lane Community College

Katie Herrington
Jones Junior College

Cathy Kennedy
Colorado State University

Mary Mock
University of South Dakota

Leonid Polyakov
Essex County College

Debra Tavasso
East Carolina University

Jennifer Thomas
Emporia State University

Martin Turnauer
Radford University

Dale Wagoner
Chabot College

Mary A. Wyandt
University of Arkansas

Beverly Zeakes
Radford University

For the Fifth Edition

John Batacan
Idaho State University

Steve Bordi
West Valley Community College

Judy Drolet
Southern Illinois University–Carbondale

Don Haynes
University of Minnesota–Duluth

Mary Iten
University of Nebraska at Kearney

Emogene Johnson Vaughn
Norfolk State University

Patricia Lawson
Arkansas State University

Rosalie Marinelli
University of Nevada

Marilyn Morton
SUNY-Plattsburgh

Trish Root
North Seattle Community College

Walt Rehm
Cuesta College

Betty Shepherd
Virginia Western Community College

Ladona Tournabene
University of South Dakota

Glenda Warren
Cumberland College

Katie Wiedman
University of St. Francis

For the Fourth Edition

S. Eugene Barnes
University of Southern Alabama

Anne K. Black
Austin Peay State University

Susan Ceriale
University of California–Santa Barbara

Bridget M. Finn
William Paterson University

Marianne Frauenknecht
Western Michigan University

Edna Gillis
Valdosta State University

Joe Goldfarb
University of Missouri–Columbia

Phil Huntsinger
University of Kansas

Gordon B. James
Weber State University

Sylvia M. Kubsch
University of Wisconsin–Green Bay

Frederick M. Randolph
Western Illinois University

Dell Smith
University of Central Arkansas

B. McKinley Thomas
Augusta State University

Chuck Ulrich
Western Illinois University

For the Third Edition

Dayna S. Brown
Morehead State University

Diane M. Hamilton
Georgia Southern University

Joe Herzstein
Trenton State College

Rebecca Rutt Leas
Clarion University

Dorinda Maynard
Eastern Kentucky University

Steven Navarro
Cerritos College

Mary Beth Tighe
The Ohio State University

For the Second Edition

James D. Aguiar
Ithaca College

Carolyn M. Allred
Central Piedmont Community College

Joan Benson
University of Utah

Daniel E. Berney
California State University–Dominguez Hills

Ronnie Carda
Emporia State University

Barbara Funke
Georgia College

William C. Gross
Western Michigan University

Richard Hurley
Brigham Young University

L. Clark McCammon
Western Illinois University

Dan Neal
Southwestern Oregon Community College

David Quadagno
Florida State University

Leslie Rurey
Community Colleges of Spokane

Scott E. Scobell
West Virginia State College

Raeann Koerner Smith
Ventura College

Karen T. Sullivan
Marymount University

Joan Tudor
Chapman University

Stuart L. Whitney
University of Vermont

For the First Edition

Sandra L. Bonneau
Golden West College

Richard A. Kaye
Kingsborough Community College

Donald Haynes
University of Minnesota–Duluth

J. Dale Wagoner
Chabot College

Special Acknowledgments

Authors do not exist in isolation. To publish successful textbooks, an entire team of professionals must work together for a significant amount of time. During the past three decades, we have worked with many talented people to publish 17 successful textbooks.

For this edition of *Focus on Health,* we used the professional expertise and writing talents of a team of four contributing authors. Leonard Kaminsky, Ph.D., Professor and Coordinator of Ball State University's Adult Fitness and Cardiac Rehabilitation Programs, took on the task of revising and updating Chapter 4 (Becoming Physically Fit) and Chapter 10 (Reducing Your Risk of Cardiovascular Disease). Chapter 7 (Making Decisions About Drug Use) and Chapter 8 (Taking Control of Alcohol Use) were revised by Alison Cockerill, M.S., Health Educator in the Ball State Student Health Center. Robert Pinger, Ph.D., Professor and Chairperson of the Department of Physiology and Health Science at Ball State, revised Chapter 16 (Protecting Your Safety). And Chapter 17, The Environment and Your Health, was written by David LeBlanc, Ph.D., Professor of Biology at Ball State University. We thank these contributors for their professional dedication to this book and their personal commitment to the health of college students with whom they work on a daily basis.

We remain grateful to Vicki Malinee, who saw us through nine book projects. This latest edition of *Focus on Health* also bears the imprint of Nick Barrett, Executive Editor, Health and Human Performance. His infectious enthusiasm for *Focus on Health* and his positive vision for the future of our personal health texts make us especially proud to be McGraw-Hill authors.

Special recognition goes to Pam Cooper, Executive Marketing Manager, who is as energetic a person as we have seen in college publishing. We are confident that her experience, expertise, and talent will allow this book to reach many of our teaching colleagues.

We are also grateful to those who worked behind the scenes at McGraw-Hill on the production of this book. Lynda Huenefeld made a major contribution to the development of both the book and its supplements package. Project Manager Mel Valentín juggled this book and its larger version simultaneously with remarkable grace and good humor, all the while keeping watch over every detail and deadline. Senior Designer Kim Menning created an exciting, dynamic new look for the seventh edition. And

Photo Research Coordinator Alexandra Ambrose culled a fine selection of colorful, thought-provoking images.

Finally, we would like to thank our families for their continued support and love. More than anyone else, they know the energy and dedication it takes to write and revise textbooks. To them we continue to offer our sincere admiration and loving appreciation.

Dale B. Hahn
Wayne A. Payne
Ellen B. Lucas

A Visual Guide to Focus on Health

Whether you're trying to get in shape, looking for sound health advice, trying to interpret the health information you see in the media, or just working toward a good grade, *Focus on Health* is designed to help you succeed. Here's a brief guide to some of the useful and eye-opening features you'll find inside.

Chapter Objectives

Each chapter opens with a set of clear learning goals; check them out before you begin reading the chapter, and use them for review once you've completed it.

Eye on the Media

Curious about all those ads you see for various drugs? Wondering about the reliability of the health information you find on the Internet? This feature investigates the way that written, broadcast, and electronic media shape our perceptions about health, health care, and wellness.

chapter seventeen

the environment and your health

Chapter Objectives

On completing this chapter, you will be able to:

▪ identify several environmental factors that can impact your personal health in either positive or adverse ways.

▪ explain how your personal health is influenced by different environmental factors on several scales, including personal environment, the community and regional environment, and the global environment.

▪ describe specific actions that you can take to minimize health risks associated with your personal environment—your home, your automobile, your workplace.

▪ describe the distinction between a "point source" versus a "nonpoint source" of community/regional air or water pollution.

▪ detail several specific actions that you can take to minimize environmental health risks at the community and regional level.

▪ describe several global environmental health issues, and offer several actions that you might take to foster change.

Eye on the Media

Hype versus Useful Information

An obscure scientist, an expert in an arcane subdiscipline of climatology, stands in front of his peers at a scientific conference and predicts a major shift in global climate. His warnings are brushed off by the powers-that-be. Within a month there are several massive polar hurricanes encircling the northern hemisphere of Earth. Within the following two weeks, the northern half of the United States is buried under ice and uninhabitable. Ten of millions of Americans are dead from storms and temperatures that dip to −150° F. The survivors have moved to Mexico, probably permanently. Within two hours, *The Day after Tomorrow* has brought the complex, long-term process of global climate change to a tidy storyline conclusion. Television pundits predict the movie will raise public awareness of this looming environmental problem. A few weeks later the issue has fallen off the public radar.

"The Media" is one of the most powerful forces in American society, and its influence extends across most of the Earth's human population. As large multinational corporations have come to control many media producers, information and news are increasingly being filtered for their entertainment value. That which is deemed sufficiently interesting to be entertaining is often hyped, with the most titillating aspects repeated over and over. Information that is deemed uninteresting is simply ignored.

The "entertainm...

time periods. For example, likely effects of global climate change include expansion of tropical diseases into more northern latitudes, increased frequency of droughts and heat waves, gradual depletion of freshwater supplies, and extinctions of many species that cannot adapt to the changes. Compared to killer super polar storms and massive glaciers that appear in two weeks, these real-life issues have entertainment value similar to watching grass grow. The U.S. population is being exposed to hundreds, if not thousands of chemicals that have not been tested for human toxicity. They are found in our air, water, and food supply. They are found in our body fluids and hair. Some have been shown to cause cancer and birth defects in experimental animals. The U.S. Environmental Protection Agency estimates that air pollution in major U.S. cities contributes to thousands of deaths due to respiratory and cardiovascular disease each year. In the last 20 to 30 years, cancer rates in the U.S. population have increased substantially, while fertility of men as measured by sperm counts has been declining by 1–3% per year. When was the last time you heard anything about these issues on the evening news or read about them in a newspaper or magazine?

On the positive s... ...ver been ...asier to obtai...

Changing for the Better

Learn to put health concepts into practice by following these useful tips. This feature provides practical advice for making positive changes and staying motivated to follow a healthy lifestyle.

Changing for the Better

Eating on the Run

I am always in a hurry and don't have time to cook, and so a lot of my meals end up being fast food. Are there better choices I can make when eating on the run?

The typical American eats about three hamburgers and four orders of French fries each week, so you aren't alone. With over 300,000 fast-food restaurants in the United States, fast food is definitely part of the American lifestyle. Here are some things to consider when eating at fast food restaurants:

• Don't supersize! Go for the "small" or "regular" size.
• Don't wait until you are starving because that leads to overeating and supersizing!
• Decide what you w... ...der ahead of time and d... ...oved

• Order grilled instead of fried chicken or fish.
• Look for the "light" choices.
• Limit your condiments. Mustard, ketchup, salsa, and low-fat or fat-free condiments and dressing are preferable to regular mayonnaise or high-fat dressings.
• For breakfast, choose cereal and milk or pancakes rather than a breakfast sandwich (which can have about 475 calories, 30 grams of fat, and 1,260 mg of sodium).
• Bring fast food from home! Buy portable foods at the grocery store to take with you that can be eaten quickly and easily, such as portable yogurt, a banana or apple, low-fat granola bar, or breakfast bar.
• Order lo... ...fat or skim milk or water inst... ...of soda.

Discovering Your Spirituality

A healthy body and a healthy mind go hand in hand. This feature will help you tap into your spiritual side to improve your self-esteem, foster good relationships with others, and jump-start your physical health.

Discovering Your Spirituality
Yoga: Creating Peaceful Time

In a typical college day that includes academic, social, and financial pressures, you can lose the sense of who you really are. Do you ever find yourself wondering why you're making certain choices and what's really important to you? Meditative practices such as yoga offer you the chance to slow down and recapture a sense of yourself.

The word *yoga* comes from a Sanskrit root meaning "union" or "joining," referring to the integration of body, mind, and spirit. Yoga has evolved from ancient beginnings in the Himalayan mountains of India. Accounts of its origin differ, and some suggest that it reaches back 6,000 years. Yoga is practiced by people of all social, economic, and religious background. many past yoga masters h   there i   or even

Each exercise, called an *asan* or *ansana*, has specific effects. The "diamond pose," for example, limbers the lower back, hips, and groin muscles. Specialized workouts—to address pregnancy, sports, weight-loss programs, and other needs—can be created by including carefully selected exercises.

Yoga requires no special equipment and can be practiced in a small space such as a bedroom. Instructors in the United States have worked to make yoga accessible to the American lifestyle by developing special   that can be pursued durin   usiness, or the   quently   ses or

Talking Points

TALKING POINTS How could you tactfully bring up a friend's weight problem to show concern for his or her health?

Throughout each chapter, you'll find these tips for starting a dialogue about sensitive health topics.

Learning from Our Diversity

These unique boxes invite you to explore the rich diversity of your own campus, and to gain perspective on the way such characteristics as age, racial/ethnic background, physical abilities, and sexual orientation can shape individuals' lives and well-being.

Learning From Our Diversity
Diverse Personalities

When we think about diversity, we may think about differences in ethnicity, culture, religion, sexual orientation, and disabilities, but we don't often consider differences in personality as part of diversity. Diversity can refer to any difference or potentially separating factor between or within groups. With respect to psychological health, there certainly are differences in personality traits—for example, outgoing vs. shy, detail oriented vs. spontaneous, flexible vs. structured. Often people value certain personality characteristics over others—for instance, being extraverted, organized, responsible, humorous, and open minded. Other traits can seem positive in one situation but negative in another. For example, being sensitive can be seen as a positive quality when you are sensitive to the feelings of other people and can relate well to other   however, it can also be   negatively if you are   ived as   sitive in   too perso

Intuitives tend to be nonconformist, creative, and divergent global thinkers. Thinking types are more analytical and logical, and they base their decisions on facts, rules, and policies. Feeling types base their decisions on how they will affect other people; they tend to be peace-keepers, conflict avoidant, and sensitive to the feelings of others. Organized, good with time management, and structured are qualities of a judging type, whereas spontaneous, adaptable, and flexible describe perceptives.

The MBTI maintains that there are no good or bad personality types, only important differences, and it uses the four scales to describe them. The MBTI talks about how you can play to your strengths and understand your weaknesses and how you can appreciate other people's   nality types. In fact, the idea beh   is instrument is that it is   opposites   a relationsh

Personal Assessment

Do you eat too much fat? What's the best method of birth control for you if you are sexually active? Are you a perfectionist? Each chapter in *Focus on Health* includes an assessment to help you learn the answers to these and many other questions.

personal assessment

how stressed are you?

A widely used life-stress scale called the Social Readjustment Rating Scale by Holmes and Rahe has been used to determine the degree of stress that you are experiencing because of life events over the past year. It also projects your chances of developing an illness- or stress-related health condition. Stress can lead to some serious health problems, and the more stress you have in your life, the more vulne

Outstanding personal achievement	28
Begin or end school	26
Partner begins/stops working	26
Change in living conditions	25
Change in personal habits	24
Trouble with supervisor	23
Change in work hours	20

Focus on Health

chapter one

Shaping Your Health

Chapter Objectives

On completing this chapter, you will be able to:

▪ understand how your health affects your lifestyle.

▪ recognize how the delivery of health care influences definitions of health.

▪ detail some of the health concerns outlined by the Institute of Medicine and Healthy People 2010.

▪ suggest additional reasons why health behavior change is difficult, beyond those outlined in your textbook.

▪ speculate on strategies for encouraging health behavior change.

▪ list Prochaska's six stages of change.

▪ describe and compare the range of traditional and nontraditional students on your campus.

▪ describe the developmental tasks of young adulthood, and assess your level of progress in mastering them.

▪ monitor your own activities, and list the dimensions of health from which resources are drawn.

▪ compare wellness and health promotion, noting both the differences and the similarities between the two concepts.

▪ describe your textbook's new definition of health, and compare it with definitions from episodic health care and health promotion.

Eye on the Media

Where Does Our Health Information Come From?

Today our health information comes from a variety of media—some more reliable than others. Eye on the Media will appear in each chapter of this text, highlighting the important issue of which ones are good (in other words, valid and reliable) sources for learning about health.

Radio and Television

When you think of radio, the first thing that may come to mind is your favorite music. But two areas of radio are especially important for news and information: talk radio and public radio networks such as National Public Radio (NPR) and Public Radio International (PRI). Talk radio raises the question of validity of information. For example, if you're listening to a talk show about HIV exposure, the perceptions and opinions of the host (which may be strong or even extreme) are an important part of the show. When this point of view is combined with the opinions of callers, whose "facts" may come from unauthoritative sources, what you're hearing is probably not solid information. It's certainly not a good basis for making your health decisions.

NPR and PRI, however, take a scholarly approach to news, featuring experts who do not always agree on an issue. In general, the news reports on NPR and PRI are long enough to present an in-depth, balanced treatment of health-related topics.

Television, too, is often an important source of health information. Coverage ranges from brief health-related segments on national or local news programs to entire cable programs devoted to health topics, such as those seen on the Learning and Discovery channels. While these programs can be timely and accurate, television also provides an array of "Infomercials" promoting health products that should be evaluated more critically.

Newspapers and Magazines

Let's assume that most people read only one or two newspapers a day—their local paper and perhaps a national newspaper such as the *New York Times* or *USA Today.* If so, the health information they are receiving is typically from wire services like the Associated Press; it is condensed and simplified but accurate within these limitations. When health-related information in newspapers is accompanied by illustrations and identification of the original source of information (such as a professional journal), it is more helpful to the reader.

Unlike newspapers, magazines are so diverse in terms of ownership, intended audience, and standards of validity that it is difficult to determine the reliability of their health-related content. In general, the national news magazines, such as *Time* and *Newsweek,* are very careful about the accuracy of their reporting, often including primary (original) sources. Their content is considered "state of the art." In contrast, the checkout-lane tabloids, such as the *Globe* and the *National Enquirer,* are known for printing stories with "health" content that few readers take seriously. Between these two extremes is a wide array of general content magazines, such as the *Saturday Evening Post,* and health-oriented magazines, such as *Prevention,* that vary greatly in validity and reliability.

Professional Journals

Your college library probably offers a broad selection of professional journals. Through these publications, the members of an academic discipline share the latest developments and issues in their field with their colleagues and other readers. Because the study of health is so multifaceted, drawing on different disciplines for information, health-related journals are plentiful. The vast majority of articles that appear in publications such as the *New England Journal of Medicine* and the *Journal of the American Dietetic Association* are peer-reviewed. This means that professionals in the particular field review and judge the content of a submitted article to determine whether or not it should be published. Then, if a study being reported was not carefully controlled, or if its underlying theory seems to be flawed, the article is returned to the author(s) for refinement. This process greatly reduces the risk of publishing invalid information. Currently, journals are beginning to appear in fields such as complementary (alternative) health care. When reading such publications, you need to consider whether they are backed by a peer-review process.

Government Documents

Each year various departments of the federal government, particularly the Department of Health and Human Services (DHHS), release the results of research being done under the oversight of its many divisions and agencies. These documents, such as the annual *Surgeon General's Report on Smoking and Health,* become the source of much of the health-related news reported by other media sources, including textbooks and professional journals. These publications generally can be purchased through the U.S. Government Printing Office. They are also available through urban public libraries and large university libraries. With few exceptions, the information in these publications is reviewed by the most respected authorities in each field.

Books

Books continue to be a vast source of information on health-related topics. Today's health books, in addition to academic health textbooks such as *Focus On Health,* fall into three categories: reference books, medical encyclopedias, and single-topic trade (retail) books.

Included in the category of reference books are important professional publications such as *The Merck Manual* and the *Physicians' Desk Reference.* These books, intended for professionals in various health fields, contain the most current information on specific aspects of health. Although these books can be purchased by the general public, their content is technical and complex, and their language is often difficult for nonprofessional readers to follow.

More valuable to the typical American household are the various medical (health) encyclopedias, such as *The Johns Hopkins Home Medical Handbook* and *The Mayo Clinic Family Health Book.* Such books usually include a wide array of medical conditions and offer valuable information about health promotion and disease prevention. Their clear writing styles and highly valid information make these books excellent home references.

Single-topic health-related trade books, such as those about diets and health problems, are readily available from retail outlets such as bookstores and Internet stores. Like magazines, these books are difficult to assess because of their quantity and the varying backgrounds of the authors. Some are very sound in terms of content and philosophy. Others may be misleading and may contain advice that could be dangerous to your health. Included in this group are self-help books, the best-selling health books of all.

The Internet

By the year 2007, according to Forrester Research, it is projected that nearly 85 percent of American households will have direct access to the Internet. Internet access is also available through libraries, educational institutions, and the workplace. With just a few clicks, you can reach many health-related Web sites that offer a wide range of health information. Chat rooms provide a forum for individuals to share their personal health experiences. Because the Internet is such an important source of health information for both professionals and the general public, this textbook highlights helpful Web sites in all chapters. To learn about criteria for assessing the validity and reliability of Internet information, see Chapter 15.

Source:
Forrester Research. *83.4% U.S. households connected by 2007,* April 23, 2004, www.itfacts.biz/index.php?id=105ml-3A.

"Take care of your health, because you'll miss it when it's gone," younger people hear often from their elders. This simple and heartfelt advice is given in the belief that young people take their health for granted and assume that they will always maintain the state of health and wellness they now enjoy. Observation and experience should, however, remind all of us that youth is relatively brief, and health is always changing—often in a downward direction. In fact, as health deteriorates, our ability to participate in meaningful life activities can be compromised or even lost. Consider, for example, how failing health might affect the following activities:

- Your ability to pursue an education or a career
- Your opportunity to socialize with friends and family
- The chance to travel—for business, relaxation, or adventure
- The opportunity to meet and connect with new people

Keys to Longer Living

Experts generally agree on basic lifestyle characteristics that support greater longevity and, we hope, a higher quality of life. Small adjustments that promote this improvement include:

- Testing your cholesterol level regularly and taking a 30-minute brisk walk every day.

- Wearing a seat belt in the car and a helmet while riding a bicycle, motorcycle, or while skating.

- Substituting olive oil instead of butter.

- Quitting smoking or at least reducing the amount of tobacco used daily. Lung cancer is the most frequent cause of cancer-related death in the United States.

- Avoiding sun exposure from 11 A.M. until 2 P.M. when UV radiation is most dangerous. Stay inside during those peak hours and always wear sunscreen outdoors.

- Asking questions of your doctor or pharmacist about concerns, test results, diagnosis, or treatments. It is often helpful to take someone with you to important appointments.

- Don't worry! Even if everyone was overly cautious, we would still not live in a risk free world—unnecessary worry can stress the mind and body.

- The ability to conceive or the opportunity to parent children
- Participation in hobbies or recreational activities
- Your enjoyment of a wide range of foods
- The opportunity to live independently

Quality of life issues such as these are your parents' and grandparents' focus when they advise you to take care of your health. As you will learn in this chapter, health is intertwined with activities such as these—indeed, your authors will present a new definition of health specifically related to accomplishing these important life tasks. But first, we review a few familiar perceptions of health, each of which is concerned primarily with illness and death, and we discuss strategies for changing health behaviors.

Definitions of Health

By the time they reach college age, most Americans are familiar with the many ways in which health care is provided. Following are some easily recognizable examples, all of which serve to reinforce our traditional definitions of health. Note that these examples involve the cure or management of illness and the extension of life, indicated by the concerns about **morbidity** and **mortality.**

We present a new definition of health near the end of the chapter. This new definition should be viewed as a partner to the following traditional examples of health care. The principal difference relates to the new definition's developmental focus rather than a focus on traditional concerns about morbidity and mortality.

Episodic Health Care

The vast majority of Americans use the services of professional health care providers during periods (*episodes*)

of illness and injury, that is, when we are "unhealthy." We consult providers seeking a diagnosis that will explain why we are not feeling well. Once a problem is identified, we expect to receive effective treatment from the practitioner that will lead to our recovery (the absence of illness) and a return to health. If we are willing to comply with the care strategies prescribed by our practitioner, we should soon be able to define ourselves as "healthy" once again.

The familiarity of episodic health care is evident in the 890 million times that Americans visited physicians during 2002. Although some of these visits were for preventive health care (see discussion on page five), the vast majority were in conjunction with illness. When viewed according to racial group, Whites averaged 3.4 visits, Blacks 2.5, and Asians 2.3 visits during that year.[1] A similar report in 2000 indicated that Native Americans made only 0.8 visits that year.[2]

 TALKING POINTS Would you be hesitant to talk to your doctor about health advice you found on the Internet? How would you approach the subject?

Preventive or Prospective Medicine

Simple logic suggests that it makes more sense to prevent illness than to deal with it through episodic health

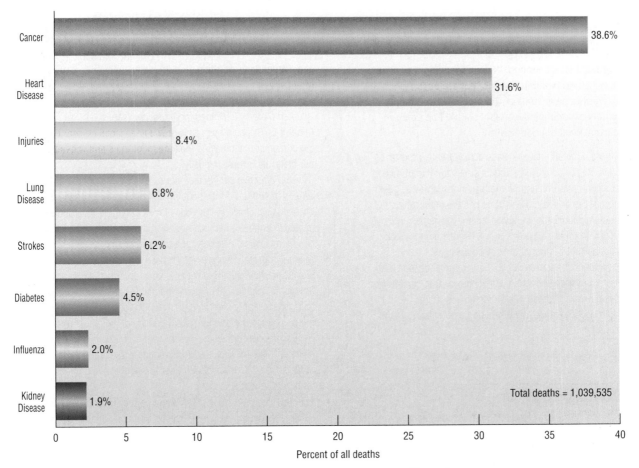

Figure 1-1 Top eight causes of death. 2004 marked the first year that cancer surpassed heart disease as the leading cause of death for Americans under the age of 80.

Sources: *Estimated Cancer Cases and Deaths by Sex, for All Sites, US, 2005,* American Cancer Society, 2005. *Deaths: Final Data for 2002.* National Vital Statistics Report. National Center for Health Statistics, October 12, 2004.

(medical) care. This philosophy characterizes **preventive** or **prospective medicine.** Unfortunately, however, many physicians say they have little time to practice preventive medicine because of the large number of episodically sick people who fill their offices every day.

When physicians do practice preventive or prospective medicine, they first attempt to determine their patient's level of risk for developing particular conditions. They make this assessment by identifying **risk factors** (and **high-risk health behaviors**) with a variety of observational techniques and screening tests, some of which may be invasive (taking tissues from the body such as a biopsy or blood draw). Additionally, an important tool in assessing risk is an accurate family health history, something that over one-third of all adults cannot adequately provide to their health care providers.[3] So important is a health history that the federal government has established a Web site to assist us in becoming familiar with our family's health history

(www.hhs.gov/familyhistory). Certainly, if you identify any of the conditions shown in Figure 1-1, share them with your primary care physician.[4]

Key Terms

preventive or **prospective medicine** physician-centered medical care in which areas of risk for chronic illnesses are identified so that they might be lowered

risk factor a biomedical index such as serum cholesterol level or a behavioral pattern such as smoking, associated with a chronic illness

high-risk health behavior a behavioral pattern, such as smoking, associated with a high risk of developing a chronic illness

---

As if being a student is not enough, I'm experiencing a growing sense of concern about health problems that are occurring in my family. I don't want to have some of the problems that family members are now experiencing, so what should I be doing to sustain my current level of good health?

Prescriptions for good health usually place considerable importance on *risk reduction.* Health care professionals stress the importance of identifying behavioral patterns and biomedical indexes that suggest the potential for illness or death. Each of us has the opportunity to receive information, counseling, behavior change strategies, and medical therapies designed to lower our risk. The extent to which we act on this opportunity is our degree of *compliance.*

Some risk factors cannot be reduced. For example, gender, race, age, and genetic predisposition make developing certain conditions more likely. Being aware of these risk factors is important.

To refocus on good health, concentrate on these actions, which can reduce risk factors:

- *Refrain from using tobacco in any form.* This rule is so critically important that the surgeon general of the United States has identified smoking as the single most important reversible factor contributing to illness and early death.
- *If you drink alcohol, do so in moderation.* This is particularly important for people who must drive or operate machinery, women who are pregnant or planning to become pregnant, and people taking certain medications.
- *Engage in regular exercise designed to train the cardiorespiratory system as well as maintain muscle strength.* You can use a wide array of exercises as the basis of a fitness program, and you can develop specific programs around recommendations about frequency, duration, and intensity of activity.
- *Familiarize yourself with the newly adopted Dietary Guidelines for Americans* (see Chapter 5). Strong emphasis is now being placed on controlling portion size, increasing the amount of fruits and vegetables in our diets, and exercising daily.
- *Develop effective coping techniques for use in moderating the effects of stress.* Effective coping can reduce the duration of physiological challenge the body faces during periods of unexpected change. Remember, however, that some forms of coping can themselves be sources of additional stress.
- *Maintain normal body weight.* Persons who are excessively overweight or underweight may experience abnormal structural or functional changes, predispose themselves to chronic illnesses, and unnecessarily shorten their lives. Lifelong weight management is preferable to intermittent periods of weight gain and loss.
- *Receive regular preventive health care from competent professionals.* This care should include routine screening and risk-reducing lifestyle management, early diagnosis, and effective treatment if needed.
- *Maintain an optimistic outlook.* Anger, cynicism, and a pessimistic outlook on life can erode the holistic basis on which high-level health is built. Several chronic conditions, including cardiovascular diseases and cancers, occur more frequently in persons who lack a positive outlook on their own lives and life in general.
- *Establish a personally meaningful belief system.* Over the course of long life the presence of such a system and the supportive spiritual community usually associated with it may prove to be the most beneficial health resource we can possess.

It is disconcerting to report that important medical information, including laboratory reports, comprehensive drug inventories, and family health histories, are often missing from medical files. A 2003 study involving primary care physician medical records suggests that perhaps one out of every seven patient files is missing information important to providing comprehensive health care.[5]

Once they have identified levels of risk in patients, health practitioners try to lower those risk levels through patient education, lifestyle modification, and, when necessary, medical intervention. Continued compliance on the part of the patients will result in a lower level of risk that will continue over the years. Note that preventive medicine is guided by practitioners, and patients are expected to be compliant with the direction they are given.

Although preventive medical care appears to be a much more sensible approach than episodic care is in reducing morbidity and mortality, third-party payers (insurance plans) traditionally have not provided adequate coverage for these services. Managed health care plans that earn a profit by preventing sickness, such as health maintenance organizations, or HMOs (see Chapter 15), should be much more receptive to the concept and practice of preventive medicine.

Health Promotion

Throughout the United States, YMCA/YWCA-sponsored wellness programs, commercial fitness clubs, and corporate fitness centers offer risk-reduction programs under the direction of qualified instructors, many of whom are university graduates in disciplines such as exercise science, wellness management, and **health promotion.** Using approaches similar to those employed in preventive medicine, these nonphysician health professionals attempt to guide their clients toward activities and behaviors that will lower their risk of chronic illness. Unlike preventive medicine, with its sometimes invasive assessment procedures and medication-based therapies, health promotion programs are not legally defined as medical practices and thus do not require the involvement of physicians. In addition, the fitness focus, social interaction, and healthy lifestyle orientation these programs provide tend to mask the emphasis on preventing chronic illness that would be the selling point of such efforts if they were undertaken as preventive medicine. In fact, it is likely that people receiving health promotion in these settings do not recognize it as such. Rather, they are submitting to assessments and listening to health-related information only as incidental parts of personal goals, such as losing weight, preparing for their first marathon, or simply meeting friends for lunch hour basketball.

Community Health Promotion

In addition to the practices just described, a group-oriented form of health promotion is offered in many communities. This approach to improving health through risk reduction is directed at empowering community groups, such as church congregations or a neighborhood association, so they can develop, operate, and financially sustain their own programs with little direct involvement of health promotion specialists.[6,7]

The key to successful community-based health promotion is **empowerment.** [8] In the context of health, empowerment refers to a process in which individuals or groups of people gain increasing control over their health. To take control over health matters, individuals and groups must learn to move beyond a variety of barriers that once were restrictions on health enhancement.

Empowerment programs have produced positive health consequences for individuals and groups that traditionally have been underserved by the health care system, such as minority populations. Once such people are given needed information, inroads into the political process, and skills for accessing funding sources, they become better able to plan, implement, and operate programs tailored to their unique health needs.

Perhaps no greater challenge in establishing health-related empowerment is that related to the devastating tsunami that occurred on December 26, 2004, in the Indian Ocean basin. In addition to coping with a death toll approaching 200,000 and the displacement of entire communities, much of the effort and resources needed to rebuild viable communities will eventually need to be transitioned from professionally staffed international relief organizations into the hands of the local people. When successful, these programs stand as excellent examples of the fact that people can make a difference when they become empowered.

Having learned about the sources of our familiar definitions of health, recall that a new and unique definition is presented later in the chapter.

Federal Programs to Improve the Health of People in the United States

To identify all the health-related concerns identified by members of the health community would be a monumental undertaking far beyond the scope of this book. However, in 2003, the Institute of Medicine released a list of priority health concerns that they believe need particular attention.[9] Among these priority concerns are[9] these:

- treatment of asthma
- coordination of care for the 60 million or more persons with chronic health conditions
- reduction in the development of diabetes
- development of evidence-based cancer screening
- enhanced rates of immunization, particularly for flu and pneumonia
- improved detection of depression, which is now inadequately diagnosed and treated
- aggressively promoted prevention of cardiovascular disease, presently the second leading killer of American adults
- reduction of tobacco dependence through cessation and prevention of smoking
- widened availability of prenatal care

Key Terms

health promotion movement in which knowledge, practices, and values are transmitted to people for use in lengthening their lives, reducing the incidence of illness, and feeling better

empowerment the nurturing of an individual's or group's ability to be responsible for their own health and well-being

---

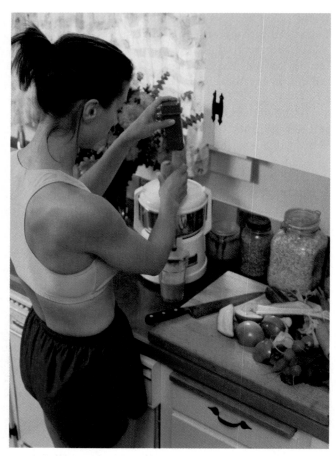

Many students have been able to change a specific health-related behavior, such as replacing poor eating habits with nutritious food choices.

While improvements in these areas are greatly needed, the Institute of Medicine has no specific programs in place at this time to address them. In comparison, well-established and ongoing programs, Healthy People 2000 and Healthy People 2010, have established specific goals and objectives to improve the health of Americans in many of these areas. A brief description of this ongoing program follows.

In 1991 the U.S. Department of Health and Human Services document titled *Healthy People 2000: National Health Promotion and Disease Prevention Objectives*[10] outlined a strategic plan for promoting the health of the American public. The plan included 300 health objectives in 22 priority areas. Forty-seven of the 300 objectives were defined as "sentinel" ones, that is, particularly significant goals that could be used to measure the progress of the 1990s health promotion objectives.

Progress toward achieving the objectives was assessed near the middle of the decade and reported in a document titled *Healthy People 2000: Midcourse Review and 1995*

Revisions.[11] Although progress was reported in some areas, little or no progress was reported in many. Subsequently, a new plan, called *Healthy People 2010: Understanding and Improving Health,*[12] was formulated, refined, and is now being implemented.[13]

Central to the design of *Healthy People 2010: Understanding and Improving Health* are two paramount goals: (1) increasing quality and years of life and (2) eliminating health disparities in areas such as gender, race, and ethnicity, as well as income and education level. These goals in turn provide 28 more focused objectives. Progress in accomplishing these objectives is anticipated through the manipulation of the behavioral, biological, and environmental determinants of health as they relate to 10 of the leading health indicators: (1) physical activity, (2) weight management, (3) tobacco use, (4) substance abuse, (5) responsible sexual behavior, (6) mental health, (7) injury and violence, (8) environmental quality, (9) immunization, and (10) access to health care.

The success of *Healthy People 2010: Understanding and Improving Health* will not be known until nearer the end of the decade. However, if its goals are ultimately reached, Americans can anticipate improved quantity and quality of life.

Changing Health-Related Behavior

Although some health concerns can be successfully addressed collectively though local, state, or national efforts such as those just outlined, most are ultimately based on the willingness and ability of persons to change aspects of their own behavior.

Why Behavior Change Is Often Difficult

Several factors can strongly influence a person's desire to change high health-risk behaviors, including these:

1. A person must know that a particular behavioral pattern is clearly associated with (or even causes) a particular health problem. For example: cigarette smoking is the primary cause of lung cancer.
2. A person must believe (accept) that a behavioral pattern will make (or has made) him susceptible to this particular health problem. For example: my cigarette smoking will significantly increase my risk of developing lung cancer.
3. A person must recognize that risk-reduction intervention strategies exist and that should she adopt these in a compliant manner she too will reduce her risk for a particular health condition. For example: smoking cessation programs exist, and following such a program could help me quit smoking.

4. A person must believe that benefits of newly adopted health-enhancing behaviors will be more reinforcing than the behaviors being given up. For example: the improved health, lowered risk, and freedom from dependence resulting from no longer smoking are better than the temporary pleasures provided by smoking.

5. A person must feel that significant others in his life truly want him to alter his high-risk health behaviors and will support his efforts. For example: my friends who are cigarette smokers will make a concerted effort to not smoke in my presence and will help me avoid being around people who smoke.

When one or more of the conditions listed above is not in place, the likelihood that persons will be successful in reducing health-risk behaviors is greatly diminished.

Stages of Change

The process of behavioral change unfolds over time and progresses through defined stages.[14,15] James Prochaska, John Norcross, and Carol DiClemente outlined six predictable stages of change. They studied thousands of individuals who were changing long-standing problems such as alcohol abuse, smoking, and gambling. While these people used different strategies to change their behavior, they all proceeded through six consistent stages of change in the process referred to as **Prochaska's Stages of Changes.**[16]

Precontemplation Stage

The first stage of change is called *precontemplation,* during which a person might think about making a change but ultimately finds it too difficult and avoids doing it. For example, during this phase a smoker might tell friends, "Eventually I will quit" but have no real intention of stopping within the next six months.

Contemplation Stage

For many, however, progress toward change begins as they move into a *contemplation* stage, during which they might develop the desire to change but have little understanding of how to go about it. Typically, they see themselves taking action within the next six months.

Preparation Stage

Following the contemplation stage, a *preparation* stage begins, during which change begins to appear to be not only desirable but possible as well. A smoker might begin making plans to quit during this stage, setting a quit date for the very near future (a few days to a month) and perhaps enrolling in a smoking-cessation program.

Action Stage

Plans for change are implemented during the *action* stage, during which changes are made and sustained for a period of about six months.

Maintenance Stage

The fifth stage is the *maintenance* stage, during which new habits are consolidated and practiced for an additional six months.

Termination Stage

The sixth and final stage is called *termination*, which refers to the point at which new habits are well established, and so efforts to change are complete.

Today's Health Concerns

To this point in the chapter we have identified some health concerns and addressed the desirability of health-related behavior change. Earlier in the chapter, we looked at those illnesses that are the major causes of death that afflict the U.S. public. However, in spite of astonishing progress on many fronts, we continue to face a number of serious health challenges from those and other illnesses. Heart disease, cancer, accidents, drug use, and mental illness all are important concerns for each of us, even if we are not directly affected by them. Also becoming increasingly troublesome are the complex problems of environmental pollution, violence, health care costs, and the international scope of the HIV/AIDS epidemic, as well as other sexually transmitted diseases. Figure 1-1 on page 5 lists the eight leading causes of death in the United States expressed as a percentage of all deaths. Table 1.1 depicts the leading causes of death at various age levels. World hunger, overpopulation, and the threat of domestic and international terrorism are other health-related issues that will affect us, as well as the generations that follow.

The health concerns just mentioned are by no means unmanageable. Fortunately, we as individuals can reduce the likelihood of encountering many of these conditions by making choices in the way we live our lives. On a personal level, we can decide to pursue a plan of healthful living to minimize the incidence of illness and disease and to extend life.

Key Terms

Prochaska's Stages of Change the six predictable stages—precontemplation, contemplation, preparation, action, maintenance, and termination—people go through in establishing new habits and patterns of behavior

---

Table 1.1 Leading Causes of Death in the United States by Age Group, 2002

In data collected by the American Cancer Society comparing 2003–2004 deaths from cancer and heart disease, cancer was found to have surpassed heart disease for the first time as the leading cause of death for Americans under 80 years of age (see Figure 1-1). However, note the preponderance of heart disease deaths over cancer deaths in persons 85 and over.

1-4 Years	Number of Deaths
Unintentional injuries	1,641
Birth defects	530
Cancer	402
5–14 Years	
Unintentional injuries	2,718
Cancer	1,017
Homicide	356
15–24 Years	
Unintentional injuries	15,912
Homicide	5,214
Suicide	4,010
25–44 Years	
Unintentional injuries	29,279
Heart disease	20,948
Cancer	19,957
45–64 Years	
Cancer	143,018
Heart disease	124,230
Unintentional injuries	23,020
65–84 Years	
Heart disease	431,486
Cancer	311,819
Stroke	76,811
85 and over	
Heart disease	339,409
Cancer	29,182
Strokes	66,412

Source: "Deaths: Final Data for 2002," *National Vital Statistics Report*, National Center For Health Statistics, October 12. 2004.

Health: More than the Absence of Illness?

What exactly is health? Is it simply the absence of disease and illness, as Western medicine has held for centuries—or does health embrace other elements we ought to consider now that the 21st century has begun?

Rather routinely national news magazines (and other media) feature articles describing advances in modern medicine.[17,18] These articles describe vividly in words and images the impressive progress being made in fields such as drug development, gene manipulation, computer-aided surgery, and the role of nutrition in health. Because of articles like this that relate health to medical care, most of us continue to hold to our traditional perception of health as (1) the virtual absence of disease and illness (low levels of morbidity) and (2) the ability to live a long life (reduced risk of mortality). However, in striving to be fully "health educated" in the new century, perhaps we need to consider a broader definition that more accurately reflects the demands associated with becoming functional and satisfied persons as we transition through each adult stage of life—*young adulthood, middle adulthood,* and, finally, *older adulthood.* With this in mind, look forward to another definition of health—one that recognizes the importance of the more familiar definitions of health but is focused on the demands of our own growth and development. However, before looking at this new perception of health and its relationship to young adulthood let's meet the readers of this book, today's college students, each of whom is or once was a young adult.

Today's College Students

Readers of this textbook are college students, but they are also young adults, middle-age adults, or even older adults. In some cases their decision to be a student has placed them in settings far different from those being experienced by other people their age. For many students, college classes are sandwiched in between other obligations—for example full-time job, parenting, community involvement, even the care of older parents. Some might be the first members of their families to pursue higher education. Many students come from economic, racial, or ethnic backgrounds quite different from those of the majority of their classmates. Thus, today there is no one type of college student, but all students are progressing through life in predictable yet unique ways.

Traditional-Age Undergraduate College Students

Statistics indicate that more than 15.8 million students were enrolled in degree-granting U.S. colleges and universities in 2002.[19] Nearly 57 percent of these students were women. In 2002, minority students made up approximately 25 percent of U.S. college students, and foreign students totaled 4 percent.[20]

Because nearly 62 percent of all undergraduates are traditional-age students,[19] this book is directed first at these students. However, because of significant growth in the proportion of older students, we also address a variety of life experiences that are appropriate to these students. Unquestionably, the nontraditional-age students in our classes help our traditional-age students understand the wide and varied role that health plays throughout the life cycle.

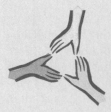

Learning from Our Diversity

Back to the Future: Nontraditional-Age Students Enrich the College Experience

To anyone who's visited a U.S. college campus in the last 15 years, it's abundantly clear that the once typical college student—White, middle class, between the ages of 18 and 24—is not always a majority on campus. In most institutions of higher learning, today's student body is a rich tapestry of color, culture, language, ability, and age. Wheelchair-accessible campuses roll out the welcome mat for students with disabilities; the air is filled with the music of a dozen or more languages spoken by students from virtually every part of the world; students in their 60s chat animatedly with classmates young enough to be their grandchildren.

Of all the trends that are changing the face of college enrollment in the United States, perhaps the most significant is the increasing diversity in the age of students now on campus. Older students today are both a common and welcome sight in colleges and universities across the country. Many women cut short their undergraduate education—or defer graduate school—to marry and raise children. Divorcees, widows, and women whose children are grown often return to college, or enroll for the first time, to prepare for professional careers. And increasingly, both men and women are finding it desirable, if not essential, to further their education as a means of either keeping their current job or qualifying for a higher position.

Just as children are enriched by the knowledge and experience of their grandparents and other older relatives, so too is today's college classroom a richer place when many of the seats are filled by students of nontraditional age. Without being didactic or preachy, older students can provide valuable guidance and direction to younger classmates who may be uncertain of their career path, or who may be wrestling with decisions about marriage and parenthood. In doing so, nontraditional-age students can gain helpful insights about young people's feelings, attitudes, challenges, and aspirations.

Among the many important benefits of today's increasingly diverse college campus, surely one of the most significant is the enhanced opportunity for intergenerational communication and understanding made possible by the growing numbers of students of nontraditional age.

In your classes, how would you characterize the interactions between traditional-age students and those of nontraditional age? In what ways are they enriching each other's college experience?

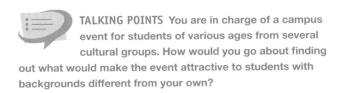

TALKING POINTS You are in charge of a campus event for students of various ages from several cultural groups. How would you go about finding out what would make the event attractive to students with backgrounds different from your own?

Nontraditional-Age Undergraduate College Students

In 2001, nearly 38.5 percent of U.S. undergraduate college students were classified as **nontraditional-age students.**[19] Included in this vast overlapping group are part-time students, military veterans, students returning to college, single parents, older adults, and evening students. These students enter the classroom with a wide assortment of life experiences and observations. Most of these students are 25 to 40 years old. (Read the Learning from Our Diversity box for a closer look at nontraditional-age students.)

Many nontraditional-age students are trying to juggle an extremely demanding schedule. The responsibilities of managing a job, a schedule of classes, and perhaps a family present formidable challenges. Performing these tasks on a limited budget compounds the difficulty. For many of these students, concerns over paying next month's rent, caring for aging parents, and finding affordable child care are among the challenges that confront them.

We want to make this textbook meaningful for both traditional-age and nontraditional-age students. Much of the information we present applies to both categories of students. We ask nontraditional-age students to do two things as you read this book: (1) reflect on your own young adult years and (2) examine your current lifestyle to see how the decisions you made as a younger adult are affecting the quality of your life now. Also, as a nontraditional-age student, you may have young adult children whose lives you can observe in light of the information you will find in this book.

Minority Students

Although enrollment patterns at colleges and universities vary, the overall number of minority students is increasing. In 2001, approximately 25 percent of all college students were minority students, with African Americans,

Key Terms

nontraditional-age students administrative term used by colleges and universities for students who, for whatever reason, are pursuing undergraduate work at an age other than that associated with the traditional college years (18–24)

Hispanic Americans and Asian Americans representing the largest groups of minority students.[19] These students bring a rich variety of cultural influences and traditions to today's college environment.

Students with Disabilities

People with reported disabilities are another rapidly growing student population, currently constituting 9.3 percent of all undergraduates.[21] Improved diagnostic, medical, and rehabilitation procedures coupled with improved educational accommodations have opened up opportunities for these students at an increasing rate. In addition to students who have evident disabilities, such as blindness, deafness, or a physical disability requiring use of a wheelchair, an increasing number of students with "hidden" disabilities are on campuses—students with learning disabilities (including attention deficit disorders), those with managed psychiatric and emotional problems, and those recovering from alcohol and substance abuse. Interestingly, many students with reported "hidden disabilities" often do not consider themselves to be disabled.[22]

 TALKING POINTS When controversial subjects are discussed in class, do you think that your opinions (or how you present them) are affected by the fact that students of different cultural backgrounds are involved in the discussion?

Developmental Tasks of Young Adulthood

Because most of today's undergraduate college students range between the ages of 18 and perhaps 40, we address several areas of growth and development (defined as *developmental tasks*) that characterize the lives of people in this age group. When people sense that they are making progress in some or all of these areas, they are likely to report a sense of life satisfaction or, as we describe it, a sense of well-being.

Forming an Initial Adult Identity

For most of childhood and adolescence, most young people are seen by adults in their neighborhood or community as someone's son or daughter. With the onset of young adulthood, that stage has almost passed; both young people and society are beginning to look at each other in new ways.

As emerging adults, most young people want to present a unique identity to society. Internally they are constructing perceptions of themselves as the adults they wish to be; externally they are formulating the behavioral patterns that will project this identity to others.

Completion of this first developmental task is necessary for young adults to establish a foundation on which to nurture identity during later stages of adulthood. As a result of their experiences in achieving an initial adult identity, they become capable of answering the central question of young adulthood: "Who am I?" Most likely, many nontraditional-age students also ask themselves this question as they progress through college and anticipate the changes that will result from completing a high level of formal education.

Establishing Independence

In contemporary society the primary responsibility for socialization during childhood and adolescence is assigned to the family and school, and less formally to the peer group. For nearly two decades these groups function as the primary contributor to a young person's knowledge, values, and behaviors. By young adulthood, however, students of traditional college age should be demonstrating the desire to move away from the dependent relationships that have existed between themselves and these socializing agents.

 TALKING POINTS What does being an adult mean to you at this point? How would you explain this to your best friend?

Travel, new relationships, marriage, military service, and, of course, college have been traditional avenues for disengagement from the family. Generally, the ability and willingness to follow one or more of these paths helps a young adult establish independence. Success in these endeavors depends on the willingness to use a variety of resources that we will explore later.

Assuming Responsibility

The third developmental task in which traditional-age college students are expected to progress is the assumption of increasing levels of responsibility. Young adults have a variety of opportunities to assume responsibility. College-age young adults may accept responsibility voluntarily, such as when they join a campus organization or establish a new friendship. Other responsibilities are placed on them when professors assign term papers, when dating partners exert pressure on them to conform to their expectations, or when employers require consistently productive work. In other situations they may accept responsibility for doing a particular task not for themselves but for the benefit of others. As important and demanding as these areas of responsibility are, a more fundamental responsibility awaits young adults: the responsibility of maintaining and improving their health and the health of others.

Why Men Die Young

The extra longevity of women in our society is well established. In fact, the difference in life expectancy for male and female infants born today is projected to be 80 years for females, but only 75 for males. This five-year difference has commonly been attributed to genetic factors. However, new evidence demonstrates that this discrepancy may be affected more by male behavior rather than genetic traits.

Men outrank women in all of the top 15 causes of death except for Alzheimer's disease. Men's death rates are twice as high for suicide, homicide, and cirrhosis of the liver. In every age group, American males have poorer health and higher risk of mortality than do females. Common increased risks include:

- More men smoke than women.

- Men are twice as likely to be heavy drinkers and to engage in other risky behaviors such as abusing drugs and driving without a seatbelt.

- More men work in dangerous settings than women do, and men account for 90 percent of on-the-job fatalities.

- More men drive SUVs that are rollover prone, and suffer fatalities in motorcycle accidents.

Perhaps some of these increased risks are associated with deep-seated cultural beliefs about men's bravery and machismo, which reward men for taking risks and facing danger head-on. This "macho" attitude seems to extend to the care that men take of their own physical and mental health. Women are twice as likely to visit their doctor on an annual basis and explore preventative medical treatments than are men. Men are more likely to ignore symptoms and less likely to schedule checkups or seek follow-up treatment. Psychologically, men tend to internalize their feelings or stressors, or even self-medicate to deal with stress, while women tend to seek psychological help. Almost all stress-related diseases are more common in men.

In the final analysis, men and women alike must be responsible for their own health and well-being. By making sound choices regarding diet, exercise, medical care, and high-risk behaviors, both genders can attempt to maximize the full potential of their life expectancy.

Broadening Social Skills

The fourth developmental task of the young adult years is broadening the range of appropriate and dependable social skills. Adulthood ordinarily involves "membership" in a variety of groups that range in size from a marital pair to community organizations or a multinational corporation. These memberships require the ability to function in many different social settings and with a wide variety of people.

The college experience traditionally has prepared students very effectively in this regard, but interactions in friendships, work relationships, or parenting may require that they make an effort to grow and develop beyond levels they achieved by belonging to a peer group. Young adults need to refine a variety of social skills, including communication, listening, and conflict management.

Nurturing Intimacy

The task of nurturing intimacy usually begins in young adulthood and continues through midlife. During this time it is developmentally important to establish one or more intimate relationships. Most people in this age group are viewing intimacy in its broadest sense as a deeply close, sharing relationship. Intimacy may unfold in the context of dating relationships, close friendships, and certainly mentoring relationships.

Involvement in intimate relationships varies, with some people having many relationships and others having only one or two. The number does not matter. From a

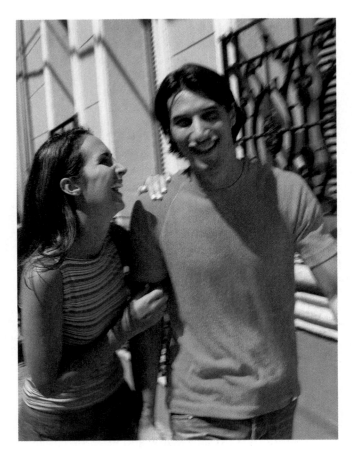

Intimacy can occur in many forms, including traditional dating relationships.

developmental standpoint, what matters is that we have others with whom to share our most deeply held thoughts and feelings as we attempt to validate our own unique approach to living. In the absence of a willingness or an ability to pursue intimacy, a sense of emotional isolation can develop.

Related Developmental Tasks of Young Adulthood

In addition to the five developmental tasks of young adulthood just described, two additional areas of growth and development seem applicable to 18- to 24-year-olds. These include obtaining *entry-level employment* and *developing parenting skills.*

For at least the last 65 years, students in increasing numbers have pursued a college education in large part to gain entry into many occupations and professions. Students of today certainly anticipate that a college degree will open doors for their first substantial employment or entry-level employment.

In many respects employment needs go beyond those associated purely with money. Employment provides the opportunity to assume new responsibilities in which the skills learned in college can be applied and expanded. Employment also involves taking on new roles (such as colleague, mentor, mentee, or partner) that may play an important part in the way we define ourselves for the remainder of our lives. In addition, employment provides a new, more independent arena in which friendships (intimacy) can be pursued. By no means least important, entry-level employment provides the financial foundation on which we can establish independence.

For many people, young adulthood also marks the entry to parenthood, one of the most important responsibilities anyone can choose to assume. The multitude of decisions associated with this commitment will, naturally, shape the remainder of one's life. Examples of these decisions are whether to parent or not and, if so, when to begin, how many children to have, how long to wait between children, and what role parenting will play in the context of overall adulthood. The ability to make sound decisions and to develop the skills and insights necessary to parent effectively may be the most challenging aspect of growth and development that confronts young adults.

The Multiple Dimensions of Health

In an earlier section of the chapter we promised to give you a new definition of health that would be less focused on morbidity (illness) and mortality (death) than most others are. However, before we present that new definition, we

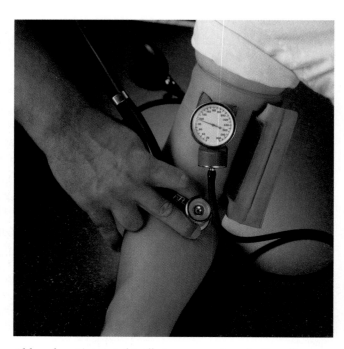

Although not interested in illness or premature death, wellness practitioners find it critically important that they inform their clients about the role of elevated blood pressure in the development of cardiovascular disease.

introduce here a *multidimensional concept of health* (**holistic health**)—a requirement for any definition of health that moves beyond the cure/prevention of illness and the postponement of death.

Although our modern health care community too frequently acts as if the structure and the function of the physical body are the sole basis of health, common experience supports the validity of a *holistic* nature to health. In this section we examine six components, or dimensions, of health, all interacting in a synergistic manner allowing us to engage in the wide array of life experiences (see Figure 1-2).

Physical Dimension

Most of us have a number of physiological and structural characteristics we can call on to aid us in accomplishing the wide array of activities that characterize a typical day and, on occasion, a not so typical day. Among these physical characteristics are our body weight, visual ability, strength, coordination, level of endurance, level of suscep-

---

Key Terms

holistic health a view of health in terms of its physical, emotional, social, intellectual, spiritual, and occupational makeup

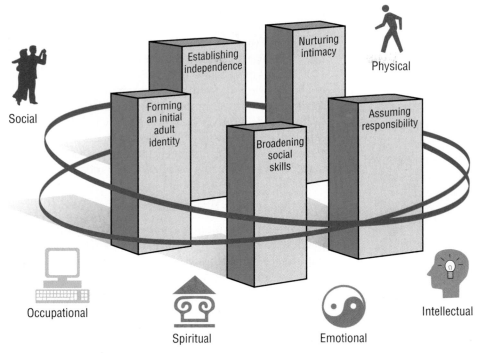

Figure 1-2 Mastery of the developmental tasks of young adulthood through a balanced involvement of the six dimensions of health leads to the enjoyment of a more productive and satisfying life.

tibility to disease, and powers of recuperation. In certain situations the physical dimension of health may be the most important. This importance almost certainly is why traditional medicine for centuries has equated health with the design and operation of the body.

Emotional Dimension

We also possess certain emotional characteristics that can help us through the demands of daily living. The emotional dimension of health encompasses our ability to see the world in a realistic manner, cope with stress, remain flexible, and compromise to resolve conflict.

For young adults, growth and development often give rise to emotional vulnerability, which may lead to feelings of rejection and failure that can reduce productivity and satisfaction. To some extent we are all affected by feeling states, such as anger, happiness, fear, empathy, guilt, love, and hate. People who consistently try to improve their emotional health appear to enjoy life to a much greater extent than do those who let feelings of vulnerability overwhelm them or block their creativity.

Social Dimension

A third dimension of health encompasses social skills and cultural sensitivity. Initially, family interactions, school experiences, and peer group interactions foster develop-

ment in these areas, but future social interactions will demand additional skill development and refinement of already existing skills and insights. In adulthood, including young adulthood, the composition of the social world changes, principally because of our exposure to a wider array of people and the expanded roles associated with employment, parenting, and community involvement.

The social abilities of many nontraditional-age students may already be firmly established. Entering college may encourage them to develop new social skills that help them socialize with their traditional-age student colleagues. After being on campus for a while, nontraditional-age students are often able to interact comfortably with traditional-age students in such diverse places as the library, the student center, and the classroom. This interaction enhances the social dimension of health for both types of students.

Intellectual Dimension

The abilities to process and act on information, clarify values and beliefs, and exercise decision-making capacity rank among the most important aspects of total health. For many college-educated persons, the intellectual dimension of health may prove to be the most important and satisfying of the six. In fact, for all of us, at least on certain occasions, this holds true. Our ability to analyze, synthesize, hypothesize, and then act on new information enhances the quality of our lives in multiple ways.

Spiritual Dimension

The fifth dimension of health is the spiritual dimension. Although certainly it includes religious beliefs and practices, many young adults would expand it to encompass more diverse belief systems, including relationships with other living things, the nature of human behavior, and the need and willingness to serve others. All are important components of spiritual health.

Through nurturing the spiritual dimension of our health, we may develop an expanded perception of the universe and better define our relationship to all that it contains, including other people. To achieve growth in the spiritual dimension of health, many people undertake a serious study of doctrine associated with established religious groups and assume membership in a community of faith. For others, however, spiritual growth is believed to occur, in the absence of a theist-based belief system, as they open themselves to new experiences that involve nature, art, body movement, or stewarding of the environment.

Interestingly, the role of the spiritual dimension of health was given an increased measure of credence when studies published in the scientific literature, including a statistical review of 42 earlier studies, demonstrated a consistently longer life for persons who regularly participated in religious practices, particularly for women.[23,24] This was true even when factors such as smoking, alcohol use, and income were statistically eliminated. Contradictory to these findings, however, was a more recent report suggesting that the association between religious attendance and survival may be weaker than earlier studies have suggested.[25]

Perhaps more relevant to college students than the spiritual dimension of health's relationship to life expectancy is spirituality's positive influence during college. In the 2003 College Student Survey conducted by UCLA's Higher Education Research Institute, college students who defined themselves as spiritual seemed less stressed during school than did those reporting a less spiritually related focus.[26]

Occupational Dimension

A significant contribution made by the currently popular wellness movement is that it defines for many people the importance of the workplace to their sense of well-being. In today's world, employment and productive efforts play an increasingly important role in how we perceive ourselves and how we see the "goodness" of the world in which we live. In addition, the workplace serves as both a testing ground for and a source of life-enhancing skills. In our place of employment we gain not only the financial resources to meet our demands for both necessities and luxuries but also an array of useful skills such as conflict resolution, experiences in shared responsibility, and intellectual growth that can be used to facilitate a wide range of nonemployment-related interactions. In turn, the workplace is enhanced by the healthfulness of the individuals who contribute to its endeavors.

Environmental Dimension

Some academics would add to the dimensions just discussed an *Environmental Dimension*. If this dimension is defined on the basis of land, air, and water, then it might be an additional dimension to consider. However, should the environmental dimension be extended to include all that is material and metaphysical surrounding each individual, such a concept seems beyond the scope of this chapter. Thus, we have elected not to expand the number of holistic dimensions of health beyond those traditionally discussed.

Wellness

Expanded perceptions of health are the basis for **wellness.** Recall that episodic health care, preventive medicine, and community health promotion are directly aligned with concerns about morbidity and mortality, whereas health

Key Terms
wellness the unlocking of our full potential through the adoption of an overall wellness lifestyle

promotion at the individual level is focused on aspects of appearance, weight management, body composition, and physical performance capabilities. Wellness differs from these kinds of health care concerns because it virtually has no interest in morbidity and mortality.

Practitioners describe wellness as a process of extending information, counseling, assessment, and lifestyle-modification strategies, leading to a desirable change in the recipients' overall lifestyle, or the adoption of a wellness lifestyle. Once adopted, the wellness lifestyle produces a sense of well-being that in turn enables recipients to unlock their full potential.

This explanation of how wellness differs from episodic health care, preventive medicine, and health promotion does, on first hearing, seem progressive and clearly devoid of interest in morbidity and mortality concerns. But in practice, wellness programs are not all that different from other kinds of health care. We have consistently noted that wellness programs, as carried out on college campuses, in local hospital wellness centers, and in corporate settings, routinely transmit familiar health-related information and engage in the same risk-reduction activities that characterize preventive medicine and health promotion. It is in the final aspect of wellness, the "unlocking of full potential," that wellness differs from other concepts of health—although the focus to which this "full potential" should be directed is not often identified.

A New Definition of Health

At the beginning of the chapter we hinted at a new way to view health—a view that would be far less centered in morbidity and mortality concerns than are traditional concepts of health and even of wellness. The definition that we propose takes into account the differences between *what health is for* (its role) and *what health is* (its composition).

The Role of Health

The role of health in our lives is very similar to the role of a car. Much as a car (or other vehicle) takes us to places we need or want to be, good health enables us to accomplish the activities that collectively transition us into and through developmental tasks associated with young adulthood (pages 12–14). Recall that the process of moving through each stage of adulthood does not occur simply because of the passage of time but rather because we actively participate, on a day-to-day basis, in demands of life appropriate to our life stage.

The Composition of Health

Now that you know what the role of health is, its composition can be seen as being more than simply having a body free of illness and apparently destined for a long life. Rather, the composition of health is that of a collection of resources, from each dimension of health (pages 14–16), determined to be necessary for the successful accomplishment of activities that you need or want to do. Some of these needed resources are already within you (intrinsic), whereas others need to come from outside (extrinsic). However, regardless of their origin, once they are accessed and applied to activities, small forward growth steps will occur. Obviously, to recognize what resources are needed, you must be a student of society's expectations for persons of your age, as well as your own highly personalized developmental aspirations.

Our Definition of Health

By combining the role of health with the composition of health, we offer a new definition of health:

> Health is a reflection of one's ability to use the **intrinsic** and **extrinsic** resources related to each dimension of health to participate fully in the activities that contribute to growth and development, with the goal of feeling a sense of well-being as one evaluates one's progress through life.

In light of this definition, do not be surprised when we ask whether you are resourceful (healthy) enough to attain the goals you wish to reach, whether you are healthy enough to sustain a particular behavioral pattern that you have adopted, or whether you are experiencing the sense of well-being to which you aspire.

Taking Charge of Your Health

- Complete the Comprehensive Health Assessment on pp. 21–30. Develop a plan to modify your behavior in the areas in which you need improvement.

- Take part in a new spiritual activity, such as meditating, creating art or music, or attending a religious service.

- To promote the social dimension of your health, try to meet one new person each week during the semester.

- Choose one developmental task you would like to focus on, such as assuming responsibility, and plan the steps you can follow to progress in this area.

- Volunteer to be an assistant in a community service program, such as a literacy project or a preschool program.

SUMMARY

- When used to define health, *morbidity* and *mortality* relate to the prevalence of particular diseases and illnesses and to death resulting from those diseases and illnesses.
- When we seek the services of health care practitioners because of symptoms of illness or disease, we are said to be seeking episodic health care.
- Preventive medical care attempts to minimize the incidence of illness and disease by identifying early indicators of risk to bring them under control.
- Individual health promotion involves risk-reduction activities similar to those used in preventive medical care, except that the techniques cannot be invasive and are directed by professionals who are not physicians. Its most visible emphasis tends to be on fitness and body composition.
- Community health promotion involves the empowerment of individuals so that they can organize and participate in their own health promotion activities.
- Healthy People 2010 is a federally funded program to improve the nation's health, increase life expectancy, and expand access to comprehensive health care.
- A decision to change a health behavior is often difficult to make because of the multiplicity of factors underlying the maintenance of the high-risk behavior.
- Health behavior change requires movement through a multistaged process, including precontemplation, contemplation, preparation, action, maintenance, and termination.
- A wide array of health problems (for example, cancer, cardiovascular disease, HIV/AIDS) persist despite today's highly sophisticated health care technology.

- Today's college campus is a dynamic blend of students of both traditional and nontraditional ages and of diverse background, cultures, and attributes.
- Young adulthood is characterized by five key developmental tasks: forming an initial adult identity, establishing independence, assuming responsibility, broadening social skills, and nurturing intimacy.
- Personal development during young adulthood involves a set of developmental tasks that are common to all yet may be undertaken differently by each individual.
- Multidimensional definitions of health, including holistic health, have existed for decades—although the primary emphasis has always been on the physical dimension.
- Current multidimensions of health may include many or all of the following dimensions: physical, emotional, social, intellectual, spiritual, and occupational.
- Wellness contends a disinterest in morbidity and mortality, rather emphasizing living a wellness lifestyle that leads to a sense of well-being.
- Our definition of health includes the role of health and the composition of health. The role of health is to enable individuals to participate in the activities that collectively constitute growth and development. The composition of health is the intrinsic and extrinsic resources on which individuals can draw to participate fully in their own growth and development.

REVIEW QUESTIONS

1. What are morbidity and mortality, and how are they involved in the more traditional definitions of health?
2. When and from whom do people seek episodic health care?
3. In preventive medical care, who determines a person's level of risk and decides what risk-reduction techniques should be implemented?
4. What does the term *empowerment* mean, and how would it appear as a component of a community-based health promotion program?
5. What are the six stages that persons pass through as they consider and then attempt to change their health behavior?
6. What are several of the more pressing health problems that confront the American people?
7. In what ways is the current U.S. college student population more diverse than any that came before?

8. What are the developmental tasks of young adulthood and how can the accomplishing of one influence the accomplishing of any of the remaining four?
9. How does the term *multidimensional* apply to the concept of holistic health?
10. What are the most frequently included dimensions within a holistically centered definition of health?
11. What is the underlying reason that proponents of wellness give for being disinterested in morbidity and mortality?
12. How does your textbook's definition of health differ from traditional definitions?
13. How does your textbook define the role of health? The composition of health?
14. Why is it necessary to understand developmental expectations before we can answer the question, "Are you healthy enough to . . . ?"

ENDNOTES

1. Woodwell DA and Cherry DK. *National Ambulatory Medical Care Survey: 2002 Summary.* Advance Data From Vital and Health Statistics. National Center for Health Statistics. Number 346. August 26, 2004.

2. Centers for Disease Control and Prevention: *National Ambulatory Medical Care Survey: 2000.* Atlanta, GA: July 2002.

3. Roper Center for Public Opinion Research (for Pfizer Women's Health), University of Connecticut. Adults know their family history. *USA Today*. May 30, 2000. p. 5D.

4. *U.S. Surgeon General's Family History Initiative.* Washington, DC: United State Department of Health and Human Services. 2004. www.hhs.gov/family history/download.html.

5. Smith PC, et al. Missing information during primary care visits. 2005. *JAMA*. Feb 2; 293(5): 565–571.

6. Cottrell RR, Girvan JT, McKenzie JF. *Principles and Foundations of Health Promotion and Education* (3rd ed.). San Francisco: Benjamin Cummings, 2005.

7. Kreuter MW, Lezin NA, Kreuter MW, Green LW. *Community Health Promotion Ideas That Work: A Field-Book for Practitioners.* Sudbury, MA: Jones and Bartlett Publishers. 2003.

8. McKenzie JF, Neiger BL, Smeltzer JL. *Planning, implementing and evaluating health promotion programs* (4th ed.). Benjamin Cummings, 2005.

9. *Priority Areas for National Action: Transforming Health Care Quality* (2003). Washington, DC: The National Academies Press, 2003.

10. *Healthy People 2000: National Health Promotion and Disease Prevention Objectives* (full report with commentary). Washington, DC: U.S. Department of Health and Human Services. Public Health Service, 1991.

11. *Healthy People 2000: Midcourse Review and 1995 Revisions.* Washington, DC: U.S. Department of Health and Human Services. Public Health Service, 1995.

12. *Healthy People 2010: Understanding and Improving Health.* Washington, DC: U.S. Department of Health and Human Services. Public Health Service, 2000.

13. *Healthy People 2010: Understanding and Improving Health* (2nd ed.). Washington, DC: U.S. Department of Health and Human Services. Public Health Service, 2000.

14. Prochaska JO, Velicer WF. The transtheoretical model of health behavior change. 1994. *Am J of Health Promotion.* 12:38–48.

15. Norcross JC, Prochaska JO. Using the stages of change. 2002. *Harv Ment Health Lett.* 18(11):507.

16. Prochaska JO, Norcross JC, Clemente CC. *Changing for Good.* New York: Willian Morrow and Company, 1994.

17. Diet and genes. *Newsweek* (with Harvard Medical School). January 17, 2005.

18. The quest for memory drugs. *Newsweek* (with Harvard Medical School). December 6, 2004.

19. College enrollment by sex, age, race, and hispanic origins: 1980 to 2001 (No. 280). Washington, DC: U.S. Census Bureau. *Statistical Abstract of the United States: 2003.*

20. Foreign (nonimmigrant) student enrollment in college: 1976 to 2002 (No. 281). Washington, DC: U.S. Census Bureau. *Statistical Abstract of the United States: 2003.*

21. Undergraduates reported disability status by selected characteristics: 1999–2000 (No. 285). Washington, DC: U.S. Census Bureau. *Statistical Abstract of the United States: 2003.*

22. U.S. National Center for Education Statistics, *Profile of Undergraduates in U.S. Postsecondary Education Institutions, 1999–2000.* Washington, DC: July, 2000.

23. Hummer RA, et al. Religious involvement and adult mortality in the United States: Review and perspective. *South Med J.* 2004. Dec: 97(12)1223–1230.

24. McCullough ME, et al. Religious involvement and U.S. adult mortality: A meta-analysis review. *Health Psychology* 2000; 19(2): 211–222.

25. Bagiella W, Hong V, Sloan RP. Religious attendance as a predictor of survival in the EPESE cohorts. *Int J Epidemiol.* 2005 Jan 19, 34, 443–451.

26. *Spirituality in Higher Education: A National Search For Meaning and Purpose* (Pilot Survey 2003). Higher Education Research Institute, University of California, Los Angeles. www.spirituality.ucla.edu.

As We Go to Press

In 1996 the U.S. Preventive Services Task Force recommended that prenatal HIV testing need not be extended beyond those women determined to have come from high-risk backgrounds. When identified as HIV positive, these women were placed on a combination drug therapy, delivered by Caesarean section, and advised not to breast-feed their infants. For those compliant with this form of pregnancy management, the risk of infecting their infants dropped below 1 percent, from the otherwise expected 25 percent infant-infection rate. Five years later, in 2001, the Centers for Disease Control and Prevention (CDC) recommended that HIV testing become a routine part of prenatal care for all pregnant women.

In spite of CDC's recommendation for universal HIV prenatal testing, many pregnant women either were not offered testing by their prenatal care providers or declined the offer when it was extended. Accordingly, in the absence of knowing their HIV status, women who were unknowingly infected failed to receive treatment, and infant-infection rates remained unacceptably higher than necessary.

Recently, and in response to the continuing risks to both new mothers and their infants, a newer U.S. Preventive Services Task Force recommended that the emphasis on universal prenatal testing for HIV infection be significantly strengthened. In the opinion of this panel, should the health care community commit themselves to this task, women will feel increasingly more comfortable with the role of HIV testing as a part of prenatal care, and the risk of infection to newborns will fall accordingly. Recall that preventive medical care is, in the final analysis, more affordable than episodic care.

Source: U.S. Preventive Services Task Force. Screening for HIV: Recommendation Statement. *Annals of Internal Medicine.* 2005 July; 143(1):32–37.

comprehensive health assessment

Now that you have read the first chapter, complete the following Comprehensive Health Assessment. We strongly suggest that you retake this assessment after you have completed your health course. Then compare your responses in each section of the assessment. Have your scores improved?

Social and Occupational Health	Not true/ rarely	Somewhat true/ sometimes	Mostly true/ usually	Very true/ always
1. I feel loved and supported by my family.	1	2	3	4
2. I establish friendships with ease and enjoyment.	1	2	3	4
3. I establish friendships with people of both genders and all ages.	1	2	3	4
4. I sustain relationships by communicating with and caring about my family and friends.	1	2	3	4
5. I feel comfortable and confident when meeting people for the first time.	1	2	3	4
6. I practice social skills to facilitate the process of forming new relationships.	1	2	3	4
7. I seek opportunities to meet and interact with new people.	1	2	3	4
8. I talk with, rather than at, people.	1	2	3	4
9. I am open to developing or sustaining intimate relationships.	1	2	3	4
10. I appreciate the importance of parenting the next generation and am committed to supporting it in ways that reflect my own resources.	1	2	3	4
11. I recognize the strengths and weaknesses of my parents' childrearing skills and feel comfortable modifying them if I choose to become a parent.	1	2	3	4
12. I attempt to be tolerant of others whether or not I approve of their behavior or beliefs.	1	2	3	4
13. I understand and appreciate the contribution that cultural diversity makes to the quality of living.	1	2	3	4
14. I understand and appreciate the difference between being educated and being trained.	1	2	3	4
15. My work gives me a sense of self-sufficiency and an opportunity to contribute.	1	2	3	4
16. I have equal respect for the roles of leader and subordinate within the workplace.	1	2	3	4
17. I have chosen an occupation that suits my interests and temperament.	1	2	3	4
18. I have chosen an occupation that does not compromise my physical or psychological health.	1	2	3	4
19. I get along well with my coworkers most of the time.	1	2	3	4
20. When I have a disagreement with a coworker, I try to resolve it directly and constructively.	1	2	3	4

Points _____

Spiritual and Psychological Health	Not true/ rarely	Somewhat true/ sometimes	Mostly true/ usually	Very true/ always
1. I have a deeply held belief system or personal theology.	1	2	3	4
2. I recognize the contribution that membership in a community of faith or spirituality can make to a person's overall quality of life.	1	2	3	4

		Not true/ rarely	Somewhat true/ sometimes	Mostly true/ usually	Very true/ always
3.	I seek experiences with nature and reflect on nature's contribution to my quality of life.	1	2	3	4
4.	My spirituality is a resource that helps me remain calm and strong during times of stress.	1	2	3	4
5.	I have found appropriate ways to express my spirituality.	1	2	3	4
6.	I respect the diversity of spiritual expression and am tolerant of those whose beliefs differ from my own.	1	2	3	4
7.	I take adequate time to reflect on my own life and my relationships with others and the institutions of society.	1	2	3	4
8.	I routinely undertake new experiences.	1	2	3	4
9.	I receive adequate support from others.	1	2	3	4
10.	I look for opportunities to support others, even occasionally at the expense of my own goals and aspirations.	1	2	3	4
11.	I recognize that emotional and psychological health are as important as physical health.	1	2	3	4
12.	I express my feelings and opinions comfortably, yet am capable of keeping them to myself when appropriate.	1	2	3	4
13.	I see myself as a person of worth and feel comfortable with my own strengths and limitations.	1	2	3	4
14.	I establish realistic goals and work to achieve them.	1	2	3	4
15.	I understand the differences between the normal range of emotions and the signs of clinical depression.	1	2	3	4
16.	I know how to recognize signs of suicidal thoughts and am willing to intervene.	1	2	3	4
17.	I regularly assess my own behavior patterns and beliefs and would seek professional assistance for any emotional dysfunction.	1	2	3	4
18.	I accept the reality of aging and view it as an opportunity for positive change.	1	2	3	4
19.	I accept the reality of death and view it as a normal and inevitable part of life.	1	2	3	4
20.	I have made decisions about my own death to ensure that I die with dignity when the time comes.	1	2	3	4

Points _____

Stress Management

		Not true/ rarely	Somewhat true/ sometimes	Mostly true/ usually	Very true/ always
1.	I accept the reality of change while maintaining the necessary stability in my daily activities.	1	2	3	4
2.	I seek change when it is necessary or desirable to do so.	1	2	3	4
3.	I know what stress-management services are offered on campus, through my employer, or in my community.	1	2	3	4
4.	When necessary, I use the stress-management services to which I have access.	1	2	3	4
5.	I employ stress-reduction practices in anticipation of stressful events, such as job interviews and final examinations.	1	2	3	4
6.	I reevaluate the way in which I handled stressful events so that I can better cope with similar events in the future.	1	2	3	4
7.	I turn to relatives and friends during periods of disruption in my life.	1	2	3	4

		Not true/ rarely	Somewhat true/ sometimes	Mostly true/ usually	Very true/ always
8.	I avoid using alcohol or other drugs during periods of stress.	1	2	3	4
9.	I refrain from behaving aggressively or abusively during periods of stress.	1	2	3	4
10.	I sleep enough to maintain a high level of health and cope successfully with daily challenges.	1	2	3	4
11.	I avoid sleeping excessively as a response to stressful change.	1	2	3	4
12.	My diet is conducive to good health and stress management.	1	2	3	4
13.	I participate in physical activity to relieve stress.	1	2	3	4
14.	I practice stress-management skills, such as diaphragmatic breathing and yoga.	1	2	3	4
15.	I manage my time effectively.	1	2	3	4

Points _____

Fitness

		Not true/ rarely	Somewhat true/ sometimes	Mostly true/ usually	Very true/ always
1.	I participate in recreational and fitness activities both to minimize stress and to improve or maintain my level of physical fitness.	1	2	3	4
2.	I select some recreational activities that are strenuous rather than sedentary in nature.	1	2	3	4
3.	I include various types of aerobic conditioning activities among the wider array of recreational and fitness activities in which I engage.	1	2	3	4
4.	I engage in aerobic activities with appropriate frequency, intensity, and duration to provide a training effect for my heart and lungs.	1	2	3	4
5.	I routinely include strength-training activities among the wider array of fitness activities in which I engage.	1	2	3	4
6.	I routinely vary the types of strength-training activities in which I participate in order to minimize injury and strengthen all of the important muscle groups.	1	2	3	4
7.	I do exercises specifically designed to maintain joint range of motion.	1	2	3	4
8.	I believe that recreational and fitness activities can help me improve my physical health and my emotional and social well-being.	1	2	3	4
9.	I include a variety of fitness activities in my overall plan for physical fitness.	1	2	3	4
10.	I take appropriate steps to avoid injuries when participating in recreational and fitness activities.	1	2	3	4
11.	I seek appropriate treatment for all injuries that result from fitness activities.	1	2	3	4
12.	I believe that older adults should undertake appropriately chosen fitness activities.	1	2	3	4
13.	My body composition is consistent with a high level of health.	1	2	3	4
14.	I warm up before beginning vigorous activity, and I cool down afterward.	1	2	3	4
15.	I select properly designed and well-maintained equipment and clothing for each activity.	1	2	3	4

	Not true/ rarely	Somewhat true/ sometimes	Mostly true/ usually	Very true/ always
16. I avoid using performance-enhancing substances that are known to be dangerous and those whose influence on the body is not fully understood.	1	2	3	4
17. I sleep seven to eight hours daily.	1	2	3	4
18. I refrain from using over-the-counter sleep-inducing aids.	1	2	3	4
19. I follow sound dietary practices as an important adjunct to a health-enhancing physical activity program.	1	2	3	4
20. My current level of fitness allows me to participate fully and effortlessly in my daily activities.	1	2	3	4

Points _____

Nutrition and Weight Management

	Not true/ rarely	Somewhat true/ sometimes	Mostly true/ usually	Very true/ always
1. I balance my caloric intake with my caloric expenditure.	1	2	3	4
2. I obtain the recommended number of servings from each of the food groups.	1	2	3	4
3. I select a wide variety of foods chosen from each of the food groups.	1	2	3	4
4. I understand the amount of a particular food that constitutes a single serving.	1	2	3	4
5. I often try new foods, particularly when I know them to be healthful.	1	2	3	4
6. I select breads, cereals, fresh fruits, and vegetables in preference to pastries, candies, sodas, and fruits canned in heavy syrup.	1	2	3	4
7. I limit the amount of sugar that I add to foods during preparation and at the table.	1	2	3	4
8. I examine food labels to determine the presence of trans-fats (trans-fatty acids) and select foods free of these fats.	1	2	3	4
9. I select primarily nonmeat sources of protein, such as peas, beans, and peanut butter, while limiting my consumption of red meat and high-fat dairy products.	1	2	3	4
10. I consume an appropriate percentage of my total daily calories from protein.	1	2	3	4
11. I select foods prepared with unsaturated vegetable oils while reducing consumption of red meat, high-fat dairy products, and foods prepared with lard (animal fat) or butter.	1	2	3	4
12. I carefully limit the amount of fast food that I consume during a typical week.	1	2	3	4
13. I consume an appropriate percentage of my total daily calories from fat.	1	2	3	4
14. I select nutritious foods when I snack.	1	2	3	4
15. I limit my use of salt during food preparation and at the table.	1	2	3	4
16. I consume adequate amounts of fiber.	1	2	3	4
17. I routinely consider the nutrient density of individual food items when choosing foods.	1	2	3	4
18. I maintain my weight without reliance on over-the-counter or prescription diet pills.	1	2	3	4

	Not true/ rarely	Somewhat true/ sometimes	Mostly true/ usually	Very true/ always
19. I maintain my weight without reliance on fad diets or liquid weight loss beverages.	1	2	3	4
20. I exercise regularly to help maintain my weight.	1	2	3	4

Points _____

Alcohol, Tobacco, and Other Drug Use

	Not true/ rarely	Somewhat true/ sometimes	Mostly true/ usually	Very true/ always
1. I abstain or drink in moderation when offered alcoholic beverages.	1	2	3	4
2. I abstain from using illegal psychoactive (mind-altering) drugs.	1	2	3	4
3. I do not consume alcoholic beverages or psychoactive drugs rapidly or in large quantities.	1	2	3	4
4. I do not use alcohol or psychoactive drugs in a way that causes me to behave inappropriately.	1	2	3	4
5. My use of alcohol or other drugs does not compromise my academic performance.	1	2	3	4
6. I refrain from drinking alcoholic beverages or using psychoactive drugs when engaging in recreational activities that require strength, speed, or coordination.	1	2	3	4
7. I refrain from drinking alcoholic beverages while participating in occupational activities, regardless of the nature of those activities.	1	2	3	4
8. My use of alcohol or other drugs does not generate financial concerns for myself or for others.	1	2	3	4
9. I refrain from drinking alcohol or using psychoactive drugs when driving a motor vehicle or operating heavy equipment.	1	2	3	4
10. I do not drink alcohol or use psychoactive drugs when I am alone.	1	2	3	4
11. I avoid riding with people who have been drinking alcohol or using psychoactive drugs.	1	2	3	4
12. My use of alcohol or other drugs does not cause family dysfunction.	1	2	3	4
13. I do not use marijuana.	1	2	3	4
14. I do not use hallucinogens.	1	2	3	4
15. I do not use heroin or other illegal intravenous drugs.	1	2	3	4
16. I do not experience blackouts when I drink alcohol.	1	2	3	4
17. I do not become abusive or violent when I drink alcohol or use psychoactive drugs.	1	2	3	4
18. I use potentially addictive prescription medication in complete compliance with my physician's directions.	1	2	3	4
19. I do not smoke cigarettes.	1	2	3	4
20. I do not use tobacco products in any other form.	1	2	3	4
21. I minimize my exposure to secondhand smoke.	1	2	3	4
22. I am concerned about the effect that alcohol, tobacco, and other drug use is known to have on developing fetuses.	1	2	3	4
23. I am concerned about the effect that alcohol, tobacco, and other drug use is known to have on the health of other people.	1	2	3	4

	Not true/ rarely	Somewhat true/ sometimes	Mostly true/ usually	Very true/ always
24. I seek natural, health-enhancing highs rather than relying on alcohol, tobacco, and illegal drugs.	1	2	3	4
25. I take prescription medication only as instructed, and I use over-the-counter medication in accordance with directions.	1	2	3	4

Points _____

Disease Prevention

	Not true/ rarely	Somewhat true/ sometimes	Mostly true/ usually	Very true/ always
1. My diet includes foods rich in phytochemicals.	1	2	3	4
2. My diet includes foods rich in folic acid.	1	2	3	4
3. My diet includes foods that are good sources of dietary fiber.	1	2	3	4
4. My diet is low in dietary cholesterol.	1	2	3	4
5. I follow food preparation practices that minimize the risk of food-borne illness.	1	2	3	4
6. I engage in regular physical activity and am able to control my weight effectively.	1	2	3	4
7. I do not use tobacco products.	1	2	3	4
8. I abstain from alcohol or drink only in moderation.	1	2	3	4
9. I do not use intravenously administered illegal drugs.	1	2	3	4
10. I use safer sex practices intended to minimize my risk of exposure to sexually transmitted diseases, including HIV and HPV.	1	2	3	4
11. I take steps to limit my risk of exposure to the bacterium that causes Lyme disease and to the virus that causes hantavirus pulmonary syndrome.	1	2	3	4
12. I control my blood pressure with weight management and physical fitness activities.	1	2	3	4
13. I minimize my exposure to allergens, including those that trigger asthma attacks.	1	2	3	4
14. I wash my hands frequently and thoroughly.	1	2	3	4
15. I use preventive medical care services appropriately.	1	2	3	4
16. I use appropriate cancer self-screening practices, such as breast self-examination and testicular self-examination.	1	2	3	4
17. I know which chronic illnesses and diseases are part of my family history.	1	2	3	4
18. I know which inherited conditions are part of my family history and will seek preconceptional counseling regarding these conditions.	1	2	3	4
19. I am fully immunized against infectious diseases.	1	2	3	4
20. I take prescribed medications, particularly antibiotics, exactly as instructed by my physician.	1	2	3	4

Points _____

Sexual Health

	Not true/ rarely	Somewhat true/ sometimes	Mostly true/ usually	Very true/ always
1. I know how sexually transmitted diseases are spread.	1	2	3	4
2. I can recognize the symptoms of sexually transmitted diseases.	1	2	3	4

	Not true/ rarely	Somewhat true/ sometimes	Mostly true/ usually	Very true/ always
3. I know how sexually transmitted disease transmission can be prevented.	1	2	3	4
4. I know how safer sex practices reduce the risk of contracting sexually transmitted diseases.	1	2	3	4
5. I follow safer sex practices.	1	2	3	4
6. I recognize the symptoms of premenstrual syndrome and understand how it is prevented and treated.	1	2	3	4
7. I recognize the symptoms of endometriosis and understand the relationship of its symptoms to hormonal cycles.	1	2	3	4
8. I understand the physiological basis of menopause and recognize that it is a normal part of the aging process in women.	1	2	3	4
9. I understand and accept the range of human sexual orientations.	1	2	3	4
10. I encourage the development of flexible sex roles (androgyny) in children.	1	2	3	4
11. I take a mature approach to dating and mate selection.	1	2	3	4
12. I recognize that marriage and other types of long-term relationships can be satisfying.	1	2	3	4
13. I recognize that a celibate lifestyle is appropriate and satisfying for some people.	1	2	3	4
14. I affirm the sexuality of older adults and am comfortable with its expression.	1	2	3	4
15. I am familiar with the advantages and disadvantages of a wide range of birth control methods.	1	2	3	4
16. I understand how each birth control method works and how effective it is.	1	2	3	4
17. I use my birth control method consistently and appropriately.	1	2	3	4
18. I am familiar with the wide range of procedures now available to treat infertility.	1	2	3	4
19. I accept that others may disagree with my feelings about pregnancy termination.	1	2	3	4
20. I am familiar with alternatives available to infertile couples, including adoption.	1	2	3	4

Points _____

Safety Practices and Violence Prevention	Not true/ rarely	Somewhat true/ sometimes	Mostly true/ usually	Very true/ always
1. I attempt to identify sources of risk or danger in each new setting or activity.	1	2	3	4
2. I learn proper procedures and precautions before undertaking new recreational or occupational activities.	1	2	3	4
3. I select appropriate clothing and equipment for all activities and maintain equipment in good working order.	1	2	3	4
4. I curtail my participation in activities when I am not feeling well or am distracted by other demands.	1	2	3	4
5. I repair dangerous conditions or report them to those responsible for maintenance.	1	2	3	4

6. I use common sense and observe the laws governing nonmotorized vehicles when I ride a bicycle.	1	2	3	4
7. I operate all motor vehicles as safely as possible, including using seat belts and other safety equipment.	1	2	3	4
8. I refrain from driving an automobile or boat when I have been drinking alcohol or taking drugs or medications.	1	2	3	4
9. I try to anticipate the risk of falling and maintain my environment to minimize this risk.	1	2	3	4
10. I maintain my environment to minimize the risk of fire, and I have a well-rehearsed plan to exit my residence in case of fire.	1	2	3	4
11. I am a competent swimmer and could save myself or rescue someone who was drowning.	1	2	3	4
12. I refrain from sexually aggressive behavior toward my partner or others.	1	2	3	4
13. I would report an incident of sexual harassment or date rape whether or not I was the victim.	1	2	3	4
14. I would seek help from others if I were the victim or perpetrator of domestic violence.	1	2	3	4
15. I practice gun safety and encourage other gun owners to do so.	1	2	3	4
16. I drive at all times in a way that will minimize my risk of being carjacked.	1	2	3	4
17. I have taken steps to protect my home from intruders.	1	2	3	4
18. I use campus security services as much as possible when they are available.	1	2	3	4
19. I know what to do if I am being stalked.	1	2	3	4
20. I have a well-rehearsed plan to protect myself from the aggressive behavior of other people in my place of residence.	1	2	3	4

Points _____

Health Care Consumerism

	Not true/ rarely	Somewhat true/ sometimes	Mostly true/ usually	Very true/ always
1. I know how to obtain valid health information.	1	2	3	4
2. I accept health information that has been deemed valid by the established scientific community.	1	2	3	4
3. I am skeptical of claims that guarantee the effectiveness of a particular health-care service or product.	1	2	3	4
4. I am skeptical of practitioners or clinics who advertise or offer services at rates substantially lower than those charged by reputable providers.	1	2	3	4
5. I am not swayed by advertisements that present unhealthy behavior in an attractive manner.	1	2	3	4
6. I can afford proper medical care, including hospitalization.	1	2	3	4
7. I can afford adequate health insurance.	1	2	3	4
8. I understand the role of government health care plans in providing health care to people who qualify for coverage.	1	2	3	4
9. I know how to select health care providers who are highly qualified and appropriate for my current health care needs.	1	2	3	4

	Not true/ rarely	Somewhat true/ sometimes	Mostly true/ usually	Very true/ always
10. I seek a second or third opinion when surgery or other costly therapies are recommended.	1	2	3	4
11. I have told my physician which hospital I would prefer to use should the need arise.	1	2	3	4
12. I understand my rights and responsibilities as a patient when admitted to a hospital.	1	2	3	4
13. I practice adequate self-care to reduce my health care expenditures and my reliance on health care providers.	1	2	3	4
14. I am open-minded about alternative health care practices and support current efforts to determine their appropriate role in effective health care.	1	2	3	4
15. I have a well-established relationship with a pharmacist and have transmitted all necessary information regarding medication and use.	1	2	3	4
16. I carefully follow labels and directions when using health care products, such as over-the-counter medications.	1	2	3	4
17. I finish all prescription medications as directed, rather than stopping use when symptoms subside.	1	2	3	4
18. I report to the appropriate agencies any providers of health care services, information, or products that use deceptive advertising or fraudulent methods of operation.	1	2	3	4
19. I pursue my rights as fully as possible in matters of misrepresentation or consumer dissatisfaction.	1	2	3	4
20. I follow current health care issues in the news and voice my opinion to my elected representatives.	1	2	3	4

Points _____

Environmental Health

	Not true/ rarely	Somewhat true/ sometimes	Mostly true/ usually	Very true/ always
1. I avoid use of and exposure to pesticides as much as possible.	1	2	3	4
2. I avoid use of and exposure to herbicides as much as possible.	1	2	3	4
3. I am willing to spend the extra money and time required to obtain organically grown produce.	1	2	3	4
4. I reduce environmental pollutants by minimizing my use of the automobile.	1	2	3	4
5. I avoid the use of products that contribute to indoor air pollution.	1	2	3	4
6. I limit my exposure to ultraviolet radiation by avoiding excessive sun exposure.	1	2	3	4
7. I limit my exposure to radon gas by using a radon gas detector.	1	2	3	4
8. I limit my exposure to radiation by promptly eliminating radon gas within my home.	1	2	3	4
9. I limit my exposure to radiation by agreeing to undergo medical radiation procedures only when absolutely necessary for the diagnosis and treatment of an illness or disease.	1	2	3	4

10. I avoid the use of potentially unsafe water, particularly when traveling in a foreign country or when a municipal water supply or bottled water is unavailable.	1		2		3		4
11. I avoid noise pollution by limiting my exposure to loud noise or by using ear protection.	1		2		3		4
12. I avoid air pollution by carefully selecting the environments in which I live, work, and recreate.	1		2		3		4
13. I do not knowingly use or improperly dispose of personal care products that can harm the environment.	1		2		3		4
14. I reuse as many products as possible so that they can avoid the recycling bins for as long as possible.	1		2		3		4
15. I participate fully in my community's recycling efforts.	1		2		3		4
16. I encourage the increased use of recycled materials in the design and manufacturing of new products.	1		2		3		4
17. I dispose of residential toxic substances safely and properly.	1		2		3		4
18. I follow environmental issues in the news and voice my opinion to my elected representatives.	1		2		3		4
19. I am aware of and involved in environmental issues in my local area.	1		2		3		4
20. I perceive myself as a steward of the environment for the generations to come, rather than as a person with a right to use (and misuse) the environment to meet my immediate needs.	1		2		3		4

Points _____

YOUR TOTAL POINTS _____

Interpretation

770–880 points

Congratulations! Your health behavior is very supportive of high-level health. Continue to practice your positive health habits, and look for areas in which you can become even stronger. Encourage others to follow your example, and support their efforts in any way you can.

550–769 points

Good job! Your health behavior is relatively supportive of high-level health. You scored well in several areas; however, you can improve in some ways. Identify your weak areas and chart a plan for behavior change, as explained at the end of Chapter 1. Then pay close attention as you learn more about health in the weeks ahead.

330–549 points

Caution! Your relatively low score indicates that your behavior may be compromising your health. Review your responses to this assessment carefully, noting the areas in which you scored poorly. Then chart a detailed plan for behavior change, as outlined at the end of Chapter 1. Be sure to set realistic goals that you can work toward steadily as you complete this course.

Below 330 points

Red flag! Your low score suggests that your health behavior is destructive. Immediate changes in your behavior are needed to put you back on track. Review your responses to this assessment carefully. Then begin to make changes in the most critical areas, such as harmful alcohol or other drug use patterns. Seek help promptly for any difficulties that you are not prepared to deal with alone, such as domestic violence or suicidal thoughts. The information you read in this textbook and learn in this course could have a significant effect on your future health. Remember, it's not too late to improve your health!

To Carry This Further . . .

Most of us can improve our health behavior in a number of ways. We hope this assessment will help you identify areas in which you can make positive changes and serve as a motivator as you implement your plan for behavior change. If you scored well, give yourself a pat on the back. If your score was not as high as you would have liked, take heart. This textbook and your instructor can help you get started on the road to wellness. Good luck!

chapter two

Achieving Psychological Health

Eye on the Media

Television Advertisements for Psychological Medications: Informative or Misleading?

"Trouble sleeping? Difficulty concentrating? Crying most of the time? You might want to talk to your physician about taking Paxil." We are barraged by these types of media message on a daily basis. In fact, a recent study showed that drug advertising increased from $800 million in 1996 to $2.7 billion in 2001. Does it work? Well, for every dollar spent on drug advertising, $4.20 was made in sales. Viewers are typically encouraged to talk to their doctors about specific symptoms and problems and to ask for a particular medication. Physicians report that an increasing number of patients are making appointments because of something they saw on television. On the positive side, this trend results in finding and treating problems more quickly: before drug ads appeared on TV, patients erroneously believed that there was no treatment for, or were avoiding, the problems they were experiencing. When the possibility of a solution was brought to their attention by the commercials, people tended to feel less embarrassed, to be more hopeful, and to recognize problems sooner than they otherwise might have done. Research published in *Prevention Magazine* cited favorable responses to drug advertising on TV. It found that 84 percent of people felt better informed of new treatments. Seventy-eight percent said that the ads helped them to be more involved in their medical care, 34 percent reported talking to their physician about a drug they saw on TV, and 79 percent remembered hearing about the risks and side effects. However, only 49 percent of these people said they paid attention to side effects, with the majority of people believing that they would not experience them. Understanding all the side effects and risks when they are rattled off at breakneck speed or displayed in the smallest print possible at the bottom of the TV screen can be difficult. Of course, some people may be scared off by the side effects and risks and, as a result, won't even talk to their doctors about their concerns.

Sometimes it is difficult to know from watching TV advertisements what condition or problem a drug is designed to treat. And some physicians may disagree with an advertisement's promises or suggest a different drug. The drugs typically being advertised are the newest ones on the market and so are often more expensive and haven't been used for very long. Some physicians are hesitant to prescribe these medications until more evidence exists to show that they work better than the older medications do. There is also a concern that there hasn't been enough time to reveal all the potential side effects or the long-term effects of these drugs. Often it is only after people have been taking them for some time that certain side effects become apparent, such as those associated with the antidepressant Serzone, which has recently

The terms *emotional wellness* and *psychological health* have been used interchangeably to describe how people function in the affective and cognitive realms of their lives. **Psychological health** relates to how people express their emotions; cope with stress, adversity, and success; and adapt to changes in themselves and their environment, as well as to cognitive functioning—the way people think and behave in conjunction with their emotions. There is some debate about whether thoughts influence feelings or feelings cause us to think and behave a certain way. However, the most accepted view is that the way we think can directly change how we feel about an event or situation. Thus, you can change your feelings about something by changing your perspective about a situation. This ability has implications for how we can increase our self-esteem and confidence level and improve interactions with others. You will learn more about psychological health in this chapter.

Psychological Health

How do you feel about yourself? When you apply the resources from the multiple dimensions of health (Chapter 1) in ways that allow you to direct your growth, assess deeply held values, deal effectively with change, and have satisfying relationships with others, you are psychologically healthy. Research in the area of health psychology has shown that there is a mind–body connection in which biological, psychological, and social factors interact to

influence health or illness. This is referred to as the **biopsychological model.** [1] We know that one's psychological state has a significant effect on physical health: stress, depression, and anxiety have been associated with how the immune system responds and can impair physical health. Studies have shown that terminally ill cancer patients who had good psychological health lived longer lives and reported having a higher quality of life than did other cancer patients.[2] Psychological health does not just refer to your emotional state but also to your cognitive and social functioning.

Psychological health has also been associated with developing and maintaining a positive **self-esteem,** positive

---

Key Terms

psychological health a broadly based concept pertaining to cognitive functioning in conjunction with the way people express their emotions; cope with stress, adversity, and success; and adapt to changes in themselves and their environment

biopsychological model a model that addresses how biological, psychological, and social factors interact and affect psychological health

self-esteem an individual's sense of pride, self-respect, value, and worth

---

self-concept, and a high level of **emotional intelligence.** However, as you will see, psychological health is much more than just the absence of mental illness.

Characteristics of Psychologically Healthy People

Psychologically healthy people are not perfect. They have their share of problems, flaws, and mistakes. However, it is how they perceive themselves and how they cope with their stress and failures that separate them from unhealthy individuals.

Psychologically healthy people:

- Accept themselves and others
- Like themselves
- Appropriately express the full range of human emotions, both positive and negative
- Give and receive care, love, and support
- Accept life's disappointments
- Accept their mistakes
- Express empathy and concern for others
- Take care of themselves
- Trust others as well as themselves
- Establish goals, both short and long term
- Can function both independently and interdependently
- Lead a health enhancing lifestyle that includes regular exercise, good nutrition, and adequate sleep

Normal Range of Emotions

Do you know people who seem to be "up" all the time? Although some people are like that, they are truly the exceptions. For most people, emotions are more like a roller coaster ride. Sometime they feel happy, confident, and positive, and other times they feel sad, insecure, or negative. This is normal and healthy. Life has its ups and downs, and the concept of the "normal range of emotions" reflects these changes.

Self-Esteem

What is self-esteem? How do you know when someone is lacking in self-esteem? Most people answer this question by saying that they define positive self-esteem as:

- Having pride in yourself
- Treating yourself with respect

- Considering yourself valuable, important, worthy
- Feeling good about yourself
- Having self-confidence, being self-assured
- Accepting yourself

People with low levels of self-esteem tend to allow others to mistreat them, don't take care of themselves, and have difficulty being by themselves. In addition, they have little self-confidence and so avoid taking risks and have trouble believing that other people care about them. People with low self-esteem tend to take things personally, are sometimes seen as "overly sensitive" and perfectionistic, criticize themselves and others, and believe that they can't do anything right. These individuals tend to have a pessimistic outlook on life, and see themselves as undeserving of good fortune. We explore the concepts of optimism and pessimism as they relate to psychological health in a later section of this chapter.

 TALKING POINTS You've noticed that one of your friends always seems to be critical of herself and allows others to take advantage of her. What might you say to help her to increase her self-esteem?

People with low self-esteem also have a poor self-concept, meaning that their internal picture of themselves, how they see themselves, is very negative. Because of this poor self-concept, people with low self-esteem are more vulnerable to allowing others to mistreat or abuse them, and fail to be assertive. Many psychological problems have their underpinnings in low self-esteem, including eating disorders, substance abuse problems, depression, and anxiety disorders.

Where do we get our self-esteem? Most people would say from their parents, teachers, peers, siblings, religious institutions and the media. While these factors certainly can positively or negatively affect our self-concept and self-esteem, they are all external factors. While we don't have much control over other people, we do have control over what we internalize or accept as true about ourselves.

Key Terms

self-concept an individual's internal picture of himself or herself; the way one sees oneself

emotional intelligence the ability to understand others and act wisely in human relations and measure how well one knows one's emotions, manages one's emotions, motivates oneself, recognizes emotions in others, and handles relationships

Self-concept refers to our *internal* self-perception. If our self-esteem and self-concept were based only on external factors, then we would need to change our environment and the people around us. This is the reason that people tend to tell themselves, "If I just made more money, had a nicer car, were married, or had a more prestigious job, I would feel better about myself." This situation can become a vicious cycle, leaving the person always seeking more and being perpetually unsatisfied with him- or herself. This can also lead to perfectionism and not accepting yourself.

It is generally accepted that self-esteem comes from within ourselves and is ultimately within each individual's control. Moreover, self-esteem is not an all-or-none commodity. Most people have varying degrees of self-esteem, depending on their stage of development, events in their lives, and their environment.[3]

Emotional Intelligence

A third aspect of psychological health is the degree of emotional intelligence you possess. Emotional intelligence refers to "the ability to understand others and act wisely in human relations."[4] Furthermore, emotional intelligence can be broken down into 5 main domains:

- **Knowing your emotions.** This is considered to be the cornerstone of emotional intelligence and relates to how much self-awareness and insight you have. How quickly you are able to recognize and label your feelings as you feel them determines the level of your emotional intelligence.

- **Managing your emotions.** How well can you express your feelings appropriately and cope with your emotions? People who have trouble coping with anxiety, distress, and failures tend to have lower levels of emotional intelligence.

- **Motivating yourself.** People who can motivate themselves tend to be more highly productive and independent than are those who rely on external sources for motivation. The more you can self-motivate and engage in goal-directed activities, the higher your emotional intelligence.

- **Recognizing emotions in others.** Another aspect of emotional intelligence is the degree of empathy you have or how sensitive you are to the feelings of others and how you come across to other people.

- **Handling relationships.** This refers to your level of social skills. The more interpersonally effective you are and able to negotiate conflict and build a social support network, the more emotional intelligence you possess.

Of course, people have differing levels of emotional intelligence and may have higher levels in one domain than in another. People with overall high levels of emotional intelligence tend to take on leadership roles, are confident, assertive, express their feelings directly and appropriately, feel good about themselves, are outgoing, and adapt well to stress.[4]

Enhancing Psychological Health

Most people have the opportunity to function at an enhanced level of psychological well-being. This state is often achieved by improving certain skills and abilities, including improving verbal and nonverbal communication, learning to use humor effectively, developing better conflict resolution skills, and taking an optimistic approach to life. This section explores each of these facets of psychological health.

Improving Verbal Communication

Communication can be viewed in terms of your role as sender or receiver. In sending messages, you can enhance the effectiveness of your *verbal* communication in several ways. First, take time before speaking to understand what needs to be said. For example, does the audience/listener need information, encouragement, humor, or something else? Focus on the most important thoughts and ideas. Talk *with*, rather than at, listeners to encourage productive exchanges. Begin verbal exchanges on a positive note, and maintain a positive environment. Use "minimal encouragers," such as short questions, to gain feedback. Avoid using sarcasm, which can be destructive to communication. Recognize when other forms of communication, such as e-mail messages or handwritten notes, would be better for transmitting information or ideas.

You also need to be a skilled listener. First, listen attentively to hear everything that is being said. In a polite way, stop the speaker at certain points and ask him or her to repeat or rephrase the information. This technique helps you to understand what the speaker really means rather than focusing on your own responses. Ask for clarification and summarize what you think you heard the speaker say to ensure you have received the message accurately. Also try to focus on one main topic and don't go off on tangents.

Nonverbal Communication

Strengthening your nonverbal communication skills may also enhance your psychological health. Nonverbal communication is what is communicated by your facial expressions, body posture, tone of voice, movements, and even the way you breathe—such as when you sigh or yawn. Nonverbal communication is a very powerful and sometimes more important aspect of the message than what is verbally communicated. In fact, people use information from facial cues more than any other source.[5] Facial cues, particularly from the eyes, are attended to more than any other type of nonverbal communication, even when information from other sources—such as from hand and body movements—may provide a more accurate picture of what the person is feeling. The following suggestions can enhance your nonverbal communication skills:

- *Facial expressions.* Facial expressions have been cited as one of the most important sources of nonverbal communication in terms of a person's emotional state.[5] When people speak with their eyebrows raised, they tend to be seen as more animated, excited, and happy. Flushing of one's face can indicate embarrassment, and crinkling one's nose can mean that you don't like something. Every part of your face can communicate some type of emotional reaction.

- *Eye contact.* Maintaining eye contact is an important component of positive nonverbal communication, while looking away or shifting your eyes can be read as seeming dishonest. But don't stare—5 to 7 seconds seems to be the maximum amount of time to look at someone's eyes before they begin to feel scrutinized.

- *Personal space.* There are cultural differences in how much personal space or distance is comfortable and acceptable when sitting or standing next to another person. For example, Americans' personal space—about 3 to 4 feet for a casual conversation—tends to be much greater than that of Arabs or Italians but less than for Japanese or Britons. Gender and age and degree of familiarity are other factors that can determine the amount of personal space you are comfortable having between you and another person.

- *Body posture.* Assertiveness is equated with people who carry themselves with their heads up, shoulders back, and maintaining eye contact. Folded arms, crossed legs, and turning your body away from the speaker can indicate defensiveness and rejection.

Enhancing Conflict-Management Skills

Communication can be especially challenging when there is a conflict or disagreement. Emotions such as anger, hurt, and fear might alter your ability to communicate as effectively as you would like. Some techniques for managing angry or upset people or conflictual situations are these:

- *Listen and acknowledge the other person's point of view, even if it differs from your own.* Sometimes people are so busy thinking of the next thing they want to say

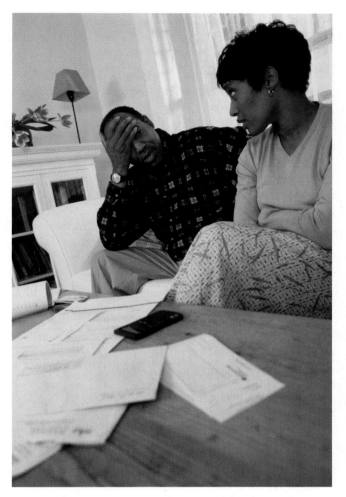

Nonverbal communication can be a powerful tool in sending messages to others through body language and posture as well as facial expressions.

that they don't pay attention to what the other person is saying. To ensure that you have heard the person accurately and to let that person know you are listening, repeat back or summarize what you heard and ask if you misunderstood something that was said.

- *Use assertive communication.* Using "I" statements rather than "You" helps to avoid putting people on the defensive and is especially helpful when negotiating conflict or disagreements. Rather than saying, "You are inconsiderate," you can say, "I feel upset when you're late and haven't called to let me know."

- *Focus not just on what you say but how you say it.* Pay attention to your tone of voice and speak in a conversational tone. People tend to talk louder because they erroneously think they will be heard if they speak louder. This can result in a shouting match in which neither person hears the other.

My partner and I have been living together for 2 years. We get along well most of the time, but when we try to talk about problems, we just can't connect. How do we learn to communicate better?

- Schedule the conversation so that you and the other person will be prepared for it.
- Choose a neutral setting to lessen the possibility of hostility.
- Set aside any preoccupations before starting the discussion.
- State your position clearly and nonaggressively.
- Keep the tone of your voice, manner of speaking, and body language respectful.
- Focus on the topic at hand.
- Be specific when you praise or criticize.

- Listen to what the other person is saying—not just the words but the feelings behind them. Don't interrupt.
- Avoid using trigger words that might turn a discussion into an argument.
- Suggest and ask for ideas about a course of action that will help resolve the problem.

If you follow these suggestions, you'll be taking into account the psychological health of the other person and yourself. This creates a sense of equality within the relationship. Since both of you will be aware of acknowledging and respecting the other person, you'll begin on a positive note.

- *Acknowledge the other person's feelings.* Use statements like "I can understand why this is so frustrating for you."

- *Watch your body posture.* Don't fold your arms in a closed, defensive posture, maintain eye contact, be aware of your facial expression so that you are not conveying hostility nonverbally. Make sure your nonverbal communication matches your verbal communication.

- *Accept valid criticism.* If you made a mistake, admit to it and apologize for whatever you think you did to contribute to the misunderstanding or conflict. This will open the door for the other person to take responsibility for their part in the conflict as well.

- *Focus on the problem at hand.* Don't bring up past hurts and problems. If you try to resolve every disagreement you have ever had with this person, you'll just wind up feeling frustrated and overwhelmed, and won't accomplish much. Stay on track by talking about the present situation.

- *Take a team approach.* Engage in mutual problem solving. This alleviates the winner-versus-loser paradigm. Look for areas of compromise and find a middle ground you can both live with.

- *Agree to disagree.* There is probably more than one right answer, and you can agree that you will not persuade the other to change his or her point of view.

- *Agree to discuss this at a later time.* Sometimes the conversation becomes too volatile and heated. Some time and distance from the problem can be beneficial.

Enhancing Psychological Health Through Humor

Having a sense of humor is another important component of psychological health. Humor helps to put things in their proper perspective, alleviating tension and pain by releasing more endorphins in our bodies. In addition, laughter reduces stress,[6] boosts the immune system,[7] alleviates pain[8] stabilizes mood,[9] decreases anxiety,[10] enhances communication,[11] and inspires creativity.[12] The research suggests that we need to laugh 30 minutes total per 24-hour period to attain these benefits. This is an easy task for children who on average laugh 250 times a day but more challenging for adults who tend to only laugh 15 times a day.[13] Employers have been putting the benefits of laughter to good use to increase productivity in factories. Factories in India have created "laughing clubs" in which workers laugh together for 20 minutes a day, resulting in less absenteeism and better performance.[14]

Recognizing the humor in everyday situations and being able to laugh at yourself will make you feel better about yourself. People who build humor into their daily lives generally feel more positive, and others enjoy being around them. Some people will say that if they don't laugh about a particular situation, they will cry, and laughing seems the better choice. In fact, humor is viewed as one of the higher-level defense mechanisms, compared to denying the problem, rationalizing or minimizing the problem, or blaming others. Some researchers have suggested that recovery from an injury or illness is enhanced when patients maintain a sense of humor.[15]

Taking an Optimistic Approach to Life

Another key to psychological health is your ability to manage and express your thoughts, feelings, and behavior in a positive manner. Do you believe that your happiness is within your control? Are people born naturally happy or sad? One important key to psychological health is the way that you think about and interpret events in your life. For example, if you say "hello" to someone and you don't get a response, do you begin to wonder if that person is angry with you? Or do you surmise that he or she didn't hear you or perhaps was distracted? Research shows that having a positive interpretation of life's events, particularly how you cope with adversity, can make a significant difference in terms of your health and academic and work performance as well as how long you will live.[16] Do you see the glass half empty, as pessimists do, or half full, as optimists do? Does it matter? Again studies overwhelmingly contend that your perspective makes a tremendous difference in your psychological health. Compared to pessimists, optimists tend to:

- Contract fewer infectious diseases
- Have better health habits
- Possess stronger immune systems
- Be more successful in their careers
- Perform better in sports, music, and academics

We do know that people can learn to be helpless and ultimately become depressed and even suicidal. Pavlov demonstrated the concept of "learned helplessness" in his classic study in which he administered an electric shock to dogs that were harnessed and couldn't escape the shocks. When he moved the dogs to another room, the dogs lay down and whimpered and didn't try to avoid the shocks. This time the dogs were not harnessed and could have easily escaped the shocks by moving to another side of the room. This reaction has been referred to as **learned helplessness.** The dogs learned that there was nothing they could do to affect their lives and they lost hope and felt trapped and powerless.[17] We have seen this same phenomenon with humans. College students volunteered for an experiment in which they were subjected to an earsplitting noise and their efforts to stop the noise were unsuccessful. Later, when they were placed in another situation in which they could have easily pulled a control lever to turn off the noise, they made no effort to do so and just suffered with the noise until the experimenter stopped it.[18] Battered women have demonstrated this same sense of powerlessness and helplessness in their inability to escape the abuse they are subjected to by their partners.

If people can learn to be helpless and pessimistic, can they also learn to feel more optimistic, powerful, and in control? Martin Seligman, a prominent psychologist, conducted studies to prove that this is possible and called this concept **learned optimism.** Learned optimism refers to your explanatory style, in other words, if you describe the glass as being half full or half empty. Seligman identified three key factors that contribute to having an optimistic or pessimistic perspective.

The first dimension of learned optimism is **permanence.** Pessimists tend to give up easily because they believe the causes of bad events are *permanent*. They say things like "Things never work out for me," "That won't ever work," or "He's always in a bad mood." Such permanent language—words like *never, always,* and *forever*—implies that these negative situations are not temporary but will continue indefinitely. Optimists tend to use temporary language—words like *sometimes, frequently,* and *often*—and they blame bad events on transient conditions. Examples of optimistic language are "It didn't work out this time," "Doing it that way didn't work," and "He's in a bad mood today." Optimists see failure as a small, transitory setback and are able to pick themselves up, brush themselves off, and persevere towards their goals.

The second aspect of learned optimism is **pervasiveness.** It refers to whether you perceive negative events as universal and generalize them to everything in your life, or if you can compartmentalize and keep them defined to the specific situation. Pessimists tend to make universal explanations for their problems, and, when something goes wrong in one part of their lives, they give up on everything. While a pessimist would say that they are not good at math, an optimist would say that they didn't perform well in that particular class with that type of math. "I'm good at algebra but not as good with geometry."

The last aspect of learned optimism is determined by whether you blame bad things on yourself or on other

---

Key Terms

learned helplessness a theory of motivation explaining how individuals can learn to feel powerless, trapped, and defeated

learned optimism how people explain both positive and negative events in their lives, accounting for success and failure

permanence the first dimension of an individual's attribution style, related to whether certain events are perceived as temporary or long-lasting

pervasiveness the second dimension of an individual's attribution style, related to whether they perceive events as specific or general

people or circumstances. Pessimism and low self-esteem tend to come from **personalization**—blaming oneself and having an internal explanatory style for negative events. An optimist might say, "The professor wrote a very poor exam and that is the reason I received a lower score," whereas the pessimist would say, "I am stupid" or "I didn't study enough." This is different from not taking responsibility for one's actions and blaming other people for your problems or mistakes. The idea is to have a balanced perspective and outlook on life. Pessimists tend to give credit to other people or circumstances when good things happen and blame themselves when bad events occur. For example, a pessimist would say, "That was just dumb luck" rather than taking credit for a success. However, if pessimists fail, they readily blame themselves, saying, "I messed up." In contrast, optimists tend to give themselves credit for their accomplishments, saying, "I worked hard and did a good job," and they don't belittle themselves when things go wrong.

Seligman conducted many studies to test how an optimistic explanatory style might be useful in daily living. For example, he worked with a swimming team from the University of California, Berkeley, to see how optimism or pessimism might affect their performance. He had their coaches tell the athletes that their times were slower than they actually were. The swimmers were then asked to swim the event again as fast as they could. The performance of the pessimists deteriorated in their 100-yard event by 2 seconds, the difference between winning the event and finishing dead last. The optimists got faster by 2 to 5 seconds, again enough to be the difference between losing and winning the race.[16] So how you interpret events, your attribution style, can make a tremendous difference in the eventual success or failure in your endeavors.

So how can you learn to be more optimistic? Albert Ellis developed a cognitive framework, called the ABC method, to become more positive in how you think and feel about things that happen in your life. When you encounter adversity, the "A" part of the formula, you try to make sense out of it and explain what has happened. For example, if you receive a notice from the bank that you have over-drawn your checking account, you start to think, "How did this happen?" These thoughts are associated with our beliefs, the "B" in ABC. You might think, "I'm irresponsible for letting this happen. I can't manage my money." Then you begin to feel bad about yourself, worthless and upset. Your beliefs affect your feelings, and so you can control your emotions by changing your beliefs and thoughts.[19] If you said, "The bank probably made a mistake" or "I might have added something incorrectly," you will most likely feel much better about yourself and the situation. The "C" aspect is the consequence of the event, how you end up feeling about the situation. When someone feels depressed, he or she feels hopeless,

trapped, and powerless. By adopting a more positive way of reframing or thinking about events, you create options, hope, and a strategy for solving problems rather than staying stuck, like the whimpering dogs lying down and putting up with being shocked. In the previously described scenario with the overdraft, you can generate ideas such as "I need to check with the bank, go over my bank statement, be more careful in recording and calculating my balances, and request overdraft protection to prevent this from becoming a problem again."

Everyone encounters adversity sometime in his or her life. You can become discouraged by these events, blame yourself, and feel hopeless, worthless, and cynical about the world. Or you can be persistent and become stronger by overcoming these obstacles, by having positive beliefs, and by seeing these problems as short-lived, specific, and not as a flaw in your character. When you embrace an optimistic perspective, you will feel more hopeful, stronger, and confident. You will be able to accept new challenges and take risks in your life.

 TALKING POINTS Think about something bad that has happened in your life recently. What were your beliefs about this event? How did you feel? Using the concepts of permanence, pervasiveness, and personalization, how can you change your beliefs about this situation? How do you feel differently about the event?

Taking a Proactive Approach to Life

In addition to the approaches already discussed, the plan that follows is intended to give you other strategies for enhancing your psychological health. The following is a four-step process that continues throughout life: constructing perceptions of yourself, accepting these perceptions, undertaking new experiences, and reframing your perceptions based on new information.

Constructing Mental Pictures

Actively taking charge of your psychological health begins with constructing a mental picture of what you're like. Use the most recent and accurate information you

---

Key Terms

personalization the final dimension of attribution style, related to whether an individual takes things personally or is more balanced in accepting responsibility for positive and negative events

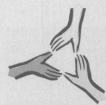

Learning from Our Diversity

Diverse Personalities

When we think about diversity, we may think about differences in ethnicity, culture, religion, sexual orientation, and disabilities, but we don't often consider differences in personality as part of diversity. Diversity can refer to any difference or potentially separating factor between or within groups. With respect to psychological health, there certainly are differences in personality traits—for example, outgoing vs. shy, detail oriented vs. spontaneous, flexible vs. structured. Often people value certain personality characteristics over others—for instance, being extraverted, organized, responsible, humorous, and open minded. Other traits can seem positive in one situation but negative in another. For example, being sensitive can be seen as a positive quality when you are sensitive to the feelings of other people and can relate well to others. However, it can also be seen negatively if you are perceived as being overly sensitive in terms of taking things too personally or overreacting to situations or criticism.

A personality test called the Myers-Briggs Type Indicator (MBTI) examines individual personality traits on four different scales and gives a score for each: extraversion vs. introversion, sensing vs. intuitive, thinking vs. feeling, and judging vs. perception. Extraverts tend to get their energy from being with other people. They do their best thinking out loud and like to talk things through, whereas introverts tend to hang back and share their thoughts once they have them fully formed and put together in their own mind. Introverts tend to get their energy from solitary or one-on-one activities. Sensing people are good with facts and details, and they are practical, traditional, and down to earth.

Intuitives tend to be nonconformist, creative, and divergent global thinkers. Thinking types are more analytical and logical, and they base their decisions on facts, rules, and policies. Feeling types base their decisions on how they will affect other people; they tend to be peacekeepers, conflict avoidant, and sensitive to the feelings of others. Organized, good with time management, and structured are qualities of a judging type, whereas spontaneous, adaptable, and flexible describe perceptives.

The MBTI maintains that there are no good or bad personality types, only important differences, and it uses the four scales to describe them. The MBTI talks about how you can play to your strengths and understand your weaknesses and how you can appreciate other people's personality types. In fact, the idea behind this instrument is that it is more helpful for opposites to work together or be in a relationship because each person can balance and complement the other. As a way to understand the diversity of people's personalities, the MBTI has been used in leadership styles, communication skills, conflict negotiation, career exploration, learning styles, and building work groups.

Psychological health entails finding a good balance between your own strengths and weaknesses as well as acknowledging and celebrating the differences among people. Knowing yourself, recognizing the impact you have on others, can help you to have more fulfilling interactions. Building relationships between diverse personality types and seeing these differences as strengthening, balancing, and enhancing is another way to celebrate diversity in our community.

---

have about yourself—what is important to you, your values, and your abilities. To construct this mental picture, set aside a period of uninterrupted quiet time for reflection.

Before proceeding to the second step, you also need to construct mental pictures about yourself in relation to *other people and material objects*, including your residence and college or work environment, to clarify these relationships.

Accepting Mental Pictures

The second step of the plan involves an *acceptance* of these perceptions. This implies a willingness to honor the truthfulness of the perceptions you have formed about yourself and other people.

Psychological development is an active process. You must be willing to be *introspective* (inwardly reflective) about yourself and the world around you and to apply these new perceptions.

Undertaking New Experiences

The next step of the plan is to test your newly formed perceptions. This *testing* is accomplished by *undertaking a new experience* or by reexperiencing something in a different way.

New experiences do not necessarily require high levels of risk, foreign travel, or money. They may be no more "new" than deciding to move from the dorm into an apartment, to change from one shift at work to another, or to pursue new friendships. The experience itself is not the goal; rather, it's a means of collecting information about yourself, others, and the objects that form your material world. The goal is to "try on" or test your perceptions to see what fits you.

Reframing Mental Pictures

When you have completed the first three steps in the plan, the new information about yourself, others, and objects becomes the most current source of information. Regardless of the type of new experience you have undertaken and its outcome, you are now in a position to modify the initial perceptions constructed during the first step. Then you will have new insights, knowledge, and perspectives. This is a continual process. As you grow and change, so will your perceptions.

Challenges to Psychological Health

In spite of their best efforts to be positive and resilient, many people have a less than optimal level of psychological health. There is some debate about how much control people actually do have over their psychological health. A general consensus is that two factors, **nature** and **nurture,** influence psychological health, but there are differing views on how much each contributes to our psychological makeup. Nature refers to the innate factors we are born with that genetically determine our degree of psychological health. Nurture is the effect that the environment, people, and external factors have on our psychological health.[20] We all know some people who are high strung or anxious by nature and others who are cheerful and naturally outgoing. We seem to be born with a predisposition toward a certain psychological health, which is often similar to our parents. "She is serious like her father" and "He is funny like his mother" are remarks people may make alluding to this genetic link. Environmental factors such as social relationships, family harmony, financial resources, job and academic concerns, and living situations or events and even the weather can influence psychological health.

Psychological Disorders

In the course of one year, an estimated 22 percent of Americans, about one in five, suffer from a diagnosable mental disorder.[21] In addition, four of the ten leading causes of disability in the United States and other developed countries are mental disorders such as depression, bipolar disorder, schizophrenia, and obsessive-compulsive disorder.[22] However, two-thirds of those suffering from psychological disorders do not receive treatment owing to the stigma and cost associated with mental health treatment.[23] Overall, minorities and Caucasians share the same prevalence rate of mental disorders; however, there are great disparities in the rate of mental health care for minorities as compared to the nonminority population.

While there are over 300 different types of mental illness that can be diagnosed, we will cover three major categories of mental disorders: mood disorders, including depression and bipolar disorder; anxiety disorders; and

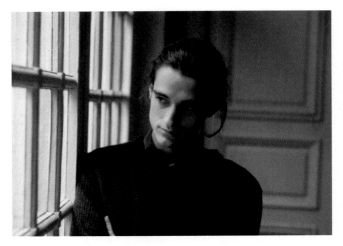

People who suffer from depression tend to feel hopeless and unmotivated, and they withdraw from others, which then increases their feelings of being trapped and stuck.

schizophrenia.[24] We will also briefly discuss Attention Deficit Disorder. Over 450 million people worldwide are affected by mental disorders at any given time, and these numbers are expected to increase in the future.[25]

Mood Disorders

Mood disorders, such as depression, seasonal affective disorder, and bipolar disorder, refer to psychological problems in which the primary symptom is a disturbance in mood.[24] You might perceive someone as moody, unable to predict if the person will be in a good or bad mood from one day to the next.

Depression

About one in ten Americans suffer some form of depression, with women experiencing **clinical depression** twice as often as men.[26] The incidence of depression

---

Key Terms

nature the innate factors that genetically determine personality traits

nurture the effect that the environment, people, and external factors have on personality

clinical depression a psychological disorder in which individuals experience a lack of motivation, decreased energy level, fatigue, social withdrawal, sleep disturbance, disturbance in appetite, diminished sex drive, feelings of worthlessness and despair

starting in childhood and adolescence has recently dramatically increased. We have already begun to see this trend, as the number of college students with depression has doubled over recent years.[27] While depression can develop at any age, the average age of onset is the mid-20s.

How can you tell the difference between having the blues and clinical depression? The symptoms of depression are as follows:

- Depressed mood most of the day, nearly every day
- Frequent crying
- Withdrawing, isolating yourself from others
- Lack of interest in activities that are typically enjoyable
- Increase or decrease in appetite resulting in significant weight loss or weight gain
- Insomnia, disturbed or restless sleep, or sleeping more than usual
- Feeling tired most of the time, regardless of how much sleep you have had
- Low self-esteem, feelings of hopelessness and worthlessness
- Difficulty concentrating, remembering things, and focusing on a task, and indecisiveness
- Frequent thoughts of suicide

Many people have experienced some of these symptoms at one point or another in their lives; however, clinically depressed individuals experience most of these symptoms every day and have felt this way for at least two weeks. Most people can find ways of pulling themselves out of feeling down, but when you have clinical depression, the normal methods you have used in the past to cope with the blues don't work. Clinical depression can range from mild to severe depression and can result in significant impairment in functioning, such as not being able to get out of bed to attend classes or go to work or have the energy or motivation to take care of your basic needs for food, hygiene, and rest. Some depressed people tend to become irritable, negative, and uncommunicative, which can cause greater stress and conflict in their relationships. Depression has been described as constantly having a black cloud over your head, and not being able to get out from underneath it no matter what you do.

There are several causes or triggers for depression to develop. Research suggests that if you have a family history of depression or any type of mood disorder, you are more prone to developing a depressive disorder. In fact, rates of depression for a child with a depressed parent are two to four times greater than for children

without this type of heredity.[28] While there is no single gene that causes depression, your genetic make-up can make you more vulnerable to depression. **Neurotransmitters** and hormone levels play a major role in the way your brain regulates your mood and emotions. Two neurotransmitters, serotonin and norepinephrine, are often found to be deficient in people with depression. (Chapter 7 includes a detailed discussion of neurotransmitters.)

However, biological processes are not the only explanation for depression. You may have a family history of depression and never develop depressive symptoms. Conversely, you may have no genetic predisposition and still become clinically depressed. Depression can be caused by many psychological factors, such as:

- Loss of a significant relationship
- Death of a family member or friend
- Physical or sexual abuse or assault
- The response to a serious illness or health problems
- Experiencing numerous setbacks and problems simultaneously

Having a support system, effective coping strategies, and a positive attributional style can make the difference between succumbing to depression or being protected during stressful and adverse times in our lives.

There are many ways to treat depression, but the most effective treatment approach is a combination of counseling and medication. Counseling can help people develop healthy coping skills, learn stress management strategies, focus on developing an optimistic explanatory style, and improve relationships and social skills. Medication, such as antidepressants, can be helpful in the treatment of depression, because they act to increase the serotonin or norepinephrine levels to a normal and functional range. Antidepressants include Prozac, Paxil, Zoloft, Celexa, Remeron, Cymbalata, Effexor, and Lexapro. It takes 4 to 6 weeks for an antidepressant to be fully effective, and there may be side effects such as dry mouth, decreased sexual drive, drowsiness, constipation, or diarrhea. Most of these will disappear after 2 weeks of taking the medication.

Most people take an antidepressant for 6 months to a year and then are able to taper off of the medication

---

Key Terms

neurotransmitters substance that transmits nerve signals; acts as chemical signals to activate or inhibit cell activity

without a reoccurrence of symptoms. If you have had three separate episodes of depression, recovering from each episode and then relapsing, this can be a sign that your depression is chemically caused and an indication that you may need to continue taking an antidepressant medication long-term.

Herbal supplements, such as St. John's Wort, have also been touted as a treatment for depression, although there is some debate as to how effective they truly are. Most health care providers agree that St. John's Wort can be somewhat effective in alleviating mild depression but not more moderate or severe types of depression. As is the case with all herbal supplements, St. John's Wort is not subject to FDA approval, and it has not been put through the clinical trials that prescription medications have undergone to establish therapeutic dose and efficacy. However, the National Institute of Mental Health, the National Center for Complementary and Alternative Medicine, and the Office of Dietary Supplements are currently conducting a $4 million collaborative four-year study to investigate the safety and the effectiveness of St. John's Wort, and so more definitive information will be available in the near future.

Exercise and activity level also play a significant role in alleviating and insulating people from depression. Again it seems that the endorphin levels and effects on brain chemistry and hormonal levels are part of the explanation for why this is a powerful antidote for depression.[29]

Electroconvulsive therapy (ECT) is another form of treatment for depression, with 100,000 Americans receiving this treatment each year. The procedure involves delivering a 90-volt burst of electricity, equal to the electricity in a 40-watt light bulb, to the brain for about a minute, causing a grand mal seizure. Proponents of ECT claim that shock treatments produce positive treatment effects for depression when no other antidepressant or treatment regime has worked. Critics of ECT say that it causes brain damage and memory loss, and that the decrease in depressive symptoms are only temporary.[31]

 TALKING POINTS Have you ever felt depressed? If so, what did you do to cope with these feelings? What did you do that worked or didn't work to make you feel better?

Suicide

Suicide is the third leading cause of death for young adults 15 to 24 years old and the eleventh leading cause of all deaths in the United States. Men commit suicide four times more often than women do, and 72 percent of all suicides are committed by white men. Suicide occurs most often among Americans age 65 and older.[30] However, women are three times more likely than men to attempt suicide. Men tend to employ more violent methods such as firearms, hanging, or jumping from high places, whereas women tend to use slower methods

The Dos and Don'ts of Suicide Intervention

Do . . .

1. **If possible, stay with the person** until you can get further assistance.
2. **Offer support and assistance.** Tell the person he or she is not alone.
3. **Remain calm.** Talk about the person's feelings of sadness and helplessness.
4. **Encourage problem solving** and taking positive steps.
5. **Emphasize the temporary nature of the problem.** Suicide is a permanent solution to a temporary problem.
6. **Seek help and don't try to handle this problem on your own.** This might involve the person's family, religious advisor,

friends, or teachers, or calling a mental health agency for consultation.

7. **Ask the person to promise not to hurt or kill him/herself.**

Don't . . .

1. **Avoid talking about suicide or dance around the topic.** Talking about suicide doesn't upset people more. In fact, often people who are thinking about killing themselves say it is a relief to talk about it and it helps them to let go of this idea, not pursue it further.
2. **Be judgmental or argumentative.** Now is not the time to debate the morality of

suicide—you will lose the debate and possibly the person.

3. **Assume that the person is not serious.** Saying "You're not serious" or "You don't mean that" may inadvertently encourage the person to show you how serious she or he truly is.
4. **Argue.** Telling a suicidal person that things aren't that bad or that other people have it worse can make him or her feel worse about himself/herself and guilty about his or her feelings of unhappiness.
5. **Promise not to tell anyone.** If you keep this promise and something happens to this person, how will you feel?

---

such as overdosing with pills or cutting their wrists, which allow more time for medical attention. Twice as many Whites complete suicide as African Americans, with Asian Americans being one of the lowest risk groups in terms of ethnicity. The suicide rate for the Hispanic population is lower than for Whites but higher than for African Americans.

Why do people attempt or commit suicide? The majority of suicidal people have depressive disorders and feel helpless and powerless over their lives. They say things like "I just want the pain to stop" and don't see any other options available to them. There are some risk factors associated with suicidal behavior such as:

- Little to no support system
- Made previous suicide attempts
- Family history of mental illness, including substance abuse
- Family history of suicide
- Problems with drugs or alcohol
- Possession of a firearm
- Exposure to suicidal behavior of others, including through the media

It is estimated that 300,000 suicide attempts occur each year in the United States, or more than one every 2 minutes. Some people say that suicidal gestures or threats are merely a cry for attention and ignore them. But left ignored, the person may go ahead and take the next step to attempt suicide because no one seems to care. It is always best to take any threats or talk

about suicide seriously and act accordingly. What should you do if a friend or family member talks to you about thoughts of suicide? See the Star box on this page for the Dos and Don'ts of Suicide Intervention.

Bipolar Disorder

Another important mood disorder is **bipolar disorder,** a condition that was previously known as manic depression. Bipolar refers to the extreme mood swings individuals with this disorder experience, from feeling euphoric, energetic, and reckless to feeling depressed, powerless, and listless. It is the least common of the mood disorders. Men and women are equally likely to develop this condition, and the average age of onset for the first manic episode typically occurs in the early 20s. This change in mood or "mood swing" can last for hours, days, weeks, or months, and it is found among all ages, races, ethnic groups, and social classes. The illness tends to run in families and appears to have a genetic link, as it is more likely to affect the children of parents who have the disorder.[24] When one parent has bipolar disorder, the risk to each

---

Key Terms

bipolar disorder a mood disorder characterized by alternating episodes of depression and mania

---

child is estimated to be 15 percent to 30 percent. When both parents have bipolar disorder, the risk increases to 50 percent to 75 percent.

We have already described depression in the previous section. Bipolar disorder involves having both depressive periods and manic episodes. **Mania** is characterized by the following:

- Excessive energy, needing little sleep
- Racing thoughts, feeling as though your mind is going 50 mph
- Rapid speech, changing from topic to topic quickly in conversation
- Irritability
- Impulsive and reckless behavior, for example, spending sprees, increased involvement in sexual activity, and drug and alcohol use
- Trying to do too much, feeling as though you can accomplish a great deal
- Being easily distracted
- Excitability

Many people with bipolar disorder will tell you that they enjoy the "highs" but dread the lows. However, manic behavior can become very destructive because when people are in a manic phase they can create enormous credit card debt, abuse drugs and alcohol, drive recklessly, and often feel invincible. They stay up all night and feel very little need for rest or food, and eventually their bodies can't function and they collapse. Mood stabilizers such as Lithium and Lithobid and anticonvulsant medications such as Depakote, Neurontin, Topomax, and Lamictal, along with psychotherapy, have been used to treat bipolar disorder.

Anxiety Disorders

Bill, a very talented and bright 26-year old, has a promising career as an executive in a large accounting firm. However, he is in jeopardy of losing his job because of his absenteeism and tardiness. He has missed several important meetings with clients and not been able to get his work done on time as a result. It can take him hours to get to work even though he lives 15 minutes away, and sometimes he doesn't go to work even though he is in the car and ready to go. Bill has a routine in the morning that involves checking the windows, doors, iron, stove, and garage door five times to ensure that things are secure and safe. Sometimes he drives away and then returns to the house to check again. He feels a need to turn the handles on doors five times, and if he loses track, he starts all over again.

Susan has been having such severe panic attacks in the car while driving to work that she has needed to pull over. Her heart races, her breathing is labored, and she sometimes feels as though she is having a heart attack and might die. She is frightened of being in the car alone and having an attack and being unable to get help, or of having a car accident. She is beginning to be afraid to leave her house and feels safer at home. She has declined invitations to go out with her friends and goes out only when absolutely necessary. She feels as though she is losing control of her life.

John worries constantly about what other people think of him. When he hears people laughing, he assumes that they are laughing at him. He has trouble having conversations with people because he believes whatever he says will sound stupid and that people will not like him. He also plays conversations over and over in his head when he is trying to go to sleep, thinking about what he should have said and worrying about how people are judging him.

Bill, Susan, and John are all suffering from *anxiety disorders*. While everyone tends to feel nervous or worry about something at some point in their lives, people with anxiety disorders feel anxious most, if not all, of the time. They also feel out of control and powerless to alleviate their anxiety, and they tend to worry about becoming anxious, so their anxiety causes them even greater anxiety. Anxiety is related to fear and is part of daily life. Some anxiety can even be helpful and motivating at times. Anxiety is a physiological, adaptive response to danger or potential threat and can enhance performance and keep us out of harm's way. In Chapter 3, Managing Stress, we discuss the fight or flight response and how the stress response is related to anxiety. Anxiety disorders are differentiated from daily stress as being:

- Intense, often debilitating, experiences during which people sometimes think they are going to die
- Long lasting, persisting after the danger or stressful event has passed
- Dysfunctional, causing significant interference in daily functioning

> ### Key Terms
>
> **mania** an extremely excitable state characterized by excessive energy, racing thoughts, impulsive and/or reckless behavior, irritability, and being prone to distraction

Anxiety disorders include **generalized anxiety disorder (GAD); obsessive-compulsive disorder (OCD),** such as Bill's problem; posttraumatic stress disorder; **panic disorder,** which describes Susan's symptoms; and phobias such as the **social phobia** John suffered from.[32] Approximately 19 million Americans have an anxiety disorder, and women are twice as likely as men to suffer from panic disorder, posttraumatic stress disorder, generalized anxiety disorder, agoraphobia, and other specific phobias.[33] There are no gender differences with obsessive-compulsive disorder or social phobia. There is a genetic component associated with developing an anxiety disorder: studies suggest that you are more likely to develop one if your parents have one. Certainly environmental stressors and events can be instrumental in whether this predisposition is activated or not.

The treatment for anxiety disorders may involve a combination of medication and counseling. There is some evidence that a deficiency in the neurotransmitter serotonin or a disturbance in metabolizing serotonin is associated with this condition, and taking an antidepressant increases the serotonin levels in the brain. Individuals suffering from anxiety disorders can also benefit from learning stress management, relaxation, and ways of coping with the stress.[32] Exercise, good nutrition, and avoidance of stimulants such as caffeine can also be helpful in alleviating anxiety.

Attention Deficit Disorder (ADD)

Once thought to be only a childhood disorder, ADD is now being diagnosed in record numbers in adults. This increase might be the result of overlooking or misdiagnosing problems in childhood that later are accurately diagnosed in adults. With symptoms that include being fidgety, disorganized, overactive, and easily distracted, a child may be seen as simply misbehaving rather than having a diagnosable disorder. It is often the child with ADD who is seen as "disruptive" in the classroom and "lazy, stupid, a day dreamer" by friends and family. Actually the truth about these individuals is often the opposite: they tend to be highly intelligent, motivated, creative, and energetic individuals.

It is currently estimated that over 15 million Americans suffer from this disorder, affecting males more than females, 3:1. There is strong evidence to support a genetic cause for ADD, although environmental factors can certainly help or hinder the problem. One of the landmark studies in ADD was conducted on adults and showed that there is a difference at the cellular level in energy consumption, between the parts of the brain that regulate attention, emotion, and impulse control in people with ADD as compared to those without.[34]

Following are the symptoms often seen in adult ADD:

- A sense of underachievement, not meeting one's goals
- Difficulty getting organized
- Chronic procrastination or trouble getting started
- Trouble with follow-through and completing tasks
- Having many tasks going on simultaneously, switching from one to another
- Easily bored and a frequent search for high stimulation
- Easily distracted, trouble focusing and sustaining attention
- Creative, intuitive, highly intelligent
- Impulsive, doesn't stop to think things through
- Impatient, low frustration tolerance
- Tendency to worry needlessly and endlessly
- Insecure
- Moody
- Restless
- Tendency toward addictive behavior
- Low self-esteem
- Inaccurate self-concept, unaware of effect on others
- Childhood history of ADD or presence of symptoms since childhood

Key Terms

generalized anxiety disorder (GAD) an anxiety disorder that involves experiencing intense and nonspecific anxiety for at least 6 months, in which the intensity and frequency of worry is excessive and out of proportion to the situation

obsessive-compulsive disorder (OCD) an anxiety disorder characterized by obsessions—intrusive thoughts, images, or impulses causing a great deal of distress—and compulsions—repetitive behaviors aimed at reducing anxiety or stress that is associated with the obsessive thoughts

panic disorder an anxiety disorder characterized by panic attacks, in which individuals experience severe physical symptoms; these episodes can seemingly occur "out of the blue" or because of some trigger and can last for a few minutes or for hours

social phobia a phobia characterized by feelings of extreme dread and embarrassment in situations in which public speaking or social interaction is involved

Psychological tests such as the Test of Variability of Attention (TOVA) and an IQ test can help substantiate a diagnosis of ADD. The TOVA tests the subject by flashing different shapes on a screen and quantifying attention, distractibility, and impulsivity based on the subject's responses. The most effective treatment for ADD involves a multimodal approach: counseling and coaching the individual to provide strategies, techniques, and structure for daily life; education, tools such as daily planners and organizers; goal setting and time management; and medication such as Concerta, Strattera, Ritalin, and Adderall. (These medications are discussed in more detail in Chapter 7).

Schizophrenia

Schizophrenia is one of the most severe mental disorders; it is characterized by profound distortions in one's thought processes, emotions, perceptions, and behavior. People with schizophrenia experience hallucinations (seeing things that are not there, hearing voices), delusions (believing that they are Jesus, the CIA is after them, or that radio waves are controlling their mind), and disorganized thinking (wearing multiple coats, scarves, and gloves on a warm day, shouting and swearing at passersby, maintaining a rigid posture and not moving for hours). The movie *A Beautiful Mind* gives a glimpse into the life of one schizophrenic, John Nash, and how he managed his symptoms.

There are several types of schizophrenia: paranoid, disorganized, catatonic, and undifferentiated. This disabling illness affects 1 percent of the U.S. population, and symptoms typically surface in people in their late teens and early 20s. Men and women are equally likely to develop schizophrenia, and it seems to run in families. Schizophrenia is often confused with multiple personality disorder, which is an entirely separate and distinct mental illness. While people with multiple personality disorder display two or more distinct identities or personalities that take control of the person's life, people with schizophrenia do not have multiple, separate, enduring personalities.

There are many theories to explain what causes schizophrenia. Some research suggests that heredity accounts for about 80 percent of the cause of schizophrenia and the other 20 percent is due to environmental stressors or situations. Researchers have also identified a number of abnormalities in the brains of diagnosed schizophrenics, including smaller temporal lobes, enlargement of the ventricles, and cerebral atrophy in the frontal lobes. Research is also being done on how the variations in chromosome-22 genes may be linked to schizophrenia. Individuals with schizophrenia also seem to have nearly double the number of dopamine receptors in their brains, leading to the theory that too much dopamine is being released into the brain pathways and causing schizophrenia symptoms.

The antipsychotic medications act to block the receptors and prevent the transmission of dopamine, reducing the amount of dopamine in the system that is creating this chemical imbalance.[1]

While there is no cure for schizophrenia, there are antipsychotic medications, such as Seroquel, Risperidone, Zyprexa, Geodon, and Abilify, that can effectively treat this illness and enable people to live functional, satisfying lives. Psychotherapy can be helpful in developing problem-solving approaches, in addition to identifying stressors and triggers, and early detection of a psychotic episode. Unfortunately some people with schizophrenia are unable to recognize that they are delusional or irrational, and so do not get treatment or take their medications on a regular basis.

Reflections of Psychological Health

What characterizes people who have developed their psychological health to their highest potential? The following discussion suggests three areas in which psychological health is evident. These include (1) movement toward fulfilling the highest level of need, (2) development of a mature level of spirituality, and (3) expression of creativity.

Maslow's Hierarchy of Needs

Abraham Maslow has been among the significant contributors to the understanding of personality and psychological health. Central to Maslow's contribution to 20th-century American psychological thought is his view of psychological health in terms of the individual's attempt to meet inner needs, what he called *the hierarchy of needs* (Figure 2-1).[20]

Maslow's theory is a positive, optimistic theory of human behavior. He believed that people are motivated to grow and fulfill their potential, referring to this phenomenon as **self-actualization.** He described self-actualization

---

> ### Key Terms
>
> **schizophrenia** one of the most severe mental disorders, characterized by profound distortions in one's thought processes, emotions, perceptions, and behavior; symptoms may include hallucinations, delusions, disorganized thinking, and/or maintaining a rigid posture and not moving for hours
>
> **self-actualization** the highest level of psychological health at which one reaches his or her highest potential and values truth, beauty, goodness, faith, love, humor, and ingenuity

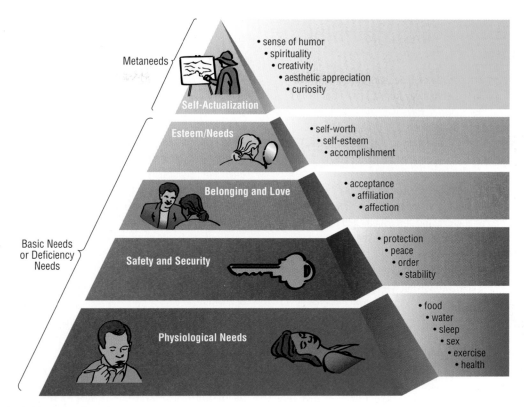

Figure 2-1 Maslow's hierarchy of needs

as "the need to become more and more what one is, to become everything that one is capable of becoming."[35] Maslow differentiated between two different categories of needs: **basic needs** and **metaneeds.** Basic needs, physiological needs, belonging and love, and esteem needs are the deficiency needs and are essential and urgent. Metaneeds come into play once the basic needs are met and include spirituality, creativity, curiosity, beauty, philosophy, and justice. Maslow's hierarchy of needs is arranged with the basic needs on the bottom, as they are the most fundamental and powerful needs. Lower level needs must be met before the next level of needs can be satisfied. Maslow believed that the fulfillment of metaneeds is needed to become a completely developed human being. Left unfulfilled, people can become cynical, apathetic and lonely.[36]

Maslow arrived at this model by examining people whom he considered to be exceptionally healthy, people he defined as having developed to their fullest potentials. Self-actualized people whom Maslow identified included Albert Einstein, Albert Schweitzer, Eleanor Roosevelt, and Abraham Lincoln. He perceived these people to share similar personality characteristics, such as being comfortable with themselves, having a strong ethical and moral code of conduct, and being innovative, compassionate, altruistic, goal oriented, and internally motivated.[37]

Spiritual Health

Having a sense of purpose, direction, and awareness is a dimension of spiritual health. This aspect of psychological health also refers to how well we integrate our beliefs and values with our behavior. People with spiritual health seek meaning and purpose in their lives and have a deep appreciation for a sense of unity and community. Spiritual health also includes one's morals, ethics, intrinsic values, and beliefs. It also refers to an awareness and appreciation of the vastness of the universe, and recognition of a dimension beyond the natural and rational, involving perhaps a belief in a force greater than oneself.[38] People who incorporate spirituality into their lives reported better psychological coping, increased well-being, increased

> **Key Terms**
>
> **basic needs** deficiency needs that are viewed as essential and fundamental, including physiological needs, belonging and love, and esteem needs
>
> **metaneeds** secondary concerns, such as spirituality, creativity, curiosity, beauty, philosophy, and justice, that can be addressed only after the basic needs are met

Mindfulness: Time to Pay Attention

Have you taken a moment today to be quiet and just be with yourself? Time alone can help you step away from a busy, fragmented world and draw inward for renewal. Having strengthened awareness of yourself in both mind and body allows you to experience the fullness of the moment, even to feel in sync with the universe. This is referred to as "mindfulness"—being aware of the present moment without judging or thinking.

Solitude can also help you establish your identity, clarify what's important to you, and strengthen your independence. Because most of our time is spent living with, caring for, or responding to others, it is only when we observe the moment that we have the opportunity to fully emerge and become ourselves.

Any time you take for this meditation will be restorative. You may start with just five minutes every morning. You will need a place where you feel comfortable to be alone with your own thoughts, whether it be at the kitchen table, in bed, in the bath, at a coffee shop, in the library, or in the garden. Go for a walk, listen to music, weed the garden, write a letter to a friend, paint, read a poem, or just be still and concentrate on your breathing. All of these are ways to reconnect you to the life force. Pretty soon you may feel that your time of mindfulness is more energizing than sleep! When you are faced with a difficult project, a household disaster, or something more serious, such as sickness or death, these reflective moments will give you mental and spiritual renewal.

It's not selfish to carve out whatever time you need alone to refresh yourself. By paying attention to your thoughts and feelings, you're reconnecting to your inner self. This nourished spirit is what you can share with others, whether family, friends, coworkers, or strangers.

satisfaction with life, lower anxiety and fewer depressive symptoms, less hostility and anger, and greater happiness in general.[39] Similarly, spirituality has also been related to better physical health. Studies have shown that no matter how spirituality was defined or measured, it has a positive effect on reducing coronary heart disease, high blood pressure, stroke, cancer, and increasing life expectancy.[40]

As a resource for the spiritual dimension of health, spirituality provides a basis on which a belief system can mature and an expanding awareness of life's meaning can be fostered. Spirituality also gives meaning to your career and helps you better understand the consequences of your vocational efforts. In addition, spirituality influences many of the experiences that you will seek throughout life and tempers your emotional response to these experiences.

In nearly all cultures, spirituality provides individuals and groups with rituals and practices that foster a sense of community—"a community of faith." In turn, the community nurtures the emotional stability, confidence, and sense of competence needed for living life fully.[40]

Creative Expression

Another characteristic of people who have developed their psychological health is creativity. Allowing yourself to express your thoughts, feelings, and individuality in a creative manner entails having self-confidence, self-esteem, and flexibility. Confidence and self-esteem are essential so that you don't feel embarrassed by your creativity and feel free to share your creative side with others. Children can easily do this when they draw a picture or make up a dance and say, "Look at me. Look at what I made." However, as we age, some of us become inhibited and don't allow ourselves to be creative or to share this part of ourselves. If you don't exercise your creative side, it can atrophy, just as unexercised muscles do.

What are some resources that you might need to develop to foster your creativity?

- *Nonconformity.* Creative individuals aren't terribly concerned about what other people think of them. They are willing to risk looking foolish or proposing ideas that are divergent from others or traditional ways of thinking.

- *Independence.* Highly creative people tend to work well alone and sometimes prefer this to working in a group. As children, they often were encouraged to solve problems on their own rather than having someone else to do so for them.

- *Motivation.* Creative people are motivated by intrinsic rather than external rewards, meaning they like to be creative for their own pleasure, not to please others or because it is expected of them. They don't fear failure, and success is not the main goal. They enjoy creativity for creativity's sake alone and not to reap rewards or praise from others.

- *Curiosity.* Creative people have a wide range of interests and a broad base of knowledge. They are open to new experiences and question things that other people ignore or take for granted.

A New Problem . . . Internet Addiction

The Internet has changed the way we work, socialize, and educate ourselves. While the Internet has provided connections that otherwise could not be made very easily with people all around the world, it has also created unique psychological problems for some individuals. There is some question about the psychological implications the Internet may be having on our society as we are moving from a world in which we used to know our neighbors and interact with people face to face to developing serious and deep relationships with people from a distance. Marriages have broken up, affairs have taken place, and teenagers have been kidnapped by people they met over the Internet. In fact, one teenager was encouraged to overdose on drugs by his Internet friends and died while communicating over the Net to this group.

There is a feeling of anonymity that is created by talking on the Web. You can be who you want to be, reveal as much or as little as you want, and not be judged by your appearance. Of course this also means people can be deceitful and dishonest about who they are and what they want from you. In addition, there is a blending of home and work and increased solitary. Studies show that greater use of the Internet is associated with less communication among family members, decreased socializing with local friends, and increased depression and loneliness.[1] One study showed that using the Internet more than 5 hours a week resulted in less time with friends, family, and social activities.[2]

In fact, there is such concern about the potential adverse effects of spending too much time on the Internet that there are mental health professionals that propose adding "Internet addiction" as a diagnosable mental disorder. How can you tell if you are addicted? Here are some warning signs:

1. Preoccupation with the Internet—planning and thinking about the next time you can get online.
2. Increased use of the Internet over time.
3. Repeatedly making unsuccessful attempts to curtail your use of the Internet.
4. Feeling irritable, restless, and moody when you attempt to cut down your use of the Internet or are prevented from getting online when you would like.
5. Unaware of how much time you are spending on the Internet, staying online more than you originally intended.
6. Lying to family members and friends about your use of the Internet.
7. Jeopardizing your job or risking losing a relationship because of the time you are spending on the Web.
8. Using the Internet as a way of escaping from problems, coping with depression.
9. Declining invitations to spend time with family and friends because you would rather be online.

Of course, answering "yes" to one of these statements does not indicate a concern. However, if you can answer "yes" to more than half of these statements, then you may want to examine your use of the Internet. Here are some ways you can avoid being an Internet addict:

- Decide how much time you want to spend on the Internet before you get online and set an alarm for that time. Stick to that time allotment and don't say "5 more minutes" which can then become an hour.

- Take frequent breaks. Spend at least 5 minutes out of every hour or 15 to 20 minutes of every 3 hours on unwired activity. Take a walk, stretch your body, eat a snack, or listen to music.

- Visit the Net with a purpose and a strategy. Surfing the Web aimlessly can lead to being online for longer than you anticipated.

- Interact with people in a nonwired world. Make a commitment to socially interact at least once a day with someone who is not online.

- Don't let the Internet be the center of your existence or the most important, enjoyable part of your day. Remind yourself of your life goals, values, and interests. What are other ways to achieve these goals besides via the Web?[3]

[1] Kraut R., Patterson M., Lundmark V., Kiesler S., Mukopadyay T. & Scherlis W., Internet Paradox: A social technology that reduces social involvement and psychological well-being? *American Psychologist*, 53(9), 1998.

[2] Streitfeld D., Study finds heavy Internet users are isolated. *Washington Post*, February 16, 2000.

[3] Goldstein D. & Flory J., Best of the Net: *Online Guide Book Series*. New York: McGraw-Hill Irwin Professional Publishing Inc. 1996.

- *Persistence.* This is seen as one of the most important traits of a creative person. As Thomas Edison said, "Genius is one-tenth inspiration and nine-tenths perspiration." Persistence requires not giving up when your first efforts are not successful and continually thinking of new ways of doing something, problem solving, or thinking "outside of the box."[41]

Some people reviewing the preceding list may recognize many of these characteristics as being already well developed in their own personalities. Others may not have demonstrated some of the traits listed, and they may appear far beyond their reach. Nevertheless, most people can increase their creativity by giving themselves permission to be creative. Some people state, "I'm not a creative person," and yet they haven't explored that part of their personality, perhaps since childhood. There are many avenues of creativity, and the first step is to experiment, to be open and spontaneous. In this way, you can gain greater psychological health from accessing your inner strengths and resources.

Psychological Health: A Final Thought

As you can see, psychological health involves how your emotions, thoughts, and behavior interplay with one another and with the world around you. There is an important mind–body connection in terms of your psychological health having a significant impact on your physical health and vice versa. Psychological health is not just the absence of mental illness, and there is a range or continuum of psychological health. Possessing a positive self-concept, developing high self-esteem, and cultivating an optimistic attitude toward life can promote psychological health and enhance relationships with others. While heredity plays a role in the development of personality and psychological health, environmental factors and stressors seem to have an equally important role. As people age and encounter developmental milestones, they also encounter new challenges, obstacles, and resources in continuing to maintain their psychological health.

Taking Charge of Your Health

Assess how effective and healthy your style of communication is by considering the following questions:

- Do you know the difference between passive, aggressive, and assertive behavior?
- Do you use assertive language such as "I" statements rather than "you" statements?
- Do you have assertive body language such as making eye contact and keeping an open body posture without crossing your arms in front of you?

- Are you aware of your nonverbal communication?
- Are you aware of the volume and tone of your voice and the message you might be conveying?
- Do you acknowledge the other person's feelings and point of view before stating your own?
- Do you feel comfortable saying "no" to requests?

- Do you feel comfortable asking for someone's help, disagreeing with someone, or giving your opinion about something?

Having a positive and effective communication style is an important aspect of psychological health and can have a significant effect on your relationships, success at work, and your self-worth. Learn to be more optimistic in your attitude and communication by considering the characteristics of an optimist on page 37.

SUMMARY

- There is a mind–body connection in which biological, psychological, and social factors interact to influence health or illness. This is referred to as the biopsychological model.
- Psychological health has also been associated with developing and maintaining a positive self-concept, positive self-esteem, and emotional intelligence.
- Psychologically healthy people display a wide range of emotions.
- People with overall high levels of emotional intelligence tend to take on leadership roles, are confident and assertive, express their feelings directly and appropriately, feel good about themselves, are outgoing, and adapt well to stress.
- Two factors, nature and nurture, influence the shaping of personality. Nature refers to the innate factors we are born with that genetically determine our personality traits. Nurture is the effect that the environment, people, and external factors have on our personality.
- Nonverbal communication is what is communicated by your facial expression, body posture, tone of voice, and movements.

- Maslow's theory is a positive, optimistic theory of human behavior. He believed that people are motivated to grow and fulfill their potential, referring to this phenomenon as self-actualization.
- People with spiritual health seek meaning and purpose in their lives and have a deep appreciation for a sense of unity and community.
- Having a positive interpretation of life's events, particularly how you cope with adversity, can make a significant difference in terms of your health and academic and work performance, as well as how long you will live.
- Clinical depression can range from mild to severe and can result in significant impairment in functioning.
- The majority of suicidal people have depressive disorders and feel helpless and powerless over their lives. It is always best to take any threats or talk about suicide seriously and act accordingly.
- Schizophrenia is one of the most severe mental disorders, characterized by profound distortions in one's thought processes, emotions, perceptions, and behavior.

REVIEW QUESTIONS

1. What are three factors that have been associated with psychological health?
2. What are the characteristics commonly demonstrated by psychologically healthy people?
3. What is the definition of self-esteem, and how can self-esteem be enhanced?
4. What characterizes people with overall high levels of emotional intelligence?
5. What relationship is there between humor and psychological health?
6. What is nonverbal communication?
7. Describe Maslow's theory of the hierarchy of needs.
8. What traits are associated with people with spiritual health?
9. How can having a positive interpretation of life's events make a significant difference in people's health?
10. How is clinical depression different from having the "blues"?
11. How should you respond to someone threatening or talking about committing suicide?

ENDNOTES

1. Papalia D, Olds S. *Psychology* (2nd ed.). New York: McGraw-Hill, 1988.
2. Seligman M. *Learned Optimism.* New York: Simon & Schuster Inc., 1990.
3. McKay M, Fanning P. *Self-Esteem* (3rd ed.). Oakland, CA: New Harbinger Publications. 1992.
4. Goleman D. *Emotional Intelligence.* New York: Bantam Books, 1997.
5. Collier G. *Emotional Expression.* Hillsdale, NJ: Lawrence Erlbaum Associates, 1985.
6. Castro B, Eshleman J, Shearer R. Using humor to reduce stress and improve relationships. *Seminar Nurse Management* 7(2), 90–92, 1999.
7. Berk LS, et al. Immune system changes during humor-associated laughter. *Clinical Research* 39, 124a, 1991.
8. Cogan R, et al. Effects of laughter and relaxation on discomfort thresholds. *Journal of Behavioral Medicine,* 139–144, 1987.
9. Martin RA, Lefcourt HM. Sense of humor as a moderator between stressors and moods. *Journal of Personality and Social Psychology,* 45, 1313–1324, 1983.
10. Nezu A, Nezu C, Blissett S. Sense of humor as a moderator of the relationship between stressful events and psychological distress. *Journal of Personality and Social Psychology* 54, 520–525, 1988.
11. Miller J. Jokes and joking: A serious laughing matter, in Durant J and Miller J (Eds). *Laughing Matters: A Serious Look at Humor.* Longman Scientific and Technical, Essex England, 1988.
12. Lefcourt HM, Martin RA. *Humor and Life Stress: Antidote to Adversity,* Springer-Verlag, New York, 1986.
13. Kuhn C. *Humor Techniques for Health Care Professionals.* Presentation at Ball Memorial Hospital, April 22, 1998.
14. Nair M. A documentary: *"The Laughing Clubs of India,"* 2001.
15. Berk L, et al. Modulation of neuroimmune parameters during the eustress of humor associated mirthful laughter. *Altern There Health Med* 7(2), 67–72, 2001.
16. Seligman M. *Learned Optimism.* New York: Pocket Books, 1990.
17. Pavlov IP. *Conditioned reflexes.* New York: Oxford University Press, 1927.
18. Hiroto D. Locus of control and learned helplessness. *Journal of Experiential Psychology* 102, 187–93, 1974.
19. Ellis A. *Reason and emotion in psychotherapy.* New York: Lyle Stuart, 1962.
20. Spear P, Penrod S, and Baker T. *Psychology: Perspective on Behavior.* New York: John Wiley & Sons, 1988.
21. *MHIC: Mental Illness and the Family,* National Mental Health Association and the Surgeon General's Report on Mental Health, 1999.
22. Murray CJL, Lopez AD (Eds.). *Summary: The Global Burden of Disease: A Comprehensive Assessment of Mortality and Disability from Diseases, Injuries, and Risk Factors in 1990 and Projected to 2020.* Cambridge, MA: Published by the Harvard School of Public Health on behalf of the World Health Organization and the World Bank, Harvard University, 2003.
23. Lehrer J. Transcript from on line news hour. *Living with Mental Illness,* December 13, 1999.
24. American Psychiatric Association. *Diagnostic and Statistical Manual on Mental Disorders* (4th ed.) (DSM-IV-TR). Washington, DC: American Psychiatric Press, 2000.
25. World Health Organization. *Mental Health,* 2003.
26. National Institute of Mental Health, 2003.
27. Dramatic increases seen in college students' mental health problems over the last 13 years. *Journal of Professional Psychology: Research and Practice,* February 2003.
28. Peterson K. Resilience, talking can help kids beat depression. *USA Today,* June 4, 2002.
29. Exercise better than drugs for depression. *British Journal of Sports Medicine* 35, 114–117, April 2001.
30. Robins L, Regier D (Eds.). *Psychiatric Disorders in America: The Epidemiologic Catchment Area Study.* New York: The Free Press, 1991.
31. Study puts spotlight on electroshock therapy. *USA Today,* March 13, 2001.
32. Bourne E. *The Anxiety and Phobia Workbook.* Oakland: CA. New Harbinger Publications Inc., 1995.
33. Narrow W, Rae D, Regier D. NIMH epidemiology note: prevalence of anxiety disorder. *One-Year Prevalence Best Estimates Calculated from ECA and NCS Data.* Population estimates based on U.S. Census estimated residential population age 18 to 54 on July 1, 1998.
34. Hallowell, E and Ratey, J. *Driven to Distraction.* New York: Simon and Schuster, 1995.
35. Maslow AH. *Motivation and Personality* (2nd ed.). New York: Van Nostrand, 1970.

36. Maslow AH. *The Farthest Reaches of Human Nature.* Magnolia, MA: Peter Smith, 1983.

37. Lindzey G, Thompson R, Spring B. *Psychology* (3rd ed.). New York: Worth Publishers, Inc. 1988.

38. Hemenway JE, et al. *Assessing Spiritual Needs: A Guide for Caregivers.* Minneapolis: Augsburg Press, 1993.

39. Ayele H, Muligan T, Gheorghiu S, Reyes-Oritiz C. Religious activity improves life satisfaction for some physicians and older patients. *Journal of the American Geriatrics Society,* 43, 453–455, 1999.

40. Levin JS. Religion and health: Is there an association, is it valid and is it causal? *Social Science Medicine* 38(11), 1475–1482, 1994.

41. Wade C, Tavris C. *Psychology.* New York: Harper & Row Publishers, 1987.

As We Go to Press

With suicide being the third leading cause of death for 10- to 20-year olds, there is reason to be concerned about how to provide effective treatment for depression in children and teenagers. The use of antidepressants to treat depression has significantly increased over the past few years. In 2004, over 1 million children were reported to take antidepressants. Thomas Insel, director of the National Institute of Mental Health stated "pediatricians write prescriptions for Prozac like it's penicillin." However, there has been mounting concern that antidepressants are increasing rather than decreasing suicidal behavior in children and adolescents. The FDA reports that "about 2 in 100 children taking antidepressants are more likely to think about or try suicide because they're on the pills." Because of recent government warnings and media coverage, there has been a sharp decline in the number of children and teens taking antidepressants.

Only Prozac has been approved by the FDA to treat children and teens with depression; however, physicians routinely prescribe other antidepressants such as Paxil, Zoloft, Celexa, Effexor, and Remeron for this population. In October 2004, the Food and Drug Administration ordered "black box" labels, the most severe warning, on all antidepressants. Researchers suggest that antidepressants may be triggering "akathisia," a rapid increase in impulsivity and energy level that might contribute to already depressed kids taking the next step and attempting suicide. Often people with depression are so lethargic, unmotivated, and tired that they don't have the energy to act on suicidal thoughts. However, when the medication starts to work, the individual's energy level increases. If the level of hopelessness has not decreased or has stayed the same, the risk of suicidal behavior increases. Also, more is known about how these medications work for adults, and medications can work differently in children and teens. The medication can change teens from lovable, friendly, bright students to hateful, angry, unmotivated kids who seem like strangers to their friends and families.

GlaxoSmithKline, makers of Paxil, has been accused of withholding information and misleading doctors about the safety of treating kids with Paxil. The company has been accused of reporting only positive results from their clinical trials and not releasing information about any negative results.

It is no wonder that physicians are becoming more reluctant to prescribe these medications for children and teens. However, this reluctance may be putting our youth at risk because they may not be receiving appropriate treatment and medication that could alleviate their depression. While some physicians perhaps were writing these prescriptions too freely, we may now have a situation that has gone to the opposite extreme in which children and adolescents are suffering needlessly, not having the quality of life they could have, which may result in losing them to depression and suicide. Work is currently underway to create national guidelines for physician treating depression in 10- to 18-year-old patients to close the gap between over- and underprescribing antidepressants.

Sources: "Spitzer Says Glaxo Withheld Paxil Info," *USA Today,* June 3, 2004. "Antidepressant Debate Takes a Delicate Turn," *USA Today,* October 18, 2004. "Questions, Answers on "Black Box" Labels," *USA Today,* October 18, 2004. "Warnings Slow Antidepressant Use," *USA Today,* February 1, 2005 "Suicide Alert Has Parents Rethinking Antidepressants," *USA Today,* February 1, 2005. "FDA Weighs Antidepressant Risk to Kids," www.intelihealth.com, January 27, 2004.

personal assessment

How does my self-concept compare with my idealized self?

Below is a list of fifteen personal attributes, each portrayed on a 9-point continuum. Mark with an X where you think you rank on each attribute. Try to be candid and accurate; these marks will collectively describe a portion of your sense of self-concept. When you are finished with the task, go back and circle where you wish you could be on each dimension. These marks describe your idealized self. Finally, in the spaces on the right, indicate the difference between your self-concept and your idealized self for each attribute.

Decisive					Indecisive				____
9	8	7	6	5	4	3	2	1	
Anxious					Relaxed				____
9	8	7	6	5	4	3	2	1	
Easily influenced					Independent thinker				____
9	8	7	6	5	4	3	2	1	
Very intelligent					Less intelligent				____
9	8	7	6	5	4	3	2	1	
In good physical shape					In poor physical shape				____
9	8	7	6	5	4	3	2	1	
Undependable					Dependable				____
9	8	7	6	5	4	3	2	1	
Deceitful					Honest				____
9	8	7	6	5	4	3	2	1	
A leader					A follower				____
9	8	7	6	5	4	3	2	1	
Unambitious					Ambitious				____
9	8	7	6	5	4	3	2	1	
Self-confident					Insecure				____
9	8	7	6	5	4	3	2	1	
Conservative					Adventurous				____
9	8	7	6	5	4	3	2	1	
Extroverted					Introverted				____
9	8	7	6	5	4	3	2	1	
Physically attractive					Physically unattractive				____
9	8	7	6	5	4	3	2	1	
Lazy					Hardworking				____
9	8	7	6	5	4	3	2	1	
Funny					Little sense of humor				____
9	8	7	6	5	4	3	2	1	

To Carry This Further . . .

1. Overall, how would you describe the difference between your self-concept and your self-ideal (large, moderate, small, large on a few dimensions)?

2. How do these differences for any of your attributes affect your sense of self-esteem?

3. How do you think someone who knows you well would rate you? Would they rate you in a similar way to how you see yourself? If not, why not?

4. Identify several attributes that you realistically believe can be changed to narrow the difference between your self-concept and your self-ideal and, thus, foster a well-developed sense of self-esteem.

chapter three

Managing Stress

Chapter Objectives

On completing this chapter, you will be able to:

▌ define stress, the stress response, and chronic stress.

▌ describe the fight or flight response.

▌ discuss the general adaptation syndrome including three stages of stress: the alarm, resistance, and exhaustion stages.

▌ discuss some of the types of student stress explored in this chapter.

▌ describe the physical aspects of stress management.

▌ describe the social aspects of stress management.

▌ describe the environmental aspects of stress management.

▌ describe the psychological aspects of stress management.

▌ describe several tools for stress management.

Eye on the Media

Spit, Spam, Spim, and Phish—The Technological Stressors

We are learning to deal with a whole new type of stress—technological stress. Destructive computer viruses; hundreds of junk mail ads sent through e-mail, instant messages, cell phones, and voicemail; and increasing worry about identity theft have brought new meaning to stress management. With over 450 new viruses discovered each month and 82,000 hacking attacks made each year, it is no wonder that 500 or more professional hacking courses now instruct people how to think like and defend against computer intruders. Hacking costs companies over $17 billion dollars a year and creates paranoia, extreme stress, and frustration in victims of these attacks. Computer attacks have become increasingly wider in scope, automated, and harder to trace.

We are often overwhelmed by the amount of information we receive on a daily basis. If you are swamped by the catalogs, junk mail, and credit card applications you receive through the U.S. mail, your stress level will probably only intensify with the deluge of junk mail received via e-mail, voicemail, and instant messaging. And Internet telephony spam, called "spit," is predicted to become a bigger problem in the future as more people make phone calls over the Internet rather than use the regular phone lines. Marketers can program their computers to send 1,000 voice messages a minute over Internet telephony. "Spim" is spam sent out as an instant message, and it has increased to 2 billion messages in 2004, four times more than was sent in 2003.

Twenty percent of Americans reported receiving commercial messages and ads on their cell phones in 2004, an increase of 13 percent from the previous year. There were 75 million spam text messages received on cell phones in 2003, 150 million in 2004, and an estimated 450 million in 2005.

Even personal web logs, or blogs, are not immune from these invasive advertisements. Spam messages masquerade as comments from readers, with some bloggers receiving 20 spam messages on their web journals each day.

Phishing is the practice of sending e-mails and using fake Web sites to lure unsuspecting customers into sharing personal and financial data such as credit card account numbers, checking account numbers, and Paypal account numbers. Phishers create Web sites that look almost identical to the real ones, such as those of financial institutions like Citibank, and then ask their customers to verify their account information, which allows phishers easy access to people's financial data. An estimated 57 million people have received phish e-mails in 2004 alone. E-mails received from phishers are convincing because phishers copy the "from" line from the real company to make them look authentic. The incidence of phishing is growing at an alarming rate. In June 2004, the Anti-Phishing Working Group (APWG), an industry group, counted 1,422 phishing attacks—more than 12 times the number of attacks reported in December. Banks, eBay, and even some government agencies, including the IRS and the FBI, have been spoofed by phishers.

What Is Stress?

How do you know when you are stressed? You might experience headaches, stomachaches, or back and neck aches, or you might feel irritable, tired, anxious, and depressed. Some people eat more, while others find eating difficult when they are stressed. **Stress** refers to physiological and psychological responses to a significant or unexpected change or disruption in one's life. It can be brought on by real or imagined factors or events.

Stress was first described in the 1930s by Hans Selye, who observed that patients suffering from a variety of illnesses all showed common symptoms, such as fatigue, appetite disturbance, sleep problems, mood swings, gastrointestinal problems, and diminished concentration and recall. He called this collection of symptoms—this stress disease—stress syndrome, or the **general adaptation syndrome (GAS).** He also described this as "the syndrome of being ill."[1] We will discuss Selye's discovery later in the chapter.

Selye defines stress as "the nonspecific response of the body to any demand whether it is caused by or results in pleasant or unpleasant conditions."[1] Stress can be both positive or negative: again, it is our response to stress— how we manage stress—that makes a difference in terms of how it affects us. Stress resulting from unpleasant events or conditions is called **distress** (from the Greek *dys*, meaning bad, as in displeasure). Stress resulting from pleasant events or conditions is called **eustress** (from the Greek *eu*, meaning good, as in euphoria). Both eustress and distress elicit the same physiological responses in the body, as noted in Selye's General Adaptation Syndrome model.

While stress may not always be negative, our responses to it can be problematic or unhealthy. Both positive and negative stressful situations place extra demands on the body—your body reacts to an unexpected change or a highly emotional experience, regardless of whether this change is good or bad. If the duration of the stress is relatively short, the overall effect is minimal, and your body will rest, renew itself, and return to normal. But, as you will learn in this chapter, long-lasting stress, experiencing multiple stressors simultaneously, and not managing stress effectively can take a toll on your body.

> **Key Terms**
>
> **stress** the physiological and psychological state of disruption caused by the presence of an unanticipated, disruptive, or stimulating event
>
> **general adaptation syndrome (GAS)** sequenced physiological responses to the presence of a stressor, involving the alarm, resistance, and exhaustion stages of the stress response
>
> **distress** stress that diminishes the quality of life; commonly associated with disease, illness, and maladaptation
>
> **eustress** stress that enhances the quality of life

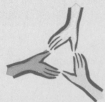

Learning from Our Diversity

Different Stressors, Different Ways to Cope

While stressful situations can affect people differently, and we all have our unique ways of coping with stress, some important cultural differences exist in the types of stress and responses to stress that ethnic groups might experience. Clearly, being of minority status can cause a great deal of stress—for example, being the victim of hate crimes, having fewer opportunities for education and employment, earning less pay for the same work done by the majority population, experiencing higher mortality rates and illness and decreased access to health care, and suffering feelings of isolation and lack of support.

Latino/a Americans, for instance, are overrepresented among the poor, have a high unemployment rate, and often live in substandard housing. Many of those who do find employment hold semiskilled or unskilled jobs. Latino/a Americans also have disproportionately high rates of tuberculosis, AIDS, and obesity. Among Latino/a farm workers, infant mortality rates are reported to be as high as 25 percent, and infants are 50 times more likely than the general population to have parasitic infections. Nearly one-third of Latino/a students drop out of high school, which is more than double the rate for African Americans and three times higher than the rate for Caucasians.

The rate of alcoholism is higher among Native Americans, with deaths owing to alcoholism being more than four times higher than those reported for the general population. Fetal Alcohol Syndrome (FAS) is nearly 33 times higher in Native American infants than in Caucasians. The suicide rate among Native Americans is 77 percent higher than the national average. High school drop-out rates and unemployment rates are also higher for this group than for any other minority population.

Elderly Chinese immigrants report higher levels of stress and depression than do members of the majority population. Obesity, substance abuse, hypertension, and depression are significantly higher for African Americans than for others.

Because different ethnic groups experience different stressors, there are also important differences to consider in the way that groups effectively manage their stress. For example, Native Americans incorporate story telling, spirituality, dreams, and visions into their stress-management strategies. A "talking circle" may be employed to help alleviate stress. This involves sitting in a circle, connecting with others by shaking hands around the circle, sharing one's innermost feelings without interruption or any response from others, burning incense and passing this around the circle, and passing a sacred object such as an eagle feather to the person who is speaking. Asian Americans commonly use yoga, meditation, and acupuncture to manage stress. Transcendental Meditation has been found to be twice as effective for African Americans than was progressive muscle relaxation.

Each of us needs to understand how we respond to stress and find strategies that work best to control stress levels. We should consider issues of diversity in order to identify the unique stressors and stress-management techniques that might best fit us.

Sources:
Hatfield, D.L. "The Stereotyping of Native Americans," *Humanist,* September 2000.
"Native Americans of North America," *Microsoft® Encarta® Online Encyclopedia 2005,* http://encarta.msn.com © 1997–2005 Microsoft Corporation.
Mui, A. C. "Living Alone and Depression among Older Chinese Immigrants, *Journal of Gerontological Social Work,* 30, 147–166, 1998.
Alexander, C., et al. "Trial of Stress Reduction for Hypertension in Older African Americans," *Hypertension,* Volume 28, 228–237, 1996.

How We Respond to Stress

When we are stressed, we react in specific ways. The **stress response** is the result of learned and conditioned habits adopted early in life as a way of coping with problems, conflict, and disruptive events. But many of our responses to stress are innate, basic human survival mechanisms left over from our primordial roots. In prehistoric times, the best response to perceived danger, such as seeing a saber-toothed tiger about to attack, might be to either fight the animal or to run away. Stress in modern times remains the same except that we are responding to 21st-century threats and dangers rather than to saber-toothed tigers. Again, it is not the events that determine how stressed we will feel but our response to these stressors. We next discuss the way that this innate stress response affects our modern lives.

Fight or Flight Response

Our response to stress involves many physiological changes that are collectively called the **fight or flight response.** In situations in which you must react immediately to danger, it is advisable to either fight off the danger or flee. For

Key Terms

stress response the physiological and psychological responses to positive or negative events that are disruptive, unexpected, or stimulating

fight or flight response the physiological response to a stressor that prepares the body for confrontation or avoidance

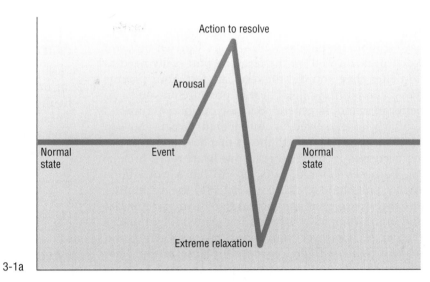

Adaptive Stress Response

Action to resolve

Arousal

Normal state   Event   Normal state

Extreme relaxation

3-1a

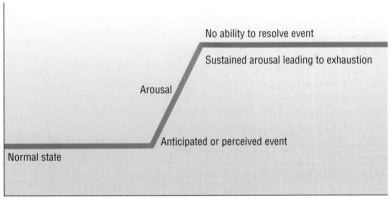

Chronic Stress Response

No ability to resolve event

Sustained arousal leading to exhaustion

Arousal

Anticipated or perceived event

Normal state

3-1b

Figure 3-1   Resolving Stress How quickly and effectively you act to resolve stress has a significant effect on how long your body remains at a high level of physiological arousal.
Source: Selye "The Stress of Life."

example, you are walking back from class at night, thinking about all the studying you need to do and you begin to cross the street. Suddenly, out of nowhere, a car's headlights are coming right at you. Since your best response is probably not to fight the car, you run as fast as you can to the other side of the road. In that split second when you see the car careening quickly toward you, your muscles tense, your heart beats faster, your adrenaline pumps faster and is released at increased levels into your bloodstream, your breathing becomes more shallow and rapid, and your pupils dilate to see the car better.

This is the fight or flight response. Again, all these changes are adaptive and helpful to your survival in getting out of harm's way. In the preceding example, when you get to the other side of the road and realize that you are okay, your body begins to relax and return to its normal state. You take a large, deep breath, expressing a big sigh of relief. Your muscles may feel even weaker than usual, your breathing may become deeper and heavier than is typical, and you may feel shaky as your body goes from extreme arousal to relaxing very quickly. Figure 3-1a depicts the changes from the normal state to an arousal state to a very relaxed state then back to normal.

Chronic Stress

Now let's consider a different situation. You have a test in a week that you are very concerned about. It seems to be preoccupying your every waking thought, and you have trouble sleeping as well. You are worried that you won't perform well on the test, and you really need to do better than you did on your last test. Your parents have been putting a great deal of pressure on you to do better in school in general. Because our bodies respond similarly to perceived or anticipated threat, you can have the same response to things that have and have not yet occurred. In other words, your heart races, breathing becomes labored, muscles are tense, your body sweats, and blood flow is constricted to the extremities and digestive organs and increases to the major muscles and brain. Your body is becoming ready to fight or flee the danger. However, you cannot take any action and make a fight or flight response, because nothing has happened yet. You haven't taken the test yet and even once you have done so, you won't know your grade. So your body remains at this high level of arousal, as depicted in Figure 3-1b.

Remaining in a continued state of physiological arousal for an extended period of time is called **chronic stress.** This high level of arousal is similar to putting your foot on the accelerator of your car while it is in park and not letting up on the gas pedal. Since the fight or flight response is meant to be a very quick, short-acting response, your body begins to wear down if kept at this physiological state of arousal for too long; eventually, you will begin to feel exhausted. This is also the reason that people cope better with anxiety by taking some action, doing something about whatever they are worried about, rather than stewing about their problems. Thus the fight or flight response can be triggered inappropriately in response to phobias, irrational beliefs, an overactive imagination, or hallucinations or delusions.

The Three Stages of Stress

Once under the influence of a stressor, people's bodies respond in remarkably similar, predictable ways. For example, when asked to give a speech for a class, your heart rate may increase, your throat becomes dry, palms sweat, and you may feel lightheaded, dizzy, and nauseous. If an individual lost her or his job or discovered that her or his partner wanted to terminate their relationship, she or he might experience similar sensations. It is clear that different stressors are able to evoke common physical reactions.

Selye described the typical physical response to a stressor in his general adaptation syndrome model[1]

discussed earlier in the chapter. Selye stated that the human body moves through three stages when confronted by stressors, as follows.

Alarm Stage

Once exposed to any event that is perceived as threatening or dangerous, the body immediately prepares for difficulty, entering what Selye called the **alarm stage.** These involuntary changes, shown in Figure 3-2, are controlled by the hormonal and the nervous systems, and they trigger the fight or flight response. For example, you realize that the final exam you thought was today was actually scheduled for yesterday. You may begin to experience fear, panic, anxiety, anger, depression, and restlessness.[2]

Resistance Stage

The second stage of a response to a stressor is the **resistance stage,** during which the body attempts to reestablish its equilibrium or internal balance. The body is geared for survival, and because staying in the alarm stage for a prolonged amount of time is not conducive to optimal functioning, it will resist the threat or attempt to resolve the problem and reduce the intensity of the response to a more manageable level. Specific organ systems, such as the cardiovascular and digestive systems, become the focus of the body's response.[2] During this phase, you might take steps to calm yourself down and relieve the stress on your body: You might deny the situation, withdraw and isolate yourself from others, and shut down your emotions. Thus, in the example above, you may not tell anyone about missing the exam, may tell yourself that you don't care about that class anyway, and go back to bed.

Key Terms

chronic stress refers to remaining at a high level of physiological arousal for an extended period of time; it can also occur when an individual is not able to immediately react to a real or a perceived threat

alarm stage the first stage of the stress response involving physiological, involuntary changes which are controlled by the hormonal and the nervous systems; the fight or flight response is activated in this stage

resistance stage the second stage of the stress response during which the body attempts to reestablish its equilibrium or internal balance

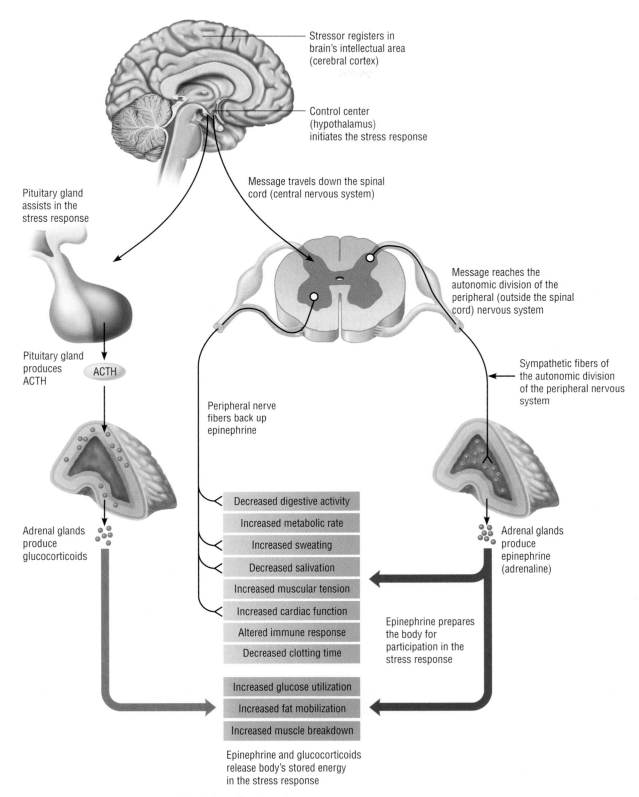

Stressor registers in brain's intellectual area (cerebral cortex)

Control center (hypothalamus) initiates the stress response

Message travels down the spinal cord (central nervous system)

Pituitary gland assists in the stress response

Pituitary gland produces ACTH

ACTH

Message reaches the autonomic division of the peripheral (outside the spinal cord) nervous system

Sympathetic fibers of the autonomic division of the peripheral nervous system

Peripheral nerve fibers back up epinephrine

Adrenal glands produce glucocorticoids

Adrenal glands produce epinephrine (adrenaline)

Decreased digestive activity

Increased metabolic rate

Increased sweating

Decreased salivation

Increased muscular tension

Increased cardiac function

Altered immune response

Decreased clotting time

Epinephrine prepares the body for participation in the stress response

Increased glucose utilization

Increased fat mobilization

Increased muscle breakdown

Epinephrine and glucocorticoids release body's stored energy in the stress response

Figure 3-2   The stress response: physiological reactions to a stressor

Exhaustion Stage

Your ability to move from the alarm stage to a less damaging resistance stage determines the effect that the stressor has on your physical and psychological health. As you gain more control and balance is reestablished, you can begin to recover from the stress.

The length of time, the energy, and the effort required to accomplish recovery determines how exhausted your body becomes as a result of the stressor. Of course, the longer your body is under stress and out of balance, the more negative the effect. Long-term exposure to a stressor or coping with multiple stressors at the same time often results in overloading your system. Specific organs and body systems that were called on during the resistance stage may not be able to resist a stressor indefinitely. When all the psychological and physical resources we rely on to deal with stress are used up, an **exhaustion stage** results, and the stress-producing hormones such as adrenaline increase again.[2] This is when chronic and serious illnesses can begin to develop, and the individual may even develop clinical depression.

Sources of Stress

There are other causes of stress besides experiencing positive or negative events in life. What events or situations trigger stress for you? For some it is financial worries, for others it might be relationship conflict, and for still others it is work-related stress. Even positive events, such as getting married, starting a new job, moving to a new place can be **stressors.** Going on vacation can be stressful as you get things done ahead of time to prepare for being away, pack your belongings, spend money on the trip, and completely change your routine. Any type of change in your life has the potential to trigger a stressful response.

Because stress involves a physiological response, it has a direct link to your physical and psychological health. The work of Thomas Holmes and Richard Rahe has found direct connections between changes in people's lives and physical illness. They developed a widely used inventory, called the Social Readjustment Rating Scale, to assess the degree of stress people experience in connection with particular life events. While one of these events alone might be tolerable, a combination of too many life changes within a short period of time may lead to illness.[3] To assess your level of stress and potential vulnerability to illness, complete the personal assessment inventory at the end of this chapter.

The Costs and Benefits of Stress

Stress can be costly, taking a toll on our physical and mental health as well as our finances.

Constant arousal and increased levels of adrenaline in your system will eventually wear down your body's immunological system. As this occurs, you will be less able to cope with stress, and so it takes less and less to cause a stress reaction. When you are chronically stressed, it takes very little to frustrate you, and you can feel easily irritated and stressed at the littlest thing. Your body is both psychologically as well as physically less able to cope with stress. This can compromise your immune system, and you may become ill more easily. It may also take longer for you to recover from illness.

A variety of medical problems have been associated with stress, such as:

- Cardiovascular problems (heart attacks, strokes, hypertension)
- Gastrointestinal problems (ulcers, irritable bowel syndrome, diarrhea, constipation, diverticulitis)
- Headaches and migraines
- Muscle spasms and cramps
- Sleep disorders
- Anxiety
- Jaw problems, (temporomandibular joint [TMJ] syndrome)
- Allergies
- Cancer
- Back pain
- Asthma
- Kidney disease
- Sexual dysfunction
- Infertility
- Alcoholism and drug abuse

As we have said, while too much stress can have a negative effect and cause some serious health problems, a moderate level of stress is positive and beneficial. Stress can be motivating and energizing. Without some stress, many of us may not get much accomplished in our day or even get out of bed! Look at the diagram in Figure 3-3. What do you notice? Too little and too much stress are not helpful. When you are not stressed at all, you can be apathetic and lethargic.

Key Terms

exhaustion stage the third stage of the stress response; the point at which the physical and the psychological resources used to deal with stress have been depleted

stressors factors or events, real or imagined, that elicit a state of stress

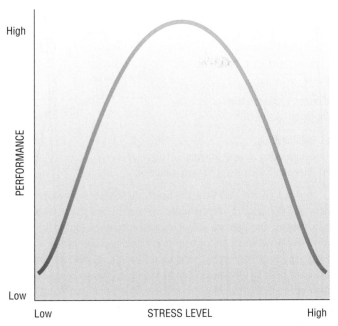

Figure 3-3 The Yerkes-Dodson Law Too little or too much stress is not helpful, but a moderate level of stress encourages peak performance. Source: Hebb DO. Drive and the CNS (central nervous system). *Psychological Review* 62(4) 243–254, 1955.

When you are too stressed, you are paralyzed with fear, like deer in the headlights. This is referred to as the **Yerkes-Dodson Law,** which uses a bell-shaped curve to demonstrate that there is an optimal level of stress for peak performance. This fact holds true for any type of performance, from academic or work activities to music or athletics.[5] Recognizing the appropriate level of stress for your ideal performance level is important in reaching your potential.

Student Stress

Going to college has been likened to "crossing into a new culture" where students face unique challenges and stressors.[6] Similarly to going to live in another country, students must learn new customs and traditions, new ways of doing things, a new language, and must leave comfortable and familiar surroundings. This can cause a high level of stress for students, many of whom have left their support system behind to live in a place where they know few people. In the sections that follow, we cover some of the specific stressors college students face and offer ways to manage these situations.

Coping with Homesickness

Homesickness is one of the most common problems facing college students—which is understandable given that they are separated from friends and family and learning to live in an entirely new environment.[6] When you are undergoing a great deal of change in your life, it is helpful to have the comfort and security of knowing that your home base remains stable and consistent. Moving from home to college can disrupt this sense of safety. While the college years can be an exciting and challenging time in your life, you may be missing your friends and family at home with whom you normally share these events. You may have also lost your sense of belonging while you struggle with finding a way to fit in with and navigate your new surroundings.

Often homesickness doesn't hit until a few weeks or maybe a month after you have moved, since the first few weeks are filled with meeting new people, social activities, and unpacking. After the dust settles, some people begin to feel lonely and alone. See Changing for the Better on page 63 for advice on how to deal with homesickness.

Relationship Problems

Along with homesickness, another very common stressor for students is relationship problems. Often students are separated by long distances from their best friends and romantic partners. While it can be difficult to maintain long-distance relationships, it is not impossible. Studies show that the key to effective long-distance relationships is communication.[7] The quality of a long-distance relationship is improved if you both are committed to each other, you can talk openly about your concerns, feelings, and fears, and you can agree on the rules of the relationship, such as dating other people. In addition, there needs to be a strong level of trust between the partners, since trust is often tested in long-distance relationships. Both of you will change, and you must share these changes so that you can grow together, not apart. Agree on how often you will see each other, call or e-mail, and focus on spending high-quality time together.

It can be beneficial to have your friends visit you at college (rather than you going home) so that they can interact with you in your new environment and meet your new friends. Often students feel as though they live in two worlds, home and school, and it can be stressful to negotiate going from one to the other. The more you

> **Key Terms**
>
> **Yerkes-Dodson Law** a bell-shaped curve demonstrating that there is an optimal level of stress for peak performance; this law states that too little or too much stress is not helpful, whereas a moderate level of stress is positive and beneficial

Yoga: The Union of Mind and Body

Yoga is often associated with Indian philosophy, such as Buddhism, but it has recently gained in popularity as a form of stress management. *Yoga* is a Sanskrit word meaning "union" of the individual soul with the universal soul. The practice of yoga directs and channels energy in a specific manner in the body. Individuals who practice yoga say they experience greater clarity in thinking and improved balance in their lives.

When individuals think of relaxation, they usually think of something that they like doing, that they find enjoyable or interesting. Such activities may include socializing, watching a movie or television, reading, going to a play or to a sporting event, or going to the beach or the mountains.

With yoga, relaxation involves slowing down the metabolism in order to let go of mental and physical tension. Many of the leisure activities mentioned above do not help us to slow down or to let go of mental and physical tension. It is purported that individuals who practice yoga experience better mental and physical health than do those who do not, because of the conscious experience of slowing down the mind and the body. The idea behind yoga is that being consciously still each day for a set period of time is the best way to become more relaxed and develop and improve concentration and energy.

The reported benefits of regular yoga relaxation are numerous. They include:

- Better overall physical and mental health
- Less fatigue and a feeling of restfulness
- "Spiritual unfoldment," which refers to an improved mind-body integration and an increased sense of harmony and peacefulness
- Enhanced concentration and focus
- A greater ability to cope with anxiety and daily stressors

It is recommended to practice yoga relaxation techniques at least once a day. Suggested times are

- Before meals
- Before going to sleep at night
- After experiencing any stressful situation

Yoga has been shown to reduce heart rate and blood pressure, increase lung capacity, improve muscle relaxation, assist with weight management, and increase overall physical endurance. Yoga may affect levels of brain or blood chemicals, including monoamines, melatonin, dopamine, stress hormones (cortisol), and GABA (gamma-aminobutyric acid). Changes in mental functions, such as improved attention, cognition, processing of sensory information, and visual perception, have been described in some research studies in humans.

In yoga, poses are held for varying lengths of time using gravity, leverage, and tension. Breathing techniques are also used. Rapid breathing (*kapalabhati*) and slow breathing (*nadi suddhi*) may be practiced along with stretching exercises. The alignment of the head with the spine is important as is inhaling and exhaling through the nose only. Focus is on breathing and not allowing the mind to wander. One usually maintains a yoga position for 5 to 20 minutes.

To learn more about yoga, find a yoga class at your college or in your local community.

Sources:
"Complementary & Alternative Medicine," *Alternative Modalities for Health and Well-Being*, www.inteliheath.com, July 8, 2005.
Kimbrough, J. *Yoga for Better Health and Living*, www.stress.about.com.

can connect these two worlds, the less stress you will experience. So it can be helpful to share what you are doing in your day—activities around campus, details of your classes, even who you ate lunch with—with your friends and family back home, and ask what they have been doing.

Balancing Work, Home, and School

It is estimated that about two-thirds of students work while going to college, and more students are working full-time to pay for the costs of tuition (see Figure 3-4). In addition, it is estimated that between 5 and 10 percent of college students also have children. This, of course, adds stress to a student's life in balancing time for school, children, work, and household responsibilities. The increase in the number of students who have children is partly a result of a nationwide trend of more women in their mid-20s or older starting or returning to college. In fact, a national study by the University of Michigan showed that the number of full-time female students over 25 years old grew by 500 percent over recent years.[8]

While some campuses offer child care, many do not, which leaves students having to coordinate schedules and juggle responsibilities, causing even more stress. Also, the cost of child care can be exorbitant for some and can certainly add to financial worries. Managing time well and having a strong support system are essential for students with children, particularly single parents. Often there is little to no time available for relaxation, socializing, or exercising, and so employing stress relief strategies can be challenging.

Test Anxiety

You have studied for the test you are about to take and are well prepared. You look at the first test question and suddenly your mind goes blank. The harder you try to think, the more nervous and distressed you feel. You just can't think clearly and feel as though you have some type of mental block—what is happening? One-fifth of students experience these feelings, referred to as **test anxiety.** Exams are one of the greatest sources of stress for college students. The physical sensations associated with test anxiety are similar to those of general anxiety, such as fidgeting; having the feeling of butterflies in your stomach; rapid heart rate; difficulty breathing; nausea; tension in your neck, back, jaw and shoulders; headaches; sweaty palms; and feeling shaky. People suffering from test anxiety make more mistakes on their tests, don't read the test accu-

rately, and tend to make simple mistakes, such as spelling errors or adding something incorrectly. Many don't pace themselves well, and have a hard time finishing exams. Test anxiety is a form of performance anxiety—people anticipate that they will perform poorly on the test.[9]

 TALKING POINTS What are some problems with stress described in this chapter that you have experienced?

Key Terms
test anxiety a form of performance anxiety that generates extreme feelings of distress in exam situations

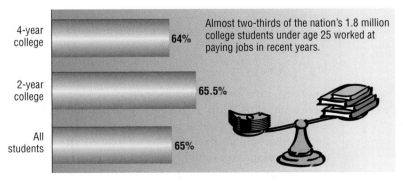

4-year college **64%**

2-year college **65.5%**

All students **65%**

Almost two-thirds of the nation's 1.8 million college students under age 25 worked at paying jobs in recent years.

Figure 3-4 Percentages of college students who also work at paying jobs
Source: Bureau of Labor Statistics, March 25, 2005.

Do You Suffer from Test Anxiety?

Test anxiety is a commonly experienced problem and can significantly impair your academic performance. Similar to managing other types of stress and anxiety, test anxiety can be coped with by using the following suggestions:

- Prepare well in advance. Don't cram at the last minute for the test. Rehearsal and repetition are the best ways of remembering information.

- Improve your odds by getting a good night's sleep before the test and eating a nutritious meal to give your brain needed energy.

- Have a positive attitude and watch your test talk. Don't talk about the test beforehand with friends, since this tends to increase anxiety. Go into the test with a confident attitude, reminding yourself that you are well prepared and have taken many tests and performed satisfactorily in the past.

- Activity reduces anxiety. If you stumble on a question, don't linger over it; go onto the next question and return to that one later.

- Ask for clarification if you don't understand a question or something on the test.

- Don't pay attention to the people around you. Focus on the test and don't allow yourself to get distracted.

- Take deep breaths, allow your breathing to help you to relax, and bring more oxygen to the brain so you can think more clearly.

- Look through the entire exam before answering the questions. Pace yourself and be aware of your time. Know when you need to be halfway through the test according to the time allotted for the exam.

Source: Newman E. *No More Test Anxiety*. Los Angeles, CA: Learning Skills Publications, 1996.

Speech Anxiety

As we have mentioned, speech anxiety, or fear of public speaking, is one of the most common anxiety disorders. Since students are frequently required to give oral presentations, expected to engage in class discussion, and graded on class-participation points, this can present a problem for some.

In addition to the basic stress-management techniques outlined in this chapter, the following strategies can be used to cope with speech anxiety:

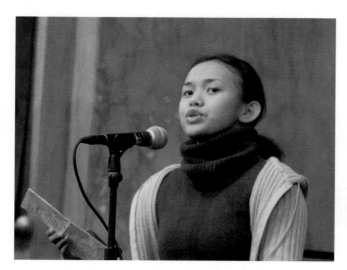

Speech anxiety or fear of public speaking is one of the most common anxiety disorders.

- Volunteer to go first. Anxiety is dealt with best by taking action. Pressure and expectations tend to mount with each person who takes a turn, so go first. Another advantage is that your performance is judged on its own merit without being compared to anyone else's.

- Practice in front of a mirror and for your friends. Solicit feedback: do you need to slow down or speak louder? Practice will also help you to remember your talk so that you don't read it word for word, which can seem less interesting to your audience.

- Engage in positive visualization. Take deep, comfortable breaths and imagine yourself giving your speech with confidence and receiving positive feedback and compliments about your performance.

- Vary your presentation style and format. Use visuals, such as slides, and engage your audience in discussion so that they are an active not a passive part of your presentation. This transfers some of the focus from you and removes some pressure, too.

Math Anxiety

Another common stressor for college students is math anxiety. Math anxiety is an intense emotional feeling of anxiety that some people have about their ability to understand mathematics. People who suffer from math anxiety feel that they are incapable of performing well in activities and classes that involve math. The incidence of math anxiety among college students has risen significantly over the last decade. Many students have even chosen their college major on the basis of how little math is required for the degree. Math anxiety has become so prevalent on college campuses that many schools have designed classes and special counseling programs to help math-anxious students. Typically, people with math anxiety have the potential to perform well in math and it is more of a psychological, rather than intellectual, problem.

Students who fear math often avoid asking questions to save embarrassment, sit in the back of the classroom, fail to seek help from the instructor, and usually put off studying math until the last moment. All these negative behaviors are intended to reduce the student's anxiety but actually result in more intense anxiety. However, there are a number of strategies that can be used to overcome math anxiety.

1. Be sure to have developed a solid arithmetic foundation. Since complex concepts build cumulatively on more simplistic ones, a remedial course or short course in arithmetic is often a significant first step in reducing the anxiety response to math.
2. Take an easier, slower math course as opposed to a faster paced, more challenging one. It is better to stack the odds in your favor than to risk reinforcing your negative experiences with math.
3. Be aware of thoughts, feelings, and actions as they are related to math. Develop a positive perspective toward math.
4. There is safety in numbers! Math anxiety is learned and reinforced over a long period of time and may take time to eliminate. You can reduce your anxiety with the help of a tutor, studying with a friend, and talking with your instructor.
5. Sit near the front of the class where you will experience fewer distractions and feel more a part of what is being discussed.
6. If you have questions or can't keep up with the instructor ask for clarification and repetition of whatever you missed.[10]
7. Review the material. As with most things, skill in math comes from practice. Make sure you review the material covered in the class, and identify questions you need to ask the instructor as soon as possible after the class. Research shows that you will remember 50 percent of what you heard in class if you review it immediately after class, but only 20 percent is retained 24 hours later if you didn't review the material right away.[11]

Stress and Learning

How does stress affect learning? Research suggests that people who are highly anxious tend to perform better than others do at simple learning tasks but less well than others do at difficult tasks, particularly those involving reasoning activities and time-limited tests. One interesting study showed that college students with average scholastic ability earned significantly better grades when they had low levels of anxiety as compared to highly anxious average students.[12] When you are more stressed or anxious, you have a diminished ability to concentrate, to recall information, and to engage in problem-solving activities. You may find yourself reading the same page in your textbook over and over again, not knowing what you read.[9]

Using Time Effectively

An overwhelming number of students identify time management as the reason for their academic success or failure. Setting priorities and goals, balancing academic life with your social life, and finding time for sleeping, eating, exercising, and working along with studying is an essential aspect of managing your stress effectively.

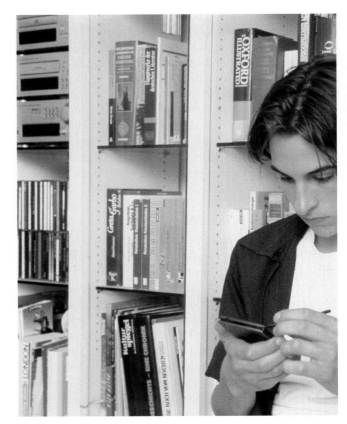

Managing your time well can greatly reduce your stress level.

Time Management

Managing your time effectively can help you cope with your stress by feeling more in control, having a sense of accomplishment, and having a sense of purpose in your life. Establishing good time management habits can take two to three weeks. By using specific systems, even the most disorganized person can make their lives less chaotic and stressful.

Assess Your Habits

The first step is to analyze how you are spending your time. What are your most productive and least productive times of day and night? Do you tend to underestimate how long something will take you to complete? Do you waste time or allow interruptions to take you off task? Carrying a notebook with you for a week and writing down how you spend your time might provide you with some insight into the answers to these questions and how you spend your time. You might find that you've been devoting most of your time to less important tasks. Perhaps it is tempting to do your laundry rather than to start writing that term paper, but this is probably not the best use of your time.

Use a Planner

Keeping a daily planner to schedule your time is the next step in managing your time more effectively. First block off all of the activities that are consistent, regular, weekly activities, such as attending classes, eating meals, sleeping, going to meetings, exercising, and working. Then look at the open, available time remaining. Schedule regular study time, relaxation time, and free time. Remember to schedule your study time during the more productive part of your waking hours. When you have a 1-hour block of time, what can you realistically get done in that time? This could be a good time to review your notes from class, pay bills, or get some reading done.

Set Goals and Prioritize

Set goals for the week as well as for each day. If something unexpected interferes with your time schedule, modify your plans but don't throw out the entire schedule.

Making a to-do list can be helpful, but it is only the first step. Breaking the large tasks into smaller, more manageable pieces and then prioritizing them is the key to effective time management. When you prioritize your tasks, try the "ABC" method of task management. The A tasks are those items that are most urgent and must be done today. Then the B tasks are those things that are important but, if need be, could wait 24 hours. The C tasks are activities that can easily wait a few days to a week. Don't fall into the C trap, which is when you do the less important tasks because they are quick and can be checked off your

list with ease. This can lead to putting off the more important A activities, leaving them until you feel stressed and overwhelmed.[13] We discuss procrastination in the next section.

Procrastination

Procrastination means postponing something that is necessary to do to reach a goal.[14] Putting things off is a common problem that plagues students and can cause stress. A survey of college students found that approximately 23 percent of students said they procrastinated about half the time, and 27 percent of students said they procrastinated most of the time.[15] Procrastination has been viewed as a time-management problem, but it is really more than that, and so time-management strategies tend to be ineffective in resolving this problem. Procrastination is also different from indecision, because people can make a decision but have trouble implementing it.

Typically there is a psychological aspect to procrastination, because we tend to delay doing things we don't want to do. Emotions such as anxiety, guilt, and dread often accompany thinking about the task. By putting the dreaded activity off, you can temporarily alleviate your anxiety and discomfort, which is a reinforcing aspect of procrastination. In the short term, procrastination seems to be a good solution and helps you to feel better. However, in the long run, procrastination usually leads to bigger problems and more work. For example putting off paying your bills may feel good at the moment, but when your electricity is turned off and you have to pay late fees, and your roommates are upset with you because they thought you had paid the bill, your pleasurable feelings soon turn sour.

Many people who procrastinate report feeling overwhelmed and highly anxious. They have difficulty tuning out external stimulation and concentrating on the task at hand. They also worry about how their performance will be judged by others and have perfectionistic standards for themselves. Students who procrastinate tend to perform less well and retain less than students who do not.[16] We discuss perfectionism in the next section.

Some techniques for combating procrastination involve time management, stress management, assertiveness training, and increasing self-esteem and self-acceptance.

> ### Key Terms
>
> **procrastination** a tendency to put off completing tasks until some later time, sometimes resulting in increased stress

My girlfriend is a perfectionist and she is driving me crazy. Nothing I do seems good enough for her as much as I try to please her. Her unrealistic expectations are causing a great deal of stress in our relationship and our friends are beginning to stay away from us because they don't like to hear us argue. What can I do?

Sometimes people who are perfectionists tend to blame others for their own sense of failure or rejection. Here are some ways to respond better to your girlfriend:

1. Communicate how you feel when she is critical of you or shows her disapproval. Suggest more positive ways that she can give you feedback or share her disappointments.
2. Give specific examples of how she may be expecting too much, and find a compromise between all or nothing.
3. Don't retaliate. It is tempting to point out her flaws when she is doing the same to you. Instead, reassure her that you think highly of her and point out her successes and accomplishments since she is probably focusing on her failures.
4. Communicate your confidence in her abilities and ask her to have the same trust in you.
5. Model acceptance of imperfection in yourself and others. Show her that everybody is flawed, no one is perfect, and this makes us human.
6. Don't focus on her mistakes or tease her when she makes an error. Instead give positive reinforcement when she doesn't do something well.
7. Help her to relax and have fun even if all the work is not yet done.
8. Talk about how she is feeling rather than the content of her message, such as saying "You sound very stressed and overwhelmed."
9. Don't fall into the perfectionist trap yourself. It is easy to think, "If I just try harder, she will be happy with me." Perfectionism is an impossible goal to reach, and so you are setting yourself up for failure and rejection.
10. Help her to see the forest rather than the trees. It is easy for perfectionists to get lost in the details and lose sight of the overall goal. It may help to alleviate her stress if you can help her to refocus on what is really important and what the overall goal is such as having fun at the party you are throwing and not having the house perfectly clean.

Procrastinators tend to both over- and underestimate how much time a task will take. When they underestimate the time, they feel justified in procrastinating because they erroneously believe they have plenty of time to complete the task. When they overestimate the time needed, they feel intimidated by the magnitude of the job, feel anxious, and so have trouble getting started. Most students explain that their anxiety stems from a fear of failure or being evaluated. Sometimes their anxiety manifests itself because they don't understand the material or what the instructor is wanting but are afraid to ask for clarification.

People also report procrastinating when they feel forced or pressured to do something they don't want to do. Rather than communicating assertively, they rebel by agreeing to do something but constantly put it off, which can be a passive-aggressive way of behaving. They fear the consequences of saying no or not fulfilling their obligations but are also angry about what they perceive as unfair expectations and demands on them. This is when some assertiveness training may be helpful. Finally, increasing self-esteem can solve problems with procrastination because feeling better about yourself relieves you of worrying about what others think of you and having constantly to prove yourself to them. Some people procrastinate because they think they need to do everything perfectly or not at all. With increased self-esteem, you are more accepting of mistakes and don't expect yourself to perform perfectly.

Perfectionism

Perfectionism leads to undue stress, because perfection is an unattainable goal. By setting the standard at perfect, you will set yourself up to fail. Perfectionists tend to be their own worst critic; they are harder on themselves than anyone else is on them, and they are also critical of others. These individuals are described as neat and organized, seeming to "have it all together" and to be able to do more than most people and do it exceptionally well. Often people envy perfectionistic people because they seem very confident and competent; however, individuals who are perfectionists never feel good enough and often feel out of control in their lives.[17] People who are perfectionists focus on what they haven't accomplished or haven't done right rather than on what they have completed or have done well. Making mistakes feels especially humiliating to persons who are perfectionistic, and they tend to feel a strong sense of shame and low self-esteem when someone catches them in error. They have difficulty with criticism or any negative feedback

Key Terms

perfectionism a tendency to expect perfection in everything one does, with little tolerance for mistakes because much of their self-esteem is based on being accurate, competent, and being the best. While striving to do your best is an admirable quality, expecting to be perfect in everything you do and never making a mistake places a great deal of stress and pressure on yourself.

To help alleviate the stress of perfectionism, base your self-esteem on who you are rather than on what you do. This involves accepting yourself and others unconditionally, including imperfections. Lowering your expectations of yourself and others and aiming for 80 percent rather than 100 percent is another strategy in battling perfectionism. Note what you are doing well and have accomplished rather than what is still left to do. Time-management strategies such as those outlined previously can be useful in managing your expectations of yourself. Push yourself to take risks and allow yourself to make mistakes. It can be useful to make mistakes on purpose in order to get accustomed to this experience and realize that people still like and accept you and nothing bad will happen. Relaxation and stress-management techniques such as the ones described at the end of this chapter can also help alleviate the stress that comes with perfectionism. You might want to take the survey at the end of this chapter to assess your level of perfectionism.

Managing Stress: Effective Coping Strategies

The research on how people cope with crisis and stress in their lives has shown that people tend to resolve problems within two weeks of experiencing a crisis.

Because stress involves a disruption in equilibrium, and the body does not function well in a chronic state of unbalance, it is human nature to seek a way to alleviate the stress the body is experiencing and return to a steady state. As we discussed previously, our bodies cannot function for very long in a sustained fight or flight response without serious damage, and so a person will naturally strive to make changes to resolve the stress for survival. However, the way that people resolve their problems and alleviate stress may be positive or negative.

A number of negative ways of dealing with stress are quite common and often quite harmful. As indicated in Figure 3-5, some people turn to alcohol and drugs to avoid their problems and numb their feelings, and cigarettes are also cited as a way of relieving stress. Many people use food to comfort themselves. Putting off distasteful tasks and avoiding stressful situations is another negative way of coping with stress. Some people use sleep as a way of escaping their problems, and certainly depression has been associated with not having the ability to effectively manage stress. In the next section, we discuss ways of effectively managing stress.

What are some positive, effective methods to cope with stress? Different strategies and methods for stress management involve the physical, social, environmental, and psychological aspects of your stress. We will review techniques and strategies within each of these dimensions, and you will need to practice and experiment to find the stress management techniques that are right for you.

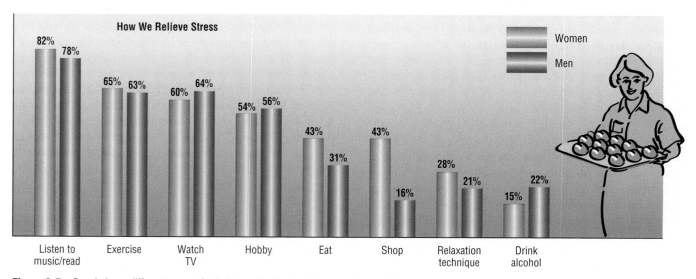

Figure 3-5 People have different ways of relaxing and relieving stress, such as cooking, reading a mystery novel, or swimming: How do you cope with stress?

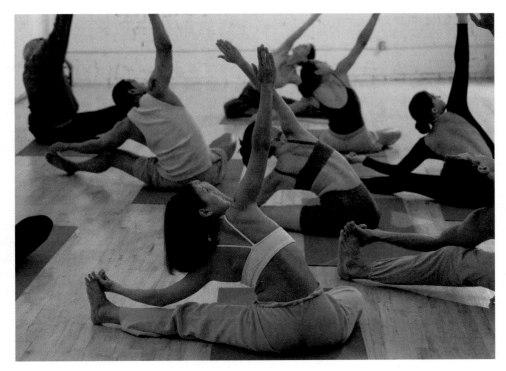

Exercising is one of the best ways to manage stress.

The Physical Aspects of Stress Management

The physical aspects of stress management involve meeting your basic needs of nutrition, sleep, and exercise as was discussed in Chapter 2 under Maslow's hierarchy of needs.[18]

Nutrition

In Chapter 5 you will learn about the nutrients that provide the necessary fuel the body needs to function. When people are stressed, they often skip meals or eat on the run. Since the fight or flight response requires more energy than is normally needed, during stressful times you must eat a balanced, nutritious diet. Without proper nutrition, the body will begin to break down its own tissues in an effort to obtain the energy required to survive. The immune system can then become compromised, making the body more susceptible to disease. It is not a coincidence that many people who are under a great deal of stress for prolonged periods of time become ill and that regaining their health takes longer than it does for those who are managing their stress well.

As we previously mentioned, people often use food to cope with stress and can overeat, typically eating high-sugar and high-fat foods such as chips, candy, and cookies. Eating too much or too little is not an effective way to manage stress and can eventually lead to serious health problems such as obesity, eating disorders, diabetes and hypertension.

Sleep

As with eating, too much sleep or too little is also an ineffective way of managing stress. Most adults require 7 to 8 hours of sleep a night.[19] Sometimes people get very little sleep during the week and try to "catch up" over the weekend, sleeping 14 hours at a time or taking naps during the day. Sleep is not like a bank account in which you can make deposits and withdrawals, and so getting an average of 7 to 8 hours a night over a week's time is not the same thing as sleeping this amount each night.

People also need uninterrupted sleep. Normal **circadian rhythms,** the biological processes related to the 24-hour light/dark cycle, are necessary for normal sleep and optimal daytime functioning. Our sleep patterns relate to these biological cycles, which also affect our patterns of hunger and eating, body temperature, and hormone release. These cycles must be in harmony for us to have a sense of well-being during our waking hours.[20]

> **Key Terms**
>
> **circadian rhythms** the internal biological clock that helps coordinate physiological processes related to the 24-hour light/dark cycle

Sleep deprivation has been found to cause losses in higher cognitive processing tasks, decline in the performance of simple tasks, memory loss, and, with prolonged sleep deprivation, temporary psychosis, such as hallucinations and delirium.[21] Research also shows that sleeping too much can result in increased depression and decreased energy levels. So getting the right amount of rest is an essential aspect of stress management.

Exercise

Exercise is another physical aspect of stress management. Exercising aerobically at least three times a week for 20 to 30 minutes has been found to manage stress effectively for several reasons. First, exercising requires you to focus on your breathing and to breath deeply, the key to stress management. By tensing and releasing the muscles through exercise, you are allowing your body to relax and unwind. Second, exercise can alleviate stress through the release of endorphins, naturally occurring chemicals in the brain. Endorphins help to counter stress, subdue pain, and increase pleasure, which is the reason people talk about the runner's high. Hitting a racquetball against the wall or playing basketball can be a great way to release the frustrations of the day and let go of tension and stress. Aerobic exercise includes walking briskly, running, bicycling, skating, and dancing. The benefits of exercise are further discussed in Chapter 4.

The Social Aspects of Stress Management

To manage stress effectively, you must also make time for fun and play. Like exercise, laughter increases the release of endorphins and requires you to breath deeply, and so having humor in your life is an essential part of stress management.[22] Research has shown that stress can be related to having inadequate social interactions.[23] Hugging and human contact has also been demonstrated as having a significant effect in reducing the harmful physical effects of stress.[24] Participating in social activities such as social organizations, sports or just talking with friends can give you the break you need to rest your mind and focus on something other than work.

Actually you don't even have to have human contact to reduce stress—just owning a pet can make a difference. Studies have shown that just petting an animal produces calming effects such as lowered blood pressure and decreased heart rate. Cardiac patients who own pets tend to live much longer than those who have no pets.[25]

The Environmental Aspects of Stress Management

To effectively manage your stress, you need to take into consideration environmental stressors such as noise level,

amount of light, and aesthetic quality of the space you inhabit. Stress has been linked to being exposed to prolonged, daily noise such as in a factory.[26] We know that depression can be related to the amount of light to which you are exposed, and this can also affect your circadian rhythms.[27] Natural light tends to elevate your mood, whereas prolonged exposure to artificial lighting can increase your stress level. Research also suggests that different colors can raise or lower your stress and energy level. Some people associate the color red with feelings of anger or hostility and blue with feeling depressed. Having plants or photos of friends and family around your living and workspace can also alleviate stress.

Smell can also play a significant role in managing stress. As the saying goes, "Stop and smell the roses." Studies have shown that aromatherapy, using different aromas or odors therapeutically, can lower stress levels. When you breathe in these oils, they send a direct message to your brain via your olfactory nerves, where they can then affect the endocrine and the hormonal systems via the hypothalamus. Odors have an amazing effect on our emotional states because they hook into the emotional or primitive parts of our brains. Aromatherapy has been used to relieve pain, enhance relaxation and stress relief, unknot tense muscles, soften dry skin, and enhance immunity. So it is wise to pay attention to your aromatic surroundings, because they may affect you much more than you may realize.

While social interaction has been shown to have positive results on lessening the effects of stress, the beneficial effect depends on the type of friends with whom you surround yourself. Spending time with negative, pessimistic people can increase your stress level rather than decrease it. It is obviously more advantageous to surround yourself with positive, optimistic friends.[28] Feeling crowded in a room and not having enough personal space can also lead to an increase in stress.[29] Interestingly, it is not being in crowds itself but how familiar you are with the people, the activity that is taking place, and how much control you feel over your personal space that makes the difference. In other words, being in a crowded room filled with your friends during a party feels subjectively different than feeling trapped in a crowded restaurant filled with strangers.

Other important aspects of managing stress in your environment include having meaningful work and challenging and interesting classes. Having work that is stimulating but not beyond your abilities helps to keep your stress response at a moderate, optimal level for performance.

The Psychological Aspects of Stress Management

Last, you can effectively cope with stress by using a variety of cognitive and psychological strategies. There are several different techniques, but as you will see, many are focused on deep breathing, which is the key to managing stress.

Relaxation and Deep Breathing

The relaxation response is a powerful weapon in ensuring you do not remain in the stress response too long. It is effective because it entails the opposite of the stress response. Rather than taking shallow breaths, you are required to breathe deeply, inhaling to a count of four and exhaling to a count of four while sitting in a comfortable position. As you breathe deeply, your muscles unwind and relax, again the opposite of the stress response. It is generally advised not to cross your legs or arms so that your muscles can relax easily. Blood flows to the extremities, and your heart rate slows. In fact, experienced users of this technique can temporarily lower their breathing rate from a typical rate of 14 to 18 breaths per minute to as few as 4 breaths per minute. Body temperature decreases, and blood pressure is lowered as well. The entire nervous system is slowed, in direct opposition to its role in the stress response. You are instructed to focus on your breathing and inner experience and become less aware of your external environment. To help to tune out the outside world, you are instructed to close your eyes and let go of the worries and concerns of the day.[31]

To try this technique, take a moment to focus on your breathing and breathe in for a count of four and out for four. After doing so a few times, tighten your body, clench your hands, teeth, and jaw, close your eyes tightly, and pull your shoulders up while you are still breathing deeply. Are you able to do so? It is virtually impossible to tense your body and breathe deeply, because they are mutually exclusive activities. Thus, the relaxation response is the foundation of most of the stress-management techniques described in this chapter. Deep breathing is the fundamental aspect of stress management.

Progressive Muscle Relaxation (PMR)

Progressive Muscle Relaxation involves learning to recognize the difference between contracted and relaxed muscles, in order to gain a sense of control over the body and the stress response. Progressive muscle relaxation enables you to intentionally put certain muscles into a controlled state of relaxation and reduce your overall stress level.

PMR is based on the use of positioning your body in a comfortable position, sitting or lying down, and concentrating on certain muscle groups. As you inhale, breathing in for a count of four, you contract your muscles starting with your forehead and count to four as you exhale and relax your muscles. Continue to clench and relax the muscles, using your breathing to help you to tighten and release, working your way down your body all the way to

your feet and toes. Concentrate on the sensations of relaxation and how different they are from the feelings of tension and stress. Fifteen minutes, twice a day, is the recommended schedule. In one to two weeks, you will have mastered the basics and will be aware of which muscles need more attention in order to relax. You will also be more sensitive to the buildup of tension in your body so that you will be able to decrease your stress level before it becomes overwhelming.[31]

Guided Imagery and Visualization

Guided imagery involves having someone describe a beautiful, relaxing scene while you focus on taking deep, comfortable breaths. While in a comfortable position, in an environment free from interruptions and distractions, you breathe deeply, relax your muscles, and imagine a pleasant scene. The imagery includes all the senses, not just what you see but pleasant smells, sounds, touch, and even taste. Guided imagery can be self-taught, or you can listen to recordings of narrated scripts.

Visualization is similar to guided imagery with the scene being more specifically focused on something you are about to do or want to accomplish, or on some performance or activity that may be causing you distress. Guided imagery and visualization techniques help you to consciously program change through positive mental images. For example, you might imagine yourself auditioning for a part in a play, seeing yourself go through your lines effortlessly and flawlessly, and feeling confident and proud of yourself. You are probably already skilled at visualization; unfortunately, we frequently engage in negative visualization and are unaware of doing so. For example, we imagine ourselves making fools of ourselves or making mistakes.

Athletes are trained in using positive visualization to improve their performance and visualize their goals.[32] Positive visualization has also been used in managing pain, especially in chronic pain management. This technique has also been effective in weight management, smoking cessation, insomnia, and for almost any type of behavior change.

Meditation and Hypnosis

Meditation allows the mind to transcend thought effortlessly when the person concentrates on a focal point. In transcendental meditation, a widely recognized approach to meditation, people repeat a mantra, or a personal word, while using deep-breathing and relaxation techniques. In other meditation approaches, alternative focal points are used to establish the depth of concentration needed to free the mind from conscious thought. Physical objects, music, and relaxing environmental sounds or breathing can be used as focal points.

Hypnosis is an artificially induced state, resembling, but physiologically distinct from, sleep. It involves a heightened state of suggestibility that creates flexible and intensified attention and receptiveness, and an increased responsiveness to an idea or to a set of ideas. The focus is on the unconscious rather than on the conscious state of mind, using deep-breathing and relaxation techniques. Hypnosis is perhaps the oldest and most misunderstood type of relaxation technique. It has been given a bad reputation by stage entertainers who use hypnosis to have unsuspecting audience members engage in embarrassing behavior.

Hypnosis is a natural state of mind that occurs spontaneously in nearly every person. It is a trancelike state, similar to those that you experience upon awakening, before falling asleep, or when you are engrossed in thought while performing other tasks—such as driving down a highway—on autopilot. It is possible to learn self-hypnosis from a trained professional or participate in hypnosis sessions with a qualified hypnotherapist.

Similar to the other techniques described, meditation and hypnosis work best when you are in a comfortable, quiet environment and practiced them at least once a day, every day, for 15 to 20 minutes.

Biofeedback

Biofeedback is a training technique in which people are taught to improve their health and performance by using signals from their own bodies. It operates on the premise that individuals can alter their involuntary responses by being "fed back" information either visually or audibly about what was occurring in their bodies. In addition, studies have shown that we have more control over so-called involuntary bodily functions than we once thought possible.

One commonly used device, for example, picks up electrical signals from the muscles and translates the signals into a form that people can detect. This device triggers a flashing light or activates a beeper every time muscles become more tense. To slow down the flashing or beeping, you need to relax your tense muscles by breathing more slowly and deeply. People learn to associate sensations from the muscle with actual levels of tension and develop a new, healthy habit of keeping muscles only as tense as is necessary for as long as necessary. After treatment, individuals are then able to repeat this response at will without being attached to the sensors. Other biological functions that are commonly measured and used in a similar way to help people gain control are skin temperature, heart rate, sweat gland activity, and brainwave activity. People can manage stress by decreasing the physiological components of the stress response.

Stress Inoculation

Working in a manner similar to a flu shot, stress inoculation involves exposing an individual to specific stressful situations, a little at a time, under controlled, safe conditions.

Stress inoculation teaches individuals to relax using deep breathing and progressive muscle relaxation while they are being exposed to stressful situations.

The first step is to construct your personal list of stressful situations and arrange the list from the least to the most stressful items, and learn how to evoke each of these situations in your mind while at the same time focusing on your breathing and relaxing your muscles. The second step is to create an arsenal of stress-coping thoughts, such as "I'm going to be all right," "I've succeeded with this before," and "Getting started is the hardest part, then it will get easier for me." The third step is to practice this *in vivo,* meaning in real-life situations, while using the relaxation and cognitive techniques to minimize the stress response.[33] In addition to stress management, stress inoculation has also been helpful in anger management.

Cognitive Self-Talk

What we tell ourselves, our self-talk, has a tremendous effect on how well we manage our stress. Stress can be generated from faulty conclusions, misinterpretations and expecting the worst. Some people claim that if they expect the worst, they won't feel disappointed or hurt, but in reality, they still feel the pain from their disappointment. We need to be careful about what we expect because we may inadvertently make it happen, a phenomenon referred to as **self-fulfilling prophecy.**[34] Self-fulfilling prophecies can work for you or against you. If you expect that work will be boring and uninteresting, you will tend to portray a negative, unmotivated attitude and will probably have a miserable time. However, if you expect to enjoy yourself at work, you are more likely to go looking for challenge and to have fun.

To change your cognitive distortions, you need to generate some rebuttals to your negative self-statements. This entails finding middle ground between all-or-nothing thinking by asking yourself what evidence proves that a statement is true and identifying some exceptions to this statement. Look for balance by asking yourself what is the opposite of this negative self-statement. Rather than telling yourself what you "should" do ask yourself what you "want" to do. Be specific instead of generalizing, and avoid labeling yourself and others. Instead of telling yourself, "I'm lazy," you might say, "I wish I would have studied a few more hours for that test," Stick to the facts without blaming yourself or others. Question yourself as to how

> ### Key Terms
>
> **self-fulfilling prophecy** the tendency to make something more likely to happen as a result of one's own expectations and attitudes

The Antidote for Anger . . . Relaxation

When we are angry, our muscles tense, we breathe shallowly, and our adrenaline level increases, similarly to how we feel when we are stressed. Expressing your anger can reduce stress. Tension tends to build with the stress of increasing frustration, worry, discomfort, or unmet needs. The greater the stress, the more tension you feel. Expressing your anger can help to get rid of this tension, but only temporarily. You may have noticed that right after you get angry, maybe even blow up, you feel more relaxed and calm. Your muscles relax, the tension leaves your body, and you breath more easily—but only briefly. Anger can create more anger because of the reinforcing effect that blowing up has in temporarily helping you to feel better. Blowing up makes it easier to react the same way the next time, and the outbursts are usually stronger and harder to control each time.

As with the stress response, the key to managing anger is to change how we respond to events and express our anger. So, instead of blowing up, should you just keep your anger inside? No; this can eventually result in an explosion similar to that caused by pressure that builds in a pressure cooker or a shaken soda can. This is the "last straw" kind of anger response. To an observer, you may seem to be overreacting to the particular situation when you are really responding to a *multitude* of situations and frustrating events. You may take your anger out on an innocent bystander or the dog. Here are some tips on effective, respectful anger management:

1. Relax, take a deep breath, count to 10.

2. Take a time out if needed. Don't continue to engage in discussion if it is getting too heated.

3. Avoid name calling. Use "I" language, as was discussed in the previous chapter.

4. Stay connected to the individual with whom you are speaking. Don't withdraw physically or psychologically unless you need a time out, and then say this directly.

5. Ask yourself what underlies your anger. Hurt, guilt, feelings of rejection and shame, and fear of abandonment may be feelings that you need to express but that come out as anger. Especially for men, anger tends to be a more comfortable emotion to express.

6. Is there a hidden agenda to your anger? Are you using your anger to control, change, or punish someone? If so, use assertive language instead, and share your thoughts and feelings directly.

7. Speak in a quieter, calmer voice than you typically do. People tend to yell, speaking more loudly than normal in order to get the other person's attention. You may feel that you don't have power or people's attention unless you yell. While anger can be attention grabbing, this kind of attention is probably not what you want. People may tend to yell back, tune you out, or agree with you without meaning it, just to stop the yelling.

8. Choose your battles wisely. Don't argue every point. Ask yourself "Is this something that is really important to me and will be as meaningful tomorrow as it is right now for me?"

9. Express your anger in a timely fashion. Don't wait a week or a month or bring up issues when you have accumulated a bunch of things that have been bothering you over time. However, it may be more productive to wait until morning to express your anger if you are tired and irritable in the evenings. Another option is to wait and arrange a specific time to talk to avoid rushing through a conversation as you get ready to leave for work or class.

10. It might feel easier or safer to redirect the anger you feel toward your boss at your best friend or partner, but that doesn't solve your conflict with your boss, and it might create conflict with your friend or partner.

After you have respectfully expressed your anger, make sure you allow time and opportunity for the other person to express his or her feelings. Tell the person you appreciate how he or she listened to you and responded to you. Share other feelings besides the primary ones of hurt and anger, so that the person knows you can be angry with him or her and still care about him or her. Remember that your way of expressing anger and resolving conflict can either be destructive or be a way of connecting with people and improving relationships.

Sources:
McKay, M., and Rogers, P. *The Anger Control Workbook*. Oakland, CA: New Harbinger Publications, Inc., 2000.
Paleg, K., and McKay, M. *When Anger Hurts Your Relationship*. Oakland, CA: New Harbinger Publications, Inc., 2001.

you know something is true and if you might be making an assumption or "mind reading." Be mindful of your self-fulfilling prophecies. It may be wiser to acknowledge that you don't know or consider many different possible outcomes rather than to expect the worst.

Changing negative self-talk requires time, practice, and patience. We develop these patterns of thinking over years, and they become almost automatic. It takes concentrated effort to be aware of and change negative thinking. Remember that your rebuttals need to be strong, nonjudgmental, and specific. Practice developing more flexible and balanced thinking about people, behavior, and situations.

As you can see, there are many different aspects to consider in managing stress, its physical, social, environmental, and psychological components. As you think about how you can more effectively manage your stress level, you will need to practice and experiment to find the stress-management techniques most beneficial for you.

 TALKING POINTS Think back to stressful times in your life. What were some positive ways you coped, and what were some negative things you did to cope?

Taking Charge of Your Health

- Analyze your past successes in resolving stressful situations, noting the resources that were helpful to you.

- Prioritize your daily goals in a list that you can accomplish, allowing time for recreational activities.

- Counteract a tendency to procrastinate by setting up imaginary (early) deadlines for assignments and rewarding yourself when you meet those dates.

- Add a new physical activity, such as an intramural team sport, to your daily schedule.

- Replace a negative coping technique that you currently use, such as smoking, with an effective alternative, such as deep breathing, relaxation exercises, or yoga.

- List the positive aspects of your life, and make them the focus of your everyday thoughts.

- Explore the stress-reduction services that are available in your community, both on and off campus.

SUMMARY

- Stress refers to physiological changes and responses your body makes in response to a situation, a real or a perceived threat.
- The fight or flight response is a physiological response to perceived, anticipated, or real threat; it causes the heart to race, breathing becomes labored, muscles are tense, the body sweats, and blood flow is decreased to the extremities and digestive organs and increased to the major muscles and brain.
- Chronic stress refers to remaining at a high level of physiological arousal too long and not being able to take immediate, effective action to alleviate the perceived or real threat.
- While too much stress can have a negative effect and cause some serious health problems, a moderate level of stress is positive and beneficial.
- Constant arousal and increased levels of adrenaline in your system will eventually wear down your body's immunological system. You will be less able to cope with stress, and so it takes less and less to cause a stress reaction.
- General Adaptation Syndrome is a sequenced physiological response to the presence of a stressor, involving the alarm, resistance, and exhaustion stages of the stress response.
- Students can experience unique types of stress such as homesickness, relationship problems, test anxiety, speech anxiety, math anxiety, problems with learning, time management, procrastination, and perfectionism.

- When you are more stressed or anxious, you have a diminished ability to concentrate, recall information, and for problem-solving activities.
- An overwhelming number of students identify time management as the reason for their academic success or failure. Setting priorities and goals, balancing academic life with social life and finding time for sleeping, eating, exercising, and working along with studying is an essential aspect of managing stress effectively.
- Procrastination means postponing something that is necessary to do to reach a goal. Typically there is a psychological aspect to procrastination, since we tend to delay doing things we don't want to do.
- While striving to do your best is an admirable quality, expecting to be perfect in everything you do and never making a mistake places a great deal of stress and pressure on yourself.
- To effectively manage your stress, you need to take into consideration environmental stressors such as the noise level, amount of light, and aesthetic quality of the space you inhabit. It is equally important to get adequate rest, nutrition, and exercise.
- Effective psychological tools for managing stress include progressive muscle relaxation, visualization, guided imagery, meditation, hypnosis, biofeedback, stress inoculation, and cognitive self-talk.

REVIEW QUESTIONS

1. What is stress? How is it linked to your physical and psychological health?
2. What is the fight or flight response?
3. What are some of the long-term effects of chronic stress?
4. Describe the Yerkes-Dodson Law.
5. Explain the three stages of the General Adaptation Syndrome.
6. List at least five unique types of stress students can experience.
7. What are some ways to cope with test anxiety? Math anxiety? Speech anxiety?
8. How does stress affect your ability to learn?

9. What do an overwhelming number of students identify as the reason for their academic success or failure?
10. Define procrastination, and explain how it relates to stress.
11. How can being perfectionistic cause stress?
12. List some environmental stressors, and explain how high levels of stress have been linked to environmental factors.
13. Describe the relaxation response and how it is effective for stress management.
14. Name five psychological tools for stress management and explain how they work.
15. What is a self-fulfilling prophecy?

ENDNOTES

1. Selye H. *Stress Without Distress.* New York: New American Library, 1975.
2. Selye H. *The Stress of Life.* New York: The McGraw-Hill Co., 1976.
3. Holmes T, Rahe R. Social Readjustment Rating Scale. *Journal of Psychosomatic Research,* 11, 1967.
4. Girdano DA, Everly GS, Dusek DE. *Controlling Stress and Tension.* Boston: Allyn & Bacon, 1996.
5. Benson H, Allen R. How much stress is too much? *Harvard Business Review,* September/October, 1980.
6. Rowh M. *Coping with Stress in College.* New York: College Board Publications, 1989.
7. Raber M, Dyck G. *Managing Stress for Mental Fitness.* Menlo Park, CA: Crisp Publications, 1993.
8. Vandenbeele J. Affordable care for kids squeezes college students. *The Detroit News,* November 23, 2001.
9. Newman E. *No More Test Anxiety.* Los Angeles, CA: Learning Skills Publications, 1996.
10. Arem C. *Conquering Math Anxiety: A Self-Help Workbook.* Pacific Grove: CA: Brooks/Cole Publishing Co., 1993.
11. Kahn N. *More Learning in Less Time.* Berkeley, CA: Ten Speed Press. 1992.
12. Lindzey G, Thompson R, Spring B. *Psychology* (3rd ed.). New York: Worth Publishers, Inc., 1988.
13. Lakein A. *How to Get Control of Your Time and Your Life.* New York: New American Library, 1973.
14. Roberts M. *Living Without Procrastination.* Oakland, CA: New Harbinger Publications, 1995.
15. Hill MB, Hill DA, Chabot AE, Barrall JF. A survey of college faculty and student procrastination. *College Student Journal* 12, 256–262, 1978.
16. Ferrari J, Johnson J, McGown W. *Procrastination and Task Avoidance; Theory, Research and Treatment.* New York: Plenum, 1995.
17. Basco M. *Never Good Enough.* New York: Simon & Schuster, 1999.
18. Maslow AH. *Motivation and Personality* (2nd ed.). New York: Van Nostrand, 1970.
19. Ferber R. *Solve Your Child's Sleep Problems.* New York: Simon & Schuster, 1985.
20. Saladin KS. *Anatomy and Physiology: The Unity of Form and Function.* New York: McGraw-Hill, 2001.
21. Spear P, Penrod S, Baker T. *Psychology: Perspectives on Behavior.* New York: John Wiley & Sons, 1988.
22. Lefcourt HM, Martin RA. *Humor and Life Stress: Antidote to Adversity.* New York: Springer-Verlag, 1986.
23. Asterita MF. *The Physiology of Stress.* New York: Human Sciences Press, 1985, p. 4–5.
24. Hugging warms the heart and also may protect it. *USA Today,* March 10, 2003.
25. Allen K, Shykoff BE, Izzo JL, Jr. Pet ownership but not ACE inhibitor therapy blunts home blood pressure responses to mental stress. *Hypertension 2001,* October, 38(4), 815–20.
26. Goliszek AG. *Breaking the Stress Habit.* Winston-Salem, NC: Carolina Press, 1987.
27. Rosenthal NE. *Winter Blues.* New York: The Guilford Press, 1998.
28. Seligman M. *Learned Optimism.* New York: Simon & Schuster, 1990.
29. Wade C, Tavris C. *Psychology.* New York: Harper & Row Publishers, 1987.
30. Benson H. *The Relaxation Response.* New York: Avon, 1976.
31. Fanning P. *Visualization for Change.* Oakland, CA: New Harbinger Publications, Inc., 1988.
32. McKay M, Davis M, Fanning P. *Thoughts and Feelings: The Art of Cognitive Stress Intervention.* Oakland, CA: New Harbinger Publications, 1981.
33. Jones RA. *Self-Fulfilling Prophecies.* Hillsdale, NJ: John Wiley & Sons, 1977.

The aftermath of a natural disaster, such as Hurricane Katrina, which hit Louisiana, Alabama, and Mississippi in 2005, can have long-lasting effects. Hurricane Katrina cost over 1,000 people their lives as well as destroying homes, businesses, schools, churches, and personal belongings. The estimated cost from this disaster was over $100 billion, making Katrina the most costly storm in U.S. history. Over 400,000 people became jobless, and 150,000 properties were lost because of Katrina. People often experience feelings of vulnerability, confusion, loss, and helplessness when faced with such widespread devastation.

As we explained in Chapter 2, many people suffer from posttraumatic stress disorder after experiencing this type of natural disaster. Individuals are faced with rebuilding their lives, some starting completely from scratch with little or no resources. It can take years to recover from such trauma; people need positive, effective coping skills to get through an extended recovery period. Sights, sounds, and smells associated with hurricanes, such as rain, wind, and thunder, can create a great deal of distress in hurricane survivors. Seeing images of hurricanes on television or any similar reminders can bring back feelings of fear, powerlessness, and exposure. Merely hearing a loud noise, such as a pan dropping on the kitchen floor, can trigger a strong, negative emotional response. Survivors may also experience nightmares and flashbacks in addition to extreme startle responses to any kind of unexpected sound. People with posttraumatic stress disorder may experience clinical depression and severe anxiety for months and even years after the event.

Losing one's pets and significant places such as home, church, school, and work can leave people feeling lost and without their usual coping strategies. As you read in the stress management chapter, talking to friends and family members is a helpful way to express feelings associated with stress and to gain support. However, some people may be separated from their support group or have lost family and friends to the disaster. With the familiar, comfortable surroundings now gone, it may be extremely hard to connect to places and environments that help people to feel safe and secure. Some people may also experience survivor guilt—guilt associated with having escaped harm or one's home being untouched while others were destroyed.

Initially, many people respond to this type of disaster by feeling numb, as if the event didn't occur or couldn't have really happened. As the reality of what did occur sinks in, individuals may begin to feel a range of emotions—depression, anxiety, anger, and hopelessness. Helpers need to instill hope, the belief that people do survive these types of tragedies and can rebuild their lives again. They should encourage survivors to express their feelings and reassure them that these feelings are normal. This type of encouragement can bring a sense of stability and calmness to people's lives. Helpers should also remember that people have good days and bad days and remind survivors that soon the good days will outnumber the bad ones. Providing opportunities for survivors to share feelings appropriately with others who can understand and relate to how they are feeling is also helpful. Focusing on what one can control rather than what one cannot control is another positive coping strategy. Connecting with community resources and statewide efforts to assist survivors can also help. Knowing that people are there to help and that people don't have to rebuild their lives alone makes a tremendous difference in the recovery process.

Sometimes people are so focused on the logistics of what they need to do to get food, shelter, and clothing that they don't have time or energy to really process what has happened to them until after these basic needs are met. So it may be months later that the emotional toll becomes apparent. Often, assistance is plentiful when a disaster first hits, but later, when the psychological distress is worsening, the rescue efforts and relief efforts have dissipated and people are not getting the aid they need at that time. Having ongoing community support groups and mental health care services available is essential. It is also helpful to reestablish a routine as soon as possible. Returning to work, school, or just having a schedule can help people to feel safe, secure, and normal.

People also respond in individual ways to disaster, with some people being more resilient than others. Those who are experienced in coping with change, crisis, and adversity may recover more quickly than those who are unaccustomed to these problems. Most human beings are geared to survival, and so people eventually will rebuild their lives—one hopes to an equal or improved quality of living. Some people might find a "silver lining" and even find some positive outcomes in the aftermath of such disasters—for example, taking the chance to start over and reconsidering what is important to them in their lives.

personal assessment

How stressed are you?

A widely used life-stress scale called the Social Readjustment Rating Scale by Holmes and Rahe has been used to determine the degree of stress that you are experiencing because of life events over the past year. It also projects your chances of developing an illness- or stress-related health condition. Stress can lead to some serious health problems, and the more stress you have in your life, the more vulnerable you are to being susceptible to illness. Let's see how you score.

Life-Stress Scale

Check off the events that have happened to you **within the last year.** Then add up your total number of stress units for each life-stress event. The number on the right hand side represents the amount, duration and severity of change required to cope with each item. See the point scale at the end of the inventory to determine the health risk associated with your stress level.

Life Event	Value	Score
Death of a partner	100	_____
Divorce	73	_____
Relationship separation	65	_____
Jail term	63	_____
Death of a family member	63	_____
Personal injury/illness	53	_____
Marriage	50	_____
Fired from job	47	_____
Reconciliation with partner	45	_____
Retirement	45	_____
Illness—family member	44	_____
Pregnancy	40	_____
Sexual difficulties	39	_____
Addition of a family member	39	_____
Change in financial situation	38	_____
Death of a close friend	37	_____
Change in job	36	_____
Frequent arguments with partner	35	_____
Mortgage over $10,000	31	_____
Foreclosure of mortgage/loan	30	_____
Change in work responsibilities	29	_____
Child leaving home	29	_____
Trouble with in-laws	29	_____
Outstanding personal achievement	28	_____
Begin or end school	26	_____
Partner begins/stops working	26	_____
Change in living conditions	25	_____
Change in personal habits	24	_____
Trouble with supervisor	23	_____
Change in work hours	20	_____
Change in residence	20	_____
Change in schools	20	_____
Change in recreation	19	_____
Change in church activities	19	_____
Change in social activities	18	_____
Mortgage/loan less than $10,000	17	_____
Change in sleeping habits	16	_____
Change in family visits	15	_____
Change in eating habits	15	_____
Vacation	13	_____
Christmas	12	_____
Minor violations of the law	11	_____
TOTAL SCORE		_____

What Is Your Health Risk?

Note that positive events such as outstanding personal achievements, vacations, and Christmas can be as stressful as negative ones. Think of events in your life that are not listed on this inventory. For example, where would you put running in a marathon or going on a diet?

⇒ If your score was 150 points or less . . .
You are on reasonably safe and healthy ground. You have about a one-in-three chance of a negative health change in the next 2 years.

⇒ If your score was between 150–300 points . . .
You have about a 50/50 chance of developing an illness related to stress in the next 2 years.

⇒ If your score was 300 points or more . . .
You have a 90% chance of developing a stress-related illness that could seriously affect your health. You need to be very watchful in how you manage your stress.

Based on Holmes and Ruhe "Social Readjustment Scale."

Am I a perfectionist?

Below are some ideas that are held by perfectionists. Which of these do you see in yourself? To help you decide, rate how strongly you agree with each of the statements below on a scale from 0 to 4.

0	1	2	3	4
I do not agree		I agree somewhat		I agree completely

_____ 1. I have an eye for details that others can miss.

_____ 2. I can get lost in details and forget the real purpose of the task.

_____ 3. I can get overwhelmed by too many details.

_____ 4. It stresses me when people do not want to do things the right way.

_____ 5. There is a right way and a wrong way to do most things.

_____ 6. I do not like my routine to be interrupted.

_____ 7. I expect a great deal from myself.

_____ 8. I expect no less of others than I expect of myself.

_____ 9. People should always do their best.

_____ 10. I am neat in my appearance.

_____ 11. Good grooming is important to me.

_____ 12. I do not like being seen before I have showered and dressed.

_____ 13. I do not like making mistakes.

_____ 14. Receiving criticism is horrible.

_____ 15. It is embarrassing to make mistakes in front of others.

_____ 16. Sharing my new ideas with others makes me anxious.

_____ 17. I worry that my ideas are not good enough.

_____ 18. I do not have a great deal of confidence in myself.

_____ 19. I'm uncomfortable when my environment is untidy or disorganized.

_____ 20. When things are disorganized it is hard for me to concentrate.

_____ 21. What others think about my home is important to me.

_____ 22. I have trouble making difficult decisions.

_____ 23. I worry that I may make the wrong decision.

_____ 24. Making a bad decision can be disastrous.

_____ 25. I often do not trust others to do the job right.

_____ 26. I check the work of others to make certain it was done correctly.

_____ 27. If I can control the process it will turn out fine.

_____ 28. I am a perfectionist.

_____ 29. I care more about doing a quality job than others do.

_____ 30. It's important to make a good impression.

_____ **TOTAL SCORE**

Scoring

Add all 30 items together to get total score. If your score was less than 30, then you are probably not a perfectionist, although you may have a few of the traits. Scores from 31 to 60 suggest mild perfectionism. When you are stressed your score may be higher. Scores of 61 to 90 suggest moderate perfectionism. This probably means that perfectionism is causing you trouble in some specific areas but is not out of control. Scores higher than 91 suggest a level of perfectionism that could cause you serious problems.

Adapted from: *Never Good Enough* by Monica Ramirez Basco.

chapter four

Becoming Physically Fit

Chapter Objectives

On completing this chapter, you will be able to:

▍ explain why cardiorespiratory fitness is more important to health than are other types of fitness, including muscular strength, muscular endurance, and flexibility.

▍ describe the effects that regular aerobic exercise has on the heart, lungs, and circulatory system.

▍ define aerobic energy production and anaerobic energy production.

▍ list and discuss the health concerns of midlife adults and of elderly adults.

▍ discuss the requirements of a suitable cardiorespiratory fitness program, including the mode of activity, frequency, intensity, duration, and resistance.

▍ explain the role of the warm-up, conditioning, and cooldown in an exercise session.

▍ explain the role exercise should play in pregnancy.

▍ discuss the role of fluid replacement in exercise, including when one should consume fluids and the best types of fluids one should consume.

▍ discuss the contribution of sleep to overall wellness.

▍ explain five principles for the prevention and care of sports injuries.

Eye on the Media

Steroids in the News

Recently, the United States Congress held hearings on the use of steroids by professional baseball players. These hearings were broadcast live on television and made headlines in newspapers and magazines. One of the major concerns raised in the hearings is that these illegal performance-enhancing drugs are becoming more widely used by college and high school students. Unfortunately, some athletes choose to cheat and use drugs to gain an unfair advantage in their physical fitness development. This approach has both ethical issues for sports and health issues for the drug user. Have you ever considered using steroids, or do you have a friend who is using steroids? Read the section on steroids on page 94. People who use steroids have to pay the price of damage to both their personal integrity and to their long-term health. Sometimes the long-term consequences are difficult to see in the glow of short-term glory.

For many people, the day begins early in the morning; continues with classes, assignments, study, a job, and/or recreational activities; and does not end until after midnight. This kind of pace demands that one be physically fit. Even a highly motivated college student must have a conditioned, rested body to maintain such a schedule.

OK, let's simplify things a bit. The paragraph above reflects how college health professors might view the value of fitness—it helps people function well enough to cope with their hectic lifestyles. But what motivates students to value **physical fitness?** Quite simply, students say that overall body fitness helps them look and feel better.

Many college students want to look in the mirror and see the kind of body they see in the media: one with well-toned muscles, a trim waistline, and no flabby tissue, especially on the arms and legs. Students become motivated to start fitness programs because they hope that they can build a better body. Through their efforts to do so, students usually start to feel better, both physically and mentally. They realize that change is possible, since they see it happening to their bodies with each passing week. "Go for it" and "Just do it" then become more than just sports marketing phrases; they become reminders that the activities that lead to fitness are a meaningful part of their lives. Fitness actually becomes fun (Figure 4-1).

Fortunately, you don't have to be a top-notch athlete to enjoy the health benefits of physical activity. In fact, even a modest increase in your daily **physical activity** level can be rewarding. The health benefits of fitness can come from regular participation in moderate **exercise,** such as brisk walking or dancing.[1]

Four Components of Physical Fitness

Physical fitness is characterized by the ability to perform occupational and recreational activities without becoming unduly fatigued and to have the capacity to handle unforeseen emergencies. The following sections focus on cardiorespiratory endurance, muscular strength, muscular endurance, flexibility, and body composition. These characteristics of physical fitness can be categorized as health-related physical fitness. Other characteristics, such as speed, power, agility, balance, and reaction time are associated with what would be called performance-related physical fitness. Although the latter type is most important for competitive athletes, it is the former type that has the most relevance to the general

Key Terms

physical fitness a set of attributes that people have or achieve that relates to the ability to perform physical activity

physical activity any bodily movement produced by skeletal muscles that results in energy expenditure

exercise a subcategory of physical activity; it is planned, structured, repetitive, and purposive in the sense that an improvement or maintenance of physical fitness is an objective

Figure 4-1 Running or working out in a gym is not for everyone. Which physical activities fit your preferences and lifestyle?

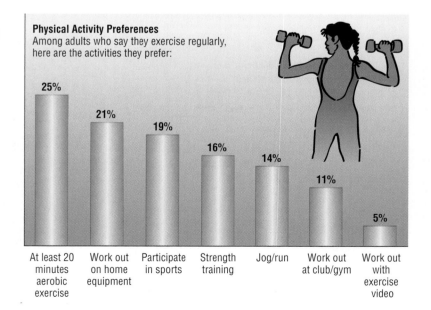

Physical Activity Preferences
Among adults who say they exercise regularly, here are the activities they prefer:

25%	21%	19%	16%	14%	11%	5%
At least 20 minutes aerobic exercise	Work out on home equipment	Participate in sports	Strength training	Jog/run	Work out at club/gym	Work out with exercise video

population. Thus, this chapter focuses on health-related physical fitness.

Cardiorespiratory Endurance

If you were limited to improving only one area of your physical fitness, which would you choose—muscular strength, muscular endurance, or flexibility? Which would a dancer choose? Which would a marathon runner select? Which would an expert recommend?

The experts, exercise physiologists, would probably say that another fitness dimension is even more important than those just listed. They regard improvement of your heart, lung, and blood vessel function as the key focal point of a physical fitness program. **Cardiorespiratory endurance** forms the foundation for whole-body fitness.

Cardiorespiratory endurance increases your capacity to sustain a given level of energy production for a prolonged period. It helps your body to work longer and at greater levels of intensity.

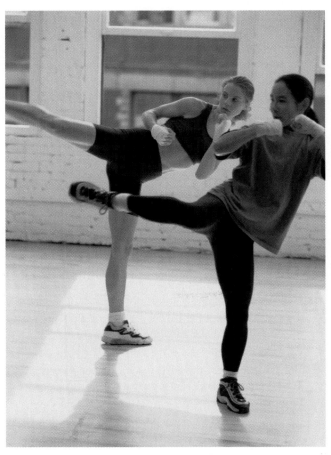

Cardiorespiratory fitness is essential for optimal heart, lung, and blood vessel function.

Your body cannot always produce the energy it needs for long-term activity. Certain activities require performance at a level of intensity that will outstrip your cardiorespiratory system's ability to transport oxygen efficiently to contracting muscle fibers. When the oxygen demands of the muscles cannot be met, **oxygen debt** occurs. Any activity that continues beyond the point at which oxygen debt begins requires a form of energy production that does not depend on oxygen.

This oxygen-deprived form of energy production is called **anaerobic** (without oxygen) **energy production,** the type that fuels many intense, short-duration activities. For example, rope climbing, weight lifting for strength, and sprinting are short-duration activities that quickly cause muscle fatigue; they are generally considered anaerobic activities. The key factor is if the energy demand of the activity exceeds the aerobic energy production capability. Thus, even activities that are typically considered to be aerobic (walking or cycling) can require anaerobic energy if the intensity is high enough.

If you usually work or play at low intensity but for a long duration, you have developed an ability to maintain **aerobic** (with oxygen) **energy production.** As long as your body can meet its energy demands in this oxygen-rich mode, it will not convert to anaerobic energy production. Thus fatigue will not be an important factor in determining whether you can continue to participate. Marathon runners, serious joggers, distance swimmers, cyclists, and aerobic dancers can perform because of their highly developed aerobic fitness. The cardiorespiratory systems of these aerobically fit people have developed a large capacity to take in, transport, and use oxygen.

Key Terms

cardiorespiratory endurance the ability of the heart, lungs, and blood vessels to process and transport oxygen required by muscle cells so that they can contract over a period of time

oxygen debt the physical state that occurs when the body can no longer process and transport sufficient amounts of oxygen for continued muscle contraction

anaerobic energy production the body's means of energy production when the necessary amount of oxygen is not available

aerobic energy production the body's means of energy production when the respiratory and circulatory systems are able to process and transport a sufficient amount of oxygen to muscle cells

Besides allowing you to participate in activities such as those mentioned, aerobic conditioning (cardiorespiratory endurance conditioning) may also provide certain structural and functional benefits that affect other dimensions of your life (see Discovering Your Spirituality below). These recognized benefits (see the Star box on page 82) have received considerable documented support. It is now well accepted that regular physical activity that produces aerobic fitness will reduce the risk of heart disease, type 2 diabetes, osteoporosis, obesity, depression, and cancer of the breast and colon.[3]

Muscular Fitness

Muscular fitness is the term used to represent the capabilities of the skeletal muscles to perform contractions. The capacity of the muscles has two distinct yet integrated characteristics: muscular strength and muscular endurance. The strength of the muscle is related to its ability to perform at or near its maximum for a short period of time. The endurance of the muscle is related to its ability to perform at submaximal levels for a long period of time.

Muscular fitness is essential for your body to accomplish work. Your ability to maintain good posture, walk, lift, push, and pull are familiar examples of the constant demands you make on your muscles to maintain or increase their level of contraction. The stronger you are, the greater your ability to contract muscles and maintain a level of contraction sufficient to complete tasks.

Muscular strength can be improved best by training activities that use the **overload principle.** By overloading, or gradually increasing the resistance (load, object, or weight) your muscles must move, you can increase your muscular strength. The following three types of training exercises are based on the overload principle.

In **isometric** (meaning "same measure") **exercises,** the resistance is so great that the contracting muscles cannot move the resistant object at all. For example, you could contract your muscles against an immovable object such as a wall. Because of the difficulty of precisely evaluating the training effects, isometric exercises are not usually used as a primary means of developing muscular strength. These exercises can be dangerous for people with hypertension.

Isotonic resistance exercises, meaning *same-tension exercises,* are currently the most popular type of strength-building exercises and include the use of traditional free

Key Terms

muscular fitness the ability of skeletal muscles to perform contractions; includes muscular strength and muscular endurance

muscular strength the component of physical fitness that deals with the ability to contract skeletal muscles to a maximal level; the maximal force that a muscle can exert

overload principle the principle whereby a person gradually increases the resistance load that must be moved or lifted; this principle also applies to other types of fitness training

isometric exercises muscular strength-training exercises in which the resistance is so great that the object cannot be moved

isotonic resistance exercises muscular strength-training exercises in which traditional barbells and dumbbells with fixed resistances are used

Structural and Functional Benefits of Cardiorespiratory (Aerobic) Fitness

Aerobic fitness can help you do the following:

- Complete and enjoy your daily activities.
- Strengthen and increase the efficiency of your heart muscle.
- Increase the proportion of high-density lipoproteins (good cholesterol) in your blood.
- Increase the capillary network in your body.

- Improve collateral circulation, the ability of nearby blood vessels to enlarge and carry blood around a blocked blood vessel.
- Control your weight.
- Stimulate bone growth.
- Cope with stressors.
- Ward off infections.
- Improve the efficiency of your other body systems.

- Bolster your self-esteem.
- Achieve self-directed fitness goals.
- Reduce negative dependence behavior.
- Sleep better.
- Recover more quickly from common illnesses.
- Meet people with similar interests.
- Obtain reduced insurance premiums.

weights (dumbbells and barbells), as well as many resistance exercise machines. People who perform progressive resistance exercises use various muscle groups to move (or lift) specific fixed resistances or weights. Although during a given repetitive exercise the weight resistance remains the same, the muscular contraction effort required varies according to the joint angles in the range of motion. The greatest effort is required at one angle (sticking point) in the range of motion.

Isokinetic (meaning "same motion") **exercises** use mechanical devices that provide resistances that consistently overload muscles throughout the entire range of motion. The resistance moves only at a preset speed, regardless of the force applied to it. For the exercise to be effective, a user must apply maximal force.[4] Isokinetic training requires elaborate, expensive equipment, so the use of isokinetic equipment may be limited to certain athletic teams, diagnostic centers, or rehabilitation clinics. The most common isokinetic machines are Cybex, Orthotron, Biodex, Mini-Gym, and ExerGenie.

Which type of strength-building exercise (machines or free weights) is most effective? Take your choice, since all will help develop muscular strength. Some people prefer machines because they are simple to use, do not require stacking the weights, and are already balanced and less likely to drop and cause injury. Other people prefer free weights because they encourage the user to work harder to maintain balance during the lift. In addition, free weights can be used in a greater variety of exercises than weight machines.

Muscular endurance can be improved by performing repeated contractions of a less than maximal level. This aspect of muscular fitness is most related to common physical activities (leaf raking, pushing a lawn mower). Although it is not as glamorous as muscular strength, muscular endurance is an important part of muscular fitness.

Amateur and professional athletes often wish to increase the endurance of specific muscle groups associated with their sports activities. This can be achieved by using exercises that gradually increase the number of repetitions of a given movement. However, muscular endurance is not the physiological equivalent of cardiorespiratory endurance. For example, a world-ranked distance runner with highly developed cardiorespiratory endurance and extensive muscular endurance of the legs may not have a corresponding level of muscular endurance of the abdominal muscles.

Flexibility

The ability of your joints to move through their natural range of motion is a measure of your **flexibility.** This fitness trait, like so many other aspects of structure and function, differs from point to point within your body and among different people. Not every joint in your body is equally flexible (by design), and, over the course of time, use or disuse will alter the flexibility of a given joint. Certainly, gender, age, genetically determined body build, and current level of physical fitness affect your flexibility.

agility - quick & easy movement

Key Terms

isokinetic exercises muscular strength-training exercises in which machines are used to provide variable resistances throughout the full range of motion

muscular endurance the aspect of muscular fitness that deals with the ability of a muscle or muscle group to repeatedly contract over a long period of time

flexibility the ability of joints to function through an intended range of motion

---

Inability to move easily during physical activity can be a constant reminder that aging and inactivity are the foes of flexibility. Failure to use joints regularly will quickly result in a loss of elasticity in the connective tissue and shortening of muscles associated with the joints. Benefits of flexibility include improved balance, posture, and athletic performance and reduced risk of low-back pain.

As seen in young gymnasts, flexibility can be highly developed and maintained with a program of activity that includes regular stretching. Stretching also helps reduce the risk of injury. Athletic trainers generally prefer **static stretching** to **ballistic stretching** for people who wish to improve their range of motion.

Body Composition

Body composition refers to what the body is made up of (muscle, bone, fat, water, minerals).[4] Of particular interest to fitness experts are percentages of body fat and fat-free weight. Health experts are especially concerned about the large number of people in our society who are overweight and obese. Increasingly, cardiorespiratory fitness trainers are recognizing the importance of body composition and are including strength-training exercises to help reduce body fat. (See Chapter 6 for further information about body composition, health effects of obesity, and weight management.)

Aging Physically

The period between 45 and 64 years of age brings with it a variety of subtle changes in the body's structure and function. When life is busy and the mind is active, these changes are generally not evident. Even when they become evident, they are not usually the source of profound concern. Your parents, older students in your class, and people with whom you will be working are, nevertheless, experiencing these changes.

- Decrease in bone mass and density
- Increase in vertebral compression
- Degenerative changes in joint cartilage
- Increase in adipose tissue—loss of lean body mass
- Decrease in capacity to engage in physical work
- Decrease in visual acuity
- Decrease in resting energy requirements
- Decrease in fertility
- Decrease in sexual function

For some midlife adults these health concerns can be quite threatening, especially for those who view aging with apprehension and fear. Some middle-aged people reject these physical changes and convince themselves they are sick. Indeed, hypochondriasis is much more common among midlife people than among young people.

Two medical conditions influenced by physical activity, osteoporosis and osteoarthritis, deserve careful examination and are discussed in the following sections.

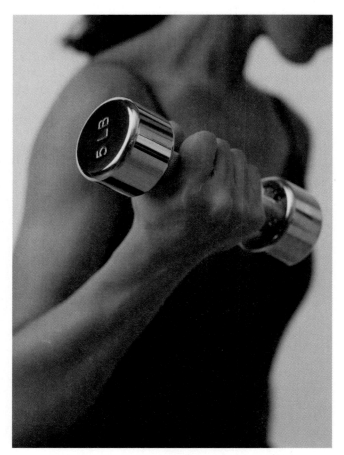

Muscular fitness is important for both good health and optimal function.

Key Terms
static stretching the slow lengthening of a muscle group to an extended stretch; followed by holding the extended position for 10 to 30 seconds
ballistic stretching a "bouncing" form of stretching in which a muscle group is lengthened repetitively to produce multiple quick, forceful stretches

Osteoporosis

Osteoporosis is a condition often seen in older middle-aged women. However, it is not fully understood why menopausal women are so susceptible to the increase in calcium loss that leads to fractures of the hip, wrist, and vertebral column. Each year over 1,500,000 fractures occur that are attributable to osteoporosis.[12]

The endocrine system plays a large role in the development of osteoporosis. At the time of menopause, a woman's ovaries begin a rapid decrease in the production of estrogen, one of two main hormones associated with the menstrual cycle. This lower level of estrogen may decrease the conversion of the precursors of vitamin D into the active form of vitamin D, the form necessary for absorbing calcium from the digestive tract. As a result, calcium may be drawn from the bones for use elsewhere in the body.

Premenopausal women have the opportunity to build and maintain a healthy skeleton through an appropriate intake of calcium. Current recommendations are for an intake of 1,200 mg of calcium per day. Three to four daily servings of low-fat dairy products should provide sufficient calcium. Adequate vitamin D must also be in the diet because it aids in the absorption of calcium.

Many women do not take in an adequate amount of calcium. Calcium supplements, again in combination with vitamin D, can be used to achieve recommended calcium levels. It is now known that calcium carbonate, a much-advertised form of calcium, is no more easily absorbed by the body than are other forms of calcium salts.

In premenopausal women, calcium deposition in bone is facilitated by exercise, particularly exercise that involves movement of the extremities. Today, women are encouraged to consume at least the recommended servings from the milk group and engage in regular physical activity that involves the weight-bearing muscles of the legs, such as aerobics, jogging, and walking.

Postmenstrual women who are not elderly can markedly slow the resorption of calcium from their bones through the use of hormone replacement therapy (HRT). When combined with a daily intake of 1,500 mg of calcium, vitamin D, and regular exercise, HRT almost eliminates calcium loss. Women need to work closely with their physicians in monitoring the use of HRT because of continuing concern over the role of HRT and the development of breast cancer and the increased risk of coronary artery disease and stroke.

Osteoarthritis

Arthritis is an umbrella term for more than 100 forms of joint inflammation. The most common form is **osteoarthritis.** It is likely that as we age, all of us will develop osteoarthritis to some degree. Often called "wear and tear" arthritis, osteoarthritis occurs primarily in the weight-bearing joints of the knee, hip, and spine. In this form of arthritis, joint damage can occur to bone ends, cartilaginous cushions, and related structures as the years of constant friction and stress accumulate.

The object of current management of osteoarthritis (and other forms) is not to cure the disease but rather to reduce discomfort, limit joint destruction, and maximize joint mobility. Aspirin and nonsteroidal anti-inflammatory agents are the drugs most frequently used to treat osteoarthritis.

It is now believed that osteoarthritis develops most commonly in people with a genetic predisposition for excessive damage to the weight-bearing joints. Thus the condition seems to "run in families." Further, studies comparing the occurrence of osteoarthritis in those who exercise and those who do not demonstrate that regular movement activity may decrease the likelihood of developing this form of arthritis.

Developing a Cardiorespiratory Endurance Program

For people of all ages, cardiorespiratory conditioning can be achieved through many activities. As long as the activity you choose places sufficient demand on the heart and lungs, improved fitness is possible. In addition to engaging in the familiar activities of swimming, running, cycling, and aerobic dance, many people today participate in brisk walking, rollerblading, cross-country skiing, swimnastics, skating, rowing, and even weight training (often combined with some form of aerobic activity). (See Learning from Our Diversity, page 86.) Regardless of age or physical limitations, you can select from a variety of enjoyable activities that will condition the cardiorespiratory system. (Complete the Personal Assessment on pages 99–100 to determine your level of fitness.)

Many people think that any kind of physical activity will produce cardiorespiratory fitness. Golf, bowling, hunting, fishing, and archery are considered to be forms

---

> **Key Terms**
>
> **osteoporosis** decrease in bone mass that leads to increased incidence of fracture, primarily in postmenopausal women
>
> **osteoarthritis** arthritis that develops with age; largely caused by weight bearing and deterioration of the joints

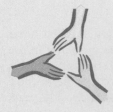

Learning from Our Diversity

A Different Kind of Fitness: Developmentally Disabled Athletes Are Always Winners in the Special Olympics

In America, as in many other countries around the world, physical fitness and athletic prowess carry a high degree of prestige, whereas lack of conditioning and poor sports performance often draw scorn and rejection. As anyone knows who's ever been picked last when sides were being chosen for a schoolyard game, few things are more damaging to youthful self-esteem than being the player nobody wants.

Some of these children blossom into accomplished athletes as they gain coordination or are inspired and guided by caring coaches. Others, lacking strong interest in sports, turn to less physical arenas in which they can excel—drama, debating, music, computers, science.

But what about people who want to be athletes at almost any cost, but who have no realistic hope of attaining the standards of athletic accomplishment set for those in top physical condition? The Joseph P. Kennedy Foundation created an arena in which these athletes could compete when it established the Special Olympics in 1968. Joseph Kennedy was the father of President John F. Kennedy, whose older sister Rosemary was virtually shut away from the world when her family discovered she was mentally disabled. Many people at that time shared the Kennedys' view that the kindest way to treat family members who were developmentally disabled was to "protect" them from stares and whispers by keeping them at home or placing them in institutions or residential facilities. Spearheaded by President Kennedy's sister Eunice Kennedy Shriver, the Special Olympics was intended to change the old attitudes toward developmentally disabled people by giving them an opportunity to compete at their own level and to celebrate their victories publicly.

Now, nearly 30 years later, the Special Olympics holds both winter and summer games and boasts participation of more than 1 million developmentally disabled athletes in 140 countries around the world. The contests are open to athletes between the ages of 8 and 63, some of whom have proved wrong the specialists who claimed they would never walk, let alone compete internationally. "Mainstream" Olympic champions such as figure-skating silver medalist Brian Orser and a host of well-known entertainers have attended opening-day ceremonies to cheer and inspire the special athletes.

But medals aren't what the Special Olympics is all about. No matter where a Special Olympian finishes in a contest, he or she is applauded and celebrated for the accomplishment of playing the game and seeing it through. The oath taken by each participant in the Special Olympics aptly states the credo of this remarkable group of athletes: "Let me win. But if I cannot win, let me be brave in the attempt."

In what ways other than physical conditioning do you think a developmentally disabled person might benefit from participating in the Special Olympics? What can the rest of us learn from these athletes' courage and perseverance?

---

of exercise. If performed regularly and for sufficient periods of time, they may enhance your health. However, they do not meet the requirements to be called exercise and would not necessarily lead to improved physical fitness. The American College of Sports Medicine (ACSM), the nation's premier professional organization of exercise physiologists and sport physicians has well-accepted guidelines for exercise training.[1,6] ~Components~

The ACSM's most recent recommendations for cardiorespiratory conditioning were published in 1999 and 2005. They include four major areas: (1) mode of activity, (2) frequency of training, (3) intensity of training, and (4) duration of training. ACSM has also made recommendations for (5) muscular fitness and (6) flexibility training. These recommendations are summarized in the following sections. You may wish to compare your existing fitness program with these standards.

Mode of Activity ~type~ ~part of cardiorespiratory Fitness~

The ACSM recommends that the mode of activity be any continuous physical activity that uses large muscle groups ~program~

and can be rhythmic and aerobic in nature. Among the activities that generally meet this requirement are continuous swimming, cycling, aerobics, basketball, cross-country skiing, rollerblading, step training (bench aerobics), hiking, walking, rowing, stair climbing, dancing, and running. Recently, water exercise (water or aqua aerobics) has become a popular fitness mode, since it is especially effective for pregnant women and elderly, injured, or disabled people.

Endurance games and activities, such as tennis, racquetball, and basketball, are fine as long as you and your partner are skilled enough to keep the ball in play; walking after the ball will do very little for you. Riding a bicycle is a good activity if you keep pedaling. Coasting will do little to improve fitness. Softball and football are generally less than sufficient continuous activities—especially the way they are played by weekend athletes.

Regardless of which continuous activity you select, it should also be enjoyable. Running, for example, is not for everyone—despite what some accomplished runners say! Find an activity you enjoy. If you need others around you to have a good time, get a group of friends to join you. Vary your activities to keep from becoming bored. You might cycle in the summer, run in the fall, swim in the winter, and play racquetball in the spring. To help you maintain your fitness program, see the suggestions in the accompanying Changing for the Better box above.

Frequency of Training

Frequency of training refers to the number of times per week a person should exercise. The ACSM recommends three to five times per week. For most people, participation in fitness activities more than five times each week does not significantly further improve their level of conditioning. Likewise, an average of only two workouts each week does not seem to produce a measurable improvement in cardiorespiratory conditioning. Thus, although you may have a lot of fun cycling twice each week, do not expect to see a significant improvement in your cardiorespiratory fitness level from doing so.

Intensity of Training

How much effort should you put into an activity? Should you run quickly, jog slowly, or swim at a comfortable pace? Must a person sweat profusely to become fit? These questions all refer to **intensity** of effort.

The ACSM recommends that healthy adults exercise at an intensity level of between 65 percent and 90 percent of their maximum heart rate (estimated by subtracting one's age from 220). This level of intensity is called the **target heart rate (THR)** or 50–85 percent of

your heart rate reserve. This rate refers to the minimum number of times your heart needs to contract (beat) each minute to have a positive effect on your heart, lungs, and blood vessels. This improvement is called the *training effect:* Intensity of activity below the THR will be insufficient to make a significant improvement in your fitness level.

Although intensity below the THR will still help you expend calories and thus lose weight, it will probably do little to make you more aerobically fit. However, intensity that is significantly above your THR will probably cause you to become so fatigued that you will be forced to stop the activity before the training effect can be achieved. For persons who are quite unfit, the 1998 ACSM recommendations permit intensity levels as low as 55 percent.

Choosing a particular THR between 65 percent and 90 percent of your maximum heart rate depends on your initial level of cardiorespiratory fitness. If you are already in relatively good physical shape, you might want to start exercising at 75 percent of your maximum heart rate. A well-conditioned person needs to select a higher THR for his or her intensity level, whereas a person with a low cardiorespiratory fitness level will still be able to achieve a training effect at a lower THR. (See Table 4.1 for examples of calculating target heart rate.)

Determining your heart rate is not a complicated procedure. Find a location on your body where an artery passes near the surface of the skin. Pulse rates are difficult to determine by touching veins, which are more superficial than arteries. Two easily accessible sites for determining heart rate are the carotid artery (one on either side of the windpipe at the front of your neck) and the radial artery (on the inside of your wrist, just above the base of the thumb).

Practice placing the front surface of your index and middle fingertips at one of these locations and feeling for a pulse. Once you have found a regular pulse, look at the second hand of a watch. Count the number of beats you feel in a 10-second period. Multiply this number by 6. This number is your heart rate. With a little practice, you can become proficient at determining your heart rate.

Key Terms

frequency the number of exercise sessions per week; for aerobic fitness 3 to 5 days are recommended

intensity the level of effort put into an activity

target heart rate (THR) the number of times per minute the heart must contract to produce a training effect

Table 4.1 Calculation of Target Heart Rate for Exercise Training

	Percentage of maximal heart rate	Heart Rate Reserve
Method:		
Information needed:	Age and desired training intensity (%)	Age, resting heart rate (HR), and desired training intensity (%)

Age-Predicted Maximal Heart Rate = 220 − age

	Percentage of maximal heart rate	Heart Rate Reserve
Example:	22-year-old, training @ 75%	45-year-old, resting HR 75 beats per minute (bpm), training at 70%
Calculation:	$(220 − 22) × .75 = 148$ bpm	$([(220 − 45) − 75] × .70) − 75 = 145$ bpm

Cardiorespiratory program

Duration of Training

The ACSM recommends that the **duration** of training be between 20 and 60 minutes of continuous or intermittent aerobic activity. Intermittent activity can be accumulated in 10-minute segments throughout the day. This is especially helpful for persons who cannot take a single large chunk of time during the day to devote to an exercise program.

However, for most healthy adults the ACSM recommends moderate-intensity activity levels with longer duration times, perhaps 30 minutes to an hour. For healthy adults who train at higher intensity levels, the duration of training will likely be shorter, perhaps 20 minutes or more.[1, 6] Adults who are unfit or have an existing medical condition should check with their fitness instructor or physician to determine an appropriate duration of training.

Resistance Training

Recognizing that overall body fitness includes muscular fitness, the ACSM recommends resistance training in its current standards. The ACSM suggests participation in resistance training two or three times a week. This training should help develop and maintain a healthy body composition—one with an emphasis on lean body mass. The goal of resistance training is not to improve cardiorespiratory endurance but to improve overall muscle strength and endurance. For some people (individuals with type 2 diabetes) resistance training with heavy weights is not recommended because it can induce a sudden and dangerous increase in blood pressure. (See the Changing for the Better box for safety precautions to observe during strength training.)

The resistance training recommended by the ACSM includes one set of 8 to 12 repetitions (10 to 15 for adults over age 50) of 8 to 10 different exercises. These exercises should be geared to the body's major muscle groups (legs, arms, shoulders, trunk, and back) and should not focus on just one or two body areas. Isotonic (progressive resistance) or isokinetic exercises are recommended. For the average person, resistance training activities should be done at a moderate-to-slow speed, use the full range of

Changing for the Better

Considering Strength Training? Think Safety . . .

I'm a 22-year-old college student thinking about starting a strength-training program. What kinds of safety precautions should I take?

- Warm up appropriately.
- Use proper lifting techniques.
- Always have a spotter if you are using free weights.
- Do not hold your breath during a lift.
- Avoid single lifts of very heavy weights.
- Before using a machine (such as Nautilus, Paramount, or Cybex), be certain you know how to use it correctly.
- Seek advice for training programs from experts (individuals with academic training and fitness training certification).
- Understand your current strength level; avoid exercises that are beyond your capacity.

motion, and not impair normal breathing. With just one set recommended for each exercise, resistance training is not very time-consuming. The ACSM, however, indicates that multiple sets could provide greater benefits, if time is available.

Flexibility Training

To develop and maintain a healthy range of motion for the body's joints, the ACSM suggests that flexibility exercises be included in one's overall fitness program. Stretching can be done in conjunction with other cardiorespiratory or muscular fitness training or can be performed separately. Note that if flexibility training is

Key Terms

duration the length of time one needs to exercise at the THR to produce a cardiorespiratory training effect

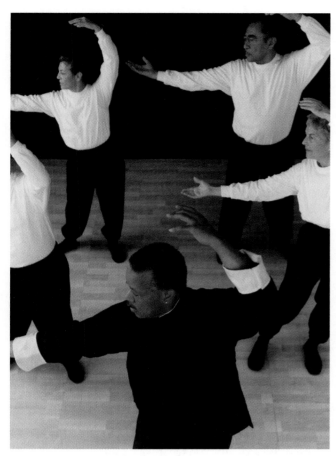

Group exercise classes can be fun and help people with their physical fitness program.

period, you should begin slow, gradual, comfortable movements related to the upcoming activity, such as walking or slow jogging. All body segments and muscle groups should be exercised as you gradually increase your heart rate. Near the end of the warm-up period, the major muscle groups should be stretched. This preparation helps protect you from muscle strains and joint sprains.

The warm-up is a fine time to socialize. Furthermore, you can mentally prepare yourself for your activity or think about the beauty of the morning sky, the changing colors of the leaves, or the friends you will meet later in the day. Mental warm-ups can be as beneficial for you psychologically as physical warm-ups are physiologically.

The second part of the training session is the conditioning phase, the part of the session that involves improving muscular fitness, cardiorespiratory endurance, and flexibility. Workouts can be tailor-made, but they should follow the ACSM guidelines discussed earlier in this chapter.

The third important part of each fitness session, the cooldown, consists of a 5- to 10-minute session of relaxing exercises, such as slow jogging, walking, and stretching. This activity allows your body to cool and return to a resting state. A cooldown period helps reduce muscle soreness.

Exercise for Older Adults

An exercise program designed for younger adults may be inappropriate for older people, particularly those over age 50. Special attention must be paid to matching the program to the interests and abilities of the participants. Often, this is best achieved by having older individuals begin their exercise program under the supervision of a certified exercise professional. The goals of the program should include both social interaction and physical conditioning.

Older adults, especially those with a personal or family history of heart problems, should have a physical examination before starting a fitness program. This examination should include a stress cardiogram, a blood pressure check, and an evaluation of joint functioning. Participants should learn how to monitor their own cardiorespiratory status during exercise.

Well-designed fitness programs for older adults will include activities that begin slowly, are monitored frequently, and are geared to the enjoyment of the participants.[5] The professional staff coordinating the program should be familiar with the signs of distress (excessively elevated heart rate, nausea, breathing difficulty, pallor, and pain) and must be able to perform CPR. Warm-up and cooldown periods should be included. Activities to increase flexibility are beneficial in the beginning and ending segments of the program. Participants should wear comfortable clothing and appropriate shoes and should be mentally prepared to enjoy the activities.

done separately, a general warm-up (walking or stationary cycling) should be performed before stretching. For most individuals, static stretching is the best type. Flexibility improvements can be obtained by training as little as two days per week; however, stretching is an activity that can be safely performed daily. ACSM recommends that a flexibility program should include all the major muscle and/or tendon groups. The intensity of each stretch should be at a position where you feel mild discomfort in the muscle. (It should not be painful; pain is an indication that something is wrong and should not be ignored.) Each stretch should be held for 10 to 30 seconds and should be repeated three to four times per training session. Remember to breathe normally (do *not* hold your breath when stretching).

Warm-Up, Conditioning, Cooldown

Each training session consists of three basic parts: the warm-up, the conditioning, and the cooldown.[4] The warm-up should last 10 to 15 minutes. During this

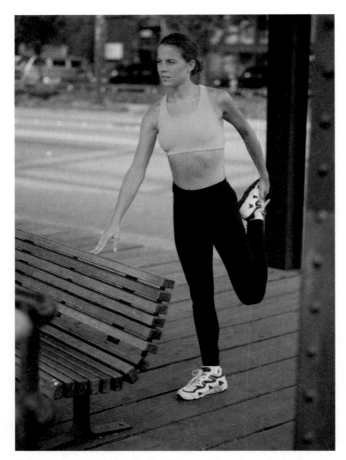

Stretching is important for flexibility and can be performed almost anywhere.

A program designed for older adults will largely conform to the ACSM criteria specified in this chapter. Certainly, specific modifications or restrictions to the exercise program may be required due to health concerns that are more frequent in older adults. Also, because of possible joint, muscular, or skeletal problems, certain activities may have to be done in a sitting position. Pain or discomfort should be reported immediately to the fitness instructor.

Fortunately, properly screened older adults will rarely have health emergencies during a well-monitored fitness program. Of course, for some older adults, individual fitness activities may be more enjoyable than supervised group activities. Either choice offers important benefits.

Low-Back Pain

A common occurrence among adults is the sudden onset of low-back pain. Four out of five adults develop this condition, at least once in their lifetime, which can be so uncomfortable that they miss work, lose sleep, and generally feel incapable of engaging in daily activities. Many of the adults who have this condition will experience these effects two to three times per year.

Although low-back pain can reflect serious health problems, most low-back pain is caused by mechanical (postural) problems. As unpleasant as low-back pain is, the symptoms and functional limitations usually subside within a week or two. The services of a physician, physical therapist, or chiropractor are not generally required.

By engaging in regular exercise, such as swimming, walking, and bicycling, and by paying attention to your back during bending, lifting, and sitting, you can minimize the occurrence of this uncomfortable and incapacitating condition. Commercial fitness centers and campus recreational programs are starting to offer specific exercise classes geared to muscular improvement in the lower back and abdominal areas.

Fitness Questions and Answers

Along with the six areas to consider in your fitness program, you should think about many additional issues when you start a fitness program.

Should I See My Doctor Before I Get Started?

This issue has probably kept thousands of people from ever beginning a fitness program. The hassle and expense of getting a comprehensive physical examination is an excellent excuse for people who are not completely sold on the idea of exercise. It is highly desirable to have regular checkups as part of your overall health plan. However, the Surgeon General has suggested that most adults can safely increase their activity level to a moderate amount without the need for a comprehensive medical evaluation. Individuals with chronic diseases should consult with their physician before increasing their activity level. If more vigorous forms of exercise are desired, then a medical exam is recommended for men over the age of 40 and women over the age of 50. It is also recommended for individuals with more than one risk factor for coronary artery disease or with any other notable health problems. The American College of Sports Medicine also recommends an exercise ("stress") test for these individuals.[6]

 TALKING POINTS If your screening tests indicate that you cannot start a vigorous fitness program, are you prepared to ask your doctor about alternative activities?

Aerobic – high intensity

How Beneficial Is Aerobic Dance Exercise?

One of the most popular fitness approaches is aerobic exercise, including aerobic dancing. Many organizations sponsor classes in this form of continuous dancing and movement. The rise in popularity of aerobic exercise video programs reflects the enthusiasm for this form of exercise. Because extravagant claims are often made about the value of these programs, the wise consumer should observe at least one session of the activity before enrolling. Discover for yourself whether the program meets the criteria outlined earlier in this chapter: mode of activity, frequency, intensity, duration, resistance training, and flexibility training.

Street dancing, swing dancing, and Latin dancing have become some of the most popular aerobic exercises. Popularized by rap music, hip-hop music, and the growth of vigorous dancing in music videos, these forms of dancing provide an excellent way of having fun and maintaining cardiorespiratory fitness. Have you experienced the exhilaration that results from an hour or two of dancing?

What Are Low-Impact Aerobic Activities?

Because long-term participation in some aerobic activities (for example, jogging, running, aerobic dancing, and rope skipping) may lead to injury of the hip, knee, and ankle joints, many fitness experts promote low-impact aerobic activities. Low-impact aerobic dancing, water aerobics, bench aerobics, and brisk walking are examples of this kind of fitness activity. Participants still conform to the principal components of a cardiorespiratory fitness program. THR levels are the same as in high-impact aerobic activities.

The main difference between low-impact and high-impact aerobic activities is the use of the legs. Low-impact aerobics do not require having both feet off the ground at the same time. Thus weight transfer does not occur with the forcefulness seen in traditional high-impact aerobic activities. In addition, low-impact activities may include exaggerated arm movements and the use of hand or wrist weights. All of these variations are designed to increase the heart rate to the THR without undo strain on the joints of the lower extremities. Low-impact aerobics are excellent for people of all ages, and they may be especially beneficial to older adults.

What Is the Most Effective Means of Fluid Replacement During Exercise?

Despite all the advertising hype associated with commercial fluid-replacement products, for an average person involved in typical fitness activities, water is still the best fluid replacement. The availability and cost are unbeatable. However, when activity is prolonged and intense, commercial sports drinks may be preferable to water because they contain electrolytes (which replace lost sodium and potassium) and carbohydrates (which replace depleted energy stores). However, the carbohydrates in sports drinks are actually simple forms of sugar. Thus sports drinks tend to be high in calories, just like regular soft drinks. Regardless of the drink you choose, exercise physiologists recommend that you drink fluids before and at frequent intervals throughout the activity particularly in warm, humid environments.

What Effect Does Alcohol Have on Sport Performance?

It probably comes as no surprise that alcohol use is generally detrimental to sport performance. Alcohol consumption, especially excessive intake the evening before a performance, consistently decreases the level of performance. Many research studies have documented the negative effects of alcohol on activities involving speed, strength, power, and endurance.[7] Lowered performance appears to be related to a variety of factors, including impaired judgment, reduced coordination, depressed heart function, liver interference, and dehydration.

What Level of Physical Activity Is Necessary to Produce Fitness?

According to the surgeon general's report on physical activity and health,[8] moderate amounts of physical activity can produce significant health benefits, including lowering the risk of premature death, coronary heart disease, hypertension, colon cancer, and diabetes. Even a variety of simple activities, such as gardening, walking, raking leaves, and dancing, that consistently increase a person's daily activity levels can be as helpful for the majority of Americans as are activities such as jogging, swimming, and cycling.

What Are the Risks and Benefits of Androstenedione?

Androstenedione ("andro") and creatine have recently received much attention for their use as possible **ergogenic aids.** Ergogenic aids are supplements taken to improve athletic performance.[9] Andro is a steroidlike precursor to the male hormone testosterone. When taken into the body, andro stimulates the body to produce more of its natural testosterone. Increased levels of testosterone help a person build lean muscle mass and recover from injury more quickly.

Andro's primary use as an ergogenic aid is to build muscle tissue, improve overall body strength, and boost performance, especially in anaerobic sports. Andro is banned by the National Football League (NFL), the National Collegiate Athletic Association (NCAA), and the IOC. The health

> ### Key Terms
>
> **ergogenic aids** supplements that are taken to improve athletic performance

Choosing an Athletic Shoe

Proper-fitting sports shoes can enhance performance and prevent injuries. The American Academy of Orthopaedic Surgeons[1] provide the following advice for consumers of athletic or exercise shoes.

- Try on athletic shoes after a workout or run and at the end of the day. Your feet will be at their largest.

- Wear the same type of sock that you will wear for that sport.

- When the shoe is on your foot, you should be able to freely wiggle all your toes.

- The shoes should be comfortable as soon as you try them on. There is no break-in period.

- Walk or run a few steps in your shoes. They should be comfortable.

- Always re-lace the shoes you are trying on. You should begin at the farthest eyelets and apply even pressure as you crisscross a lacing pattern to the top of the shoe.

- There should be a firm grip of the shoe to your heel. Your heel should not slip as you walk or run.

- If you participate in a sport three or more times a week, you need a sports-specific shoe.

It can be hard to choose from the many different types of athletic shoes available. There are differences in design and variations in material and weight. These differences have been developed to protect the areas of the feet that encounter the most stress in a particular athletic activity. Specific recommendations for choosing selected types of shoes are presented below.

Aerobic Shoes

Flexibility: more at ball of foot than running shoes; less flexible than court shoes or running shoes; sole is firmer than running shoes. Uppers: most are leather or leather-reinforced nylon. Heel: little or no flare. Soles: rubber if you dance on wood floors; polyurethane for other surfaces. Cushioning: more than court shoes; less than running shoes. Tread: should be fairly flat, especially on forefoot; may also have "dot" on the ball of the foot for pivoting.

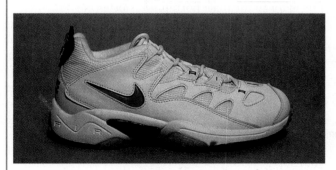

Court Shoes (Basketball, Tennis, Volleyball)

Soles: can be made from rubber for durability, EVA for lightweight cushioning, or polyurethane, which is both lightweight and durable. Flexibility: should be most flexible in the forefoot, for making jump shots. Cushioning: should absorb shock in the ball of the foot, for land-

ing from jump shots. Heel: a snug-fitting heel cup is essential to keep the ankle in place; the shoe can be high-, mid-, or low-cut, depending on the amount of ankle support desired. Tread: for playing outdoors, the sole should be harder and the tread deeper; a smoother tread works well for playing on a court. Uppers: can be made of leather for durability or nylon or other synthetics for breathability.

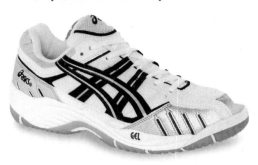

Running Shoes

Heel: flare gives foot broader, more stable base. Soles: usually carbon-based for longer wear. Cushioning: more than court shoes, especially at heel. Tread: "waffle" or other deep-cut tread for grip on many surfaces.

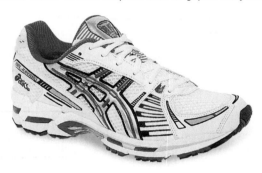

Walking Shoes

Cushioning: can be forefoot and heel, or primarily forefoot or heel. Heel: may have some flare, similar to running shoes. Soles: typically polyurethane for durability. Tread: some tread for traction, but slightly flatter than running shoes.

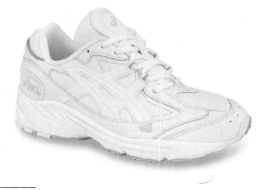

---

[1]http://orthoinfo.aaos.org/fact/thr_report.cfm?Thread_ID=32&topcategory=Foot

continued

Cross-Training Shoes
Cushioning: can be forefoot and heel, or primarily forefoot or heel.
Tread: can be moderate to aggressive.

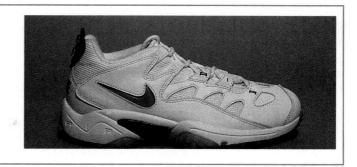

concerns that most physicians attribute to andro are similar to those of anabolic steroids (see Figure 4-2).

St. Louis Cardinal baseball player Mark McGwire's admitted use of andro put this supplement in the national spotlight in the summer of 1998. That was the season when McGwire rocked the baseball world by surpassing Roger Maris's home run record by hitting 70 home runs. It is interesting, though, that during the 1999 baseball season McGwire opted to stop using andro but still managed to hit nearly 70 home runs.

What Are the Risks and Benefits of Creatine?

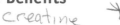

Creatine is an amino acid found in meat, poultry, and fish. In a person's body, creatine is produced naturally in the liver, pancreas, and kidneys. Typically, people get one to two grams of creatine each day from their food intake.[9] As an ergogenic aid, creatine performs its work in the muscles, where it helps restore the compound adenosine triphosphate (ATP). ATP provides quick energy for muscle contractions. It also helps to reduce the lactic acid buildup that occurs during physical exertion. This buildup causes a burning sensation that limits the amount of intense activity one can perform.

Early studies suggest that creatine can help athletes in anaerobic sports, which require short, explosive bursts of energy. However, the increase in performance has been small, the long-term health effects are unknown, studies have been restricted to highly trained subjects (not recreational athletes), and damage to kidneys is possible with high dosages. Users are cautioned to consume ample amounts of water to prevent cramping and dehydration.

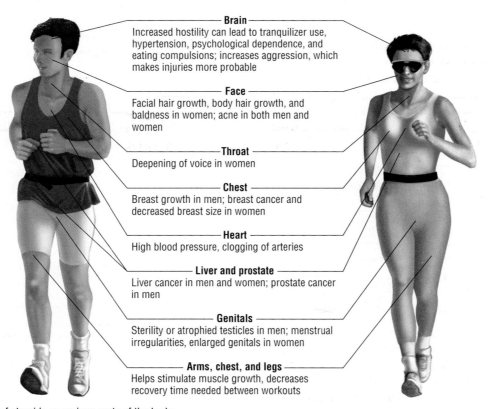

Brain
Increased hostility can lead to tranquilizer use, hypertension, psychological dependence, and eating compulsions; increases aggression, which makes injuries more probable

Face
Facial hair growth, body hair growth, and baldness in women; acne in both men and women

Throat
Deepening of voice in women

Chest
Breast growth in men; breast cancer and decreased breast size in women

Heart
High blood pressure, clogging of arteries

Liver and prostate
Liver cancer in men and women; prostate cancer in men

Genitals
Sterility or atrophied testicles in men; menstrual irregularities, enlarged genitals in women

Arms, chest, and legs
Helps stimulate muscle growth, decreases recovery time needed between workouts

Figure 4-2 Effects of steroids on various parts of the body

All in all, creatine is unlikely to prove as potentially dangerous as androstenedione. If additional studies should indicate that creatine can consistently improve performance, this substance might be banned by many sports federations. For now, the safest, most prudent recommendation is for athletes to spend their time and energy improving their training programs rather than looking for a solution in a bottle.

How Worthwhile Are Commercial Health and Fitness Clubs?

The health and fitness club business is booming. Fitness clubs offer activities ranging from free weights to weight machines to step walking to general aerobics. Some clubs have saunas and whirlpools and lots of frills. Others have course offerings that include wellness, smoking cessation, stress management, time management, dance, and yoga. The atmosphere is friendly, and people are encouraged to have a good time while working out.

If your purpose in joining a fitness club is to improve your cardiorespiratory fitness, measure the program offered by the club against the ACSM standards. If your primary purpose is to meet people and have fun, request a trial membership for a month or so to see whether you like the environment.

Before signing a contract at a health club or spa, do some careful questioning. Find out when the business was established, ask about the qualifications of the employees, contact some members for their observations, and request a thorough tour of the facilities. You might even consult your local Better Business Bureau for additional information. Finally, make certain that you read and understand every word of the contract.

What Is Cross-Training?

Cross-training is the use of more than one aerobic activity to achieve cardiorespiratory fitness. For example, runners may use swimming, cycling, or rowing periodically to replace running in their training routines. Cross-training allows certain muscle groups to rest and injuries to heal. Also, cross-training provides a refreshing change of pace for the participant. You will probably enjoy your fitness program more if you vary the activities.

What Are Steroids, and Why Do Some Athletes Use Them?

Steroids are drugs that can be legally prescribed by physicians for a variety of health conditions, including certain forms of anemia, inadequate growth patterns, and chronic debilitating diseases. Steroids can also be prescribed to aid recovery from surgery or burns. **Anabolic steroids** are

drugs that function like the male sex hormone testosterone. They can be taken orally or by injection. Anabolic steroids are used by athletes who hope to gain weight, muscular size and strength, power, endurance, and aggressiveness. Over the last few decades, many bodybuilders, weightlifters, track athletes, and football players have chosen to ignore the serious health risks posed by illegal steroid use.

The use of steroids is highly dangerous because of serious, life-threatening side effects and adverse reactions. These effects include heart problems, certain forms of cancer, liver complications, and even psychological disturbances. The side effects on female steroid users are as dangerous as those on men. Figure 4-2 shows the adverse effects of steroid use.

Steroid users have developed a terminology of their own. Anabolic steroids are called "roids" or "juice." "Roid rage" is an aggressive, psychotic response to chronic steroid use. "Stacking" is a term that describes the use of multiple steroids at the same time.

Most organizations that control athletic competition (for example, the NCAA, The Athletics Congress, the NFL, and the IOC) have banned steroids and are testing athletes for illegal use. Many athletes finally seem to be getting the message and are steering clear of steroids.

TALKING POINTS If you suspected that a young person you know was using steroids, what strategies would you use to encourage the person to change his or her behavior?

Are Today's Children Physically Fit?

Major research studies published during the last 10 years have indicated that U.S. children and teenagers lead very sedentary lives. Children ages 6 to 17 score extremely poorly in the areas of strength, flexibility, and cardiorespiratory endurance. In many cases, parents are in better shape than their children are. A major consequence of these sedentary habits in children is obesity. The 1999–2000 National Health and Nutrition Examination Survey (NHANES) indicates that 15 percent of children and adolescents ages 6 to 19 years are overweight. Indeed, from NHANES II (1976-80) to NHANES III (1988–1994), the prevalence of overweight nearly doubled among children and adolescents and has continued

---

Key Terms

anabolic steroids drugs that function like testosterone to produce increases in weight, strength, endurance, and aggressiveness

to rise. The seriousness of these data is revealed by the fact that most obese children become obese adults.

This situation presents a challenge to educators and parents to emphasize the need for strenuous play activity. Television watching and parental inactivity were implicated as major factors in these studies.

 TALKING POINTS What can you do to encourage children to become more active participants in physical activities?

How Does Sleep Contribute to Overall Fitness?

Although sleep may seem to be the opposite of exercise, it is an important adjunct to a well-planned exercise program. Sleep is so vital to health that people who are unable to sleep sufficiently (those with insomnia) or who are deprived of sleep experience deterioration in every dimension of their health. Fortunately, exercise is frequently associated with improvement in sleeping.

The value of sleep is apparent in a variety of positive changes in the body. Dreaming is thought to play an important role in supporting the emotional dimension of health. Problem-solving scenarios that occur during dreams seem to afford some carryover value in actual coping experiences. A variety of changes in physiological functioning, particularly a deceleration of the cardiovascular system, occurs during sleep. The feeling of being well rested is an expression of the mental and physiological rejuvenation one feels after a good night's sleep.

The amount of sleep needed varies among people. In fact, for any person, sleep needs vary according to activity level and overall state of health. As we age, the need for sleep appears to decrease from the six to eight hours young adults require. Elderly people routinely sleep less than they did when they were younger. This decrease may be offset by the short naps older people often take during the day. For all people, however, periods of relaxation, daydreaming, and even an occasional afternoon nap promote electrical activity patterns that help regenerate the mind and body.

How Do I Handle Common Injuries That May Be Caused by My Fitness Activities?

For the most part, emergency care for injuries that pertain to the bones or muscles should follow the RICE acronym.[10] Depending on the type and severity of the injury, the importance of rest (R), ice (I) or cold application, compression (C), and elevation (E) cannot be overstated. Each type of injury identified in Table 4.2 has a particular RICE protocol to follow. Any significant injury should be reported to your college student health center, an athletic trainer, a physical therapist, or a physician.

The major signs and symptoms of exercise injury include:

- A delay of over one hour in your body's return to a fully relaxed, comfortable state after exercise
- A change in sleep patterns
- Any noticeable breathing difficulties or chest pains
- Persistent joint or muscle pain
- Unusual changes in urine composition or output (marked color change)
- Anything unusual (for example, headaches, nosebleeds, fainting, numbness in an extremity, and hemorrhoids)

If any of these signs or symptoms appear, stop exercise and contact your physician.

What Is the Female Athlete Triad?

In the early 1990s, the American College of Sports Medicine identified a three-part syndrome of disordered eating, **amenorrhea** (lack of menstruation), and osteoporosis as the female athlete triad.[11] The conditions of this syndrome appear independently in many women, but among female athletes they appear together. The female athlete triad is most likely to be found in athletes whose sport activities emphasize appearance (for example, diving, ice skating, or gymnastics).

Parents, coaches, athletic trainers, and teammates should be watchful for signs of the female athlete triad. This syndrome has associated medical risks, including inadequate fuel supply for activities, inadequate iron intake, reduced cognitive function, altered hormone levels, reduced mental health, early onset of menopause, increased likelihood of skeletal trauma, altered blood fat profiles, and increased vulnerability to heart disease.[11] Vitally important is an early referral to a physician who is knowledgeable about the female athlete triad. The physician will likely coordinate efforts with a psychologist, a nutritionist, and an athletic trainer to improve the health of the athlete and prevent recurrences.

Key Terms

amenorrhea cessation or lack of menstrual periods

Table 4.2 Common Injuries Associated with Physical Activity

Injury	Condition
Achilles tendinitis	A chronic tendinitis of the "heel cord," or muscle tendon, located on the back of the lower leg just above the heel. It may result from any activity that involves forcefully pushing off with the foot and ankle, such as in running and jumping. This inflammation involves swelling, warmth, tenderness to touch, and pain during walking and especially running.
Ankle sprains	Stretching or tearing of one or several ligaments that provide stability to the ankle joint. Ligaments on the outside or lateral side of the ankle are more commonly injured by rolling the sole of the foot downward and toward the inside. Pain is intense immediately after injury, followed by considerable swelling, tenderness, loss of joint motion, and some discoloration over a 24- to 48-hour period.
Groin pull	A muscle strain that occurs in the muscles located on the inside of the upper thigh just below the pubic area and that results from either an overstretch of the muscle or from a contraction of the muscle that meets excessive resistance. Pain will be produced by flexing the hip and leg across the body or by stretching the muscles in a groin-stretch position.
Hamstring pull	A strain of the muscles on the back of the upper thigh that most often occurs while sprinting. In most cases, severe pain is caused simply by walking or in any movement that involves knee flexion or stretch of the hamstring muscle. Some swelling, tenderness to touch, and possibly some discoloration extending down the back of the leg may occur in severe strains.
Patellofemoral knee pain	Nonspecific pain occurring around the knee, particularly the front part of the knee, or in the kneecap (patella). Pain can result from many causes, including improper movement of the kneecap in knee flexion and extension; tendinitis of the tendon just below the kneecap, which is caused by repetitive jumping; bursitis (swelling) either above or below the kneecap; and osteoarthritis (joint surface degeneration) between the kneecap and thigh bone. It may involve inflammation with swelling, tenderness, warmth, and pain associated with movement.
Quadriceps contusion "charley horse"	A deep bruise of the muscles in the front part of the thigh caused by a forceful impact or by some object that results in severe pain, swelling, discoloration, and difficulty flexing the knee or extending the hip. Without adequate rest and protection from additional trauma, small calcium deposits may develop in the muscle.
Shin splints	A catch-all term used to refer to any pain that occurs in the front part of the lower leg or shin, most often caused by excessive running on hard surfaces. Pain is usually caused by strain of the muscles that move the ankle and foot at their attachment points in the shin. It is usually worse during activity. In more severe cases it may be caused by stress fractures of the long bones in the lower leg, with the pain being worse after activity is stopped.
Shoulder impingement	Chronic irritation and inflammation of muscle tendons and a bursa underneath the tip of the shoulder, which results from repeated forceful overhead motions of the shoulder, such as in swimming, throwing, spiking a volleyball, or serving a tennis ball. Pain is felt when the arm is extended across the body above shoulder level.
Tennis elbow	Chronic irritation and inflammation of the lateral or outside surface of the arm just above the elbow at the attachment of the muscles that extend the wrist and fingers. It results from any activity that requires forceful extension of the wrist. Typically occurs in tennis players who are using faulty techniques hitting backhand ground strokes. Pain is felt above the elbow after forcefully extending the wrist against resistance or applying pressure over the muscle attachment above the elbow.

Taking Charge of Your Health

- Assess your level of fitness by completing the National Fitness Test on pages 99–100.

- Start a daily stretching program based on the guidelines in this chapter.

- Implement or maintain a cardiorespiratory fitness program that uses the most recent American College of Sports Medicine recommendations.

- Examine your athletic shoes to determine their appropriateness for the fitness activities you do (see Choosing an Athletic Shoe on page 92–93).

- Monitor your physical activities for potential danger signs indicating that you should consult an athletic trainer, physical therapist, or physician.

- For 2 weeks, keep track of the amount of sleep you are getting. Determine whether this is enough sleep, and make adjustments accordingly.

SUMMARY

- Physical fitness allows one to engage in life's activities without unreasonable fatigue.
- The health benefits of exercise can be achieved through regular moderate exercise.
- Fitness comprises four components: cardiorespiratory endurance, muscular fitness, flexibility, and body composition.
- The American College of Sports Medicine's program for cardiorespiratory fitness has four components: (1) mode of activity, (2) frequency of training, (3) intensity of training, and (4) duration of training. ACSM now recommends that everyone also include (5) resistance training and (6) flexibility training.

- The target heart rate (THR) refers to the number of times per minute the heart must contract to produce a training effect.
- Training sessions should take place in three phases: warm-up, conditioning, and cooldown.
- Fitness experts are concerned about the lack of fitness in today's youth.
- Static stretching is the recommended type of stretching.
- Low-impact aerobic activities have a lower risk of muscle and joint injuries than do high-impact activities.
- College students who are interested in fitness should understand the important topics of steroid use, cross-training, fluid replacement, the female athlete triad, and proper sleep.

REVIEW QUESTIONS

1. Identify the four components of fitness described in this chapter. How does each component relate to physical fitness?
2. What is the difference between anaerobic and aerobic energy production? What types of activities are associated with anaerobic energy production? With aerobic energy production?
3. List some of the benefits of aerobic fitness.
4. Describe the various methods used to promote muscular strength. How do "andro" and creatine differ?
5. What does the principle of overload mean in regard to fitness training programs?

6. Identify the ACSM's six components of an effective cardiorespiratory conditioning program. Explain the important aspects of each component.
7. Under what circumstances should you see a physician before starting a physical fitness program?
8. Identify and describe the three parts of a training session.
9. Describe some of the negative consequences of anabolic steroid use.
10. How does adequate sleep help improve one's fitness?

ENDNOTES

1. American College of Sports Medicine. Position stand on the recommended quantity and quality of exercise for developing and maintaining cardiorespiratory and muscular fitness and flexibility in healthy adults. *Med Sci Sports Exerc* 30(6):975–991, 1998.
2. American Heart Association, Councils on Clinical Cardiology and Nutrition, Physical Activity and Metabolism. *Exercise and Physical Activity in the Prevention and Treatment of Atherosclerotic Cardiovascular Disease.* Circulation; 107:3109, 2003.
3. Casperson C, et al. *Public Health Reports* 100:126, 1985.
4. Brubaker PH, Kaminsky LA, Whaley MH. Coronary artery disease. *Human Kinetics,* 2002.
5. An exercise prescription for older people. *Harvard Heart Letter* 8(10): 1–4, 1998.
6. American College of Sports Medicine. *Guidelines for Exercise Testing and Prescription* (7th ed.). New York: Lippincott, Williams, and Wilkins, 2005.

7. Williams MH. Alcohol and sport performance, *Sports Science Exchange* 4(40): 1–4, 1992.
8. U.S. Department of Health and Human Services. *Physical Activity and Health: A Report of the Surgeon General,* 1996, Centers for Disease Control and Prevention, National Center for Chronic Disease Prevention and Health Promotion.
9. The creatine craze, *UC Berkeley Wellness Letter* 14(3):6, 1998.
10. Arnheim DD, Prentice WE. *Essentials of Athletic Training.* New York: McGraw-Hill, 1999.
11. Stevens WC, Brey RA, Harris JE, Fowlkes-Godek S. The dangerous trio: A case study approach to the female athletic triad, *Athletic Therapy Today,* 2(2):30–36, 1997.
12. National Osteoporosis Foundation. Physician's Guide to Prevention and Treatment of Osteoporosis. Washington, DC: 2005.

personal assessment

What is your level of fitness?

You can determine your level of fitness in thirty minutes or less by completing this short group of tests based on the National Fitness Test developed by the President's Council on Physical Fitness and Sports. If you are over 40 years old or have chronic medical disorders such as diabetes or obesity, check with your physician before taking this or any other fitness test. You will need another person to monitor your test and keep time.

Three-Minute Step Test

Aerobic capacity. Equipment: 12-inch bench, crate, block, or stepladder; stopwatch. Procedure: face bench. Complete 24 full steps (both feet on the bench, both feet on the ground) per minute for 3 minutes. After finishing, sit down, have your partner find your pulse within 5 seconds, and take your pulse for 1 minute. Your score is your pulse rate for 1 full minute.

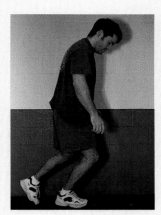

Scoring standards (heart rate for 1 minute)

Age	18–29		30–39		40–49		50–59		60+	
Gender	F	M	F	M	F	M	F	M	F	M
Excellent	<80	<75	<84	<78	<88	<80	<92	<85	<95	<90
Good	80–110	75–100	84–115	78–109	88–118	80–112	92–123	85–115	95–127	90–118
Average	>110	>100	>115	>109	>118	>112	>123	>115	>127	>118

Sit and Reach

Hamstring flexibility. Equipment: yardstick; tape. Positioned parallel to your legs and between them, tape a yardstick to the floor. Sit with legs straight and heels about 5 inches apart, heels even with the 15-inch mark on the yardstick.

While in a sitting position, slowly stretch forward as far as possible. Your score is the number of inches reached.

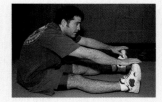

Scoring standards (inches)

Age	18–29		30–39		40–49		50–59		60+	
Gender	F	M	F	M	F	M	F	M	F	M
Excellent	>22	>21	>22	>21	>21	>20	>20	>19	>20	>19
Good	17–22	13–21	17–22	13–21	15–21	13–20	14–20	12–19	14–20	12–19
Average	<17	<13	<17	<13	<15	<13	<14	<12	<14	<12

Arm Hang

Upper body strength. Equipment: horizontal bar (high enough to prevent your feet from touching the floor); stopwatch. Procedure: hang with straight arms, palms facing forward. Start watch when subject is in position. Stop when subject lets go. Your score is the number of minutes and seconds spent hanging.

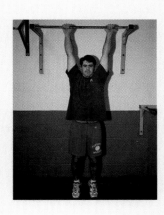

Scoring standards (heart rate for 1 minute)

Age	18–29		30–39		40–49		50–59		60+	
Gender	F	M	F	M	F	M	F	M	F	M
Excellent	>1:30	>2:00	>1:20	>1:50	>1:10	>1:35	>1:00	>1:20	>:50	>1:10
Good	:46–1:30	1:00–2:00	:40–1:20	:50–1:50	:30–1:10	:45–1:35	:30–1:00	:35–1:20	:21–:50	:30–1:10
Average	<:46	<1:00	<:40	<:50	<:30	<:45	<:30	<:35	<:21	<:30

Curl-Ups

Abdominal and low back strength. Equipment: stopwatch. Procedure: Lie flat on upper back, knees bent, shoulders touching the floor, arms extended above your thighs or by your sides, palms down. Bend knees so that the feet are flat and 12 inches from the buttocks. Curl up by lifting head and shoulders off the floor, sliding hands forward above your thighs or the floor. Curl down and repeat. Your score is the number of curl-ups in 1 minute, without breaking a beat.

Scoring standards (number in 1 minute)									
Age	18–29		30–39		40–49		50–59		60+	
Gender	F	M	F	M	F	M	F	M	F	M
Excellent	>45	>50	>40	>45	>35	>40	>30	>35	>25	>30
Good	25–45	30–50	20–40	22–45	16–35	21–40	12–30	18–35	11–25	15–30
Average	<25	<30	<20	<22	<16	<21	<12	<18	<11	<15

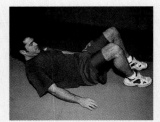

Push-Ups (Men)

Upper body strength. Equipment: stopwatch. Assume a front-leaning position. Lower your body until chest touches the floor. Raise and repeat for 1 minute. Your score is the number of push-ups completed in 1 minute, without breaking a beat.

Scoring standards (number in 1 minute)					
Age	18–29	30–39	40–49	50–59	60+
Excellent	>50	>45	>40	>35	>30
Good	25–50	22–45	19–40	15–35	10–30
Average	<25	<22	<19	<15	<10

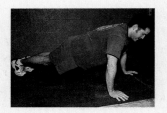

Modified Push-Ups (Women)

Upper body strength. Equipment: stopwatch. Assume a front-leaning position with knees bent up, hands under shoulders. Lower your chest to the floor, raise, and repeat. Your score is the number of push-ups completed in 1 minute, without breaking a beat.

Scoring standards (number in 1 minute)					
Age	18–29	30–39	40–49	50–59	60+
Excellent	>45	>40	>35	>30	>25
Good	17–45	12–40	8–35	6–30	5–25
Average	<17	<12	<8	<6	<5

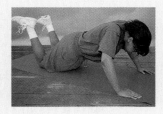

To Carry This Further . . .

Note your areas of strengths and weaknesses. To improve your fitness, become involved in a fitness program that reflects the concepts discussed in this chapter. Talking with fitness experts on your campus might be a good first step.

chapter five

Understanding Nutrition and Your Diet

Chapter Objectives

On completing this chapter, you will be able to:

- name and describe the seven types of nutrients.

- describe saturated, monounsaturated, and polyunsaturated fats, and explain their effects on the human body.

- discuss the recent growth in fat-free foods and their possible advantages and disadvantages.

- define complete protein foods and incomplete protein foods, and give examples of each.

- describe three processes that vitamins help perform in the body.

- discuss the roles of minerals and water in the body.

- describe the benefits of soluble and insoluble fiber.

- describe the Food Guide Pyramid and the number of recommended servings for each food group in the pyramid.

- discuss new recommendations in the USDA's *Dietary Guidelines for Americans*.

- describe foodbourne illnesses and strategies for preventing them.

- name three types of vegetarian diets and describe the advantages and disadvantages of each.

Eye on the Media

How Low Is Low Carb?

We see advertising for "low carbs" on candy bars, chips, peanut butter, and even on beer. Restaurants have jumped on the low-carb bandwagon by putting low-carb choices on their menus. But what does "low carb" mean? Well, if you ask 10 different people, you may get 10 different answers, because there is no one answer. Currently there is no standard definition as to how few carbohydrates a product must contain to qualify as low carb. With the recent low-carb craze, the FDA has been subject to increased pressure to issue guidelines for what can be called "low carb." We saw a similar phenomenon with the low-fat and low-calorie craze; these terms were not defined by the FDA until foodmakers started using them on packaging, creating confusion and misinformation. The FDA eventually standardized the use of "low-fat" for advertising and packaging.

Many gimmicks are used to advertise and portray foods as having few carbohydrates, including phrases such as carb smart, carb aware, carb sense, low-carb lifestyles, carb free, carb conscious, and carb wise. Note the words linked with a low carbohydrate level—wise, smart, free, intelligent. Does this make a difference to the consumer or the manufacturer? Absolutely; sales have tripled for products that remain unchanged except for adding something on their packaging that suggests low carbs.

Actually, this type of advertising is illegal, because the FDA prohibits any nutrient claim that it hasn't defined. However, this fact doesn't seem to have stopped the tidal wave of low-carb advertising. "Net carb" is another phrase commonly being tossed around that has not been standardized or defined by the FDA. This term has been used to refer to the net effect that carbs have after one subtracts from the product the sugar, alcohol, fiber, and other carbohydrates that supposedly have a minimal effect on blood sugar. This approach is misleading and confusing to the consumer as well as being illegal, because it has not been approved by the FDA.

For now, the FDA is sending warnings to companies such as Russell Stover Candies and Peak Performance about mislabeling their products as low carb. Many companies are becoming more creative in the way they package their foods, using terms such as "good for a low-carb lifestyle" or "great for low-carb diets." Foodmakers are also limiting how much they are packaging so that they can be ready to change their advertising quickly, with little loss in revenue, in anticipation of the FDA's ruling. It's probably only a matter of time before the FDA defines what can be called "low carb"; in the meantime, in the absence of FDA regulation it would be prudent for consumers to be wary of anything that claims to be low carb.

Sources: "What Does It Mean to Be Low Carb?" *USA Today,* May 25, 2004.
"Cashing In on the Low-Carb Craze," *Nutrition Action,* March 2004.
"FDA Recommends Changes to Food Labels," *USA Today,* March 12, 2004.

Mealtime—A Chance to Share and Bond

Food is important to your physical well-being—for energy, growth, repair, and regulation of your body and its function. But it's also important to the well-being of your spirit. The sharing of food nourishes our spiritual sense of community. This happens through the type of foods selected, the method of preparation, the uniqueness of presentation, and the people involved. From a spiritual perspective, the sharing of food can be a highly satisfying activity.

When food is shared in the company of those who care about us in the deepest and most personal ways, we experience a sense of community and well-being. The simple act of being together and engaged in a familiar and comfortable practice is reassuring. Meals that involve family or friends, especially dinners for special occasions or important holidays, can be particularly rewarding.

Food is often at the center of the celebration of special occasions. Weddings, birthdays, anniversaries, graduations, promotions, retirements, and funerals take on a special meaning when people come together to share food and drink. From the first birthday cake through the retirement dinner to the lunch provided by neighbors after the funeral of a loved one, food can help to symbolize and acknowledge these events in our lives.

Food has been part of many religious practices and customs for centuries. Some foods have symbolic meanings related to major life experiences, and ceremonies and religious rites. Food can take on symbolic and spiritual meaning, such as bread representing the body of Christ in the Christian religion.

The use of food in spirituality helps to bring groups together to build a stronger sense of community. For example, Ramadan, the ninth month of the Islamic calendar, is considered one of the holiest months of the year in Islam, and from dawn to sunset Muslims abstain from food. The fast is broken at sunset when families and friends come together and enjoy traditional dishes such as fattoushi, a salad. For Jews, the Seder is the most important event in the Passover celebration. Gathering family and friends together, the Seder maintains long-held traditions and customs involving food. The home is cleaned and cleared of all leavened food (foods containing yeast) and grains, and only foods that are kosher are consumed. In the Christian religion, family and friends celebrate Easter by having a meal together on Easter Sunday, usually including lamb, which represents Christ and is seen as a good omen.

Finally, food connects people on a spiritual level by allowing them to share traditions, religious practices, and beliefs. These customs help people build a sense of fellowship and can unify them in times of joy and sorrow.

Healthy eating is important throughout life, in order to maintain a high level of wellness. Food provides the body with the **nutrients** required to produce energy, repair damaged tissue, promote tissue growth, and regulate physiological processes.

Physiologically, these nutrients—carbohydrates, fat, protein, vitamins, minerals, dietary fiber, and water—are essential in adequate quantity. In addition, the production, preparation, serving, and sharing of food enrich our lives in other ways (see Discovering Your Spirituality).

Types and Sources of Nutrients

Let's discuss the familiar nutrients first: carbohydrates, fats, and proteins. These three nutrients provide our bodies with **calories.*** Calories are used quickly by our bodies in energy metabolism, or they are stored in the form of glycogen or adipose (fatty) tissue. The other nutrient groups, which are not sources of energy for the body, will be discussed later.

---

*The term "calorie" is used here to mean a kilocalorie (kcal), which is the accepted scientific expression of the energy value of a food.

Carbohydrates

Carbohydrates are various combinations of sugar units, or saccharides, and are the major energy source for the body. Each gram of carbohydrate contains 4 calories. Since the average person requires approximately 2,000 calories per day and about 45–65 percent of our calories come from carbohydrates, approximately 1,200 calories per day come from carbohydrates.[1] However, age, gender, and activity level affect the number of calories an individual requires each day (Table 5.1).

Key Terms

nutrients elements in foods that are required for the energy, growth, and repair of tissues and regulation of body processes

calories units of heat (energy); specifically, 1 calorie is the amount of heat required to raise the temperature of 1 gram of water by 1°C

carbohydrates chemical compounds composed of sugar units; the body's primary source of energy

Table 5.1 Find Your Calorie Count

The number of calories your body needs daily is based on age, gender, and lifestyle. While many people structure their diets around a 2,000-calorie plan, the actual number of calories an individual needs to maintain energy and health could be more or less than that amount. Look for your daily calorie requirements on the chart below.

		ACTIVITY LEVEL		
Gender	Age	Sedentary	Moderately active	Active
Child	2–3	1,000	1,000–1,400	1,000–1,400
Female	4–8	1,200	1,400–1,600	1,400–1,800
	9–13	1,600	1,600–2,000	1,800–2,200
	14–18	1,800	2,000	2,400
	19–30	2,000	2,000–2,200	2,400
	31–50	1,800	2,000	2,200
	51+	1,600	1,800	2,000–2,200
Male	4–8	1,400	1,400–1,600	1,600–2,000
	9–13	1,800	1,800–2,200	2,000–2,600
	14–18	2,200	2,400–2,800	2,800–3,200
	19–30	2,400	2,600–2,800	3,000
	31–50	2,200	2,400–2,600	2,800–3,000
	51+	2,000	2,200–2,400	2,400–2,800

Sedentary means a lifestyle that includes only the light physical activity associated with typical day-to-day life.
Moderately active means a lifestyle that includes physical activity equivalent to walking about 1.5 to 3 miles per day at 3 to 4 miles per hour, in addition to the light physical activity associated with typical day-to-day life.
Active means a lifestyle that includes physical activity equivalent to walking more than 3 miles per day at 3 to 4 miles per hour, in addition to the light physical activity associated with typical day-to-day life.

Source: Dietary Guidelines For Americans 2005

Carbohydrates occur in three forms, depending on the number of saccharide (sugar) units that make up the molecule. Monosaccharides are carbohydrates with one saccharide unit. Disaccharides are carbohydrates with two saccharide units, one of which is always a glucose unit. Polysaccharides, or starches, are carbohydrates with more than two saccharide units. Starches are found primarily in vegetables, fruits, and grains. Starches provide much overall nutrition benefit since most starch sources also contain significant amounts of vitamins, minerals, protein, and water. Dietary fiber is also a polysaccharide. Starches play an important role in all the dietary recommendations discussed later in the chapter.

The average adult American consumes about 150 pounds of sweeteners each year—usually in sodas, candies, and pastries, which offer few additional nutritional benefits.[2] For years, excess sugar intake was blamed for a number of serious health problems, including obesity, mineral deficiencies, behavioral disorders, dental cavities, diabetes, and cardiovascular disease. However, with the exception of dental cavities, current scientific data do not confirm that sugar itself directly causes any of these health problems. Today, the USDA recommends a limit of 10 teaspoons of sugar per day for a 2,000 calorie diet.

Much of the sugar we consume is hidden. For example, it is an ingredient in ketchup, salad dressings, cured meat products, and canned vegetables and fruits. High-fructose corn syrup, often found in these items, is a highly concentrated sugar solution.

Starches are complex carbohydrates composed of long chains of sugar units. However, these starches should not be confused with the adjective "starchy." When people talk about starchy foods, they usually mean complex carbohydrates, or "heavy" foods. True starches are among the most important sources of dietary carbohydrates. Starches are found primarily in vegetables, fruits, and grains. Eating true starches is overall nutritionally beneficial because most starch sources also contain much-needed vitamins, minerals, plant protein, and water.

Fats

Fats (lipids) are an important nutrient in our diets because they provide a concentrated form of energy (9 calories per gram). Fats provide a feeling of **satiety** and keep us from feeling hungry. Because fats take longer to leave the stomach than either carbohydrates or proteins do, our stomachs feel full for a longer period of time, decreasing our appetite. Fats also help give food its pleasing taste, and they carry the fat-soluble vitamins A, D, E, and K. Without fat, these vitamins would quickly pass through the body. Fat also insulates our bodies to help us retain heat.

Dietary sources of fat are often difficult to identify. The visible fats in our diet, such as butter, salad oils, and the layer of fat on some cuts of meat, represent only about 40 percent of the fat we consume. Most of the fat we eat is hidden in food.

At the grocery store, the fat content of some foods is expressed as a percentage of the product's weight. For example, the different types of milk available include skim milk (no fat), low-fat milk (½ percent), reduced-fat milk (1–2 percent), and whole milk (3–4 percent).

Key Terms

satiety (suh **tie** uh tee) the feeling of no longer being hungry; a diminished desire to eat

The labeling term "reduced-fat" for 1 percent and 2 percent milk was introduced in 1997 to indicate that these types of milk are no longer considered low-fat. The new dietary guidelines recommend that no more than 20–35 percent of our calories come from fat. In addition it is suggested that people:

- Consume less than 10 percent of calories from saturated fatty acids and less than 300 mg/day of cholesterol, and keep trans-fatty acid consumption as low as possible.
- Get most fats from sources of polyunsaturated and monounsaturated fatty acids, such as fish, nuts, and vegetable oils.
- Make choices that are lean, low fat, or fat free when selecting and preparing meat, poultry, dry beans, and milk or milk products.

Children 2–3 years of age, however, need 30–35 percent fat in their diets for growth.[3]

All dietary fat is made up of a combination of three forms of fat: saturated, monounsaturated, and polyunsaturated, based on chemical composition. Paying attention to the amount of each type of fat in our diet is important because of the known link to heart disease (see Chapter 10). Not all fats are created equal. **Saturated fats,** including those found in animal sources and vegetable oils to which hydrogen has been added (hydrogenated), becoming *trans-fatty acids,* need to be carefully limited in a healthy diet.

Concern over the presence of trans-fatty acids (an altered form of a normal vegetable oil molecule) is associated with changes detrimental to the cell membrane, including those cells lining the artery wall. Among the changes being suggested is an increase in calcium deposits.[4] This could result in a rough surface, leading to plaque formation (see Chapter 10).

Processing can change the structure of fat, making it more saturated. As a result, the oils become semisolid and more stable at room temperature. The term *trans* describes the chemical makeup of a fatty acid. Most trans-fatty acids come from hydrogenated oil, which is found in foods such as stick margarine, peanut butter, and crackers. They are popular in food manufacturing because they can extend the shelf life of the food: the oil stays mixed in the food and doesn't rise to the top, and the food doesn't become too soft at room temperature. Many foods are fried with these fats in the fast-food industry.[5]

Tropical Oils

Although all cooking oils (and fats such as butter, lard, margarine, and shortening) have the same number of calories by weight (9 calories per gram), some oils contain high percentages of saturated fats. All oils and fats contain varying percentages of saturated, monounsaturated, and polyunsaturated fats. However, the tropical oils—coconut, palm, and palm kernel—contain much higher percentages of saturated fats than do other cooking oils. Coconut oil, for example, is 92 percent saturated fat. Tropical oils can still be found in some brands of snack foods, crackers, cookies, nondairy creamers, and breakfast cereals, although they have been removed from most national brands. Do you check for tropical oils on the ingredients labels of the foods you select?

Cholesterol

There has been a great deal of focus and concern over cholesterol levels. **Cholesterol** is a white, fatlike substance found in cells of animal origin. It is not found in any vegetable product, so products such as peanut butter and margarine that claim they are cholesterol free never had it in the first place. Cholesterol is used to synthesize cell membranes and also serves as the starting material for the synthesis of bile acids and sex hormones. Although we consume cholesterol in our diet—in such foods as shrimp and other shellfish, animal fat, and milk—we don't need to obtain cholesterol from external sources. The human liver can synthesize enough of the substance to meet the body's needs. Note that some foods high in cholesterol may provide other important nutrients and could remain in a healthy diet on a modest basis. A high level of cholesterol has been reported to be a risk factor in the development of cardiovascular disease (see Chapter 10).

A number of medical conditions can give rise to high blood cholesterol, such as liver disease, kidney failure, hypothyroidism, and diabetes. Certain medications, (some diuretics, for example) can also raise blood cholesterol, irrespective of diet. Considerable evidence suggests that increased intake of saturated fats may increase serum (blood) cholesterol levels. Nutritionists recommend that people restrict their dietary intake of cholesterol to 300 mg or less per day. In other words, no more than 20–35 percent of your total caloric intake should

---

Key Terms

saturated fats fats that promote cholesterol formation; they are in solid form at room temperature; primarily animal fats

cholesterol a primary form of fat found in the blood; lipid material manufactured within the body and derived from dietary sources

come from fat, with most fats being monounsaturated and polyunsaturated. Trans fat should be limited as much as possible.

Trans fats can act like saturated fat, potentially raising LDL blood cholesterol levels and decreasing HDL cholesterol. This is the reason nutritionists encourage us to use butter rather than stick margarine. To reduce your intake of trans fat, make sure you check the labels on foods to see if they list "partially hydrogenated vegetable oil" as one of the ingredients. Foods such as cakes, cookies, crackers, snack foods, stick margarine, vegetable shortening, and fried foods are most likely to have hydrogenated vegetable oil as one of the ingredients.

Low-Fat Foods

Low fat and *low calorie* do not mean the same thing, but often people confuse the two. Fat-free, low-fat, and reduced-fat foods have been popular for many years with people thinking they can eat as much as they want of these foods. This is far from true; a fat-free or reduced-fat product may have as many if not more calories per serving than do regular products. For example, 2 tablespoons of fat-free caramel topping have 103 calories, the same amount as homemade-with-butter caramel topping.[6] Fatty foods make people feel fuller longer than do fat-free foods; thus people tend to eat more of the fat-free foods and so consume *more* calories. In general, the lower the fat, the higher the price tag, because the food industry recognizes that Americans are willing to pay more for reduced-fat and fat-free labels. However, this situation may be changing, since people have realized that lower fat with potentially higher calories doesn't equal weight loss or healthy weight management. With Subway trading in cookies for a fruit roll and soda for a 100 percent juice carton in its kids-pak meals and McDonald's offering a piece of fresh fruit in lieu of French fries for its Happy Meals and touting salads for adult fare, the fast-food tide seems to be turning from supersized and superfat to include some healthier choices. This will be discussed in more depth later in this chapter.

Proteins

Proteins are found in every living cell. They are composed of chains of **amino acids.** Of the 20 naturally occurring amino acids, the body can synthesize all but 9 *essential amino acids** from the foods we eat. A food that contains all 9 essential amino acids is called a *complete*

protein food. Examples are animal products, including milk, meat, cheese, and eggs. A food source that does not contain all 9 essential amino acids is called an *incomplete protein* food. Vegetables, grains, and legumes (peas or beans—including chickpeas, butter beans, soybean curd [tofu], and peanuts) are principal sources of incomplete protein. Vegan vegetarians (see page 130), people with limited access to animal-based food sources, and those who have significantly limited their meat, egg, and dairy product consumption, need to understand how essential amino acids can be obtained from incomplete protein sources. This requires the careful selection of plant foods in combinations that provide all the essential amino acids:

- Sunflower seeds/green peas
- Navy beans/barley
- Green peas/corn
- Red beans/rice
- Sesame seeds/soybeans
- Black-eyed peas/rice and peanuts
- Green peas/rice
- Corn/pinto beans

When even one essential amino acid is missing from the diet, a deficiency can develop. Soybeans provide the same high-quality protein as animal protein.[7] Furthermore, soybeans contain no cholesterol or saturated fat and can actually lower blood lipid levels, reducing the risk of heart disease.[8]

Protein primarily promotes growth and maintenance of body tissue. However, when caloric intake falls, protein is broken down and converted into glucose. This loss of protein can impede growth and repair of tissue. Protein also is a primary component of enzyme and hormone structure. It helps maintain the *acid-base balance* of our bodies and is a source of energy (4 calories per gram consumed). Nutritionists recommend that 12–15 percent of our caloric intake be from protein, particularly that of plant origin. The RDA for adults is 58 grams of dietary protein for men and 46 grams for women each day.

---

*Eight additional compounds are sometimes classified as amino acids, so some nutritionists believe that there are more than 20 amino acids.

> **Key Terms**
>
> **proteins** compounds composed of chains of amino acids; the primary components of muscle and connective tissue
>
> **amino acids** the chief components of protein; can be manufactured by the body or obtained from dietary sources

Vitamins

Vitamins are organic compounds that are required in small amounts for normal growth, reproduction, and maintenance of health. Vitamins differ from carbohydrates, fats, and proteins because they do not provide calories or serve as structural elements for our bodies. Vitamins are *coenzymes*. By facilitating the action of **enzymes,** vitamins help initiate a wide variety of body responses, including energy production, use of minerals, and growth of healthy tissue.

Vitamins can be classified as *water soluble* (capable of being dissolved in water) or *fat soluble* (capable of being dissolved in fat or lipid tissue). Water-soluble vitamins include the B-complex vitamins and vitamin C. Most of the excess of these water-soluble vitamins is eliminated from the body in the urine. The fat-soluble vitamins are vitamins A, D, E, and K. Excessive intake of these vitamins causes them to be stored in the body in the adipose (fat) tissue. It is therefore possible to consume and retain too many of these vitamins, particularly vitamins A and D. Because excess fat-soluble vitamins are stored in the body's fat, organs that contain fat, such as the liver, are primary storage sites.

Because water-soluble vitamins dissolve quickly in water, it's important not to lose them during the preparation of fresh fruits and vegetables. One method is not to overcook fresh vegetables. The longer vegetables are steamed or boiled, the more water-soluble vitamins will be lost. Some people save the water in which vegetables were boiled or steamed and use it for drinking or cooking. More vitamins are retained with microwave cooking than with stove-top cooking.

To ensure adequate vitamin intake, a good approach is to eat a variety of foods. Unless there are special circumstances, such as pregnancy, lactation, infancy, or an existing health problem, nearly everyone who eats a reasonably well-rounded diet consumes enough vitamins to prevent deficiencies. People often think taking megadoses of vitamins such as vitamin C can be health-enhancing, but actually the reverse is true. Taking large doses of vitamin C from a dietary supplement can put a strain on your kidneys, causing kidney stones and diarrhea. Too much niacin, vitamin B6, and folate can also be harmful.[5]

 TALKING POINTS What would you say to a friend who is following a low-carbohydrate, high-fat weight loss diet to help that person see its potential pitfalls?

Some professionals recommend that supplements be taken with food, since they're really components of food and help the body metabolize other food components.

The fat-soluble nutrients should be taken with a little oil or fat to enhance absorption. The water-soluble nutrients are easily absorbed without food but may work better when taken with meals. In addition, some people complain of stomach upset when they take vitamins on an empty stomach.

Unfortunately, not all people eat a balanced diet based on a variety of foods. Recent studies suggest that a somewhat higher intake of vitamins A, C, and E for adults might reduce the risk of developing cancer, atherosclerosis, and depressed levels of high-density lipoprotein (HDL) cholesterol; however, several unanswered questions remain, including the amounts needed for effectiveness (see Chapter 10).[9]

Consuming an adequate amount of folic acid before and during pregnancy has been shown to reduce the incidence of birth defects. To ensure adequate folic acid intake (400 micrograms/day), in 1997 the Food and Drug Administration (FDA) began to require that bread and cereal products be supplemented with folic acid. The goal of this requirement is for pregnant women and women of childbearing age to receive at least 140 micrograms/day through dietary intake. Taking a daily multivitamin before and during pregnancy would easily provide the remaining amount of folic acid necessary to promote fetal neural tube closure (thus preventing spina bifida). Folic acid is also considered important in the prevention of cardiovascular disease.[10]

At the same time that many health experts are recommending some vitamin supplementation, the FDA has prohibited manufacturers of food supplements, including vitamins, from making *unsubstantiated claims* for the cure and prevention of disease. Supplement manufacturers fought against the implementation of this regulation by suggesting to the public that vitamins might become available only by prescription. This did not happen. Today, manufacturers of folic acid supplements may make claims about the product's ability to prevent neural tube defects in infants.

Key Terms

vitamins organic compounds that facilitate the action of enzymes

enzymes organic substances that control the rate of physiological reactions but are not themselves altered in the process

---

Phytochemicals

Certain physiologically active components are believed to deactivate carcinogens or function as antioxidants. Among these are the carotenoids (from green vegetables), polyphenols (from onions and garlic), indoles (from cruciferous vegetables), and the allyl sulfides (from garlic, chives, and onions). These **phytochemicals** may play an important role in sparking the body to fight and slow the development of some diseases such as cancer. At this time, however, the exact mechanisms through which the various phytochemicals reduce the formation of cancer cells is not understood. Although it is generally agreed that these foods are important in planning food selections, no precise recommendations regarding the amounts of various phytochemical-rich plants have been made.

Minerals

Nearly 5 percent of the body is composed of inorganic materials, the *minerals.* Minerals function primarily as structural elements (in teeth, muscles, hemoglobin, and hormones). They are also critical in the regulation of body processes, including muscle contraction, heart function, blood clotting, protein synthesis, and red blood cell formation. Approximately 21 minerals have been recognized as essential for good health. Unlike vitamins, minerals are inorganic and can't be destroyed by heat or food processing.

Major minerals are those that exist in relatively high amounts in our body tissues. The RDAs include 250 mg of each one daily. Examples are calcium, phosphorus, sulfur, sodium, potassium, and magnesium. Examples of **trace elements,** minerals seen in relatively small amounts in body tissues, include zinc, iron, copper, selenium, and iodine. Trace elements are required only in small quantities, fewer than 20 mg daily of each, but they are essential for good health. As with vitamins, the safest, most appropriate way to prevent a mineral deficiency is to eat a balanced diet. However, calcium, a major mineral, can be taken as a supplement to help prevent osteoporosis.

Water

Water may well be our most essential nutrient, since without water most of us would die from the effects of **dehydration** in less than a week. We could survive for weeks or even years without some of the essential minerals and vitamins, but not without water. More than half our body weight comes from water. Water provides the medium for nutrient and waste transport, controls body temperature, and functions in nearly all of our body's biochemical reactions.

Most people seldom think about the importance of an adequate intake of water and fluids. The average adult loses about 10 cups of water daily through perspiration, urination, bowel movements, and breathing. Adults require about 6–10 glasses a day, depending on their activity level and environment. People who drink beverages that tend to dehydrate the body (tea, coffee, and alcohol) should increase their water consumption. To see if you're drinking enough fluid, check your urine. A small amount of dark-colored urine can be an indication that you are not consuming enough fluid and need to drink more. Urine that is pale or almost colorless means you are most likely taking in enough fluids. Needed fluids are also obtained from fruits, vegetables, fruit and vegetable juices, milk, and noncaffeinated soft drinks. Excessive water consumption by infants, however, can dilute sodium stores in the body to dangerously low levels, possibly causing death.[11] Also, dentists are increasingly concerned about the abnormally high number of dental cavities seen in children who have consumed bottled water rather than fluoridated tap water.[12]

Fiber

Although not considered a nutrient by definition, **fiber** is an important component of sound nutrition. Fiber consists of plant material that is not digested but moves through the digestive tract and out of the body. Cereal, fruits, and vegetables all provide us with dietary fiber.

Fiber can be classified into two large groups on the basis of water solubility. *Insoluble* fibers are those that can absorb water from the intestinal tract. By absorbing water, the insoluble fibers give the stool bulk and decrease the time it takes the stool to move through the digestive tract. In contrast, *soluble* fiber turns to a "gel" in the intestinal tract and binds to liver bile, to which cholesterol is attached. Thus the soluble fibers may be valuable in removing cholesterol, which lowers blood cholesterol levels. How much fiber do you need? Adults should eat from 25 to 35 g of fiber each day; however, most American adults eat only 11 g per day.

Key Terms

phytochemicals physiologically active components believed to deactivate carcinogens and to function as antioxidants

trace elements minerals present in very small amounts in the body; micronutrient elements

dehydration the abnormal depletion of fluids from the body; severe dehydration can be fatal

fiber plant material that cannot be digested; found in cereal grains, fruits, and vegetables

---

Fiber has many benefits, including helping to curb your appetite and prevent overeating because it is filling, requires more chewing, stays in the stomach longer, and absorbs water, adding to the feeling of fullness. Fiber also helps to slow the absorption of sugar from the intestines, thus steadying the blood sugar and slowing down the absorption of fat from the foods you eat. Consuming adequate amounts of fiber has an important effect on reducing serious medical problems because soluble fiber lowers LDL cholesterol and protects against cardiovascular disease while insoluble fiber protects against developing colon cancer.[13]

In recent years, attention has been given to three forms of soluble fiber—oat bran, psyllium (from the weed plantain), and rice bran—because of their ability to lower blood cholesterol levels.

Oat bran can lower cholesterol levels by five to six points in people whose initial cholesterol levels are moderately high. To accomplish this reduction, a daily consumption of oat bran equal to a large bowl of cold oat bran cereal or three or more packs of instant oatmeal would be necessary. Oatmeal can also be eaten as a cooked cereal or used in other foods, such as hamburgers, pancakes, or meatloaf.

The New Dietary Guidelines for Americans 2005

The Dietary Guidelines for Americans is science-based and summarizes the analysis of new scientific information regarding nutrition, health, physical activity, and food safety. The goal of these guidelines is to lower the risk of chronic disease and promote health through diet and physical activity.

The United States Department of Agriculture (USDA) releases a revision of their dietary guidelines for Americans every five years. However, the food pyramid has not undergone a revision since it was created in 1992. The most recent revision, announced in 2005, has some significant changes to the food pyramid, including its name. It's now called My Pyramid to reflect a personalized approach to healthy eating. These changes are based on evidence that found that Americans are consuming too many calories and yet are not meeting the recommended intake for some nutrients. It was determined that Americans have too much saturated and trans fats, cholesterol, and added sugar and salt in their diets and not enough calcium, potassium, fiber, magnesium, and vitamins A, C and E. There are also some special recommendations for specific population groups. For people over 50, consuming vitamin B_{12} in its crystalline form (such as fortified foods or supplements) is recommended. Women of childbearing age need to eat iron-rich plant food or iron-fortified food with an enhancer for iron absorption, such as vitamin-C-rich foods. Taking in adequate amounts of folic acid daily from fortified foods or supplements is important for pregnant women and women who may become pregnant. Older adults, people with dark skin, and those not exposed to enough sunlight need to consume extra vitamin D from vitamin-D-fortified foods and/or supplements.

These findings were used to formulate the new USDA Food Guide for Americans, which focuses on overall caloric intake rather than on one particular food group, such as fats or carbohydrates. Portion sizes are emphasized, and the recommendations are made in cups rather than in serving sizes, to help people have better portion control. There is also an increased emphasis on consuming **nutrient-dense foods,** which provide substantial amounts of vitamins and minerals and comparatively few calories. Junk foods typically are not nutrient-dense, since they are high in sugar and saturated and trans fats, high in calories, and low in vitamins and minerals.

Americans are advised to consume more whole grains, milk products, fruits, and vegetables as well. Another key aspect is the focus on daily exercise, with 60 to 90 minutes of moderate exercise as the recommended amount. Restricting salt, alcohol, and trans fat are other important aspects of the dietary guidelines.

The new food pyramid, MyPyramid, takes a more personalized approach to healthy eating (see Figure 5-1). The pyramid has been tipped onto its side, and the colors and size of the bands reflect the proportion of each food group people generally need to consume each day. The steps signify the importance of daily exercise. The food pyramid acknowledges that people have different dietary needs based on age, gender, and physical activity level. There are 12 different recommendations based on these factors, and you can find the one that best fits you through the USDA's Web site at www.mypyramid.gov. People can also assess their activity level and food intake through www.mypyramidtracker.gov.

Some of the specific key recommendations for a healthy pattern of eating, physical activity, and handling food on a daily basis that have been suggested by these new guidelines include:[26]

1. Choose a variety of fruits and vegetables. Select from all five vegetable subgroups (dark green, orange, legumes, starchy vegetables, and other vegetables).
2. Eat 2 cups of fruit and 2½ cups of vegetables.
3. Consume 3 1-ounce equivalents of whole-grain products per day, with at least half of the grains coming from whole grains.

Key Terms

nutrient-dense foods foods that provide substantial amounts of vitamins and minerals and comparatively few calories

---

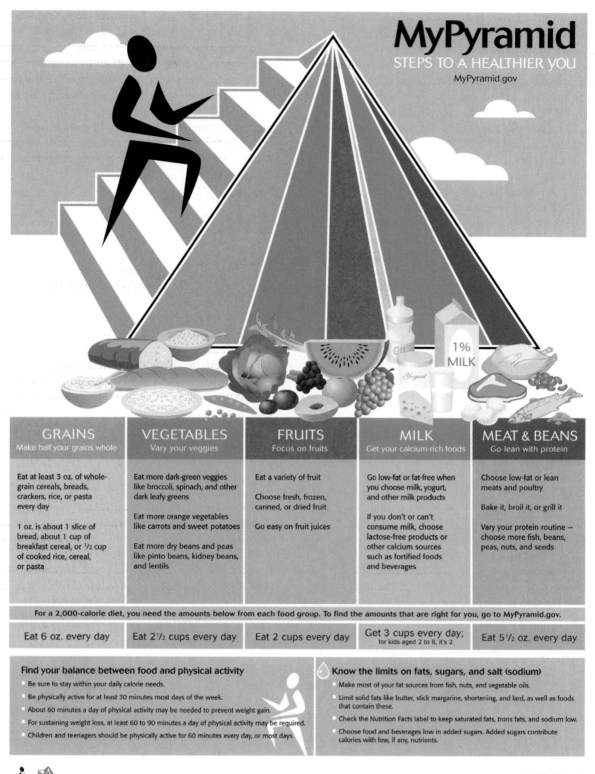

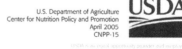

Figure 5-1 The new look for the food pyramid takes a personal approach to healthy eating.

4. Drink 3 cups of fat-free or low-fat milk or the equivalent.
5. Engage in at least 30 minutes of moderate intensity physical activity on most days of the week to reduce the risk of chronic disease. Engage in 60 to 90 minutes of physical activity for weight management.
6. Those who choose to drink alcoholic beverages should consume no more than 1 drink per day for women and 2 drinks per day for men.
7. Consume less than 10 percent of calories from saturated fats and less than 300 mg/day of cholesterol. Keep trans fats at a minimum.
8. Keep total fat intake between 20–35 percent of calories, with most fats coming from polyunsaturated and monounsaturated fats.
9. Choose low-fat, fat-free, or lean meat, poultry, milk, and bean products.
10. Consume less than 2,300 mg (approximately 1 teaspoon) of sodium daily.
11. Clean hands, food-contact surfaces, and fruits and vegetables. Meat and poultry shouldn't be washed or rinsed.
12. Separate raw, cooked, and ready-to-eat foods while shopping, preparing, and storing foods.
13. Cook foods to a safe temperature, and chill perishable food promptly.
14. Avoid unpasteurized milk and milk products, raw or partially cooked eggs, and foods containing raw eggs or undercooked meat and poultry, unpasteurized juices, and raw sprouts.

The most effective way to take in adequate amounts of nutrients is to eat a balanced diet as outlined by the USDA's most current guidelines. (See Table 5.2.) The USDA particularly focuses on meeting these dietary needs by consuming food, not dietary supplements. In addition, the USDA advises consuming a variety of nutrient-dense foods and beverages (discussed later in the

Table 5.2   Adult Recommended Dietary Allowances (RDAs): Four Different Calorie Levels

Food Groups	1,600 Calories	2,000 Calories	2,600 Calories	3,100 Calories	Serving Sizes
Grains	6 servings	7–8 servings	10–11 servings	12–13 servings	1 slice bread, 1 oz dry cereal, ½ cup cooked rice, pasta, or cereal
Vegetables	3–4 servings	4–5 servings	5–6 servings	6 servings	1 cup raw leafy vegetable ½ cup cooked vegetable 6 oz vegetable juice
Fruits	4 servings	4–5 servings	5–6 servings	6 servings	6 oz fruit juice 1 medium fruit ¼ cup dried fruit ½ cup fresh, frozen, or canned fruit
Low-fat or fat-free dairy foods	2–3 servings	2–3 servings	3 servings	3–4 servings	8 oz milk 1 cup yogurt 1½ oz cheese
Meat, poultry, fish	1–2 servings	2 or less servings	2 servings	2–3 servings	3 oz cooked meats, poultry, or fish
Nuts, seeds, legumes	3–4 servings	4–5 servings	1 serving	1 serving	⅓ cup or 1½ oz nuts 2 Tbsp or ½ oz seeds ½ cup cooked dry beans or peas
Fat and oils	2 servings/ week	2–3 servings/ week	3 servings	4 servings	1 tsp soft margarine 1 Tbsp low-fat mayonnaise 2 Tbsp light salad dressing 1 tsp vegetable oil
Sweets	0 servings	5 servings/week	2 servings	2 servings	1 Tbsp sugar 1 Tbsp jelly or jam ½ oz jelly beans 8 oz lemonade

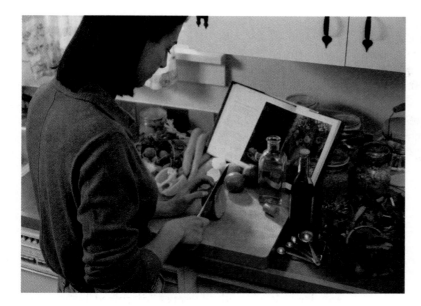

Eating a healthy diet including fruits and vegetables is the best way to get the necessary vitamins and minerals.

chapter). To determine whether you are eating a healthful diet balanced with choices from each food group, complete the personal assessment entitled "Rate Your Plate" on page 135.

Fruits

As previously mentioned, the new guidelines suggest eating 2 cups of fruits per day for a 2,000 calorie/day adult diet. One medium-sized fruit, ¼ cup dried fruit, or 1 cup of fresh, frozen, or canned fruit is equivalent to 1 serving or 1 cup. Orange fruits such mango, cantaloupe, apricots, and red or pink grapefruit provide sources of vitamin A. Kiwi, strawberries, guava, papaya, and cantaloupe and citrus fruits are good sources of vitamin C. Oranges and orange juice also provide folate. Some good sources for potassium are bananas, plantains, dried fruits, oranges and orange juice, cantaloupe and honeydew melons, and tomato products. For the majority of your fruit intake, it is generally recommended to consume whole fruits and avoid fruit juices to ensure adequate fiber and to avoid the high sugar content associated with fruit juices. The American Cancer Society indicates that this food group may play an important role in the prevention of certain forms of cancer.

Vegetables

Two and one-half cups of vegetables per day is the new recommendation for adults following a 2,000 calorie diet. As with the fruit group, the important function of this group is to provide vitamin A, vitamin C, complex carbohydrates, and fiber. Because Americans tend to eat only a few vegetables, such as potatoes, corn, and carrots, the new guidelines give specific recommendations about the types of vegetable. One general rule is to "eat your colors," meaning you should consume a variety of vegetables over the course of a week. The USDA recommends:

- Dark green vegetables—3 cups/week
- Orange vegetables—2 cups/week
- Legumes (dry beans)—3 cups/week
- Starchy vegetables—3 cups/week
- Other vegetables—6½ cups/week

Again, avoid drinking vegetable juices as a way of meeting these requirements because they can be high in salt and sugar and don't provide the fiber intake that whole vegetables do. **Cruciferous vegetables,** such as broccoli, cabbage, brussels sprouts, and cauliflower, may be particularly helpful in the prevention of certain forms of cancer.[24] It has also been determined that antioxidants in vegetables and fruits may slow the age-related changes in cognitive function.[25] Decreased risk of heart disease has also been associated with the consumption of fruits and vegetables.

Key Terms

cruciferous vegetables vegetables, such as broccoli, whose plants have flowers with four leaves in the pattern of a cross

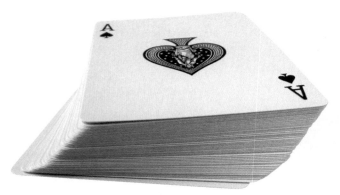

To get an idea of portion sizes—a stacked deck of cards is equivalent to 3 ounces.

Milk and Milk Products

The new dietary guidelines recommend increasing the consumption of milk to 3 cups of fat-free or low-fat milk each day, or its equivalent in another milk product. Milk consumption has been associated with higher bone density and can help fight osteoporosis. Calcium and high-quality protein, required for bone and tooth development, are two primary nutritional benefits provided by this food group. The guidelines further suggest that children 2 to 8 years old should consume 2 cups per day of fat-free or low-fat milk, or equivalent milk products, whereas children 9 years of age and older should consume 3 cups per day of fat-free or low-fat milk, or equivalent milk products. Milk, cheese, yogurt, and ice cream are included in this food group.

Meat, Poultry, Fish, Dry Beans, Eggs, and Nuts

Our need for selections from this protein-rich group is based on our daily need for protein, iron, and the B vitamins. Meats include all red meat (beef, pork, and game), fish, and poultry. It is strongly recommended that we choose lean meats and low-fat or fat-free foods in this group. Meat substitutes include dry beans, eggs, tofu, peanut butter, nuts and seeds. For individuals who are lactose intolerant (lactose upsets their intestines) or are vegan (vegetarians who don't consume any animal products, including dairy products), soybeans, tofu, spinach, kale, okra, beet greens, and oatmeal are good alternative sources of calcium. The 2005 USDA guidelines recommend that adults eat 5½ ounces of meat or protein foods each day. One ounce is equivalent to:

- 1 ounce cooked lean meat, poultry, or fish
- 1 egg
- ¼ cup cooked dry beans
- ¼ cup tofu
- 1 tablespoon peanut butter
- ½ ounce nuts or seeds

The fat content of meat varies considerably. Some forms of meat yield only 1 percent fat, whereas others may be as high as 40 percent fat. Poultry and fish are generally significantly lower in overall fat than are red meats. Interestingly, the higher the grade of red meat, the more fat is marbled throughout the muscle fiber. Indeed, people usually find that higher-grade steak usually tastes better, but that is because of its higher fat content.

Meats are generally excellent sources of iron. Iron is present in much greater amounts in red meats and organ meats (liver, kidney, and heart) than in poultry and fish. Iron plays a critically important role in hemoglobin synthesis on red blood cells and thus is an important contributor to physical fitness (see Chapter 4) and overall cardiovascular health (see Chapter 10). However, meat and fish should be fresh, stored appropriately, and cooked adequately to reduce the likelihood of serious foodborne illnesses.

Breads, Cereals, Rice, and Pasta

The nutritional benefit from the breads, cereals, rice, and pasta group lies in its contribution of B-complex vitamins and energy from complex carbohydrates. Some nutritionists believe that foods from this group promote protein intake, since many of them are prepared as complete-protein foods—for example, macaroni and cheese, cereal and milk, and bread and meat sandwiches.

This group is referred to as the "grain group" by the USDA, and there is a particular emphasis on consuming at least 3 of the 6 ounces of this group from whole grains. Whole grains can reduce the risk of chronic disease and help with weight maintenance.

Whole grains consist of the entire grain seed, or the kernel, and can't be identified by the color of the food. The FDA requires that food contain 51 percent or more whole-grain ingredients by weight and be low fat in order to be called "whole grain." On food labels, "whole grain" should be the first ingredient listed. It is further advised to avoid refined grains, because the grain-refining process typically removes most of the bran and some of the germ, resulting in the loss of dietary fiber, minerals, vitamins, and other important nutrients. Wheat flour, enriched flour, and degerminated cornmeal are *not* whole grains.

Anatomy of MyPyramid

One size doesn't fit all

USDA's new MyPyramid symbolizes a personalized approach to healthy eating and physical activity. The symbol has been designed to be simple. It has been developed to remind consumers to make healthy food choices and to be active every day. The different parts of the symbol are described below.

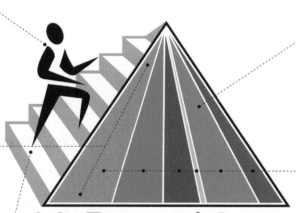

Activity
Activity is represented by the steps and the person climbing them, as a reminder of the importance of daily physical activity.

Moderation
Moderation is represented by the narrowing of each food group from bottom to top. The wider base stands for foods with little or no solid fats or added sugars. These should be selected more often. The narrower top area stands for foods containing more added sugars and solid fats. The more active you are, the more of these foods can fit into your diet.

Personalization
Personalization is shown by the person on the steps, the slogan, and the URL. Find the kinds and amounts of food to eat each day at MyPyramid.gov.

Proportionality
Proportionality is shown by the different widths of the food group bands. The widths suggest how much food a person should choose from each group. The widths are just a general guide, not exact proportions. Check the Web site for how much is right for you.

Variety
Variety is symbolized by the 6 color bands representing the 5 food groups of the Pyramid and oils. This illustrates that foods from all groups are needed each day for good health.

Gradual Improvement
Gradual improvement is encouraged by the slogan. It suggests that individuals can benefit from taking small steps to improve their diet and lifestyle each day.

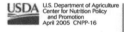

U.S. Department of Agriculture
Center for Nutrition Policy
and Promotion
April 2005 CNPP-16

USDA is an equal opportunity provider and employer.

GRAINS	VEGETABLES	FRUITS	OILS	MILK	MEAT & BEANS

Some products are labeled **enriched,** meaning that some of nutritional elements that were removed during processing are returned to the food; however, only three B vitamins (thiamine, niacin, riboflavin) and iron are replaced.

The USDA recommends 6 ounces of grains daily, with at least 3 ounces coming from whole grains. One ounce is equivalent to:

- 1 slice of bread
- 1 cup dry cereal
- ½ cup cooked rice, pasta, cereal

The food industry has risen to the challenge of providing nutritious whole-grain foods with improved taste and texture. For example, ConAgra has spent millions of dollars over the past five years to develop "white wheat" made from a naturally occurring albino variety of flour. It has 3½ times more dietary fiber, 11 times more vitamin E, 5 times more magnesium, and 4 times more niacin than does refined, unenriched wheat flour. It also tastes milder and sweeter than most whole grains do. It combines the best of both worlds—the nutrition of whole wheat with the taste of white flour.[27]

> ### Key Terms
>
> **enriched** the process of returning to foods some of the nutritional elements (B vitamins and iron) removed during processing

Fats, Oils, and Sweets

Where do such items such as beer, butter, candy, colas, cookies, corn chips, and pastries fit into your diet? Most of these items contribute relatively little to healthful nutrition; they provide additional calories, generally from sucrose and significant amounts of salt and fat. The new dietary guidelines make specific recommendations about fats, salt, sugar, and alcohol intake.

The USDA refers to the fats and oils group as the "Oil group" on the food pyramid. The recommended total daily fat intake should be 20–35 percent of your total calories, with most fats coming from sources of polyunsaturated and monounsaturated fatty acids, such as fish, nuts, and vegetable oils. Canola oil and olive oil are preferred over other types of oils. Less than 10 percent of total calories should be from saturated fats, and less than 300 mg/day should come from cholesterol. Trans-fatty acid consumption is to be kept "as low as possible." A limit of 24 grams, or 6 teaspoons of oils, is the daily recommendation. One teaspoon is equivalent to:

- 1 teaspoon soft margarine
- 1 tablespoon low-fat mayonnaise
- 2 tablespoons light salad dressing
- 1 teaspoon vegetable oil

The USDA also suggests that we choose and prepare foods and beverages with little added sugars or caloric sweeteners. The new food guide recommends no more than 8 teaspoons of added sugars per day, which is equivalent to a ½ ounce of jelly beans or an 8-ounce glass of lemonade. Eating too much sugar has been thought to be a major contributor to the increase in obesity in Americans.

Something new to the USDA guidelines is the limitation on salt intake. They advise consuming less than 2,300 mg, or 1 teaspoon, of sodium each day and to choose and prepare foods with little salt. Most of our salt intake comes from processed or prepared foods. Many people are unaware of the high sodium content in prepared foods, sauces, soups, and canned foods, and so reading the labels for ingredients is extremely important. You might be surprised by some of the foods that contain salt—cookies, minute rice, canned green beans, soft drinks, and cereal. It is also difficult to know how to make healthy choices when eating out if you don't know the sodium content in the menu items. Too much sodium is linked to hypertension, and about 30 percent of Americans have sodium-sensitive high blood pressure, which can lead to heart attack or stroke. It is estimated that about 150,000 deaths each year are caused by too much salt.

Table 5.3 Sample 2,000-Calorie Menu Based on the New Dietary Guidelines for Americans, 2005

Breakfast
1 cup oatmeal
1 cup low-fat vanilla yogurt
½ cup blackberries

Snack
1 medium banana

Lunch
2 whole wheat tortillas each filled with 1 ounce of cooked chicken breast, ¼ cup refried beans, ¼ cup onion and tomato, 2 tablespoons shredded light cheese, and ¼ cup shredded romaine lettuce
16 ounces water

Snack
¼ cup unsalted peanuts
1 medium apple

Dinner
1½ cups cooked whole wheat pasta topped with ½ cup low-fat pasta sauce, ½ cup cooked mushrooms, ¼ cup cooked onions, and 2 ounces cooked extra-lean ground turkey breast
1 cup skim milk

Snack
6 ounces fat-free yogurt
1 cup grapes

Another difference in the new dietary guidelines is the recommendation concerning alcohol consumption. The USDA states that "those who choose to drink alcoholic beverages should do so sensibly and in moderation." *Moderation* is defined as the consumption of up to 1 drink per day for women and up to 2 drinks per day for men. One drink is defined as either 12 fluid ounces of regular beer, 5 fluid ounces of wine, or 1½ fluid ounces of 80-proof distilled spirits. Since alcoholic beverages tend to contribute calories but little nutrition, they are counterproductive to taking in sufficient nutrients while not going over the daily caloric allotment. However, there are some indications that moderate alcohol consumption, such as having a glass of red wine each day, assists in decreasing the risk of coronary heart disease.

Table 5.3 provides a sample 2,000-calorie menu based on the new USDA dietary guidelines.

Fast Foods

Fast foods deliver a high percentage of their calories from fat, often associated with their method of preparation (for example, frying in saturated fat). **Fat density** is a serious limitation of fast foods. In comparison with the recommended standard (20–35 percent of total calories from fat), 40 percent to 50 percent of the calories in fast foods come from fats. Although many fast-food restaurants are now using vegetable oil instead of animal fat for frying (to reduce cholesterol levels), this change has not lowered the fat density of these foods. One average fast-food meal supplies over one-half the amount of fat needed in a day. In addition, fast foods are often high in sugar and salt. Table 5.4 shows how many fast foods are high in sodium and saturated and trans fat.

Although many fast-food restaurants have broadened their menus to include whole-wheat breads and rolls, salad bars, fruit, and low-fat milk, a recent study showed that those who said they ate out at fast-food restaurants at least twice a week or more gained 10 pounds more than those who did not. Also, sit-down chain restaurants such as Applebees, Outback Steakhouse, Chili's, Cracker Barrel, Denny's, Olive Garden, and Red Lobster offer children's meals that are adult sized in calories and fat content. For example, the boomerang cheeseburger with fries at Outback Steakhouse has 840 calories and 31 grams of saturated-plus-trans fat. Applebee's grilled cheese sandwich with fries has 900 calories and 14 grams of saturated fat in the grilled cheese alone.

Some of the fast-food restaurants seem to be turning away from their healthy food offerings and reinstating high-fat and high-calorie meals. For example, Burger King recently introduced its Enormous Omelet Sandwich, which comprises one sausage patty, two eggs, two American cheese slices, and three strips of bacon on a bun. This adds up to a whopping 730 calories and 47 grams of fat. It has a suggested retail price of $2.99, or $3.49 for the value meal, which comes with fried potatoes and coffee or juice. The hash browns add 230 calories and 15 grams of fat to the meal.

Hardee's has also bucked the "health trend" in fast-food restaurants by offering a burger it dubbed the "Monster Thickburger," with 1,400 calories and 107 grams of fat. The Grand Slam breakfast at Denny's, which comes with two pancakes, two eggs, two strips of bacon, and two sausage links, has 665 calories and 49 grams of fat, according to the Denny's Web site. The Fabulous French Toast Platter—with three slices of French toast,

Key Terms

fat density the percentage of a food's total calories that are derived from fat; above 30% is considered to be a high fat density

Table 5.4 The Fast Lane

Within each section, foods are ranked from least to most bad fat (saturated + trans), then calories.

	Calories	Total Fat (grams)	Saturated + Trans Fat (grams)	Sodium (milligrams)
Burgers, etc.				
Burger King BK Veggie	380	16	3	930
McDonald's Hamburger	260	9	4	530
Wendy's Jr. Hamburger	280	9	4	600
McDonald's McVeggie*	350	8	4	1,200
Burger King Hamburger	310	13	6	550
McDonald's Cheeseburger	310	12	7	740
Burger King Whopper Jr.	390	22	8	550
McDonald's Quarter Pounder	420	18	8	730
Wendy's Classic Single	430	20	8	890
Burger King The Angus Steak Burger	570	22	9	1,270
McDonald's Big N' Tasty	520	29	11	730
McDonald's Big Mac	560	30	12	1,010
McDonald's Quarter Pounder with Cheese	510	25	14	1,150
Wendy's Big Bacon Classic	580	29	14	1,390
Burger King Whopper	700	42	14	1,020
Wendy's Classic Double with Cheese	700	39	19	1,470
Burger King Whopper with Cheese	800	49	20	1,450
McDonald's Double Quarter Pounder with Cheese	730	40	22	1,330
Burger King Double Whopper	970	61	24	1,110
Wendy's Classic Triple with Cheese	970	59	29	2,060
Burger King Double Whopper with Cheese	1,060	69	30	1,540
Chicken & Fish Sandwiches				
Wendy's Ultimate Chicken Grill	360	7	2	1,090
McDonald's Chicken McGrill	400	16	3	1,010
McDonald's Filet-O-Fish	400	18	5	640
Wendy's Spicy Chicken Fillet	510	19	5	1,480
Burger King Chicken Whopper	570	25	5	1,410
McDonald's McChicken	420	22	6	760
McDonald's Crispy Chicken	500	23	6	1,090
Wendy's Homestyle Chicken Fillet	540	22	6	1,320
Burger King Chicken	560	28	8	1,270
Burger King TenderCrisp Chicken	780	45	11	1,730
Burger King BK Fish Filet	520	30	NA	840
French Fries				
McDonald's, small (2½ oz)	230	11	5	140
Burger King, small (2½ oz)	230	11	6	410
Wendy's, small (3 oz)	280	14	6	270
McDonald's, medium (4 oz)	350	16	7	220
Wendy's, medium (5 oz)	440	21	9	430
Burger King, medium (4 oz)	360	18	10	640
Wendy's, Biggie (5½ oz)	490	24	10	480
McDonald's, large (6 oz)	520	25	11	330
Wendy's, Great Biggie (6½ oz)	590	29	12	570
Burger King, large (5½ oz)	500	25	13	880
Burger King, king (7 oz)	600	30	16	1,070
Chicken Nuggets (no. pieces—weight)				
McDonald's McNuggets (6–3½ oz)	250	15	5	670
Burger King Tenders (5–2½ oz)	210	12	6	530
McDonald's Selects (3–4½ oz)	380	20	6	930
Wendy's Homestyle Strips (3–5½ oz)	410	18	7	1,470
McDonald's McNuggets (10–5½ oz)	420	24	8	1,120
Burger King Tenders (8–4½ oz)	340	19	9	840
McDonald's Selects (5–8 oz)	630	33	11	1,550
McDonald's McNuggets (20–11½ oz)	840	49	16	2,240
McDonald's Selects (10–15½ oz)	1,270	66	21	3,100
Entrée Salads				
Burger King Fire-Grilled Chicken or Shrimp Garden Salad, Vinaigrette[1]	310	18	4	1,770
Wendy's Mandarin Chicken Salad, Oriental Sesame dressing	550	26	4	1,210
Burger King Fire-Grilled Chicken or Shrimp Caesar Salad, Caesar dressing[1]	320	20	5	1,600
McDonald's California Cobb Salad with Grilled Chicken, Cobb dressing	380	20	7	1,500
McDonald's Caesar Salad with Grilled Chicken, Caesar dressing	390	24	7	1,330
McDonald's Bacon Ranch Salad with Grilled Chicken, Ranch dressing	410	24	7	1,470
Wendy's Spring Mix Salad, Low Fat Honey Mustard dressing	420	27	8	630
McDonald's California Cobb Salad with Crispy Chicken, Cobb dressing	480	27	9	1,580

Table 5.4—continued

	Calories	Total Fat (grams)	Saturated + Trans Fat (grams)	Sodium (milligrams)
McDonald's Bacon Ranch Salad with Crispy Chicken, Ranch dressing	510	31	9	1,560
McDonald's Caesar Salad with Crispy Chicken, Caesar dressing	490	32	10	1,410
Burger King TenderCrisp Garden Salad, Ranch dressing	530	32	10	1,780
Wendy's Spring Mix Salad, House Vinaigrette	500	42	11	1,040
Burger King TenderCrisp Caesar Salad, Caesar dressing	520	33	11	1,870
Wendy's Chicken BLT Salad, Honey Mustard dressing	680	47	13	1,320
Wendy's Homestyle Chicken Strips Salad, Ranch dressing	670	45	15	1,760
Wendy's Taco Supremo Salad	680	31	17	1,700
Baked Potatoes & Chili				
Burger King Chili (7½ oz)	190	8	3	1,040
Wendy's Chili, small (8 oz)	220	6	3	780
Wendy's Broccoli & Cheese Potato	440	15	3	540
Wendy's Chili, large (12 oz)	330	9	4	1,170
Wendy's Sour Cream & Chives Potato	340	6	4	40
Wendy's Bacon & Cheese Potato	560	25	7	850
Desserts & Shakes				
Wendy's Fresh Fruit Bowl with Yogurt	220	1	0	90
McDonald's Apple Dippers with Dip (3 oz)	100	1	1	40
McDonald's Fruit 'n Yogurt Parfait (5½ oz)	160	2	1	90
McDonald's Ice Cream Cone (3 oz)	150	4	2	60
Wendy's Frosty, small (12 oz)	330	8	5	150
Burger King Dutch Apple Pie (4 oz)	340	14	6	470
McDonald's Triple Thick Shake (12 oz)[2]	430	10	7	150
McDonald's Baked Apple Pie (3 oz)	250	11	8	150
Burger King Shake, small (9 oz)[2]	410	14	8	250
Wendy's Frosty, large (20 oz)	540	13	9	250
Burger King Shake, medium (13 oz)[2]	580	18	12	360
McDonald's McFlurry (12 oz)[2]	590	18	12	220
McDonald's Triple Thick Shake (21 oz)[2]	750	18	12	270
Burger King Shake, large (19 oz)[2]	830	27	18	520
McDonald's Triple Thick Shake (32 oz)[2]	1,130	26	18	410

	Calories	Total Fat (grams)	Saturated + Trans Fat (grams)	Sodium (milligrams)
McDonald's Extra Value Meals				
(includes medium fries and medium Coke, unless noted)				
Chicken McGrill Sandwich	960	32	10	1,250
Filet-O-Fish Sandwich	960	34	12	880
Crispy Chicken Sandwich	1,060	39	13	1,330
Chicken McNuggets (10 pieces)	980	40	15	1,360
Big N' Tasty	1,080	45	18	970
Chicken Selects (5 pieces)	1,190	49	18	1,790
Big Mac	1,120	46	19	1,250
Quarter Pounder with Cheese	1,070	41	21	1,390
Double Quarter Pounder with Cheese, large Fries, large Coke	1,560	65	33	1,680
Burger King Value Meals				
(includes medium fries and medium Coke, unless noted)				
Chicken Whopper	1,130	43	14	2,050
Chicken Tenders (8 pieces)	900	37	18	1,480
Chicken Sandwich	1,120	46	18	1,910
TenderCrisp Chicken Sandwich	1,340	63	21	2,370
Whopper	1,260	60	24	1,660
Whopper, king fries, king Coke	1,690	72	30	2,090
Whopper with Cheese, large Fries, large Coke	1,590	74	33	2,330
Double Whopper with Cheese, king fries, king Coke	2,050	99	46	2,610
Wendy's Combo Meals				
(includes Biggie fries and medium cola, unless noted)				
Ultimate Chicken Grill Sandwich, Salad with Low Fat Honey Mustard, Iced Tea	510	10	2	1,450
Homestyle Chicken Fillet Sandwich	1,150	46	16	1,800
Homestyle Chicken Strips (3 pieces)	1,020	42	17	1,950
Classic Single	1,040	44	18	1,370
Big Bacon Classic	1,190	53	24	1,870
Classic Double with Cheese, Great Biggie Fries, Biggie Cola	1,480	68	31	2,040
Classic Triple with Cheese, Great Biggie Fries, Biggie Cola	1,750	88	41	2,630

*Limited availability. [1]Average of the items listed. [2]Average of all flavors. NA Number not available.

Daily Values (daily limits for a 2,000-calorie diet): *Total Fat:* 65 grams. *Saturated + Trans Fat:* 20 grams. *Sodium:* 2,400 milligrams.

Sources: McDonald's, Burger King, Wendy's.

The use of information from this article for commercial purposes is strictly prohibited without written permission from CSPI.

Source: Nutrition Action Health Letter, "Fast Food in '05," March 2005.

Table 5.5 Making Better Fast Food Choices

Fast food meals can be high in calories, fat, cholesterol, and sodium. But it is still possible to eat fast food occasionally and follow a sensible diet. Take a look at how a few sample meals stack up against one another, and against the recommended daily intake for calories (2,000–2,700 per day), fat (no more than 50–80 g), cholesterol (no more than 300 mg), and sodium (no more than 1,100–3,300 mg).

	Poor choice	Sensible choice
Burger (McDonald's)	Double quarter-pound burger with cheese, large fries, 16 oz soda	Hamburger, small fries, 16 oz diet soda
	1,560 calories *65 g fat* *98 mg cholesterol* *1,680 mg sodium*	*490 calories* *20 g fat* *30 mg cholesterol* *670 mg sodium*
Pizza (Domino's)	4 slices sausage and mushroom pizza, 16 oz soda	3 slices cheese pizza, 16 oz diet soda
	1,000 calories *28 g fat* *62 mg cholesterol* *2,302 mg sodium*	*516 calories* *15 g fat* *29 mg cholesterol* *1,470 mg sodium*
Chicken (KFC)	2 pieces fried chicken (breast and wing), buttermilk biscuit, mashed potatoes with gravy, corn-on-the-cob, 15 oz soda	1 piece fried chicken (wing), mashed potatoes with gravy, cole slaw, 15 oz diet soda
	1,232 calories *57 g fat* *157 mg cholesterol* *2,276 mg sodium*	*373 calories* *19 g fat* *46 mg cholesterol* *943 mg sodium*
Taco (Taco Bell)	Taco salad, 16 oz soda	3 light tacos, 16 oz diet soda
	1,057 calories *55 g fat* *80 mg cholesterol* *1,620 mg sodium*	*420 calories* *15 g fat* *60 mg cholesterol* *840 mg sodium*

SOURCE: Adapted from "Fast Food Facts" from the office of the Minnesota Attorney General: *www.olen.com/food/book.html*.

two bacon strips, and two sausage links—contains 1,261 calories and 79 grams of fat. Many of the "meal deals" offered by restaurants, such as Burger King's King Value Meal (a Double Whopper with Cheese) and Wendy's Classic Triple with Cheese plus Great Biggie Fries and a Biggie Cola, supply more than a day's worth of calories and sodium and two days of saturated and trans fat.

Who are these restaurants appealing to with these menu items? Research shows that men ages 18 to 24 make fast-food choices based on getting the most for the least amount of money, not on nutritional value. And don't be fooled by thinking that if it's salad it's healthy, because that can be far from the truth. Wendy's Garden Sensations Salads, for example, have half the daily fat allowance and one third of the day's sodium. Burger King's TenderCrisp salads have 500 calories and 11 grams of fat, and McDonald's salads have 500 calories, 19 grams of fat, and half the day's allotment of sodium.

On the other side of the coin, some healthy fast-food choices are Burger King's veggie burger with 380 calories (although it contains 930 mg of sodium), Wendy's Ulti-

mate Chicken Grill (360 calories), McDonald's Chicken McGrill (400 calories), McDonald's Hamburger (260 calories,) and McDonald's fruit and yogurt (160 calories).

Table 5.5 shows some other healthy food choices you can make at several fast-food restaurants.

Functional Foods

At the forefront of healthful nutrition is the identification and development of foods intended to affect a particular health problem or to improve the functional capability of the body. **Functional foods** contain not

> **Key Terms**
>
> **functional foods** foods capable of contributing to the improvement/prevention of specific health problems

What Does "Organically Grown" Really Mean?

The new USDA organic food labels went into effect in October 2002 to standardize regulations for foods grown without synthetic pesticides or other chemicals. Under the new USDA rules, organic means:

- Meat, poultry, and eggs are from animals given no growth hormones or antibiotics. Vitamin and mineral supplements are allowed. Livestock are given organic feed and live in conditions that allow for "exercise, freedom of movement and reduction of stress."

- Products are not genetically engineered or irradiated to kill germs.

- Crops are grown on land that has not been fertilized with sewage sludge or chemical fertilizers.

- Pests and plant disease are treated primarily with insect predators, traps, natural repellants, and other nonchemical methods.

- Weeds are controlled by mulching, mowing, hand weeding, or mechanical cultivation, not chemical herbicides.

There are different types of organic foods: "100% organic," meaning the food contains all organic ingredients; "organic," which means at least 95% of the product is organic; and "made with organic ingredients," which means at least 70% of the food is organic as defined above.

only recognized nutrients but also new or enhanced elements that impart medicine-like properties to the food. Alternative labels also exist for various subclasses of functional foods, such as *nutraceuticals,* or food elements that may be packaged in forms appearing more like medications (for example, pills or capsules), and *probiotics.*[18] **Probiotics** are living bacteria (good bugs) that are thought to help prevent disease and boost the immune system. They make the environment in the digestive system inhospitable for harmful bacteria (the bad bugs). More than 400 types of bacteria reside in and on our bodies and outnumber human cells 10 to 1. Yogurt is one example of a food that gives you a dose of these good bugs—lactobacillus bulgaris.

Examples of functional foods include garlic (believed to lower cholesterol), olive oil (thought to prevent heart disease), foods high in dietary fiber (which prevent constipation and lower cholesterol), and foods rich in calcium (which prevent osteoporosis). In addition, foods that contain high levels of vitamins A, C, and E—primarily fruits and vegetables—and provide the body with natural sources of antioxidants are functional foods.

Other functional foods are those that contain or are enriched with folic acid. These vitamin B–family foods aid in the prevention of spina bifida and other neural tube defects and the prevention of heart disease. Foods

that are rich in selenium are sometimes categorized as functional foods because of selenium's potential as an agent in cancer prevention. Most recently, the FDA has approved a "heart healthy" label for foods that are rich in soy protein.[19] All of the functional foods discussed here are approved to carry **health claims** on the basis of current FDA criteria.[20]

One category of functional foods being researched is vegetables that are genetically engineered to produce a specific biological element that is important to human health. An example is tomatoes that are high in lycopene. Another example, as described earlier, is a new type of margarine that can lower the level of and change the properties of blood cholesterol. Food technologists are interested in expanding the functional food family to include a greater array of health-enhancing food items.

 TALKING POINTS What fast-food restaurants are your favorites? Are you surprised at any of the information in this chapter regarding your favorite meals? Will you change your order next time you visit a fast-food restaurant?

Food Additives

Today many people believe that the food they consume is unhealthy because of the 2,800 generally recognized as safe (GRAS) **food additives** that can be put into food during production, processing, and preparation. But should these additives be banned?

Food additives refer to substances added to food to provide color or flavor, replace sugar or fat, or improve nutritional content, texture, or shelf life. Food additives must undergo FDA testing and approval to ensure that the benefits outweigh any risks associated with these additives. For example, emulsifiers help to give peanut butter a more consistent texture and prevent separation

---

Key Terms

probiotics living bacteria (good bugs) that help to prevent disease and strengthen the immune system

health claims liability statements attesting to a food's contribution to the improvement/prevention of specific health problems

food additives chemical compounds intentionally added to the food supply to change some aspect of the food, such as its color or texture

I am always in a hurry and don't have time to cook, and so a lot of my meals end up being fast food. Are there better choices I can make when eating on the run?

The typical American eats about three hamburgers and four orders of French fries each week, so you aren't alone. With over 300,000 fast-food restaurants in the United States, fast food is definitely part of the American lifestyle. Here are some things to consider when eating at fast food restaurants:

- Don't supersize! Go for the "small" or "regular" size.
- Don't wait until you are starving because that leads to overeating and supersizing!
- Decide what you want to order ahead of time and don't be swayed by "value meal" or what "looks good."
- Ask for a nutritional guide for the menu. Look at the calories, fat grams, and sodium when making your selection.

- Order grilled instead of fried chicken or fish.
- Look for the "light" choices.
- Limit your condiments. Mustard, ketchup, salsa, and low-fat or fat-free condiments and dressing are preferable to regular mayonnaise or high-fat dressings.
- For breakfast, choose cereal and milk or pancakes rather than a breakfast sandwich (which can have about 475 calories, 30 grams of fat, and 1,260 mg of sodium).
- Bring fast food from home! Buy portable foods at the grocery store to take with you that can be eaten quickly and easily, such as portable yogurt, a banana or apple, low-fat granola bar, or breakfast bar.
- Order low-fat or skim milk or water instead of soda.
- Go to a variety of different kinds of fast-food restaurants so you aren't eating hamburgers every day, and set a limit on how many meals you are going to eat out each week.

while stabilizers and thickeners can give ice cream a smooth, uniform texture. Preservatives such as antioxidants prevent apples from turning brown from exposure to air and fats and oils in baked goods from spoiling. The three most common additives are sugar, salt, and corn syrup.[21]

Food Labels

Since 1973, the FDA has required food manufacturers to provide nutritional information (labels) on products to which one or more nutrients have been added or for which some nutritional claim has been made. Originally, there was concern about whether the public could understand the labels and whether additional information would be required. So the FDA, in consultation with individual states and public interest groups, developed new labeling regulations. Revised labels began appearing on food packages in May 1993. The currently used label is shown in Figure 5-3. Specific types of information contained on this label are highlighted.

Foods that were not initially covered by the 1993 food-labeling guidelines are gradually being assigned labels. For example, many single-ingredient meats are now being labeled. Processed meat, fish, and poultry products, such as hot dogs and chicken patties, must bear labels. Fresh fruits and vegetables are not required to be labeled, but many stores label them voluntarily.

Recent additions to the 1993 requirements include the labeling of fruit juices for pasteurization (unpasteurized

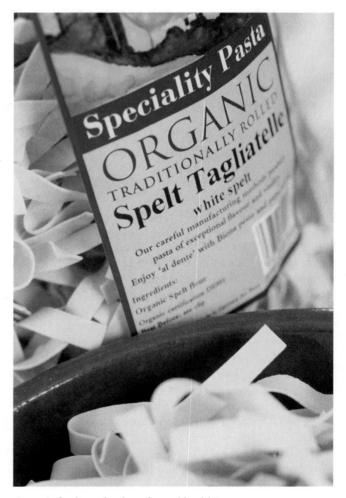

Organic foods tend to be safer and healthier.

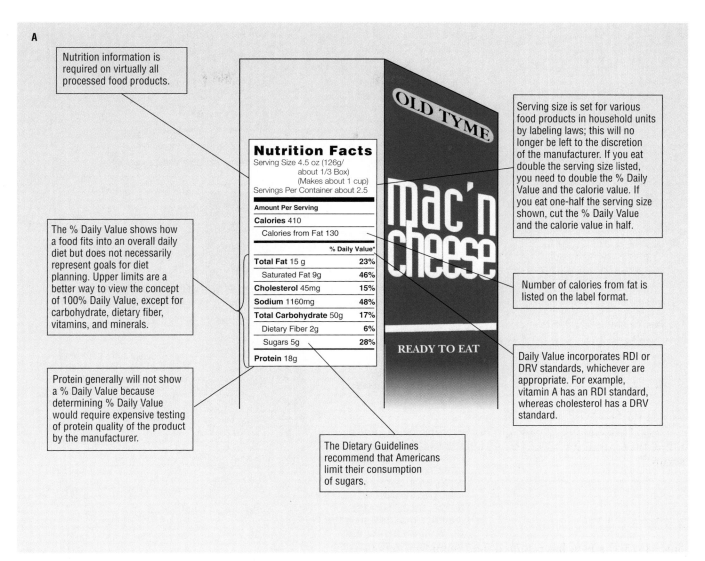

Figure 5-3   The Nutrition Facts panel on a food label

juices can be a source of *Escherichia coli [E. coli]* contamination), the identification of milk from cows whose food has been enhanced with bovine growth hormone, and the issuing of specific criteria for legal use of the term "organic." Some supermarkets also label fresh and frozen poultry and seafood with information about how it was prepared and stored. This point-of-purchase labeling is voluntary.

Beginning January 1, 2006, foodmakers have been required by the FDA to put the amount of trans fat on food labels, sparking some companies such as Frito-Lay and Kraft to start reducing and even eliminating trans fat from its products. The FDA has further recommended that food labels list calories in larger type print, list the percentage of the consumer's daily allotment of calories, and list the total amount of calories in the con-

tainer, not just the calories per serving. For example, pretzels might be listed as having 100 calories per serving and approximately 15 servings per bag and so it is up to you to compute how many servings and calories you have consumed. The FDA is also urging restaurants to list calories on their menus. The FDA prohibits any nutrient claim that it has not defined. For example, the FDA recently defined *low fat* as containing 3 grams or less of fat per serving (see the Star Box on page 115 for more on this). The FDA has not yet defined what can be considered to be low carb even though many foodmakers and restaurants use this term in their advertising. Consumers need to know what is meant by claims such as *low calorie, low fat,* and *low carb;* having a standard definition makes it much easier to make healthy and informed nutritional choices.

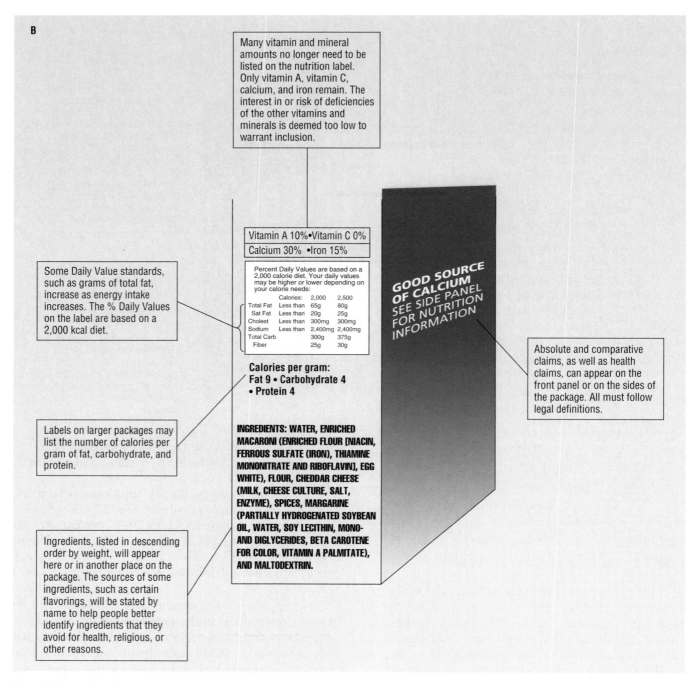

B

Many vitamin and mineral amounts no longer need to be listed on the nutrition label. Only vitamin A, vitamin C, calcium, and iron remain. The interest in or risk of deficiencies of the other vitamins and minerals is deemed too low to warrant inclusion.

Some Daily Value standards, such as grams of total fat, increase as energy intake increases. The % Daily Values on the label are based on a 2,000 kcal diet.

Labels on larger packages may list the number of calories per gram of fat, carbohydrate, and protein.

Ingredients, listed in descending order by weight, will appear here or in another place on the package. The sources of some ingredients, such as certain flavorings, will be stated by name to help people better identify ingredients that they avoid for health, religious, or other reasons.

Vitamin A 10% • Vitamin C 0%
Calcium 30% • Iron 15%

Percent Daily Values are based on a 2,000 calorie diet. Your daily values may be higher or lower depending on your calorie needs:

		Calories:	2,000	2,500
Total Fat	Less than		65g	80g
Sat Fat	Less than		20g	25g
Cholest	Less than		300mg	300mg
Sodium	Less than		2,400mg	2,400mg
Total Carb			300g	375g
Fiber			25g	30g

Calories per gram:
Fat 9 • Carbohydrate 4
• Protein 4

INGREDIENTS: WATER, ENRICHED MACARONI (ENRICHED FLOUR [NIACIN, FERROUS SULFATE (IRON), THIAMINE MONONITRATE AND RIBOFLAVIN], EGG WHITE), FLOUR, CHEDDAR CHEESE (MILK, CHEESE CULTURE, SALT, ENZYME), SPICES, MARGARINE (PARTIALLY HYDROGENATED SOYBEAN OIL, WATER, SOY LECITHIN, MONO- AND DIGLYCERIDES, BETA CAROTENE FOR COLOR, VITAMIN A PALMITATE), AND MALTODEXTRIN.

GOOD SOURCE OF CALCIUM SEE SIDE PANEL FOR NUTRITION INFORMATION

Absolute and comparative claims, as well as health claims, can appear on the front panel or on the sides of the package. All must follow legal definitions.

Figure 5-3 *continued*

There is also a push for the FDA to make food labels clearer, more understandable to children as well as to adults, and uniform. This is especially important for people with food allergies, whose health may depend on the clarity of a food label. For example "whey, casein, and lactoglobulin" can be used to indicate the presence of milk in a product, but some people who are lactose intolerant, may not realize that they are consuming a milk product. Additionally, some restaurant menus now state the nutritional content of some selections and provide cautionary notes about their safe cooking.

Dietary Supplements

In 2004 it was estimated that Americans spent 19 billion dollars on a wide array of over-the-counter (OTC) products known collectively as *dietary supplements.*

These nonprescription products are legally described as:[22]

- Products (other than tobacco) that are intended to supplement the diet, including vitamins, amino acids, minerals, glandular extracts, herbs, and other plant products such as fungi
- Products that are intended for use by people to supplement the total daily intake of nutrients in the diet
- Products that are intended to be ingested in tablet, capsule, softgel, gelcap, and liquid form
- Products that are not in themselves to be used as conventional foods or as the only items of a meal or diet

Unlike prescription medications (see Chapter 15), dietary supplements have been available in the marketplace for years almost without restriction. However, dietary supplements now must be deemed safe for human use on the basis of information supplied to the FDA by the manufacturers. In addition, the labels on these products cannot make a direct claim, with the exception of calcium and folic acid supplements, that they can cure or prevent illnesses. However, other materials with such claims may be displayed close to the dietary supplements themselves. Further, the labels on dietary supplements must remind consumers that the FDA has not required these products to undergo the rigorous research required

of prescription medications, and so the FDA cannot attest to their effectiveness. Beyond this, consumers are left to themselves to decide whether to purchase and use dietary supplements.

Probiotic products, dietary supplements with live bacteria, are gaining in popularity. The U.S. sales of probiotic supplements have increased 10–15 percent over the past 5 years, reaching $170 million in 2002. Actimel is one of the biggest sellers, claiming to "help to strengthen your body's natural defenses" and enhance your immune system.[23]

Easily accessible to anyone, over 15,000 different dietary supplements can be purchased in grocery stores, drugstores, and discount stores, through mail-order catalogs, and over the Internet. Because of the great demand for these products, major pharmaceutical companies are now entering the dietary supplement field. Whether this trend leads to the development of more effective products, or to a greater effort on the part of the FDA to demand proof of effectiveness, remains to be seen. By definition, supplements are not foods but simply "supplements." Therefore they remain free from requirements to substantiate their claims of effectiveness (as now required for functional foods).

TALKING POINTS A friend asks you about the advantages and disadvantages of taking a dietary supplement. What would you point out to your friend?

Food Safety

Technological advances in food manufacture and processing have done much to assure that the food we eat is fresh and safe. Yet concern is growing that certain recent developments may also produce harmful effects on humans. For example the preparation, handling, and storage of food, irradiation of foods, and genetic engineering of foods all contribute to the safety of our food in terms of food contamination.

Foodborne Illness

Foodborne illness or food poisoning is the result of eating contaminated food. The symptoms of food poisoning can be easily mistaken for the flu—fatigue, chills, mild fever, dizziness, headaches, upset stomach, diarrhea, and severe cramps. Illness develops within 1 to 6 hours following ingestion of the contaminated food and recovering is fairly rapid.[24] Bacteria are the culprits in most cases of food poisoning, which can be the result of food not being cooked thoroughly to destroy bacteria or not keeping food cool enough to slow their growth. In addition, nearly half of all cases of food poisoning can be prevented with proper hand washing so as to not contaminate food by viruses, parasites, or toxic chemicals. Food safety is such an important issue that the USDA incorporated it into the new dietary guidelines. (Some of the guidelines are included in Changing for the Better on page 131.) Food should be refrigerated below 40° Fahrenheit or kept warm above 140° Fahrenheit. Between 40 and 140° Fahrenheit, bacteria can double in number in as little as 20 minutes, so it is important to keep food at safe temperatures. (See Figure 5-4 on temperature rules for safe cooking and handling of foods.)

Most of us know that we must wash our hands before handling food; however, do you use the USDA's recommended protocol for hand washing? They recommend washing your hands often during food preparation, wetting your hands, applying soap, rubbing your hands for 29 seconds, rinsing hands thoroughly under clean, warm, running water and drying your hands completely using a clean disposable or cloth towel.

It is estimated that 76 million Americans are the victims of food poisoning each year, and about 5,000 of these people die.

Salmonella is the most common foodborne illness and is found mostly in raw or undercooked poultry, meat, eggs, fish, and unpasteurized milk. *Clostridium perfringens,* also called the "buffet germ," grows where there is little to no oxygen and grows fastest in large portions held at low or room temperatures. For this reason, buffet table servings should be replaced often and leftovers should be refrigerated quickly. Refrigerated leftovers may become harmful to eat after 3 days. The old adage "if in doubt, throw it out" applies to any questionable leftovers. A third type of food

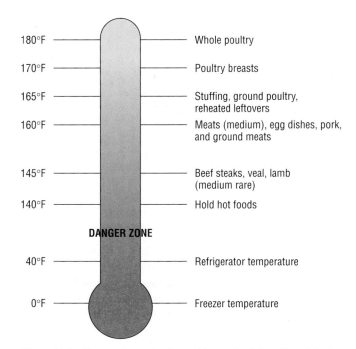

Figure 5-4 Temperature rules for cooking and safe handling of food

poisoning is botulism which is rare but often fatal. It is caused from home-canned or commercially canned food that hasn't been processed or stored properly. Some warning signs are swollen or dented cans or lids, cracked jars, loose lids, and clear liquids turned milky.

The Center for Science in the Public Interest found that fruits and vegetables account for the majority of foodborne illnesses. Salads are by far the biggest culprit. The reason for this seems to be because some of the water used to irrigate and wash produce is contaminated with human and animal feces. This problem can be difficult to regulate or correct, because produce comes from all over the world, not just from the United States.

Safe Handling of Food

It is important to handle food properly to avoid food poisoning. Frequent hand washing is at the top of the list of food safety tips. Bacteria live and multiply on warm, moist hands, and hands can inadvertently transport germs from one surface to another. It is also important to clean work surfaces with hot, soapy water and keep nonfood items such as the mail, newspapers, and purses, off the countertops. Some people advocate the use of antibacterial products, whereas others maintain that if they are overused, these products can lose their effectiveness, and bacteria then become resistant to them. Utensils, dishes, cutting boards, cookware, and towels and sponges need to be washed in hot, soapy water and rinsed well.[25]

Irradiation of Food

Because of the increasing concern about contaminated meat and meat products, the first irradiated meat, ground beef, arrived in American supermarkets in early 2000. Irradiated frozen chicken was introduced more recently. Irradiation is a process that causes damage to the DNA of disease-causing bacteria such as salmonella and E. coli as well as of insects, parasites, and other organisms so that they can't reproduce. While irradiated meat has much lower bacteria levels than regular meat does, irradiation doesn't destroy all bacteria in meat. In fact, irradiation actually destroys fewer bacteria than does proper cooking.[24] There is also some concern that irradiation will lull consumers into a false sense of security so that they erroneously believe that they don't have to take the usual precautions in food handling and preparation. For example, undercooking, unclean work surfaces, unwashed cooking utensils, and improper storage can still contaminate meat. Some also claim that irradiated meat has a distinct off-taste and a smell, like "singed hair."

Safe Farming Techniques

In recent decades, there has been an increased push toward ensuring better treatment of animals raised for slaughter and for dairy production in the United States. As a result of recent reforms, more than half of beef cattle in North America meet their end at slaughterhouses based on innovative designs that consider the fears and inclinations of herd animals. The cages of laying hens are nearly one third larger than the old ones were, and the practice of starving hens for weeks at a time to stimulate egg production is beginning to be phased out. These reforms are important to ensure more humane treatment of these animals, but they are also proving beneficial to human health and food quality. It has been suggested that there is an increase in the quality of meat when animals are treated humanely, with less bruising, improved tenderness, lower incidence of (dark-cutting beef,) and lessened occurrence of pale, soft, and dry pork. Furthermore, the taste of eggs is said to be significantly better if they come from humanely treated hens.

One important component in these reforms—some of which have been government mandated and others voluntarily adopted by the agricultural industry—relates to the feed given to beef cattle. The spread of bovine spongiform encephalopathy, more commonly known as Mad Cow Disease, has largely been attributed to the use of animal feed containing the protein-rich by-products of slaughtered cows, including nerve tissue, the tissue most likely to harbor the disease. Such feed—which is believed to be the primary, if not the only, way the disease can be transmitted—was banned in the United States and Canada

in August 1997.[26] While the disease had been restricted to European cows, a number of cases of Mad Cow detected in American cattle in late 2003 encouraged the U.S. government to impose even stricter rules to protect the nation's beef supply from the disease, including banning the butchering of sick or injured cows, banning certain animal parts from the food supply, and increasing testing on suspect animals.[27]

Eliminating animal products from feed has also proven beneficial in hens. Many consumers choose only to eat poultry and eggs from free-range, vegetarian-fed chickens, for health and safety reasons. Several companies (such as Eggland's Best) claim that their vegetarian-fed hens produce eggs that have seven times more vitamin E, are lower in cholesterol, have a higher unsaturated/saturated fat ratio, and contain more omega-3 fatty acids than do factory-farmed eggs.[28]

Interestingly, McDonald's Corporation has been one of the champions for animal welfare reform. Since 1997, the fast-food leader has required all of its meat producers to undergo animal welfare audits; in 1999 they conducted 100 audits in the United States, and in 2002, they did 500 worldwide. Because McDonald's makes up such a formidable part of the meat industry, few companies could afford to lose its business by not complying with its animal welfare standards. Thus McDonald's has been instrumental in pushing the entire industry to change its production techniques.[29] The state of Florida has also been a forerunner in pushing for animal welfare in its recent passage of a measure outlawing slow stalls, where pregnant pigs are confined in stalls 2 feet wide and 7 feet long, unable to turn around or walk for much of their 115-day pregnancy.

Genetically Modified Foods

Biotech crops increased 20 percent in 2004, with the United States, Argentina, and Canada being the front-runners.[30] The success of American agriculture, in terms of food quality and marketability, has been based on the ability to genetically alter food sources to improve yield, reduce production costs, and introduce new food characteristics. Today, however, genetic technology is so sophisticated that changes are being introduced faster than scientists can fully evaluate their effects. Concerned individuals and agencies in the United States and abroad called for more extensive longitudinal research into safety issues and stricter labeling requirements for genetically modified foods. In January of 2001, the FDA determined that food companies did not need to label foods as having genetically modified components, although they could inform consumers that they are "derived through biotechnology." They had argued that without these measures consumers would have been at risk for unrecognized problems. Read more about genetically modified foods at the end of the chapter.

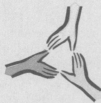

Learning from Our Diversity

Diverse Food Pyramids

Besides the new food pyramid discussed earlier in this chapter, other food pyramids exist. The Mediterranean food pyramid (Figure 5-5) emphasizes fruits, beans, legumes, nuts, vegetables, whole grains, and breads. In fact, the new food pyramid recommended by the USDA looks similar to the existing Mediterranean food pyramid. Many of the changes from the old to the new USDA food pyramid are in keeping with what had already been suggested by the Mediterranean food pyramid—for example, using more olive oil, limiting consumption of alcohol, eating more whole grains, fruits, and vegetables, choosing lean meat, and exercising daily.

The Asian food pyramid (Figure 5-6) limits meat consumption even more by recommending consumption of meat on a monthly basis and daily consumption of fish, shellfish, and dairy products. The Asian diet, like the Mediterranean diet, encourages daily intake of fruit, legumes, vegetables, and whole grains. In addition, the Asian diet includes rice and noodles and suggests eating poultry, eggs, and sweets only once a week.

The Latin American food pyramid (Figure 5-7) also advises consumption of meat, sweets, and eggs only once a week. Like the Asian diet, it encourages eating fish and shellfish on a daily basis, and, unlike the Mediterranean and Asian diets, it advises consumption of poultry on a daily basis. As in the other food pyramids, fruit, vegetables, beans, and whole grains are to be consumed every day, and physical exercise is emphasized by all three food pyramids.

The changes the USDA made to its new dietary guidelines appear to have some similarities to the Mediterranean, Asian, and Latin American pyramids in the emphasis on fruit, vegetables, whole grains, limited alcohol consumption, and increased physical activity.

Source: Nowack, D & Sarnoff, J (2003). *Food for Thought*, National Multiple Sclerosis Society, www.nationalmssociety.org/pdf/brochures/food.pdf.

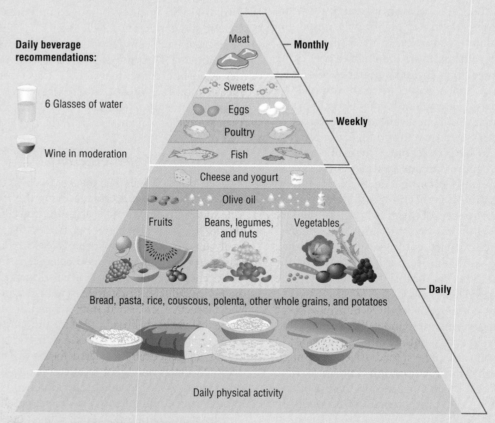

Figure 5-5   The Mediterranean Diet Pyramid

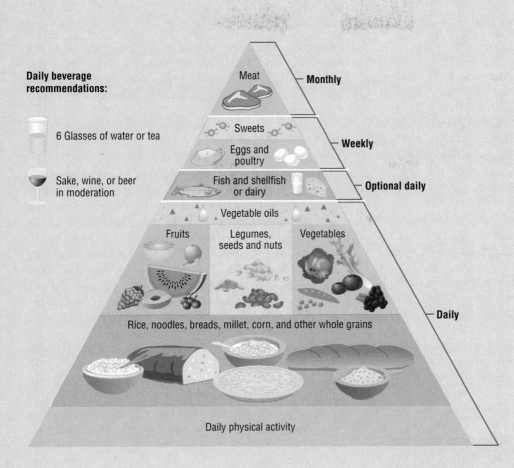

6 Glasses of water or tea

Sake, wine, or beer in moderation

Meat — Monthly

Sweets
Eggs and poultry — Weekly

Fish and shellfish or dairy — Optional daily

Vegetable oils

Fruits | Legumes, seeds and nuts | Vegetables

Rice, noodles, breads, millet, corn, and other whole grains — Daily

Daily physical activity

Figure 5-6 The Asian Diet Pyramid

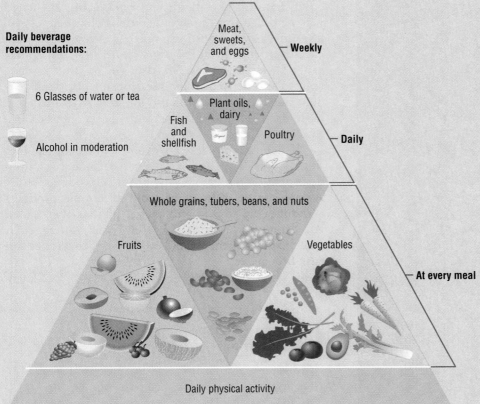

Daily beverage recommendations:

6 Glasses of water or tea

Alcohol in moderation

Meat, sweets, and eggs — Weekly

Plant oils, dairy

Fish and shellfish | Poultry — Daily

Whole grains, tubers, beans, and nuts

Fruits | Vegetables — At every meal

Daily physical activity

Figure 5-7 The Latin American Diet Pyramid

Vegetarian Diets

A *vegetarian diet* relies on plant sources for all or most of the nutrients needed by the body. This approach includes a range of diets from those that allow some animal sources of nutrients to those that exclude all animal sources. Studies show that vegetarians who eat a balanced diet don't seem to have any more iron-deficient problems than do meat eaters. Although the iron in plant food is not as well absorbed as the iron in animal food is, vegetarians tend to eat more of iron-containing foods and more vitamin C foods, which help with the absorption of the iron.[22] In addition, vegetarians tend to get enough calcium from dairy foods, tofu, beans, soybeans, calcium-fortified cereals, and vegetables such as broccoli. There has been some concern about a vitamin B_{12} deficiency, because animal foods are the best source for B_{12} and plant foods don't naturally contain the vitamin. However, soy foods such as some form of tempeh may contain vitamin B_{12}, although it is not as biologically active as the source in animal foods. Many soy products are fortified with vitamin B_{12} as well. It is

important also to note that the liver stores so much B_{12} that it would take years to become deficient in this vitamin.[22] Three types of vegetarian diets, beginning with the least restrictive, are summarized in the following sections.

Ovolactovegetarian Diet

Depending on the particular pattern of consuming eggs (*ovo*) and milk (*lacto*) or using one but not the other, an **ovolactovegetarian diet** can be a very sound approach to healthful eating for adults (see Figure 5-8 for an Ovolactovegetarian Food Guide Pyramid). Ovolactovegetarian diets provide the body with the essential amino acids and limit the high intake of fats involved in more conventional diets. The exclusion of meat as a protein source lowers the total fat intake, and the consumption of milk or eggs allows an adequate amount of saturated fat to remain in the diet. The consistent use of vegetable products as the primary source of nutrients complies with the current dietary recommendations for an increase in overall carbohydrates, complex carbohydrates, and fiber. Most vegetarians in the United States fit into this category. Vegetarians who do consume dairy products face challenges when making food choices if they wish to avoid other animal products in their food. Because most cheese is made with rennet, a coagulating agent that usually comes from stomachs of slaughtered newly born calves, many vegetarians eliminate cheese from their diet or opt for rennetless cheese. Vegetarian cheeses are manufactured using rennet from either fungal or bacterial sources. Similarly, yogurt is often made with gelatin derived from animal ligaments, skins, tendon, and bones (gelatin is also found in marshmallows, candy such as jelly beans and candy corn, poptarts, and a variety of other foods).

It has become easier to follow a vegetarian diet since stores have begun offering organic vegetarian items that do not contain these animal products. However, it can be difficult to avoid all animal products without being an avid and knowledgeable label reader. For example, McDonald's recently acknowledged it failed to disclose the use of beef flavoring in its fries and hash browns.

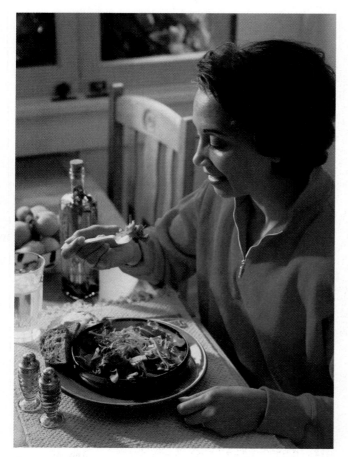

Over 12 million Americans are vegetarian.

Key Terms

ovolactovegetarian diet a diet that excludes all meat but does include the consumption of eggs and dairy products

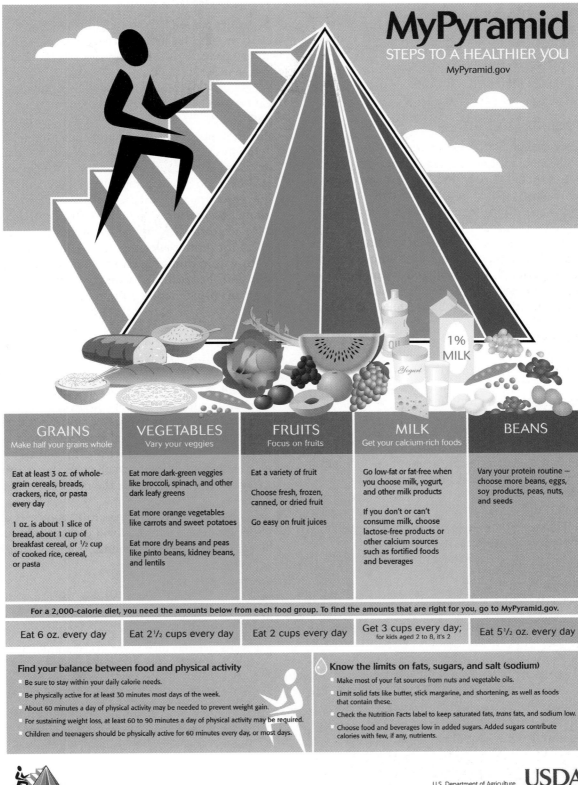

MyPyramid
STEPS TO A HEALTHIER YOU
MyPyramid.gov

GRAINS	VEGETABLES	FRUITS	MILK	BEANS
Make half your grains whole	Vary your veggies	Focus on fruits	Get your calcium-rich foods	
Eat at least 3 oz. of whole-grain cereals, breads, crackers, rice, or pasta every day	Eat more dark-green veggies like broccoli, spinach, and other dark leafy greens	Eat a variety of fruit	Go low-fat or fat-free when you choose milk, yogurt, and other milk products	Vary your protein routine — choose more beans, eggs, soy products, peas, nuts, and seeds
1 oz. is about 1 slice of bread, about 1 cup of breakfast cereal, or ½ cup of cooked rice, cereal, or pasta	Eat more orange vegetables like carrots and sweet potatoes Eat more dry beans and peas like pinto beans, kidney beans, and lentils	Choose fresh, frozen, canned, or dried fruit Go easy on fruit juices	If you don't or can't consume milk, choose lactose-free products or other calcium sources such as fortified foods and beverages	

For a 2,000-calorie diet, you need the amounts below from each food group. To find the amounts that are right for you, go to MyPyramid.gov.

| Eat 6 oz. every day | Eat 2½ cups every day | Eat 2 cups every day | Get 3 cups every day; for kids aged 2 to 8, it's 2 | Eat 5½ oz. every day |

Find your balance between food and physical activity
- Be sure to stay within your daily calorie needs.
- Be physically active for at least 30 minutes most days of the week.
- About 60 minutes a day of physical activity may be needed to prevent weight gain.
- For sustaining weight loss, at least 60 to 90 minutes a day of physical activity may be required.
- Children and teenagers should be physically active for 60 minutes every day, or most days.

Know the limits on fats, sugars, and salt (sodium)
- Make most of your fat sources from nuts and vegetable oils.
- Limit solid fats like butter, stick margarine, and shortening, as well as foods that contain these.
- Check the Nutrition Facts label to keep saturated fats, *trans* fats, and sodium low.
- Choose food and beverages low in added sugars. Added sugars contribute calories with few, if any, nutrients.

MyPyramid.gov
STEPS TO A HEALTHIER YOU

U.S. Department of Agriculture
Center for Nutrition Policy and Promotion
April 2005
CNPP-15

USDA is an equal opportunity provider and employer.

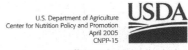

Figure 5-8 The new food pyramid for ovolactovegetarians (vegetarians who include eggs and dairy products in their diet)

Lactovegetarian Diet

People who include dairy products in their diet but no other animal products, including eggs, are *lactovegetarians*. A **pesco-vegetarian** eats fish, dairy products, and eggs along with plant foods.

Vegan Vegetarian Diet

A **vegan vegetarian diet** is one in which not only meat but also other animal products, including milk, cheese, and eggs, are excluded from the diet. When compared with the ovolactovegetarian diet, the vegan diet requires a higher level of nutritional understanding to avoid nutritional inadequacies.

One potential difficulty is that of obtaining all the essential amino acids. Since a single plant source does not contain all the essential amino acids, the vegan must learn to consistently employ a complementary diet. By carefully combining various grains, seeds, and legumes, amino acid deficiency can be prevented.

In addition to the potential amino acid deficiency, the vegan could have some difficulty in maintaining the necessary intake of vitamin B_{12}. Possible ramifications of inadequate B_{12} intake include depression, anemia, back pain, and menstrual irregularity. Vegans often have difficulty maintaining adequate intakes of iron, zinc, and calcium.[1] Calcium intake must be monitored closely by the vegan. In addition, vitamin D deficiencies can occur. Supplements and daily exposure to sunshine will aid in maintaining adequate levels of this vitamin.

> **TALKING POINTS** What do you think about vegetarian diets? If you were to follow a vegetarian diet, which one would you be more likely to choose?

Food Allergies

Being intolerant to certain foods is not the same as being allergic to particular foods. **Food intolerance** means that a food upsets your intestines, usually because of an enzyme deficiency. A lactase deficiency, for example, causes lactose intolerance. Lactose intolerance affects 20 percent of Caucasian Americans, 75 percent of African Americans, and 50 percent of Hispanic Americans. Intolerance of gluten (found in wheat, rye, barley, and perhaps oats) affects 1 of every 150 Americans and can cause malnutrition, premature osteoporosis, colon cancer, thyroid disease, diabetes, arthritis, miscarriage, and birth defects.

A **food allergy** mistakenly calls the body's disease fighting immune system into action, creating unpleasant and sometimes life-threatening symptoms. Peanuts, milk,

eggs, shellfish, tree nuts, fish, soy, and wheat account for 90 percent of food allergies. Eight percent of children and 2 percent of adults have food allergies. For some members of this group, food-based allergies may be serious or even life threatening.

Because food allergies generally develop slowly, initial symptoms may not be fully recognized or even associated with the food. It takes three exposures to the allergic food to obtain a significant food allergy reaction. The first time a person eats a food she is allergic to, she may have little or no reaction. The second time she eats this food, she will most likely have a more observable reaction, such as breaking out in hives, itching, runny nose, burning in the mouth, and wheezing. The third exposure can bring on a full-blown reaction, which for peanut allergies, among others, can result in death within minutes. There is no cure for food allergies, and the treatment is to avoid these foods and to carry an epi-pen (epinephrine) at all times.

Nutrition and the Older Adult

Nutritional needs change as adults age. Age-related changes to the structure and function of the body are primarily responsible for such altered nutritional requirements. These changes can involve the teeth, salivary glands, taste buds, oral muscles, gastric acid production, and peristaltic action. In addition, chronic constipation resulting from changes in gastrointestinal tract function can decrease the older adult's interest in eating.

The progressive lowering of the body's basal metabolism is another factor that will eventually influence the dietary patterns of older adults. As energy requirements

---

Key Terms

pesco-vegetarian diet a vegetarian diet that includes fish, dairy products, and eggs along with plant foods

vegan vegetarian diet a vegetarian diet that excludes all animal products, including eggs and dairy products

food intolerance an adverse reaction to a specific food that does not involve the immune system; usually caused by an enzyme deficiency

food allergy a reaction in which the immune system attacks an otherwise harmless food or ingredient; allergic reactions can range from mildly unpleasant to life threatening

fall, the body gradually senses the need for less food. In addition a tendency to decrease activity levels also occurs with aging. Because of this decreased need for calories, nutrient density—the nutritional value of food relative to calories supplied—is an important consideration for older adults. The new USDA dietary guidelines make some specific suggestions for people over 50. They include consuming more vitamin B_{12}, because older people tend to have difficulty absorbing this vitamin. Older adults are also encouraged to consume extra vitamin D-fortified foods, since this vitamin may be lacking in this group.

Psychosocial factors also alter the role of food in the lives of many older adults. Social isolation, depression, chronic alcohol consumption, loss of income, transportation limitations, and housing are lifestyle factors that can lessen the ease and enjoyment associated with the preparation and consumption of food. Consequently, a person's food intake might decrease.

International Nutritional Concerns

Nutritional concerns in the United States are centered on overnutrition, including fat density and excessive caloric intake. In contrast, in many areas of the world the main concern is the limited quantity and quality of food. Reasons for these problems are many, including the weather, the availability of arable land, religious practices, political unrest, war, social infrastructure, and material and technical shortages. Underlying nearly all of these factors, however, is unabated population growth.

To increase the availability of food to countries whose demand for food outweighs their ability to produce it, a number of steps have been suggested, including the following:

- Increase the yield of land currently under cultivation.
- Increase the amount of land under cultivation.
- Increase animal production on land not suitable for cultivation.
- Use water (seas, lakes, and ponds) more efficiently for the production of food.
- Develop unconventional foods through the application of technology.
- Improve nutritional practices through education.

Little progress is being made despite impressive technological breakthroughs in agriculture and food technology (such as a wide array of genetically modified seeds and soybean-enhanced infant foods), the efforts of governmental programs, and the support of the Food and Agricultural Organization of the United Nations and the U.S. Department of Agriculture. Particularly in Third World countries, where fertility rates are two to four times higher than those of the United States, annual food production needs to increase between 2.7 percent and 3.9 percent to keep up with population needs. With the world population now at 6.6 billion, and projected to reach 9 billion by 2070 before dipping to 8.4 billion in 2100,[31] food production in the coming decades may need to be increased beyond these estimates.

Taking Charge of Your Health

Smart Supermarket Shopping

- Make a shopping list before you go and stick to it!

- Don't go grocery shopping when you are hungry.

- Shop just once a week, don't make special trips.

- Read the food labels and check for the percentage of fat, sodium, sugar, and so on.

- Take note of the "sell by" or expiration date. The items stocked toward the back are usually the newest.

- For the single shopper, look for foods sold in single servings: juice, yogurt, frozen meals, soup, and pudding, for example.

- Buy fresh fruits and vegetables over canned and frozen. If buying canned or frozen fruits and vegetables, look for ones without added sugar, fats, salt, and sodium.

- Choose brown rice over white, whole wheat over white bread.

- Skip the ramen noodle soups. The noodles are usually flash-cooked in oil and high in fat and sodium.

- Avoid giant muffins, bagels, and donuts, and select the smaller ones.

- Meat labeled "select" is leaner than meat graded "choice."

- Leaner cuts of beef are flank, sirloin, and tenderloin. The leanest pork is fresh, canned, cured, or boiled ham, Canadian bacon, pork tenderloin, rib chops, and roast.

- Ground turkey and chicken can contain the skin, which makes it higher in fat and calories. For a lower-fat option, look for ground turkey or chicken meat. Ground turkey breast is lower still.

- Buy water-packed tuna and sardines rather than those packed in oil.

- Buy low-fat or fat-free milk rather than 2% or whole milk.

- Look for low-fat cheeses, sour cream, mayonnaise, and cream cheese that are labeled "part skim," "reduced fat," or "fat free."

- Buy canola or olive oil rather than corn oil, or use nonstick cooking spray.

- Consider buying cholesterol-free or reduced-cholesterol egg substitutes, especially if you don't use eggs very often, because they tend to last longer than fresh eggs do.

Source: Kirby J. *Dieting for Dummies.* New York: Wiley Publishing Co., 1998.

SUMMARY

- Carbohydrates, fat, and protein supply the body with calories.
- Fat is important for nutritional health beyond serving as the body's primary means of storage of excess calories.
- Saturated fats, including trans-fatty acids and cholesterol, should be carefully limited because of their association with chronic diseases.
- The food pyramid provides important dietary guidelines for a healthy diet.
- Protein supplies the body with amino acids needed to construct its own protein.
- Vitamins serve as catalysts for body responses and are found in water-soluble and fat-soluble forms.
- Minerals are incorporated into various tissues of the body and participate in regulatory functions within the body.
- An adequate amount of water and other fluids is required by the body daily and is obtained from a variety of food sources, including beverages.
- Fiber is undigestible plant material and has two forms, water soluble and water insoluble.

- Food allergies can be life threatening, and currently there is no cure for them. The most common food allergies are peanut, milk, egg, shellfish, tree nuts, fish, soy, and wheat.
- Fat-free or low-fat foods can be more calorie dense than anticipated.
- Fast foods should play only a limited role in daily food intake because of their high fat density and their high levels of sugar and sodium.
- Controversy exists about the application of new food technologies such as irradiation, genetic engineering, and animal welfare.
- Current dietary recommendations focus on the role of trans fat, saturated fat, sodium, and physical activity in health and disease.
- Nutrient density plays an important role in the management of caloric intake for people of all ages, particularly older adults.

REVIEW QUESTIONS

1. Which nutrients supply the body with calories?
2. What is the function of fat in nutritional health besides serving as the body's primary means of storage for excess calories? What is the basis of our current concern about saturated fats, cholesterol, and trans-fatty acids?

3. What is the principal role of protein in the body? How can complete protein be obtained by people who eat few or no animal products?
4. Which vitamins are water soluble and which are fat soluble? What is the current perception regarding the need for

vitamin supplementation? Which vitamins are regarded as antioxidants?

5. What are food allergies, and which are the most common?

6. What functions do minerals have in the body? What is a trace element?

7. What are the two principal forms of fiber, and how does each of them contribute to health?

8. How many glasses of water per day are currently recommended?

9. What method of grouping foods is now used?

10. What are the current dietary recommendations regarding trans fat, saturated fat, and sodium intake?

11. How can fat-free or low-fat foods be both low in nutritional density and high in caloric density?

12. What are functional foods, and how are they different from dietary supplements? Which has been empowered by the FDA to make health claims?

13. What information can be obtained from our current food labels?

14. What are an ovolactovegetarian diet and semivegetarianism, and how do they differ from a vegan diet?

15. What is nutrient density?

ENDNOTES

1. Wardlaw GM, Kessel M. *Perspective in Nutrition* (5ᵗʰ ed.). New York: McGraw-Hill, 2002.

2. Wardlaw GM. *Contemporary nutrition: Issues and insights.* New York: McGraw-Hill, 1999.

3. *Caring for Your School-Age Child: 5–12,* American Academy of Pediatrics, 2001.

4. Kummerow FA, Zhou Q, Mahfouz MM. Effect of trans-fatty acids on calcium influx into human arterial endothelial cells, *Am J Clin Nutr* 70(5):832–838, 1999.

5. Duyff R. *American Dietetic Association Complete Food and Nutrition Guide* (2ⁿᵈ ed.). Hoboken, NJ: John Wiley & Sons, Inc. 2002.

6. National Institutes of Health. *Practical Guide to the Identification, Evaluation and Treatment of Overweight and Obesity in Adults,* 2001.

7. Young VR. Soy protein in relation to human protein and amino acid nutrition, *J Am Diet Assoc* 91, 828–835, 1991.

8. Anderson J, Johnstone R, Cook-Newell M. Meta-analysis of the effects of soy protein intake on serum lipids, *N Engl J Med* 333, 276–282, 1995.

9. Greenberg ER, Sporn MB. Antioxidant vitamins, cancer, and cardiovascular disease, *N Engl J Med* 334(18):1189–1190, 1996.

10. Jacques PF, et al. The effect of folic acid fortification on plasma folate and total homocysteine concentrations, *N Engl J Med* 340(19):1449–1454, 1999.

11. Scariati PD, et al. Water supplementation of infants in the first month of life, *Arch Pediatr Adolesc Med* 151(8):830–832, 1997.

12. Children, water, and fluoride: AAPD parent information, American Academy of Pediatric Dentistry.

13. Sears W, Sears M. *The Family Nutrition Book,* New York: Little, Brown and Co., 1999.

14. American Cancer Society. *Cancer facts and figures*—The Association, 2001.

15. Marcus, E. On the Fast Track to Health. *Newsday,* p. B14, January 7, 2004.

16. Willett W. *Eat, Drink and Be Healthy,* New York: Free Press, 2001.

17. Waladkhani AR, Clemens MR. Effect of dietary phytochemicals on cancer, *Int J Mol Med* 1(4): 747–753, 1998.

18. Fransworth ER. What we are trying to do? *Medicinal Food News* 1(1):1–6, 1999.

19. FDA approves new health claim for soy protein and coronary heart disease [FDA talk paper], U.S. Food and Drug Administration Center for Food Safety and Applied Nutrition, October 20, 1999.

20. Kurtzweil P. Staking a claim to good health, *FDA Consumer,* November–December 1998.

21. Insel P, Turner E, Ross D. *Nutrition,* Sudbury, MA: Jones and Barlett Publishers, 2002.

22. Dietary Supplement Health and Education Act of 1994, U.S. Food and Drug Administration, Center for Food Safety and Applied Nutrition, 1 December 1995.

23. A bug for what's bugging you, in *USA Today,* D-1, July 9, 2003.

24. The Truth about Irradiated Meat, *Consumer Reports,* 34–37, August, 2003.

25. Williams S and Schlenker E. *Essentials of Nutrients and Diet Therapy* (8ᵗʰ ed.). St. Louis, MO: Mosby Inc., 2003.

26. Oppel RA, Jr. Infected cow old enough to have eaten now-banned feed. *The New York Times,* December 30, 2003.

27. Grady D. U.S. imposes stricter safety rules for preventing mad cow disease. *The New York Times,* December 31, 2003.

28. Corporate Website, *www.eggland.com.*

29. Food sellers push animal welfare, *USA Today,* August 13, 2003.

30. Biotech crops gained ground across globe, *USA Today,* January 13, 2005.

31. Lutz W, Sanderson W, Scherbov S. The end of the world population growth, *Nature* 412(6846): 543–545, 2001.

Is Cookie Monster Going on a Diet?

"C" is not for cookie anymore. C is for carrots. With the increase in childhood obesity, the ever-popular children's television show, *Sesame Street,* has decided to focus on teaching children about healthy foods and physical activity. According to Sesame Street's spokesperson, each show will open with a health tip for kids about nutrition, exercise, hygiene, and rest. There will be talking eggplants and carrots and new songs about the importance of physical activity. The Cookie Monster's new song is "A Cookie Is a Sometimes Food," as he learns the difference between sometimes foods (sweets) and anytime foods (fruits). Senator Hillary Clinton teaches him about the various textures and tastes of food, and Elmo learns to exercise with the help of Senate Majority Leader Bill Frist.

Of course, sitting in front of the television is probably not conducive to children increasing their activity level. Sixty percent of children reported that they don't participate in sports, and 25 percent say that they engage in no physical activity outside school. Researchers from the Harvard School of Health suggested that the more television children watch, the fewer fruits and vegetables they eat. This study found that, over the course of a year, children lack 13 percent of recommended nutrition from fruits and vegetables, owing to increased television viewing.

However, we can't hold the Cookie Monster solely responsible for the rising obesity rates in children. Surely Ronald McDonald, Burger King's Burgermeister, and that larger-than-life mouse Chuck E. Cheese have to shoulder some of the responsibility for children eating burgers, fries, pizza, and soft drinks. Junk food accounts for one-third of all calories consumed by all Americans, so adults are not necessarily good role models for children regarding healthy eating. Most school vending machines are filled with junk food such as sodas, chips, and candy bars. Sixty-seven percent of adolescents say they buy junk food from vending machines at school on a regular basis.

Legislation is being considered on a national level to regulate food sales in schools in order to restrict the types of foods and drinks sold there. School cafeterias are also under scrutiny as to how healthy the choices are for students. Some schools have eliminated the sale of soft drinks entirely and may eliminate other junk foods as well.

It is increasingly apparent that a number of factors contribute to the rising obesity rates among children. It will be interesting to see what kind of effect the Sometimes Cookie Monster and the All-the-Time Carrot Monster will have on children's eating habits.

Sources: "Cookie Monster Eating Less Cookies," *USA Today,* April 7, 2005. "School Vending Rated as Junk," *USA Today,* May 12, 2004.

personal assessment

Rate your plate

Take a closer look at yourself—your current food decisions and your lifestyle. Think about your typical eating pattern and food decisions.

Do You . . .

	Usually	Sometimes	Never
Consider nutrition when you make food choices?	❑	❑	❑
Try to eat regular meals (including breakfast), rather than skip or skimp on some?	❑	❑	❑
Choose nutritious snacks?	❑	❑	❑
Try to eat a variety of foods?	❑	❑	❑
Include new-to-you foods in meals and snacks?	❑	❑	❑
Try to balance your energy (calorie) intake with your physical activity?	❑	❑	❑

Now for the Details

Do You . . .

Eat at least 6 ounces of grain products daily?	❑	❑	❑
Eat at least 2½ cups of vegetables daily?	❑	❑	❑
Eat at least 2 cups of fruits daily?	❑	❑	❑
Consume at least 3 cups of milk, yogurt, or cheese daily?	❑	❑	❑

Go easy on higher-fat foods?	❑	❑	❑
Go easy on sweets?	❑	❑	❑
Drink 8 or more cups of fluids daily?	❑	❑	❑
Limit alcoholic beverages (no more than 1 daily for a woman or 2 for a man)?	❑	❑	❑

Score Yourself

Usually = 2 points
Sometimes = 1 point
Never = 0 points

If you scored . . .

24 or more points—Healthful eating seems to be your fitness habit already. Still, look for ways to stick to a healthful eating plan—and to make a "good thing" even better.

16 to 23 points—You're on track. A few easy changes could help you make your overall eating plan healthier.

9 to 15 points—Sometimes you eat smart—but not often enough to be your "fitness best."

0 to 8 points—For your good health, you're wise to rethink your overall eating style. Take it gradually—step by step!

Whatever your score, make moves for healthful eating. Gradually turn your "nevers" into "sometimes" and your "sometimes" into "usually."

Adapted from *The American Dietetic Association's Monthly Nutrition Companion: 31 Days to a Healthier Lifestyle,* Chronimed Publishing, 1997.

personal assessment

Are you feeding your feelings?

Sometimes people use food as a way of coping with their emotions and problems. To identify how you might be using food as a coping strategy and what feelings you tend to associate with eating, complete the following inventory.

1 = Never

2 = Rarely

3 = Occasionally

4 = Often

5 = Always

1. _____ Do you eat when you are angry?
2. _____ When you feel annoyed, do you turn to food?
3. _____ If someone lets you down, do you eat to comfort yourself?
4. _____ When you are having a bad day, do you notice that you eat more?
5. _____ Do you eat to cheer yourself up?
6. _____ Do you use food as a way of avoiding tasks you don't want to do?
7. _____ Do you view food as your friend when you are feeling lonely?
8. _____ Is food a way for you to comfort yourself when your life seems empty?
9. _____ When you are feeling upset, do you turn to food to calm yourself down?
10. _____ Do you eat more when you are anxious, worried, or stressed?
11. _____ Does eating help you to cope with feeling overwhelmed?
12. _____ Do you eat more when you are going through big changes or transitions in your life?
13. _____ Do you reward yourself with food?
14. _____ When you think you have done something wrong, do you punish yourself by eating?
15. _____ When you are feeling badly about yourself, do you eat more?
16. _____ When you feel discouraged about your efforts to improve yourself, do you eat more, thinking "what's the use of trying"?

_____ **TOTAL SCORE**

Interpretation

If you scored between . . .

0–13   You don't eat to cope with your emotions. Your eating may not be related to your emotional state. However, you may avoid eating when you are upset or having trouble coping with your feelings. You may run away from food rather than running to food to cope.

14–66   Although you fall in the average range, you may use food to deal with specific situations or feelings such as anger, loneliness, or boredom. See the breakdown of scores below to identify how you may be using food to cope with particular feelings.

67 and above   You run to food to cope with your emotions, and you may want to consider developing other ways of appropriately expressing your feelings.

If you answered "4" or "5" to most of questions #1 – #4, this can be indicative of eating when you are angry.

If you answered "4" or "5" to most of questions #5 – #8, this can be indicative of eating when you are lonely or bored.

If you answered "4" or "5" to most of questions #9 – #12, this can be an indication that you are a stress eater.

If you answered "4" or "5" to most of questions #13 – #16, this can be an indication that you are using food to cope with feelings of low self-esteem and self-worth.

chapter six

Maintaining a Healthy Weight

Chapter Objectives

On completing this chapter, you will be able to:

▪ describe the role of the media and entertainment industry in defining the ideal body image.

▪ define overweight and obesity.

▪ discuss how effective body mass index, electrical impedance, skin fold measurements, hydrostatic weighing, and appearance are as methods of assessing body weight.

▪ discuss the causes of obesity, including genetics, metabolism, physiological and hormonal changes, environmental factors, dietary practices, sociocultural factors, and psychological factors.

▪ describe the body's use of food in activity requirements, in basal metabolism, and in the thermic effect.

▪ discuss the primary types of weight-management techniques, including dietary alterations, surgical interventions, medications, weight loss programs, and physical activity.

▪ provide evidence supporting physical exercise as the most important component of a weight-loss program.

▪ define anorexia nervosa, bulimia nervosa, binge eating disorder, chewing and spitting food syndrome, night-time eating syndrome, body dysmorphic disorder, and bigorexia.

▪ discuss the at-risk groups for eating disorders and factors to consider for males with eating disorders.

▪ discuss ways of treating eating disorders.

Eye on the Media

Weight Loss and Reality

The Biggest Loser, The Swan, and *America's Next Top Model*—we are bombarded by television programs that tell us how we should be focused on our appearance, particularly on losing weight. Since the majority of adult Americans are overweight, weight loss would seem appealing to most television viewers. However, this preoccupation with appearance and weight sends a perilous message—that to feel good about yourself, you must be thin and beautiful. The shows also create an expectation of achieving the perfect body, which is an impossible goal.

The Biggest Loser is described as a "weight-loss drama" in which contestants follow comprehensive diet and exercise plans, supervised by physicians and personal trainers. They compete to see which team can lose the most weight. There are temptations and physical challenges along the way to make the endeavor even more difficult and perhaps more like real life. All the contestants from the first season continued to lose weight after the show ended, by continuing to exercise regularly and monitoring their caloric intake. Most of the contestants also refer to the support of their families and friends as another key factor in continuing to manage their weight. Some of the more positive components of the show are

- *Realization*—You must realize where you are so that you can figure out where you want to be. As Kirstie Alley from the show *Fat Actress* stated, "I didn't really realize I was fat until I saw the first show."

- *Coaching*— Many of the contestants continued to work with a personal trainer or exercised with a friend.

- *Accountability*—With millions of television viewers watching, along with family and friends, contestants feel some accountability. It is important to broadcast your weekly progress toward your goals. This is the reason many people find keeping a food diary to be helpful.

- *Rewards*—A healthier body, a grand prize of $250,000, book and television offers, tours, interviews, and notoriety are some of the obvious rewards mentioned by the contestants. They also talk of additional rewards, such as increased sense of self-esteem and self-worth, taking new risks, having more energy, and experiencing less stress.

- *Goals*—The contestants set weight goals during the show and continued to set weight management goals after the show ended. They also set goals such as helping others to manage their weight, wearing a swimsuit, or developing relationships.

- *Support*—Team members supported one another during the show, which seems to be a significant factor in continued success in managing their weight. Support from friends, family, and fans also helped to inspire and motivate these individuals to stay on course.

Of course you don't have to be on a television show to incorporate these factors into your own life. *USA Today* conducted a "Weight Loss Challenge" in 2004 and looked at what it takes to be a successful loser. They reported that according to 126 registered dieticians, the key factors are being honest with yourself, setting goals and priorities, having a positive attitude, and being organized. These factors sound remarkably similar to the weight-loss components identified in *The Biggest Loser* and *The Swan*.

On *The Swan*, a nine-episode series, 18 women get plastic surgery and a full makeover over a three-month time. The premise of the show is that women are transformed from "ugly ducklings" to "beautiful swans." The contestants are not permitted to see their new look until the end of their three-month makeover. The final episode consists of a two-hour beauty pageant with all the episodes' "winners." Their transformations include exercising with a personal trainer, following a commercial diet plan, having therapy sessions, and undergoing extensive cosmetic surgery such as brow-lift, chin implant, lower-eye-lift, face-lift, fat transfer to lips and cheek folds, tummy tuck, breast-lift, rhinoplasty, hair implants, dental surgery, and liposuction. The winners of the beauty pageants have been awarded such prizes as a contract as a spokesperson for NutriSystem, continued educational opportunities, a $100,000 necklace, a new car, a mink coat, and vacations to Las Vegas, Hawaii, and Thailand. As with *The Biggest Loser*, this program utilizes the important positive components of realization, account-ability, coaching, rewards, and support. However, this show also presents a dangerous message in linking self-esteem to beauty and setting some unrealistic goals (discussed later in this section).

American's Next Top Model shows the transformation of everyday young women who train to become supermodels. With supermodel Tyra Banks as their mentor, the participants learn how to model on catwalks, engage in intense physical-fitness exercises, and do fashion photo shoots and learn publicity skills. The Grand Prize package includes the opportunity to receive a Revlon modeling contract and to be managed by Wilhelmina Models, in addition to a guaranteed appearance in *Marie Claire* magazine.

The goals of these contestants are a par-ticularly important factor to consider. Most of the people on these shows are not just looking to lose weight and change their appearance; they believe that, by focusing on their appearance and weight, they will save their marriages, increase their self-esteem and self-confidence, become better mothers, have more successful careers—in essence become different people. For example, one of the contestants on *The Swan* beauty pageant said that one of the reasons she applied to be on the show was to save her marriage (which ended before the show did). Another contestant said she wanted to reinvent herself by changing her appearance so that she could stand up to her abusive husband. How realistic are these goals? Tiffany, a contestant on *Top Model* said that it was "one of the most humiliating experiences of my life."

What is the message to viewers? One of the contestants on *The Biggest Loser* said, "When you feel good, you look good," but these programs are sending the opposite message—that you need to look good to feel good, and looking good means being thin and fitting the cultural ideal of beauty.

The other component of these reality television makeover shows is the extensive use of plastic surgery costing tens of thousands of dollars for each contestant. How many of us have the money or the desire to undergo extensive plastic and reconstructive dental surgery? Actually, the numbers are rising to epidemic proportions. From 1996 to 2001, the number of Americans undergoing cosmetic surgery increased 1,125 percent. According to the American Society for Aesthetic Plastic Surgery, nearly 6.9 million cosmetic procedures occurred in the United States in one year, with women undergoing 88 percent of them. In this quick-fix society, some Americans are no longer willing to wait for the results they want. However, these fixes come with costs of their own, such as complications from surgeries and having to have repeated surgeries.

In addition, medical problems such as hypertension, heart attacks, gastrointestinal problems, osteoporosis, and kidney problems can result from unhealthy diets and taking diet supplements. These dangers would seem to outweigh the benefits of trying to reach the unrealistic goal of having the perfect body.

Rather than undergoing a series of diet programs, surgeries, and pills to manage your weight, you will be much healthier if you follow a balanced diet and engage in regular exercise. Shows like *The Swan, The Biggest Loser,* and *America's Next Top Model* prey on people's low self-esteem and exploit their fears about appearance. As was discussed in Chapter 2, there is much more to self-esteem than external factors such as how people see us and our outer appearance. In addition, the research shows that physical attractiveness does not predict self-esteem. In other words, some people who didn't think they were physically attractive had higher self-esteem than those who did see themselves as attractive.

Sources:
Attansai, K. "Anti-Aging Options Require Balanced Approach to Health, Beauty," *Today's Pentecostal Evangel,* August 10, 2003.
www.realitytvcalendar.com/shows/swan/html 2005.
www.nbc.com/The Biggest Loser/.

Weight management has become an obsession in American culture as well as a significant health problem. In the United States, obesity has risen at an epidemic rate during the past 20 years. One of the national health objectives for the year 2010 is to reduce the prevalence of obesity among adults to less than 15 percent.[1] Research indicates that the situation is worsening rather than improving. According to the National Center for Chronic Disease Prevention and Health Promotion, an estimated 65 percent of adult Americans are either overweight or obese.[2] Currently 30 percent, or 60 million, adult Americans are obese with more women (33 percent) than men (28 percent) meeting the criteria for obesity. Up 74 percent since 1991, the number of overweight children and adolescents has tripled in the past 20 years.[2]

When the body is supplied with more energy than it can use, the result is an excess of energy (or a **positive caloric balance**) stored in the form of fat. This continuous buildup of fat can eventually lead to obesity. Women eat 335 more calories and men eat 168 more calories per day than they did 30 years ago. Additionally, nearly two-thirds of Americans are not physically active on a regular basis, and 25 percent are completely sedentary.[3] In fact, in a study conducted by the RAND Institute, it was found that in terms of chronic conditions, obesity is a more powerful risk factor than poverty, heavy drinking, or smoking.[4]

Regardless of this issue, few experts question the real dangers to health and wellness from obesity. Among the health problems caused by or complicated by obesity are increased surgical risk, hypertension, various forms of heart disease, stroke, type 2 diabetes, several forms of cancer, deterioration of joints, complications during pregnancy, gallbladder disease, and an overall increased risk of mortality[5] (see Star box on page 144). Obesity is so closely associated with these chronic conditions that medical experts now recommend that obesity itself be defined and treated as a chronic disease.

Body Image and Self-Concept

Although physicians focus on obesity, in our image-conscious society, being overweight is also a problem. The media tell people that being overweight is undesirable and that they should conform to certain ideal **body images** (such as being tall, thin, and "cut" with muscular definition). For example, the average actress and model is thinner than 95 percent of the female population and weighs 23 percent less than the average woman.[6] The average American woman is 5'4", 143 pounds, and wears a size 10–12. The average model is 5'10" and 110 pounds.[7] Today's lean but muscular version of perfection is a very demanding standard for both women and men to meet.

People may become dissatisfied and concerned about their inability to achieve these ideals. The scope of this dissatisfaction is evident in a study of over 800 women, which revealed that nearly half were unhappy with their weight, muscle tone, hips, thighs, buttocks, and legs.[8] When this type of dissatisfaction exists, people begin to question their attractiveness, and their self-esteem tends to decline.

Overall, men report feeling more comfortable with their weight and perceive less pressure to be thin than women do. A national survey showed that 41 percent of men were dissatisfied with their weight, with many of these men wanting to gain weight and increase muscle mass. While the average American women wants to lose 11 pounds, the average American man wants to lose 1 pound or is happy with his weight.[11]

However, men do tend to have the desire to be more muscular, more "cut," bigger, and stronger. An increasing number of men have become obsessed with being bigger and more muscular, referred to as the "Adonis Complex."[12] This term comes from Greek mythology, which depicted Adonis as half man and half god, considered to be the ultimate in masculine beauty. Men with this preoccupation obsessively lift weights for hours a day, sometimes sacrificing important social relationships, jobs, or physical health.

In many cases, these men take anabolic steroids or diet supplements to get bigger. They manifest a sort of "reverse anorexia nervosa", also referred to as **bigorexia**. The main characteristic of bigorexia is the thought that no matter how hard you try, your body is never muscular enough.[12] Some men with the Adonis complex become preoccupied with fat as opposed to muscle and, hence, may develop eating disorders (discussed later in this chapter).

Research suggests that 2 to 3 million American men have used steroids or other supplements to increase muscle mass, often starting as teenagers. Steroid use can result in side effects such as psychiatric symptoms, including manic and aggressive symptoms while using steroids and depressive symptoms from withdrawal. Remarkably,

---

Key Terms

positive caloric balance caloric intake greater than caloric expenditure

body image our subjective perception of how our body appears

bigorexia the obsession with getting bigger and more muscular, and thinking that your body is never muscular enough

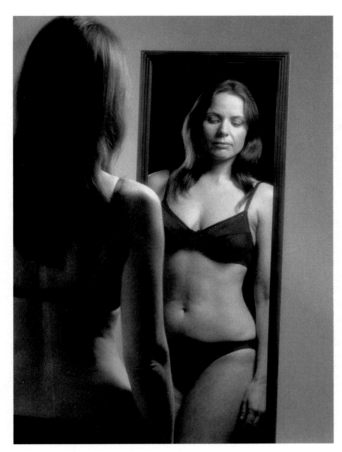

Studies show that mirrors can make us more self conscious, critical, and conforming.

parents, teachers, and even trained clinicians often remain unaware of steroid use despite these obvious physical and personality changes.

Dietary supplements such as creatine, glutamine, and androstenedione products have been advertised as "muscle and strength builders," as aids in recovering from workouts more quickly, and as immunity boosters. Baseball player Mark McGuire came under fire for his use of androstenedione, called *andro,* and brought increased attention to the use of these supplements among athletes and bodybuilders. McGuire publicly discouraged young people from taking andro and discontinued taking it himself. As with all dietary supplements, there is no regulation or standardization among these drugs, so the safe and effective dosage is not known. There is no research proving that these supplements actually do enhance athletic performance or increase muscle mass. What is known is that the side effects associated with taking these dietary supplements include shrinkage of testicles, growth of breast tissue, and impotence for men. Side effects for all youth include acne, early start of puberty, and stunted growth.

For this reason, the FDA has announced a crackdown on products containing androstenedione and is requesting companies to stop distributing dietary supplements containing androstenedione. The FDA is also encouraging Congress to consider legislation to classify these products as a controlled substance.

In comparison with being overweight, little media attention has been paid to being underweight. However, the body image problems experienced by some extremely thin people can be equally distressing.

Overweight and Obesity Defined

What's the difference between overweight and obesity? Doctors usually define **overweight** as a condition in which a person's weight is 1–19 percent higher than normal, as defined by a standard height-weight chart. **Obesity** is usually defined as a condition in which a person's weight is 20 percent or more above normal weight. "Morbid obesity" refers to being 50–100 percent above normal weight, more than 100 pounds over normal weight, or sufficiently overweight to interfere with health or normal functioning.[10]

Some clinicians and laymen continue to use standard height-weight tables to determine when weight is excessive. However, more precise techniques to determine body composition are currently available. Several of these techniques, including waist-to-hip ratio (*healthy body weight*), body mass index, "BOD POD" assessment, electrical impedance, skinfold measurements, and hydrostatic weighing, are described in the following section.

Determining Weight and Body Composition

Some of the techniques used to determine overweight and obesity are common and are routinely used by the general public. Others are expensive and of limited availability.

Key Terms

overweight a condition in which a person's excess fat accumulation results in a body weight that exceeds desirable weight by 1–19 percent

obesity a condition in which a person's body weight is 20 percent or more above desirable weight as determined by standard height/weight charts

Table 6.1 Body Mass Index Table

	Normal						Overweight					Obese						
BMI	19	20	21	22	23	24	25	26	27	28	29	30	31	32	33	34	35	36
Height (inches)									Body Weight (pounds)									
58	91	96	100	105	110	115	119	124	129	134	138	143	148	153	158	162	167	172
59	94	99	104	109	114	119	124	128	133	138	143	148	153	158	163	168	173	178
60	97	102	107	112	118	123	128	133	138	143	148	153	158	163	168	174	179	184
61	100	106	111	116	122	127	132	137	143	148	153	158	164	169	174	180	185	190
62	104	109	115	120	126	131	136	142	147	153	158	164	169	175	180	186	191	196
63	107	113	118	124	130	135	141	146	152	158	163	169	175	180	186	191	197	203
64	110	116	122	128	134	140	145	151	157	163	169	174	180	186	192	197	204	209
65	114	120	126	132	138	144	150	156	162	168	174	180	186	192	198	204	210	216
66	118	124	130	136	142	148	155	161	167	173	179	186	192	198	204	210	216	223
67	121	127	134	140	146	153	159	166	172	178	185	191	198	204	211	217	223	230
68	125	131	138	144	151	158	164	171	177	184	190	197	203	210	216	223	230	236
69	128	135	142	149	155	162	169	176	182	189	196	203	209	216	223	230	236	243
70	132	139	146	153	160	167	174	181	188	195	202	209	216	222	229	236	243	250
71	136	143	150	157	165	172	179	186	193	200	208	215	222	229	236	243	250	257
72	140	147	154	162	169	177	184	191	199	206	213	221	228	235	242	250	258	265
73	144	151	159	166	174	182	189	197	204	212	219	227	235	242	250	257	265	272
74	148	155	163	171	179	186	194	202	210	218	225	233	241	249	256	264	272	280
75	152	160	168	176	184	192	200	208	216	224	232	240	248	256	264	272	279	287
76	156	164	172	180	189	197	205	213	221	230	238	246	254	263	271	279	287	295

Source: Adapted from *Clinical Guidelines on the Identification, Evaluation, and Treatment of Overweight and Obesity in Adults: The Evidence Report, National Institutes of Health.*

Body Mass Index

Another method for assessing healthy body weight is the **body mass index (BMI).** BMI is calculated metrically as weight divided by height squared (kg/m^2). The BMI does not reflect body composition (fat versus lean tissue) or consider the degree of fat accumulated in the central body cavity. It is, nevertheless, widely used in determining obesity. Overweight is defined as a BMI between 25 and 29.9. Individuals are considered obese with a BMI of 30 or above. Severe or morbid obesity is when the BMI is greater than 40. See Table 6.1 to determine the healthy BMI range for your height.

An alternative method of determining the BMI is to use a **nomogram,** such as that shown in Figure 6-1. Like the BMI, the nomogram requires information about both weight and height.

Once you have determined your BMI, you can find out whether it falls within a healthy range by using Tables 6.1 and 6.2.

Height-Weight Tables

Height and weight tables were originally developed in 1983 to assist people in determining the relationship

Table 6.2 Healthy and Unhealthy BMIs

BMI	Weight Status
Below 18.5	Underweight
18.5–24.9	Normal
25.0–29.9	Overweight
30.0 and Above	Obese

between their weight and desirable standards. Nearly every version of these tables has come under criticism for not considering variables such as gender, age, frame size, and body composition. Some versions were

Key Terms

body mass index (BMI) a mathematical calculation based on weight and height; used to determine desirable body weight

nomogram a graphic means of finding an unknown value

							Extreme Obesity										
37	38	39	40	41	42	43	44	45	46	47	48	49	50	51	52	53	54
177	181	186	191	196	201	205	210	215	220	224	229	234	239	244	248	253	258
183	188	193	198	203	208	212	217	222	227	232	237	242	247	252	257	262	267
189	194	199	204	209	215	220	225	230	235	240	245	250	255	261	266	271	276
195	201	206	211	217	222	227	232	238	243	248	254	259	264	269	275	280	285
202	207	213	218	224	229	235	240	246	251	256	262	267	273	278	284	289	295
208	214	220	225	231	237	242	248	254	259	265	270	278	282	287	293	299	304
215	221	227	232	238	244	250	256	262	267	273	279	285	291	296	302	308	314
222	228	234	240	246	252	258	264	270	276	282	288	294	300	306	312	318	324
229	235	241	247	253	260	266	272	278	284	291	297	303	309	315	322	328	334
236	242	249	255	261	268	274	280	287	293	299	306	312	319	325	331	338	344
243	249	256	262	269	276	282	289	295	302	308	315	322	328	335	341	348	354
250	257	263	270	277	284	291	297	304	311	318	324	331	338	345	351	358	365
257	264	271	278	285	292	299	306	313	320	327	334	341	348	355	362	369	376
265	272	279	286	293	301	308	315	322	329	338	343	351	358	365	372	379	386
272	279	287	294	302	309	316	324	331	338	346	353	361	368	375	383	390	397
280	288	295	302	310	318	325	333	340	348	355	363	371	378	386	393	401	408
287	295	303	311	319	326	334	342	350	358	365	373	381	389	396	404	412	420
295	303	311	319	327	335	343	351	359	367	375	383	391	399	407	415	423	431
304	312	320	328	336	344	353	361	369	377	385	394	402	410	418	426	435	443

thought to be too rigorous in establishing cutoff points for ideal or **desirable weight,** and others were deemed too generous. Although still available, these tables are being gradually replaced by other assessment techniques.

 TALKING POINTS If a friend or close family member were dangerously overweight or obese, how would you express your concern?

Healthy Body Weight

You can determine your **healthy body weight** by using the weight guidelines found in the 2005 *Dietary Guidelines for Americans.* This assessment involves converting two body measurements, the waist and the hip circumferences, into a waist-to-hip ratio (WHR) that can then be applied to weight ranges for people of particular ages and heights. An acceptable WHR, for women is near the lower end of each weight range, and for men it is at the higher end of each weight range.

To make a WHR determination, follow these steps:

1. Measure around your waist near your navel while you stand relaxed (not pulling in your stomach).

2. Measure around your hips, over the buttocks where the hips are largest.
3. Divide the waist measurement by the hip measurement.

Women with a WHR of less than .80 generally have a body weight that falls within the healthy range for their age and height; men with a WHR of less than .90 will also probably fall within the range considered healthy for their age and height.

This system was developed because of the growing concern over the relationship between the amount of fat located around the waist, the spare tire, and the

Key Terms

desirable weight the weight range deemed appropriate for people, taking into consideration gender, age, and frame size

healthy body weight body weight within a weight range appropriate for a person with an acceptable waist-to-hip ratio

Health Risks of Obesity

Each of the diseases listed below is followed by the percentage of cases for which obesity is a contributing factor:

Colon cancer 10%

Breast cancer 11%

Hypertension 33%

Heart disease 70%

Diabetes (type 2, non-insulin-dependent) 90%

As these statistics show, being obese greatly increases your risk of many serious, and even life-threatening, chronic conditions.

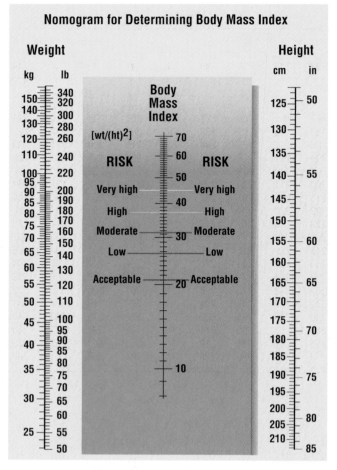

Figure 6-1 To use this nomogram, place a ruler or other straightedge between the body weight in kilograms or pounds (without clothes) located on the left-hand column and the height in centimeters or in inches (without shoes) located on the right-hand column. The BMI is read from the middle of the scale and is in metric units.

development of several serious health problems. As a point of interest, the 2005 *Dietary Guidelines for Americans* do not use WHR as a clinical marker for the treatment of obesity; instead they use only waist circumference. The risk of health problems such as heart disease and diabetes increases at a waist measurement of 35 inches for women and 40 inches for men, regardless of height.[12]

Research shows that women who have more fat concentrated around the waist, as opposed to their hips, have a greater risk of cardiovascular disease and diabetes. This has been referred to as the "apple versus pear shape" phenomenon. Whether you're an apple or pear depends on where your body stores its excess fat. If fat tends to gather high around your abdomen, you're an apple. If it collects more around your hips and thighs, you're a pear.

BOD POD (Body Composition System)

The newest method of determining body composition involves the use of the **BOD POD,** an egg-shaped chamber that uses computerized pressure sensors to determine the amount of air displaced by the person's body (larger people displace more air than smaller people). From this measure, you can then calculate the person's body density and percentage of body fat.[14] Additional techniques in which highly accurate but expensive technology is used to determine body composition, including *computed tomography (CT) scans, magnetic resonance imaging (MRI), infrared light transmission,* and *neutron activation,* may become common ways of measuring body composition in the future.[15]

Skinfold Measurements

Skinfold measurements are another way to measure body composition. In this assessment procedure, constant-pressure **calipers** are used to measure the thickness of

the layer of fat beneath the skin's surface, the *subcutaneous fat layer.* These measurements are taken at key places on the body. Through the use of specific formulas, skinfold measurements can be used to calculate the percentage of body fat. The percent body fat value can also be used in determining desirable weight.[15] There are some drawbacks to this type of measure: First, a second

Key Terms

BOD POD body composition system used to measure body fat through air displacement

caliper a device used to measure the thickness of a skinfold from which percentage of body fat can be calculated

Dieting and Religion

As was discussed in Chapter 5, spirituality guides some of our eating habits and traditions. Many stories from medieval times tell of female saints who ate almost nothing or fasted as a way of purifying the body. Catherine of Siena is said to have eaten a handful of herbs each day and occasionally shoved twigs down her throat to bring up any other food she was forced to eat. Fasting was a way of demonstrating female holiness; it was thought that prayer provided sustenance.[1] Fasting is part of other religions besides Christianity—for example, the Islamic celebration of Ramadan (Chapter 5).

Some modern diets promote spiritual components, and some food has been referred to as sinful. *The Weigh Down Diet* by Gwen Shamblin approaches weight loss from a religious perspective, advising people to feed the human soul with a relationship with God rather than with food. Holding meetings in local churches, Shamblin teaches you "God's rules for eating." She advocates allowing your stomach to become empty before eating and to give your appetite to God to control. In fact, she suggests waiting to eat until your stomach is growling and to focus on making the desire for eating go away. This is counter to what many nutritionists, physicians, and psychologists suggest in terms of healthy eating. She states that exercise is not important for weight management, writing in her book that "the only exercises we insist on are getting down on your knees to pray and getting the muscle of your will to surrender some of the extra food you have been eating."[2] Again, this advice is not consistent with the USDA's guidelines of engaging in daily physical exercise for 30–90 minutes.

There are a number of other religious or spiritually based approaches to weight loss. For example, the *Hallelujah Diet* by Rev. George Malkmus suggests that we eat a vegan diet. He states, "the Lord gave us everything we need in the Garden of Eden; fruits, vegetables, nuts, and seeds." He calls this the "Hallelujah diet" to "celebrate its true creater [sic]." Dr. Don Colbert wrote a book based on a similar philosophy called *What Would Jesus Eat?*, which encourages the consumption of non-animal-derived living foods rather than dead or processed foods. One of the newest Christian weight-management books is *The Maker's Diet* by Jordan S. Rubin. He warns against a vegan diet and suggests eating meat and dairy products instead. He further recommends eating foods in their most organic and least-processed states and consuming food in the form the body was designed by God to eat them. For example, he doesn't think milk should be pasteurized nor should the fat be removed to make skim or low-fat milk.[3]

While Shamblin is a registered dietician and has a master's degree in food and nutrition, most of the diet ministries are led by people without these types of degrees and credentials. There has been some concern raised about food safety issues with unprocessed dairy products, meat, and other foods as well as how these diets contradict the new dietary guidelines released by the USDA, particularly those concerning exercising daily and eating a balanced diet. Some critics say that God is being used as a gimmick to get in on the $50 billion dollar diet industry, while others view giving dietary advice as part of God's ministry.

[1]Brumberg, J. *Fasting Girls*. Cambridge, MA: Harvard University Press, 1989.
[2]Shamblin, G. *The Weigh Down Diet*. New York: Bantam Doubleday Dell Publishing Group, 1997.
[3]What Would Jesus Eat? Diets Grapple with God's Gastronomic Will," *Muncie Star Press*, Volume 105, No. 364, June 2004.

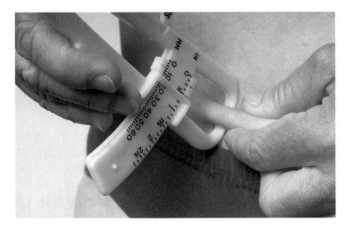

Body fat determination using skinfold calipers. Skinfold measurements are used in equations that calculate body fat density and percent body fat.

person may be required to perform the test, because it is sometimes difficult to get an accurate measurement on yourself. Second, skinfolds are notoriously hard to locate precisely, and being just a few millimeters off can make a significant difference.[16]

Young adult men normally have a body fat percentage of 10–15 percent. The normal range for young adult women is 22–25 percent. The higher percentage of fat typically found in women is related to preparation for pregnancy and breastfeeding. When a man's body fat is higher than 20 percent and a woman's body fat is above 30 percent, these people are considered to be obese.

Hydrostatic Weighing

Hydrostatic (underwater) *weighing* is another precise method of determining the relative amounts of fat and lean body mass that make up body weight. A person's percentage of body fat is determined by comparing the underwater weight with the body weight out of water and dry. The need for expensive facilities (a tank or pool) and experienced technicians makes the availability and cost of this procedure limited to small-scale applications, such as at a large research university or teaching hospital.

Appearance

While it may seem as though the simplest method of determining one's body size is to look in the mirror, for most people this is not an accurate measure. Research shows that most women are dissatisfied with their appearance or body image and perceive themselves as needing to lose an average of 10–15 pounds when in actuality they are in a healthy weight range. Body dissatisfaction is endemic to young women in Western culture as evidenced by the rate of dieting in the United States, starting at a young age. In fact, on any given day, 50 percent of 10-year-olds are on a diet, and two-thirds of high school women, and a third of all adult women are dieting.[17] There is also an important difference between one's internal concept of one's body and actual body perception, and this is particularly problematic for people with eating disorders.

Home Scale

Most people use scales at home or in a gym to determine their weight, but scales can be highly inaccurate, as evidenced by weighing yourself on a variety of scales and weighing different amounts. Also, you will probably weigh less in the morning when you first wake up and more in the evening, after having eaten during the day. So, if you are using a scale to monitor your weight, you need to do so on the same scale, at the same time of day, and with approximately the same weight of clothing. Also, remember that muscle weighs more than fat, which explains why some toned and muscular athletes can weigh as much as someone who is sedentary and overweight. In general, risk of disease increases with a higher percentage of body fat, not weight.

Causes of Obesity

Debate continues as to the causes of obesity. Genetic, physiological, metabolic, environmental, psychological, and other factors may all play a part. In the past decade, the overall prevalence of obesity has increased so that currently one-third of all Americans are obese. Moreover, in the last 20 years, the number of overweight children in the United States has tripled to one in five children.[18] Genetics,

dietary practice, and activity level seem to all play a role in this dramatic increase.

Four additional factors seem to play a significant role in the prevalence of obesity: sex, age, socioeconomic status, and race. Biology accounts for only 33 percent of the variation in body weight, so the environment can also exert an enormous influence. According to the Centers for Disease Control, prevalence rates for obesity in women is 35 percent and 31 percent among men and is found mainly in the 20–55 age group. Among women, obesity is strongly associated with socioeconomic status, being twice as common among those with lower socioeconomic status as it is among those with higher status.[19] Although prevalence among black and white men does not differ significantly, obesity is far more common among black than among white women, affecting 66 percent of black women compared with 49 percent of white women.

While the precise cause of obesity remains unclear, we do know that obesity is a complex condition caused by a variety of factors. Until we are sure what causes obesity, it will remain difficult to develop effective ways of managing weight.

Genetic Factors

Through years of research, we do know that heredity plays a major role in the development of body size and obesity. Based on studies comparing both identical and fraternal (nonidentical) twins raised together and separately, it's evident that both environment and genetics influence obesity. In fact, it is estimated that heredity accounts for 25 percent to 40 percent of the development of obesity.[10] Women have a higher percentage of body fat than do men, and this seems stable across cultures and dietary habits.[20]

There is also some speculation about population differences and prevalence of obesity suggesting that some groups possess a "thrifty genotype."[21] For example, the differences in diabetes and obesity rates in Native Americans compared with European Americans prompted some researchers to consider that some groups of people have survived periods of feast and famine by increased efficiency in energy storage and expenditure through a particular genotype. However, no specific thrifty gene or genotype has been identified.

A complex interplay of genetic factors very likely influence the development of obesity, since more than 250 genes may play a role in obesity. Promising research has explored how the leptin gene influences obesity. Discovered in the mid 1990s, the leptin gene, referred to as the "fat gene," was thought to influence satiety or the feeling of fullness in mice.[22] When the leptin gene was faulty in mice, it produced lower leptin levels, and the mice experienced excessive weight gain. However, when the leptin gene was normal, the leptin levels were higher and the mice were able to maintain normal weight. It has been theorized that leptin resistance may be involved in weight gain and the maintenance of excessive weight, but much more research needs to be conducted in this area.[23]

Physiological and Hormonal Factors

Building on the new information about the genetic and neuropsychological basis of obesity, researchers have identified centers for the control of eating within the hypothalamus of the central nervous system (CNS). These centers—the feeding center for hunger and the satiety center for fullness—tell the body when it should begin consuming food and when food consumption should stop. It takes 20 minutes on average for these signals to go from the stomach to the brain to relay the message "stop eating."

Hormonal factors also influence obesity. Obesity can be caused by a condition called **hypothyroidism,** in which the thyroid gland produces an insufficient amount of thyroxin, a hormone that regulates metabolism. Over five million Americans have this common medical condition, and as many as 10 percent of women may have some degree of thyroid hormone deficiency. In such individuals, the underactive thyroid makes burning up food difficult, and so weight gain is common. As we acquire greater understanding of the hormones and neurotransmitters that influence hunger and satiety, drugs designed to influence their actions will be developed. Some of these drugs already exist and will be described later in this chapter.

The effects of hormonal changes on eating can be seen each month just before a woman's menstrual cycle; many women say that they crave salty and sugary foods during this time. Pregnancy brings about another host of hormonal and metabolic changes. During a normal pregnancy, a woman requires an extra 300 calories a day to support the developing fetus and supportive tissues, and to fuel her elevated maternal metabolic rate. In addition, pregnant women will develop approximately 9 extra pounds of adipose tissue that will be used as an energy source during lactation. The average woman is expected to gain 25–35 pounds during pregnancy.[10] Many women express concern about their ability to lose this weight following the birth of the child, and some women do gain much more than the recommended amount of weight. However, the majority of women lose their pregnancy weight within 6 months to a year after having a baby. Nevertheless, obesity is one of the most frequent causes for complications in pregnancy. Women who are obese during pregnancy have a much higher risk of hypertension and gestational diabetes. Obesity has also been associated with infertility, poor pregnancy outcomes and miscarriage.[10]

Typically, breast-feeding can help women to burn more calories and return to their prepregnancy weight, although extra fat may linger, since nature intended this to be a store of energy for breast-feeding. Breast-feeding requires an additional 500 calories a day.[10] Mothers who breast-feed tend to lose more weight when their babies are 3 to 6 months old than do formula-feeding mothers who consume fewer calories.[24]

Metabolic Factors

Traditional theory has suggested that the energy expenditure and energy storage centers of the body possess a genetically programmed awareness of the body's most physiologically desirable weight, called **set point.**[25] However, the term *set point* is somewhat misleading in that it does not refer to a certain number or point but a weight range that the body is genetically programmed to maintain. When the body falls below its natural set point, one's metabolism reacts by slowing down the body's functioning in order to conserve energy. In other words, the body senses that it is not receiving enough calories to maintain healthy functioning and so it sends calories to essential areas of the body and uses the energy as efficiently as possible. Alternatively, when someone consumes more calories than is needed, the body begins to increase the rate of metabolism in an effort not to gain weight above the set point. The process of storing or burning more energy to maintain the body's "best" weight is called **adaptive thermogenesis.** This process also explains the reason that 90 percent of people who go on any diet gain all their weight back plus more within a year of going off the diet. When dieting, people reduce their caloric intake, which in turn lowers their metabolism. When they discontinue the diet, they typically eat more calories and foods with higher fat content on a lowered metabolism. This is a good formula for weight gain. In addition, dieters tend to lose muscle and regain their weight as fat.

There is a great deal of debate on how an individual's set point can be altered. The number of fat cells in the

---

Key Terms

hypothyroidism a condition in which the thyroid gland produces an insufficient amount of the hormone thyroxin

set point a genetically programmed range of body weight, beyond which a person finds it difficult to gain or lose additional weight

adaptive thermogenesis the physiological response of the body to adjust its metabolic rate to the presence of food

body, the blood level of insulin, and regions of the brain such as the hypothalamus all seem to play a role in determining set point. Certain drugs such as amphetamines and other diet pills and herbal supplements can act on the brain to temporarily lower the set point. However, once these drugs are discontinued, the set point returns to the previous level or perhaps an even higher level and weight increases as a result. Healthier and more permanent methods of changing one's set point are through regular exercise and healthy eating patterns. In fact, a recent study of 8,000 successful dieters found that the majority of them used "my own diet and exercise regimen" and did not follow any formal weight reduction program.[26]

The body's requirement for energy to maintain basic physiological processes decreases progressively with age. This change reflects the loss of muscle tissue as both men and women age. This loss of muscle mass eventually alters the ratio of lean body tissue to fat. As the proportion of fat increases, the energy needs of the body are more strongly influenced by the lower metabolic needs of the fat cells.[27] This excess energy is then stored in the fat cells of the body. A gradual decrease in caloric intake and a conscious effort to expend more calories can effectively prevent this gradual increase in weight leading to obesity.

Social and Cultural Factors

Ethnic and cultural differences also relate to the incidence of obesity and what is considered to be a healthy weight. African American, American Indian, and Hispanic American women have the highest risk of becoming overweight, according to the Centers for Disease Control. In fact, the results of a national study showed that more than half of all African American and Hispanic women in the United States are above what is considered a healthy body weight. The statistics are startling: 66 percent of African American women are overweight, and 33 percent are obese. For Caucasian women, 49 percent are considered overweight and 24 percent obese. Only one minority group, Asian Americans, has a lower rate of obesity than does the general population.

Obesity is second only to tobacco as the leading cause of premature deaths and disproportionately affects women of color and women of lower socioeconomic classes. On the positive side, African American women report less pressure to be thin than their white counterparts and tend to be less self-conscious about their weight.[28] Acculturation also has a significant effect on the rates of obesity—the more an ethnic group has adapted to and absorbed Western culture, the higher the rate of obesity within that group.[29]

Socioeconomic status is also an important influence on obesity, particularly in women. Upper socioeconomic women tend to be thinner than lower socioeconomic women, while among men there is not such a pattern.[30] Limited access to health care, lower education levels, lower income levels, and increased stress are some of the reasons cited for this disparity. Interestingly, higher obesity levels are also related to marriage, parenthood, and geographical location; married men, parents, and people living in rural areas tend to have a higher incidence of obesity.[31]

Environmental Factors

Certainly environmental factors such as the smell or sight of freshly made cookies, or an advertisement for a candy bar, can affect your eating habits. Even the clock signaling it is "time to eat" can encourage us to eat even when we aren't hungry. While this may seem adaptive and helpful in regulating our food intake, Dr. Kelly D. Brownell, a professor of psychology at Yale and an expert on eating disorders, has gone so far as to label American society a "toxic environment" when it comes to food. Researchers contend that the local environment has a powerful effect on eating. Factors such as portion size, price, advertising, the availability of food, and the number of food choices presented all can influence the amount the average person consumes. For example, moviegoers will eat 50 percent more popcorn if given an extra-large tub of popcorn instead of a container one size smaller, even if the popcorn is stale. If a tabletop in the office is stocked with cookies and candy, coworkers tend to nibble their way through the workday, even if they are not hungry. One study showed that when the candy was in plain sight on workers' desks, they ate an average of nine pieces each. Storing the candy in a desk drawer reduced consumption to six pieces, as compared to putting the candy a couple of yards from the desk, cutting the number to three pieces per person.[32] In response to these and other findings, many public schools have begun offering only healthy foods in their cafeterias, replacing soft drinks, candy, and chips with juice, milk, fruit, and granola bars.

Packaging and price can also influence the amount people consume, a concept of which advertisers, restaurants, and grocery stores are well aware. Dropping the price of the low-fat snacks by even a nickel resulted in dramatically increased sales. In contrast, stickers signaling low-fat content or cartoons promoting the low-fat alternatives had little influence over which snacks were more popular. This is true not only of food but also of beverages: people tend to drink *more* from short, wide glasses than from thin, tall ones, thinking they are drinking less.[32]

Having more choices also appears to make people eat more. In one study, people ate more when offered sandwiches with four different fillings than they did when they were given sandwiches with their single favorite filling. In another study, participants who were served a four-course meal with meat, fruit, bread, and a pudding, ate 60 percent more food than did those served an equivalent meal of only their favorite course. Even the cup holders in automobiles have grown larger to make room for giant drinks. Note that these findings apply to people of all body sizes not just people who are overweight or obese, as is often the misconception. However, one difference seems to relate to the age of the individuals studied. One study found that 3-year-olds who were served three different portion sizes of macaroni and cheese for lunch on three different days ate the same amount each time. Five-year-olds, however, ate more when more was put in front of them.[32]

 TALKING POINTS Do you think there should be more regulation of the food industry? If so, what recommendations would you make? What food would you include for regulation and how should this be determined?

Psychological Factors

Psychological factors related to overeating concern the reasons people eat other than physiological hunger. Individuals with eating disorders often report that they don't know when they are hungry and often eat when they are not hungry and don't eat when they have a biological reason for doing so. Why do people eat if not in response to hunger? Frequently people eat in response to their emotions—for example, to comfort themselves or when bored, tired, stressed, or depressed. Some people say they use food as a way of coping with hurt, sadness, and anger, "swallowing" their feelings and putting food on top of them. Others eat out of habit and associate food with certain activities, such as eating popcorn at a movie, eating chips in front of the television, and having dessert after dinner. Certainly many people think of chocolate when they want to cheer themselves up. Food is also part of celebrations, holidays, family bonding, and a mainstay of socialization. It is difficult to think about social activities we engage in that don't involve food in some way.

Some people develop relationships with food that substitute for real human relationships. Comments such as "Food is my best friend" and "A great meal is better than sex" are indicative to the degree to which many people rely on food to fill their needs. As we'll learn in our discussion of eating disorders later in the chapter, psychological issues with food can become serious, even life-threatening problems.

Dietary Practices

Many researchers believe that the number of fat cells a person has is initially determined during the first two years of life. Babies who are overfed develop a greater number of fat cells than do babies who receive a balanced diet of appropriate, infant-sized portions. When these children reach adulthood, they will have more fat cells; this increase can result in five times as many fat cells in obese people as in people of normal weight. Dieting reduces only the size of fat cells, not the number of fat cells. People who have an abnormally high number of fat cells are biologically limited in their ability to lose weight.

Another way people can become obese is with a pattern of overeating over a long period of time. If an infant's cries for food are immediately responded to, that child will be more likely to learn what the sensation of hunger is and what the appropriate response is. If crying unrelated to hunger is responded to by the offer of a cookie or candy, the child will learn to soothe himself or herself with food. Studies show that children become confused about what hunger is and how to satisfy it if their hunger needs are neglected or overindulged in infancy.[33]

Some of the first power struggles between parents and their children revolve around issues of food. A child who has little power in her life can exert some power and control through refusing to eat certain foods and demanding other foods and determining when she wants to eat. Parents who use food as a reward for good behavior ("If you get an 'A' on your test, I will treat you to ice cream"); as punishment ("You weren't behaving so you can't have dessert"); or as a guilt trip ("Don't waste food. Clean your plate. Children are starving in the world") may inadvertently be creating negative dietary practices that will continue throughout the child's life. Interestingly, research has shown that children are extraordinarily adept at meeting their nutritional needs when left to their own devices. One study allowed children to eat whatever they wanted for a week. Did they always pick high-fat, high-sugar foods? No. Actually, when we look at each day's intake, they didn't eat a balanced diet. However, when one takes the full week into consideration, they met their nutritional needs perfectly.

What your parents say to you not only has a tremendous influence on your eating behavior; what they do, their own eating practices, can have even a greater impact. Children are exposed to different foods and model what their parents eat. If a parent makes comments such as, "I shouldn't eat that because I will get fat" or doesn't eat fruits or vegetables, or sits down with a bag of chips in front of the television every night, the child will probably do the same. In the same vein, when parents exercise regularly, eat a balanced diet, and

The Growing Problem of Obesity

Children are 9 pounds heavier today, and teens are 12–16 pounds heavier than they were in the early 1960s. This can lead to greater chances of developing type 2 diabetes, high cholesterol, and a host of other health problems. The trend doesn't stop with the adolescent years. Obesity doubles from the teen years to the mid-20s. Though college students fear "the Freshman 15," the rumored tendency for first-year college students to gain 15 pounds, researchers have found that freshmen women gained an average of 4 pounds, and men gained 6 pounds.

One of the reasons American children and adolescents gain weight over the generations is that children expend significantly less energy on a daily basis than their parents or grandparents did at their age. Today's youth spend endless hours engaged in sedentary play—watching television and playing computer and handheld electronic games. Schools have not helped the situation by cutting back on physical education classes and recess.

In our fast-paced society, we are eating more and more fast food and vending machine food than we have in the past. Again, schools have come under attack for providing high-sugar and high-fat foods, as well as sodas, in the cafeterias and vending machines. College students frequently complain about the food at the college dining hall being loaded with fat and sugar; however, it is often the midnight delivery of pizza or study breaks to the vending machines that lead to weight gain. College students also say that they have trouble finding time to exercise regularly and rely on walking to and from classes and on physical education classes to provide their exercise. Unfortunately this does not typically add up to at least 30 minutes of daily physical activity as suggested by the new USDA dietary guidelines.

Americans are working more hours than they have in the past, usually well beyond the 40-hour work week, leaving little to no time for daily exercise. Many adults perceive themselves as working hard at their jobs and have no energy reserves left for exercise when they come home. They also mistakenly believe that they have already expended enough energy on the job to count toward fulfilling the daily requirement for physical activity. For some, this is an accurate assumption, but the vast majority of Americans' jobs are sedentary and don't involve manual labor or have great physical demands.

So, what can we do to curb the growing trend toward obesity? One of the most important steps to take is to get parents to role-model healthy eating to their children and to reward behavior with activities, not food. When a child's parents maintain a healthy weight, this increases the likelihood that the child will do the same. Other factors that seem important are to

1. *Go outside and play!* Parents need to encourage their children to play outside. Play with them! Go for a bike ride, play ball, take a walk.
2. *Limit screen time.* Decrease television, computer, and electronic game time to one to two hours a day maximum. Don't hit the couch or the computer as soon as you get home, because it is likely you will spend the evening there. Plan to do something active when you first get home from work or school.
3. *Avoid vending machines and fast food restaurants.* Pack nutritious snacks such as apples, carrots, nuts, and yogurt.
4. *Downsize your dishes.* Studies have repeatedly shown that we eat more when we are offered more food. Use narrower glasses, and smaller bowls and plates.
5. *Quit the clean plate club!* Researchers have also shown that we tend not to feel more full even if we eat more. In one study, a bowl automatically refilled itself with soup, unbeknownst to the subjects, and they ate almost double the amount as the group with normal bowls, and yet they didn't report feeling more full.
6. *Eat weighty food.* We tend to eat the same amount or weight in food each day. Eating food that is high in fiber and water, such as fruits and vegetables, helps us to consume fewer calories. Nutrient-dense food fills you up faster, so you eat fewer calories but get more nutrition compared to eating foods that are less nutrient dense.
7. *Water yourself.* Drink water instead of juice and sodas.

If we look at the lifestyles Americans led 40 years ago, we can see why they didn't struggle with overweight and obesity in the way we do today. Perhaps a lesson to learn from the past is to not take advantage of every convenient way to accomplish our daily living but to make choices based on a healthy lifestyle.

make positive comments about their weight, children tend to mimic this behavior.

Inactivity

When weight management experts are asked to identify the single most important reason that obesity is so high in today's society, they are most certain to point to inactivity. People of all ages tend to be less active and burn fewer calories than did their ancestors only a few generations ago. Both adults and children spend less time devoted to exercise as a result of longer work hours at sedentary jobs, a decline in physical education programs in school, and increased participation in sedentary recreational activities, such as browsing the Internet, playing video games, and watching television. In addition, many of the labor-saving devices and increased automation in the home and workplace have contributed to increased inactivity. According to some studies, nearly two-thirds of Americans are not physically active on a regular basis, and 25 percent are completely, sedentary.[3] It is not surprising that as inactivity becomes the norm so does overweight.

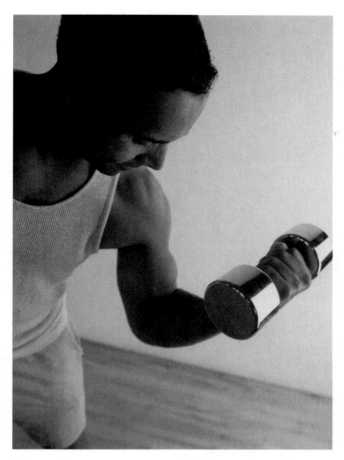

The most important component of weight management is regular exercise.

 TALKING POINTS What were the messages you received in childhood regarding food? What positive and negative eating habits have you learned from your family?

Caloric Balance

Any calories consumed in excess of those that are used by the body are converted to fat. We gain weight when our energy input is greater than our energy output. On the other hand, we lose weight when our energy output is greater than our energy input (Figure 6-2). Weight remains constant when caloric input and output are equal. In such situations, our bodies are said to be in *caloric balance.*

Energy Needs of the Body

What are our energy needs? How many calories should we consume (or burn) to achieve a healthy weight? The new USDA dietary guidelines are based on consuming

2,000 calories a day (see Chapter 5). We all vary in our specific energy needs, depending on our (1) basal metabolic rate (also referred to as resting energy expenditure, or REE), (2) activity requirements, and (3) the thermic effect of food. Gender also plays a role in caloric intake requirements; men tend to need more calories than women. We also need fewer calories as we age because our metabolism is slowing down, and we tend to become less active.

Basal Metabolism

Of the three factors that determine energy needs, basal metabolism uses the highest proportion (50% to 70%) of the total calories required by each person. **Basal Metabolic Rate (BMR)** is a measure of resting energy expenditure that is taken upon awakening, 10–12 hours after eating, or 12–18 hours after significant physical activity. A closely related construct, resting metabolic rate (RMR), is often used interchangeably with BMR. In comparison with the BMR, the RMR is measured at rest, without the stringent control on physical activity required as with measuring BMR. RMR measures the calories needed for functioning such as blood circulation, respiration, brain activity, muscle function, body temperature, and heartbeat.[34]

Basal metabolism changes as people age. For both males and females, the BMR is relatively high at birth and continues to increase until the age of 2. Except for a slight rise at puberty, the BMR then gradually declines throughout life.[35] If people fail to recognize that their BMR decreases as they grow older (2 percent per decade), they might also fail to adjust their food intake and activity level accordingly. Thus they may gradually put on unwanted pounds as they grow older.

Activity Requirements

Each person's caloric *activity requirements* vary directly according to the amount of their daily physical activity. For example, sedentary office workers require a smaller daily caloric intake than construction workers, lumberjacks, or farm workers do.

Physical activity that occurs outside the workplace also increases caloric needs. Sedentary office workers may be quite active in their recreational pursuits. Active

---

Key Terms

basal metabolic rate (BMR) the amount of energy, expressed in calories, that the body requires to maintain basic functions

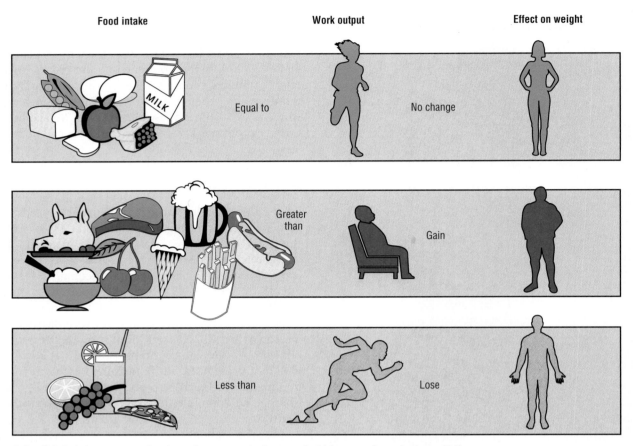

Food intake	Work output	Effect on weight
Equal to		No change
Greater than		Gain
Less than		Lose

Figure 6-2 Caloric balance: energy input equals energy output, some of which comes from physical activity.

employees may spend their off hours lounging in front of the TV. It's important to closely examine the total amount of work or activity an individual engages in to accurately estimate that person's caloric requirements. Physical activity uses 20 percent to 40 percent of caloric intake. See Table 6.4 for a breakdown of caloric expenditures for various activities.

Thermic Effect of Food

Thermic effect of food (TEF) refers to the amount of energy our bodies require for the digestion, absorption, and transportation of food. This energy breaks down the bonds that hold complex food molecules together, resulting in smaller nutritional units that can be distributed throughout the body. The amount of TEF burned varies for different types of food, with some food such as fat requiring less energy to convert to energy stores and others such as protein and carbohydrates requiring more. The TEF peaks in about 1 hour after eating and accounts for approximately 10 percent of total energy expenditure.[36]

Lifetime Weight Control

Obesity and frequent fluctuation in weight are thought to be associated with higher levels of morbidity and mortality. So it is highly desirable to maintain your weight and body composition at or near optimum levels. Although this may be a difficult goal to achieve, it is not unrealistic when approached consistently. The following are some keys to success:

- *Exercise:* Caloric expenditure through regular exercise, including cardiovascular exercise and strength training, is a key to maintaining a healthy weight and body composition (see Chapter 4).

Table 6.4 Calories Expended during Physical Activity

To determine the number of calories you have spent in an hour of activity, simply multiply the *calories per hour per pound* column by your weight (in pounds). For example after an hour of archery a 120-pound person will have expended 209 calories; a 160-pound person, 278 calories; and a 220-pound person, 383 calories.

Activity	Calories/Hour/Pound	Activity	Calories/Hour/Pound
Archery	1.74	Marching (rapid)	3.84
Basketball	3.78	Painting (outside)	2.10
Baseball	1.86	Playing music (sitting)	1.08
Boxing (sparring)	3.78	Racquetball	3.90
Canoeing (leisure)	1.20	Running (cross-country)	4.44
Climbing hills (no load)	3.30	Running	
Cleaning	1.62	11 min 30 sec per mile	3.66
Cooking	1.20	9 min per mile	5.28
Cycling		8 min per mile	5.64
5.5 mph	1.74	7 min per mile	6.24
9.4 mph	2.70	6 min per mile	6.84
Racing	4.62	5 min 30 sec per mile	7.86
Dance (modern)	2.28	Scrubbing floors	3.00
Eating (sitting)	0.60	Sailing	1.20
Field hockey	3.66	Skiing	
Fishing	1.68	Cross-country	4.43
Football	3.60	Snow, downhill	3.84
Gardening		Water	3.12
Digging	3.42	Skating (moderate)	2.28
Mowing	3.06	Soccer	3.54
Raking	1.44	Squash	5.76
Golf	2.34	Swimming	
Gymnastics	1.80	Backstroke	4.62
Handball	3.78	Breaststroke	4.44
Hiking	2.52	Free, fast	4.26
Horseback riding		Free, slow	3.48
Galloping	3.72	Butterfly	4.68
Trotting	3.00	Table tennis	1.86
Walking	1.14	Tennis	3.00
Ice hockey	5.70	Volleyball	1.32
Jogging	4.15	Walking (normal pace)	2.16
Judo	5.34	Weight training	1.90
Knitting (sewing)	0.60	Wrestling	5.10
Lacrosse	5.70	Writing (sitting)	0.78

- *Dietary modification:* Plan meals around foods that have moderate levels of fat and are low in total fat and saturated fat and high in complex carbohydrates. Many nutritionists are concerned about the safety of high-fat diets and ultra-low-fat diets for long-term weight management.

- *Lifestyle support:* In addition to committing yourself to a lifestyle that features regular physical activity and careful food choices, build a support system that nurtures your efforts. Inform your family, friends, classmates, and coworkers that you intend to rely on them for support and encouragement.

- *Problem solving:* Reevaluate your current approaches to dealing with stressors. Replace any reliance on food as a coping mechanism with nonfood options, such as exercise or talking with friends or family members.

- *Redefinition of health:* Think about health and wellness (see Chapter 2) in a manner that reinforces the importance of prevention and self-care, rather than waiting to become sick or incapacitated before paying attention to your diet and activity level.

These suggested lifestyle choices will make a significant contribution to preventing a weight problem later.

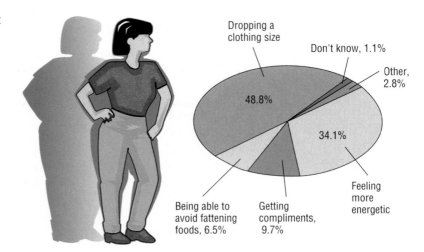

Figure 6-3 How do Americans measure success when it comes to losing weight? Most say dropping a clothing size is the best indicator that their diet is working.

Dropping a clothing size

Don't know, 1.1%

Other, 2.8%

48.8%

34.1%

Feeling more energetic

Being able to avoid fattening foods, 6.5%

Getting compliments, 9.7%

Weight-Management Techniques

Weight loss occurs when the calories consumed are fewer than required by the body for physiological maintenance and activity. This may sound overly simplified, and certainly the $50 billion-a-year weight loss industry would like us to think it is much more complicated than this.

Weight loss followed by weight gain may be less healthy and certainly more frustrating than maintaining body weight, even at weight above the desirable levels. When a diet or weight loss strategy fails, the person, not the diet, is blamed. This causes people to jump to another weight loss method and then another, and a vicious cycle has begun. However, a commitment to a lifestyle change of eating in healthy ways and engaging in regular exercise seems to be the most effective strategy for weight loss and weight maintenance. Set a goal to lose not more than 2 pounds a week, because the body tends to lose muscle rather than fat if the weight loss occurs too rapidly.[34] Many people also complain of "hanging skin" after a rapid, drastic weight loss, which can then require cosmetic surgery to rectify.

A number of approaches to weight loss can be pursued. How do dieters know when they have succeeded? Figure 6-3 shows how Americans measure their progress at losing weight. The Personal Assessment at the end of this chapter will help you evaluate your food habits in relation to healthy weight (page 171) and how you feel about your body image (page 173).

Dietary Alterations

A diet that reduces caloric intake is the most common approach to weight loss. The choice of foods and the amount of food are the two factors that distinguish the wide range of diets currently available. Note, however, that dieting alone usually does not result in long-term weight loss. Effective

and lasting weight loss requires a lifestyle change, not just going on a diet for a specific time period only to return to your old patterns of eating. This is the problem many people face when they go on strict diets and overly restrict their calories. Because the diet is so restrictive and demanding, they are unable to continue to follow it for very long and return to their previous eating patterns. In addition, people tend to overeat the foods they denied themselves while dieting, because they feel deprived and the forbidden food seems even more alluring (see Figure 6-4). This can also lead

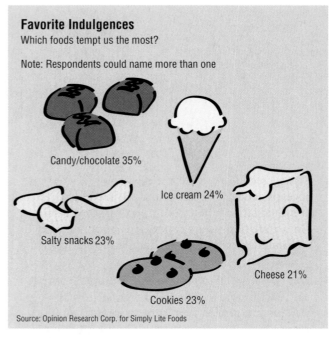

Favorite Indulgences
Which foods tempt us the most?

Note: Respondents could name more than one

Candy/chocolate 35%

Ice cream 24%

Salty snacks 23%

Cheese 21%

Cookies 23%

Source: Opinion Research Corp. for Simply Lite Foods

Figure 6-4 Late-night kitchen raids and too many daytime snacks can compromise a healthy diet. Which foods are the most difficult for you to resist?

to binge eating. Thus diets tend not to work in the long run. (See Changing for the Better on page 159.)

Balanced Diets Supported by Portion Control

For nutritional health, a logical approach to weight loss and subsequent weight maintenance is to establish a nutritionally sound balanced diet (see Chapter 5) that controls portions. Many people are confused about the difference between a portion size and a serving size. Food scales or food models can assist in gaining an understanding of portion sizes.

The new food pyramid outlines the breakdown of daily caloric intake for each food group. You can get a personalized dietary guideline by inputting your gender, age, and activity level at www.mypyramid.gov. One study showed that people cut 256 calories a day just by trimming their portion sizes by 25 percent.

Maintaining a balanced diet and watching your portion sizes is especially important on the weekends. Many people throw their good eating habits out the window on the weekends, as evidenced by a recent study that found that Americans eat an average of 115 extra calories per day from Friday to Sunday as compared to the rest of the week. Most of these calories came from alcohol and increased fat consumption. The extra calories can result in a gain of 5 pounds over the course of a year.

 TALKING POINTS Have you ever tried to lose weight? What methods were effective for you? What is the longest time you have stuck to a particular weight management strategy?

Fad Diets

Many people use fad diets in an attempt to lose weight quickly. Currently there are over 150 popular diets, often promoted by people who claim to be nutrition experts. With few exceptions, these approaches are both ineffective and potentially dangerous. In addition, some involve significant expense. A brief assessment of a variety of popular diet plans is presented in Table 6.5.

High-Protein/Low-Carbohydrate Diets

Currently, the most popular diets are those that reduce carbohydrate intake to an extremely low level while permitting an almost unlimited consumption of animal protein (meat), with its accompanying high fat content. As indicated in Table 6.5, these diets, such as *Dr. Atkins' New Diet Revolution; The Zone; The South Beach Diet; Good Carbs, Bad Carbs;* and *Dr. Phil's Ultimate Weight Solution* involve potential problems, particularly if followed for long periods.

The restriction of calories is the basis of all diets. Some suggest limiting the consumption of fat, others sugar, or the caloric intake is dangerously low for all food groups. Many diet plans, such as the South Beach Diet and the Atkins' Diet, advocate the restriction of carbohydrates, which can cause ketosis. When the carbohydrate calories are limited, intake of fat usually increases. This high-fat diet can cause an increase in blood ketones from fat breakdown and too few carbohydrates. Ketosis can cause the blood to become too acidic, and dehydration can occur. The body requires a minimum of 50–100 grams of carbohydrate per day to avoid ketosis.[34] Low-carbohydrate diets are characterized by initial rapid weight loss which is appealing to most people, but this loss is primarily due to water and not fat loss. Complications associated with low-carbohydrate, high-protein diets include dehydration, hypertension, cancer, electrolyte loss, calcium depletion, weakness due to inadequate dietary carbohydrates, nausea due to ketosis, vitamin and mineral deficiencies, and possible kidney problems. The risk of coronary heart disease may be higher in those who stay on the diet a long time, due to the increased consumption of foods high in saturated fat and cholesterol.

Controlled Fasting

In cases of extreme obesity, some patients are placed on a complete fast in a hospital setting. The patient consumes only water, electrolytes, and vitamins. Weight loss is substantial because the body is forced to begin **catabolism** of its fat and muscle tissues. Inadequate protein and sodium and potassium loss are particular health concerns.

Today, some people regularly practice unsupervised modified fasting for short periods. Solid foods are removed from the diet for a number of days. Fruit juice, water, protein supplements, and vitamins are used to minimize the risks associated with total fasting. However, unsupervised short-term fasting that is done too frequently can be dangerous and is not recommended.

Weight-Reduction Programs

In virtually every area of the country, at least one version of the popular weight-reduction programs, such as TOPS (Take Off Pounds Sensibly), Jenny Craig, Nutri Sure Losers, and Weight Watchers, can be found. These programs generally feature a format consisting of (1) a well-balanced diet emphasizing portion control and moderate fat, low–saturated fat, and high–complex carbohydrate foods, (2) specific weight loss goals to be attained over a set period of time, (3) encouragement from supportive

---

Key Terms

catabolism the metabolic process of breaking down tissue for the purpose of converting it to energy

Table 6.5 Advantages and Disadvantages of Selected Diets

Type of Diet	Advantages	Disadvantages	Examples
Limited food choice diets	Reduce the number of food choices made by the users Limited opportunity to make mistakes Almost certainly low in calories after the first few days	Deficient in many nutrients, depending on the foods allowed Monotonous—difficult to adhere to Eating out and eating socially are difficult Do not retrain dieters in acceptable eating habits Low long-term success rates No scientific basis for these diets	Good Carbs, Bad Carbs Banana and milk diet Fitonics for Life diet Kempner rice diet The New Beverly Hills Diet Fit for Life Summer sizing
Restricted-calorie, balanced food plans	Sufficiently low in calories to permit steady weight loss Nutritionally balanced Palatable Include readily available foods Reasonable in cost Can be adapted from family meals Permit eating out and social eating Promote a new set of eating habits May employ a point system	Do not appeal to people who want a "unique diet" Do not produce immediate and large weight losses	Eat Right for your Type Weight Watchers Diet Prudent Diet (American Heart Association) Eating Thin for Life Take Off Pounds Sensibly (TOPS) Overeaters Anonymous Jenny Craig
Fasting starvation diet	Rapid initial loss	Nutrient deficient Danger of ketosis > 60% loss is muscle < 40% loss in fat Low long-term success rate	ZIP Diet 5-Day Miracle Diet Hollywood Diet
High-carbohydrate diet	Emphasizes grains, fruits, and vegetables High in bulk Low in cholesterol	Limits milk, meat Nutritionally very inadequate for calcium, iron, and protein	Eat More, Weigh Less Quick Weight Loss Diet Pritikin Diet Hilton Head Metabolism Diet
High-protein, low-carbohydrate diets	Rapid initial weight loss because of diuretic effect Very little hunger Usually include all the meat, fish, poultry, and eggs you can eat Occasionally permit milk and cheese in limited amounts Limits fruits, vegetables, and bread or cereal products	Too low in carbohydrates Deficient in many nutrients—vitamin C, vitamin A (unless eggs are included), calcium, and several trace elements High in saturated fat, cholesterol, and total fat Extreme diets of this type could cause death Impossible to adhere to these	South Beach Diet Dr. Stillman's Quick Weight Loss Diet Dr. Atkins' New Diet Revolution The Zone Diet The Carbohydrate Addict's Diet Sugar Busters Dr. Phil's Ultimate Weight Solution The New Glucose Revolution

leaders and fellow group members, (4) emphasis on regular physical activity, and (5) a maintenance program (follow-up program).

In theory, these programs offer an opportunity to lose weight for people who cannot or will not participate in a physical activity program. But their effectiveness is very limited. In fact, the limited success of these programs and the difficulty that working people have in attending meetings have resulted in falling enrollment and the development of home-based programs, such as hospital-based wellness programs, YMCA and YWCA programs, and Weight Watchers. All these programs are costly when compared with self-directed approaches,

especially when the program markets its own food products (see Table 6.7).

Diet and Physical Activity

Most Americans attempting to lose weight fail to include a physical activity component in their dietary approach. How much exercise is enough? The new USDA dietary guidelines (Chapter 5) advise American adults to engage in at least 30 minutes of moderately intense aerobic exercise almost every day for weight maintenance and 60–90 minutes of this type of exercise for weight loss. Weight training has become a more important factor in weight management. As with most things, too much or too little exercise is not beneficial.

Type of Diet	Advantages	Disadvantages	Examples
		diets long enough to lose any appreciable amount of weight Dangerous for people with kidney disease Weight lost, which is largely water, is rapidly regained Expensive Unpalatable after first few days Difficult for dieter to eat out Unattractive side effects (e.g., bad breath) May require potassium and calcium supplements	Protein Power The Fat or Flush Plan
Low-calorie, high-protein supplement diets	Usually a premeasured powder to be reconstituted with water or a prepared liquid formula Rapid initial weight loss Easy to prepare—already measured Palatable for first few days Usually fortified to provide recommended amount of micronutrients Must be labeled if > 50% protein	Usually prescribed at dangerously low calorie intake of 300 to 500 cal Overpriced Low in fiber and bulk—constipating in short amount of time	Metracal Diet Cambridge Diet Liquid Protein Diet Last Chance Diet Oxford Diet Genesis New Direction
High-fiber, low-calorie diets	High satiety value Provide bulk	Irritating to the lower colon Decreases absorption of trace elements, especially iron Nutritionally deficient Low in protein	Pritikin Diet F Diet Zen Macrobiotic Diet
Protein-sparing modified fast < 50% protein: 400 Cal	Safe under supervision High-quality protein Minimize loss of lean body mass	Decreases BMR Monotonous Expensive	Optifast Medifast
Premeasured food plans	Provide prescribed portion sizes—little chance of too small or too large a portion Total food programs Some provide adequate calories (1,200) Nutritionally balanced or supplemented	Expensive Do not retrain dieters in acceptable eating habits Preclude eating out or social eating Often low in bulk Monotonous Low long-term success rates	NutriSystem Carnation Plan

As will be discussed in the next chapter, some people with eating disorders tend to overexercise which results in diminishing returns and possible medical problems.

Physical Intervention

A second approach to weight loss involves techniques and products designed to change basic eating patterns. Some are self-selected and self-applied, and others must be administered in an institutional setting by highly trained professionals.

Hunger- and Satiety-Influencing Products

Many overweight people want to lessen their desire to eat or develop a stronger sense of when they have eaten enough. Today, many dieters are confused about the safety of pharmaceutical approaches to weight loss, including both over-the-counter (OTC) and prescription drugs.

Until recently, **phenylpropanolamine (PPA)** was incorporated into many OTC weight-loss products. Discontinuation of its use is based on its adverse effects

> **Key Terms**
>
> **phenylpropanolamine (PPA)** (fen ill pro pan **ol** ah meen) the active chemical compound still found in some over-the-counter diet products

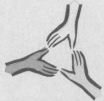

Learning from Our Diversity

Different Clothing Sizes around the World?

You are in London, England, and decide to buy some of the latest English fashions. You find a pair of pants you like and try them on. They don't fit. In fact nothing in your size fits. Why not? Because not all sizes are the same for women.

As you can see from Table 6.6, if you wear a size 12 in American stores, you will need to find a size 14 in the British stores or an 11 in Japanese stores or a 40 in the Parisian boutiques.[1] Is this true for men's clothing? No, you will find that a waist size of 38 is the same in American, British, and Japanese clothing. Why is this? Well, it is the same reason that you will find that not all women's size-12 clothing is the same even in the same country! What you will find is that the more expensive the clothing, the smaller the size compared to its true size. In other words, you can compare a pair of jeans from a discount store to the identical pair of pants in an expensive department store and find that the expensive pants are labeled one to two sizes smaller than the pants in the discount store. You will also discover that the smaller-size pants have a much larger-size price tag. Again, does this hold true for men's clothing? No, it doesn't. The reason is that women will pay more for a smaller size, a lot more, while most men will not. There is not a market for smaller-size clothing for men the way there is for women.

Women feel much more pressure to comform to the popular size. The popular size can vary from generation to generation and between different cultures. Whereas a size 6 was the desired size for women in the 1980s, size 4 in the early 1990s, size 2 in the late 1990s, now size 0 is the size to be for American women. When size 4 was popular in the United States, size 6 was the British size to strive for, whereas in Japan it was size 3. This situation reflects the changing cultural ideal for female beauty, which can lead to unhealthy eating, dangerous dieting, and the development of eating disorders in order to fit into the current fad size. Women are increasingly succumbing to this pressure and going to greater lengths to achieve perfection. This includes undergoing plastic surgery because they can't achieve the perfect body naturally and so turn to unnatural methods to try to meet the perception of perfection.

Men, however, are not immune to the trend of rising obesity around the world. In Cyprus, the Czech Republic, Finland, Germany, Greece, Malta, and Slovakia, more men are overweight or obese than American men are. Although the Mediterranean diet has been touted as a healthy diet, obesity is also higher in the Mediterranean countries.[2]

Eating disorders and distorted eating are more prevalent in cultures adopting Westernized values. One startling example of how quickly and significantly Western ideals of beauty can influence others was seen when television first came to the island of Fiji in 1995. Before the introduction of television, a common compliment given to someone was "you've gained weight," and dieting was almost nonexistent. Telling someone that he or she looked thin was a way of saying that the person didn't look well. Within three years of having television, the number of teenagers at risk for eating disorders more than doubled; 74 percent of teens said they felt too big or too fat, and 62 percent reported that they had been dieting in the past month.[3]

In the United States and other Westernized societies, the cultural ideal for beauty is becoming thinner and thinner. A generation ago, a model weighed 8 percent less than the average woman did, but she now weighs 23 percent less. With the ideal dress size for women now at a size 0, there is a message for women to aspire to nothingness. What can be done about this alarming trend? Women can refuse to buy more expensive clothing just because they are labeled with smaller sizes, as men have done for years. We can glorify all sizes and shapes of women. As Angel, a 17-year-old high school basketball player from West Los Angeles stated, "I'm 5'8" and 165 pounds. I'm not a size 4. I'm tall. I'm muscular. I'm a thick girl. I accept that."[4]

Table 6.6 Size Comparisons

Women's Clothing

UK	6	8	10	12	14	16	18	20	22
USA	4	6	8	10	12	14	16	18	20
Russia	40	42	44	46	48	50	52	54	56
Spain/France	34	36	38	40	42	44	46	48	50
Italy	38	40	42	44	46	48	50	52	54
Germany	32	34	36	38	40	42	44	46	48
Japan	3	5	7	9	11	13	15	17	19
Dominican Republic	10	12	14	16	18	20	22	24	26

Men's Clothing

Suits, Sweaters, and Jackets

UK	34	36	38	40	42	44	46	48
USA	34	36	38	40	42	44	46	48
Europe	44	46	48	50	52	54	56	58
Japan	S	–	M	–	–	L	–	–

Shirt Collars

UK	14	14½	15	15½	16	16½	17	17½
USA	14	14½	15	15½	16	16½	17	17½
Europe	36	37	38	39	40	41	42	43
Japan	36	37	38	39	40	41	42	43

Source: www.hostelscentral.com/hostels-article-34.html.

[1]"International Clothes Sizes Compared," www.hostelscentral.com.

[2]"Some European Countries More Obese Than in U.S.," *USA Today,* March 28, 2005.

[3]Kilbourne, J. *Can't Buy My Love.* New York: Simon & Schuster Inc., 1999.

[4]"The New Girls," *Oprah Magazine,* May 2004.

Table 6.7 The Real Cost of Dieting

Plan	Annual Cost
Weight Watchers	$709
Over-the-counter diet pills	$500
Nutritional counseling	$450–$1200
Physician-supervised weight loss program	$2,000–$3,500
Prescription diet pills	$1,090–$1,343
Gastric bypass surgery	$20,000–$25,000

Source: Chatzky JS. The real costs of diets, *USA Weekend*, December 2002.

on conditions such as hypertension, diabetes, glaucoma, and thyroid disease. PPA can also be found in some OTC and prescription cold and cough medications. The FDA recommends that consumers not use any products containing PPA because of its association with higher risk for stroke.

The FDA also continues to advise against using OTC weight loss products containing ephedrine (*ma huang* and Chinese ephedra), which was banned due to health risks. Because they are categorized as dietary supplements, the FDA can't regulate these products to ensure that they meet certain standards or are safe and effective. Many people see these supplements as safe because they are "natural," and yet they can be more dangerous and deadly than prescription medications because they are not inspected as to the purity and accuracy of the contents or the potency of the ingredients. Recently, more than $5 billion was spent on herbal supplements in the United States, with one of every three Americans reporting using them.

Ephedrine, found in most herbal diet pills, has been linked to heart attacks, strokes, hepatitis, headache, tremors, anxiety, extreme irritability, and insomnia in consumers of all ages. Metabolife, an herbal diet supplement that contains ephedra has sold 50 million bottles over the past few years, about 225,000 pills an hour. In 2003 the death of 23-year-old Baltimore Orioles pitcher Steve Bechler was linked to an ephedra supplement, prompting the FDA to reexamine the supplement. Ephedra was banned by the FDA in late 2003.[37]

Some prescription medications have been shown to produce serious side effects. Two such medications, phentermine and fenfluramine, have been prescribed for patients who wanted to lose weight. Both drugs affect levels of serotonin, the neurotransmitter associated with satiety. This popular combination, referred to as *phenfen,* gradually raised concern among health experts because of the side effects it produced in people with angina, glaucoma, and high blood pressure. In addition, reports began to surface that some patients had developed a rare but potentially lethal condition called *pulmonary hypertension.*

During the mid-1990s, a new serotonin-specific weight loss drug, *dexfenfluramine* (Redux), was approved for use in the United States. Results among patients who used the drug, in combination with dietary modification and exercise, seemed impressive during the initial months of its widespread use. However, some patients began to take dexfenfluramine with fenfluramine in an attempt to find a new combination that would be even more effective than phenfen or Redux used alone, and death resulted in some cases.

Thus, two combinations of three serotonin-specific drugs were in vogue in early 1997. However, by May of 1997, there were reports of weight loss patients with newly diagnosed heart valve damage who had been using these drug combinations. In some cases, damage was correctable only by valve-replacement surgery. Accordingly, in September 1997, the FDA requested voluntary withdrawal of fenfluramine and dexfenfluramine from the market.[38] Manufacturers responded by ceasing all distribution of the drugs. Phentermine remains on the market and is used in combination with various antidepressants, such as Prozac, Zoloft, and Paxil.

Soon after reports of the initial concern over the use of phentermine and fenfluramine, the FDA approved another serotonin-specific obesity drug, sibutramine (Meridia) even though an advisory committee within the FDA recommended against approving it. Meridia acts on serotonin in the body similarly to how phenfen and Redux functioned and, like its predecessors, has been linked to heart attacks, high blood pressure, strokes, and death; however, it still remains on the market in the United States. Italy recently pulled Meridia from the market following reports of deaths linked to this drug.

A non-serotonin-influencing drug, *orlistat* (Xenical), has recently been approved. Unlike the serotonin-specific drugs, orlistat reduces fat absorption in the small intestine by about 30 percent. The drug is intended for use among people who are 20 percent or more above ideal weight. It could cause a 10 percent loss of body weight without significant dietary restriction. Some concern exists about the lack of absorption of fat-soluble vitamins among people taking the drug. Additionally, anal leakage may accompany the drug's use, particularly following meals with high fat content.

Surgical Interventions

It used to be that surgical measures were undertaken only if the person's weight was severely endangering his or her health and other less invasive methods had been unsuccessful. Now surgeries such as liposuction, tummy tucks, gastric bypass surgery, and gastric band surgeries are becoming increasingly popular and commonplace, especially among teenagers. Insurance companies are approving these expensive surgeries because the cost of obesity and its related medical problems are even more costly. Gastric bypass surgery, vertical banded gastroplasty, and laparoscopic adjustable gastric banding all involve major surgery. All three operations limit the amount of food a person can eat at one time, because overeating results in vomiting or severe diarrhea. Because the stomach is made smaller, individuals who have undergone these procedures must limit their food intake to half a cup to a cup of food at each "meal." However, it is possible to regain weight by eating small portions of high-calorie foods on a consistent basis. Individuals lose weight because this type of surgery limits the amount of food that can be digested, therefore decreasing the amount of calories that you can eat at one time.

Gastric Bypass Surgery

This is the most common type of weight loss surgery, and it has gained interest since celebrities such as singer Carnie Wilson, American Idol judge Randy Jackson, and weatherman Al Roker have gone public about their experiences with this surgery. It is a major operation and involves dividing the stomach into two compartments to create a pouch, the size of a thumb, for food to enter. The small intestine is cut below the stomach and connected to a smaller portion of the stomach, bypassing the larger stomach and a section of the intestine, which are no longer used (see Figure 6-5). In 2003, 103,200 gastric bypass surgeries (also referred to as *bariatric surgery*) were performed, compared to 16,800 in 1993. The average cost per surgery is $25,000, and the average death rate is 1 in 200. Candidates for this surgery typically have a BMI above 40 or are 100 pounds or more (men) or at least 80 pounds (women) overweight. People with a BMI between 35 and 40 who suffer from type 2 diabetes or life-threatening cardiopulmonary problems may also be candidates for surgery.

Gastric bypass surgery tends to result in greater weight loss (93.3 pounds on average) than does gastroplasty (67 pounds on average) after one year. Over two years, gastric bypass surgery patients have been shown to lose two-thirds of excess weight. These surgeries are not without their risks: hernias, ulcers, liver damage, infection, internal leaks, and even death. These surgeries are not a cure-all for weight management; individuals who have these operations must continue to exercise regularly, take nutritional supplements, eat small portions very slowly, and decrease intake of high-sugar foods in order to maintain their weight loss.

Gastric Band Surgery

There are two types of gastric band surgery: vertical banded gastroplasty and laparoscopic adjustable gastric banding. Vertical banded gastroplasty uses both a band and staples to create a small stomach pouch, limiting the passage of food into the rest of the stomach. This results in a feeling of fullness after only a few mouthfuls of food. This used to be the most common weight loss surgery, but it has decreased in popularity with the rise of gastric bypass surgery. Laparoscopic adjustable gastric banding, a less invasive procedure, involves an inflatable band being placed around the upper end of the stomach, again creating a small pouch. A narrow passage is also made into the rest of the stomach. The band is inflated with a salt solution through a tube that connects the band to an access port positioned under the skin. In this way, the band can be tightened or loosened over time to change the size of the passageway into the stomach.

Three types of obesity surgery

The success depends on how good a candidate the patient is, how skilled the surgeon is, and how much support follows the operation. Risks range from death, to a hernia or ulcer, to surgical failures such as internal leaks. Although the surgery limits the amount of food the patient can eat in one sitting, it's possible to gain the weight back by eating small but continuous portions of high-calorie junk food. the following techniques are becoming increasingly popular for treating severely obese patients:

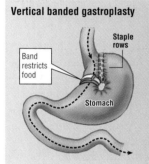

Gastric bypass surgery

Small intestine connected to stomach compartment

Staple rows

Stomach

Done by an open surgery or laparoscopically. The stomach is divided into two compartments, each closed by several rows of staples, creating a thumb-size pouch at the top. A small outlet is created in the smaller portion of the stomach, and the small intestine is connected to it. Food entering the small stomach causes a sensation of fullness, then slowly empties into the intestine through the small outlet.

Vertical banded gastroplasty

Band restricts food

Staple rows

Stomach

Four rows of staples are placed vertically in the upper part of the stomach. The outlet at the lower end of the pouch created by these staples is restricted by a ring that limits the passage of food into the rest of the stomach. The person feels full after a few bites of food.

Laparoscopic adjustable gastric banding

Golf-ball size pouch

Band restricts food

Stomach

An inflatable band is placed around the outside of the upper stomach to create a small pouch with a narrow outlet to the rest of the digestive tract.

Sources: USA TODAY research; the American Society for Bariatric Surgery, May 5, 2004

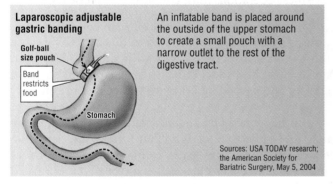

Figure 6-5 Three types of obesity surgery

Liposuction and Abdominoplasty

Liposuction is the most frequent cosmetic operation in the United States in which fat tissue is removed. Liposuction involves removing unwanted fat from specific areas, such as the abdomen, hips, buttocks, thighs, knees, upper arms, chin, cheeks, and neck. A small tube is inserted through the skin, and adipose tissue is vacuumed out. This is more of a sculpting or contouring operation than a weight loss surgery, because little weight is lost. Potential risks and outcomes include infection; the formation of fat clots or blood clots, which may travel to the lungs and cause death; excessive fluid loss, which can lead to shock or fluid accumulation that must be drained; friction burns or other damage to the skin or nerves; numbness; skin discoloration; irregular body contours; and sagging skin.

Abdominoplasty, known more commonly as a tummy tuck, is a major surgical procedure to remove excess skin and fat from the middle and lower abdomen and to tighten the muscles of the abdominal wall. It leaves a permanent scar, which can extend from hip to hip. Infection and blood clots are some of the potential risks.

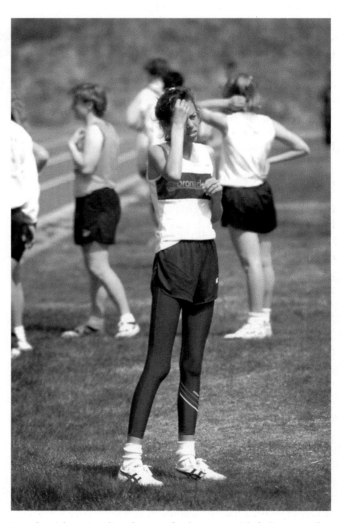

People with eating disorders use food to cope with feeling out of control, stressed, upset, or bored.

A balanced diet and regular exercise are required to maintain the results from this surgery.

Body Wraps

Although not a surgical procedure or a weight loss technique, *body wrapping* is another form of body contouring. In this procedure, various areas of the body are tightly wrapped with 6-inch strips of materials soaked in a solution of amino acids, which is claimed to draw toxins out of the underlying tissue, shrink fatty deposits, diminish cellulite, lighten stretch marks, and eliminate inches of fat. Once the wrapping is removed, the newly contoured body area may remain this way for 4 to 10 weeks. Although the secret to the success of a particular spa's body wrapping approach is supposed to lie in its uniquely formulated soaking solution, the contouring effect probably results from dehydration of underlying tissue and redistribution of extracellular fluids through pressure from the wrapping.

Eating Disorders

Some people have medically identifiable, potentially serious difficulties with body image, body weight, and food selection. Among these disorders are two that are frequently seen among college students—anorexia nervosa and bulimia nervosa. In addition, binge eating and disordered eating are also found in college populations. These topics are included in this chapter because most eating disorders begin with dieting. However, most eating disorders also involve inappropriate food choices and psychological issues (discussed in Chapters 2 and 5).

In the United States, conservative estimates indicate that after puberty 5 to 10 million females and 1 million males are struggling with eating disorders such as anorexia, bulimia, or binge eating disorder. It is estimated that approximately 8 percent of college women will develop an eating disorder, and the population most at risk for developing bulimia is college freshmen women. Ninety to 95 percent of people with eating disorders are women, although the prevalence of eating disorders in men is on the rise. Athletes such as dancers, gymnasts, swimmers, runners, and wrestlers are at risk for developing eating disorders because of the focus on weight and appearance for successful performance. In fact, any group in which success is influenced by weight or attractiveness is at risk for the development of an eating disorder, such as those involved in the performance arts, theatre, television, and modeling.

Recognizing Anorexia Nervosa and Bulimia Nervosa

The American Psychological Association uses the following diagnostic criteria to identify anorexia nervosa and bulimia

Anorexia	Bulimia
• Body weight is 15% or more below desirable weight	• Binge eating two or more times a week for at least 3 months
• Fear of weight gain	• A lack of control over bingeing
• Distorted body image	• Engaging in inappropriate compensatory behavior purging two or more times a week for at least 3 months to prevent weight gain
• In women, the absence of 3 or more menstrual periods (younger girls may not start); In men, sex hormones decrease	• Overly concerned about body image

Characteristic symptoms include the following. Note that it is unlikely that all the symptoms will be evident in any one individual.

Anorexia	Bulimia
• Looks thin and keeps getting thinner	• Bathroom use immediately after eating
• Skips meals, cuts food into small pieces, moves food around plate to appear to have eaten	• Eating in secret
• Loss of menstrual periods and possible infertility	• Excessive time (and money) spent food shopping
• Wears baggy clothes in an attempt to disguise weight loss and to keep warm	• Shopping for food at several stores instead of one store
• Significant hair loss	• Menstrual irregularities and possible fertility problems
• Extreme sensitivity to cold	• Excessive constipation
• Dizziness, lightheadedness, headaches	• Swollen and/or infected salivary glands, sore throat
• Withdrawn, irritable, depressed	• Bursting blood vessels in the eyes
• Insomnia	• Dental erosion in teeth and gums
• Decreased sex drive	• Dehydration and kidney dysfunction
• Dehydration, kidney dysfunction	• Significant hair loss; dry, brittle hair and nails
• Fatigue, loss of energy	• Increased acne and skin problems
• Fatigue, loss of energy	• Heart irregularities, heart failure
• Decreased concentration	
• Lanugo (fine downy body hair)	
• Heart irregularities, heart failure	

Anorexia Nervosa

Anorexia nervosa is an eating disorder in which a person denies his or her own feelings of hunger and avoids food, with marked weight loss occurring. Anorexics tend to run from food in the relentless pursuit of thinness, although they perceive themselves as never thin enough. To meet the diagnostic criteria for anorexia nervosa, the individual has an intense fear of gaining weight, even though he or she weighs less than 85 percent of the expected weight for his/her age, gender, and height, and, in females, menstruation ceases for at least three consecutive months.[40] In addition, people with anorexia perceive themselves as overweight and much larger than they really are. Anorexics lose their ability to recognize when they are hungry and have difficulty eating even if they want to do so. Depression, irritability, withdrawal, perfectionism, and low

> **Key Terms**
>
> **anorexia nervosa** an eating disorder in which the individual weighs less than 85 percent of the expected weight for his or her age, gender, and height, has an intense fear of gaining weight, and, in females, ceases to menstruate for at least 3 consecutive months. People with anorexia perceive themselves as overweight, even though they are underweight

self-esteem are some of the psychological problems associated with anorexia. In addition, anorexics tend to feel cold most of the time because they have very little body fat (2–10 percent) and also suffer from lightheadedness, dizziness, insomnia, hair loss, muscle cramps, stress fractures, fatigue, decreased memory and concentration, and gastrointestinal problems. More serious complications include heart and kidney failure, hypothermia, osteoporosis, infertility, and, in 25 percent of cases, death.

As with other eating disorders, anorexia nervosa also involves a sense of feeling out of control in one's life and attempting to find control through food and weight loss. It is not a coincidence that anorexia nervosa typically begins around puberty: most individuals with anorexia have a fear of growing up and all that goes with being an adult, such as financial responsibility, sexual relationships, leaving one's family, and becoming more autonomous and independent.

Anorexia often begins with dieting but may also begin as a result of an illness such as the stomach flu, a relationship that breaks up, or after dental surgery, when it might be expected that one would temporarily eat less. However, anorexics will tell you that the disorder begins to take on a life of its own after what started as wanting to lose a few pounds turns into losing 15 percent or more of body weight and still not feeling satisfied with one's appearance. Friends and family might initially encourage the person on his or her weight loss and say complimentary things about his or her appearance but soon become concerned when the person's weight continues to dramatically decrease.

Anorexia has become more common as changing cultural ideals for beauty have changed. Our standards have gone from Marilyn Monroe who was a voluptuous 5'5", 128-pound woman to Kate Moss who has been reported to be 5'7" and 105 pounds.[7] Now the "lollipop look" is considered the "in look" in Hollywood, with actresses and models having stick-thin bodies, making their heads seem huge. More attention has been drawn to this disorder since Mary-Kate Olsen went public with her battle with anorexia in the summer of 2004. She is not alone; other stars have admitted to having anorexia—for example, Tracey Gold (*Growing Pains* sitcom), fashion model Carrie Otis, Spice Girl Victoria Beckem, singer Whitney Houston, Courtney Thorne-Smith (from *Alley McBeal*), and actress Christina Ricci. Because many of these stars are seen as the standard for the American body ideal, they may be inadvertently increasing the number of women with eating disorders.

Denial of problems plays a major role in eating disorders in that the individual refuses to acknowledge that there is anything wrong, even though she is becoming thinner and wasting away, and family and friends are expressing great concern. Anorexia nervosa is considered a serious medical and psychological disorder; however, some anorexics argue that "Anorexia is a lifestyle not a disorder." Heated debates and discussions often occur on pro-anorexia Web sites. With names like "Thinspiration," "Stick Figures," and "Anorexic and Proud," these pro-anorexia forums have become very popular and deadly in the past few years. These Web sites show computer-enhanced pictures of models and actresses such as Calista Flockhart and Lara Flynn Boyle, making them appear thinner and more skeletal than they really are.[41]

Messages on these Web sites include tips on how to starve, how to purge, and ways of hiding one's disorder, as well as encouragement to lose more weight. There has been a push among health providers, educators, and health organizations to eliminate these types of Web sites, and they have been somewhat successful. However, these sites still do exist, although somewhat disguised and underground.[42]

The three groups that have traditionally been overlooked in the incidence of anorexia are women of color, female athletes (see the Female Athlete Triad in Chapter 4), and men. The research shows a significant increase in the incidence of anorexia among these three groups. More focus has been given to anorexia among women of color, and it has been proposed that this group might be more vulnerable to developing eating disorders than Caucasian women are because of ethnocultural identity issues. It has been suggested that the more pressure women of color feel to fit into the dominant culture's standards of beauty and thinness, the more likely they are to develop eating disorders.

Often female athletes are not diagnosed with eating disorders because the symptoms of anorexia—absence of menses, low body fat and weight, and osteoporosis—are referred to as the female athletic triad and are not uncommon among athletes and don't necessarily signify the presence of an eating disorder.

The incidence of anorexia nervosa (as well as bulimia nervosa, which we'll cover later) has traditionally been much lower in men than in women. Today, however, the incidence of both conditions is increasing in men as they begin to feel some of the same pressures that women feel to conform to the weight and body composition standards imposed by others. The "lean look" of young male models serves as a standard for more and more young men, whereas the requirements to "make weight" for various sports drives others. Runners, jockeys, swimmers, and gymnasts frequently must lose weight quickly to meet particular standards for competition or the expectations of coaches and trainers. Researchers report that men are less inclined than women are to admit that they may have an eating disorder, thinking it is a "woman's illness." Thus they are less likely to seek treatment. In addition, physicians tend not to suspect men of having eating disorders, and so they go untreated.

Resources for Anorexia and Bulimia Treatment

Local Resources

- College or university health centers
- College or university counseling centers
- Comprehensive mental health centers
- Crisis intervention centers
- Mental health associations

Organizations and Self-Help Groups

American Anorexia/Bulimia Association, Inc.
418 East 76th St. New York, NY 10021
www.aabainc.org
(212) 501-8351

Anorexia Nervosa and Associated Disorders, Inc. (ANAD)
P.O. Box 7, Highland Park, IL 60035
(847) 831-3438
E-mail: anad20@aol.com
www.anad.org

Anorexia Nervosa and Related Eating Disorders, Inc. (ANRED)
P.O. Box 5102, Eugene, OR 97405
(541) 344-1144
E-mail: jarinor@rio.com
www.anred.com

Eating Disorders Awareness and Prevention, Inc.
www.edap.org

Academy for Eating Disorders
60 Revere Dr. #500
Northbrook, IL 60062-1577
(847) 498-4274
www.aedweb.org

National Eating Disorder Association
603 Stewart St., Suite 803
Seattle, WA 98101
(206) 382-3587
www.nationaleatingdisorders.org

Fortunately, psychological treatment in combination with medical and dietary interventions can return the person with anorexia nervosa to a more life-sustaining pattern of eating. The person with anorexia needs to receive the care of professionals experienced in the treatment of this disorder. It is not uncommon for this treatment to take 3 to 5 years. If others, including friends, coworkers, roommates, and parents, observe this condition, they should consult a health care provider for assistance.

 TALKING POINTS What would you do if you suspected a friend of yours had an eating disorder? Would you share your concern with him or her? If so, what would you say?

Bulimia Nervosa

Whereas anorexics are underweight, people with **bulimia nervosa** often are of a normal weight. These individuals use food and weight as a way of coping with stress, boredom, conflict in relationships, and low self-esteem. It is not uncommon in our society to comfort ourselves with food, to have social activities based on food, and to eat as a way of procrastinating a dreaded activity. However, people with bulimia take this to the extreme, engaging in recurrent bingeing, consuming unusually large amounts of food and feeling out of control with their eating.[40]

While anorexics run away from food, bulimics run to food to cope with their emotions, problems, and stress. Because they feel so guilty, ashamed, and anxious about the food they have consumed, people with bulimia **purge** by self-induced vomiting, taking an excessive number of laxatives and diuretics, excessively exercising or fasting. There is a strong preoccupation with weight, calories, and food

among sufferers of bulimia. Most people with bulimia constantly count calories, weigh themselves throughout the day, and frequently make negative statements concerning different parts of their bodies, primarily focusing on the thighs, stomach, and waist. As with anorexia, bulimia is associated with depression, isolation, anxiety, perfectionism, and low self-esteem. Dental erosion, hair loss, esophageal lesions, blood in the vomit and stools, loss of voluntary gag reflex, kidney damage, heart failure, gastrointestinal problems, ketosis, edema, infertility, parotid gland swelling, depression, and insomnia are just some of the medical problems associated with bulimia nervosa.

The recent publicity surrounding Terri Schiavo's death highlights the lethality of this disorder—she entered a persistent vegetative state following a heart attack possibly caused by bulimia. She had developed a potassium deficiency that was reportedly caused by bulimia nervosa. Many public figures have acknowledged struggling with this disorder, including Jane Fonda, Paula Abdul, Sally Field, Justine Bateman, Joan Rivers, and the late

> ### Key Terms
>
> **bulimia nervosa** an eating disorder in which individuals engage in episodes of bingeing, consuming unusually large amounts of food and feeling out of control, and engaging in some compensatory purging behavior to eliminate the food
>
> **purging** using vomiting, laxatives, diuretics, enemas, or other medications, or means such as excessive exercise or fasting to eliminate food

Princess Diana. All these individuals have talked about the pressures to be thin in order to be successful in their careers and how they succumbed to this pressure by developing an eating disorder.

As mentioned previously, bulimia often begins around age 17 to 18 years of age when young adults are separating from their families and are forging lives of their own; some conflict arises around issues of independence, autonomy, and relationships with family. There is a higher incidence of bulimia than anorexia, although some bulimics may have had anorexia in the past. There is also a higher rate of bulimia among female college students as compared to their peers who are not attending college. Treatment for bulimia nervosa involves nutritional counseling, psychological counseling, and consultation with a physician. Often people with bulimia recover from this disorder within a year of beginning treatment.

Binge Eating Disorder

Binge eating disorder is the newest term for what was previously referred to as compulsive overeating. Binge eaters use food to cope in the same way that bulimics do and also feel out of control and unable to stop eating during binges. People with this disorder report eating rapidly and in secret or may snack all day. They tend to eat until they feel uncomfortably full, sometimes hoarding food and eating when they aren't physically hungry.[40] Like people with bulimia, they feel guilty and ashamed of their eating habits and have a great deal of self-loathing and body hatred. People who have binge eating disorder do not engage in purging behavior, which differentiates it from bulimia nervosa. Typically, binge eaters have a long history of diet failures, feel anxious, are socially withdrawn from others, and are overweight. Heart problems, high blood pressure, joint problems, abnormal blood sugar levels, fatigue, depression, and anxiety are associated with binge eating. The treatment of this eating disorder involves interventions similar to those described for treating bulimia nervosa.

Chewing and Spitting Out Food Syndrome

Chewing and spitting out one's food without swallowing it has also been used as a method for weight loss or weight management. This is a common eating disorder and falls within the "Eating Disorder Not Otherwise Specified" diagnosis. It differs from bulimia nervosa, and researchers contend that chewing and spitting out food without swallowing may indicate a more severe eating disorder.[43]

Night Eating Syndrome

Night eating syndrome has not yet been formally defined as an eating disorder. The signs and symptoms of this syndrome include eating more than half of one's daily food intake after dinner and before breakfast; feeling tense, anxious, and guilty while eating; difficulty falling or staying asleep at night; and having little to no appetite in the morning. Unlike binge eating, night eating involves eating throughout the evening hours rather than in short episodes. Note that there is a strong preference for carbohydrates among night eaters. Some researchers speculate that night eating may be an unconscious attempt to self-medicate mood problems because eating carbohydrates can trigger the brain to produce so-called "feel good" neurochemicals. Research is underway in examining the underlying causes of this syndrome and developing subsequent treatment interventions. It seems likely that a combination of biological, genetic, and psychological factors contribute to this problem.

Body Dysmorphic Disorder

Body dysmorphic disorder (BDD) is a secret preoccupation with an imagined or slight flaw in one's appearance. Sometimes, people become almost completely fixated on concerns regarding body image, leading to repeatedly weighing themselves and checking mirrors throughout the day, compulsively dieting, exercising, and undergoing cosmetic surgery.[58] Perceptions of an imperfect body may lead to psychological dysfunction, such as not wanting to leave the house because of imagined defects.

Treatment for Eating Disorders

The treatment for eating disorders is multimodal and multidimensional involving nutritionists, psychologists, physicians, family, and friends. There are different treatment modalities, such as individual, group, and family counseling. Sometimes treatment requires inpatient hospitalization to medically stabilize the individual. In extreme cases, a feeding tube may be inserted to treat starvation, especially if the person refuses to eat. Behavioral modification and cognitive therapy are utilized in counseling people with eating problems. Medications such as antidepressants are often used to decrease

---

Key Terms

binge eating disorder an eating disorder formerly referred to as compulsive overeating disorder; binge eaters use food to cope in the same way that bulimics do and also feel out of control, but do not engage in compensatory purging behavior

body dysmorphic disorder a secret preoccupation with an imagined or slight flaw in one's appearance

obsessive-compulsive behavior, reduce anxiety, alleviate depression, and improve mood. Some medications can stimulate or reduce appetite as well. There is some debate over the efficacy of using an addictions model, similar to the 12-step Alcoholics Anonymous philosophy, with eating disorders. Overeaters Anonymous utilizes this model in helping people with eating problems, and many hospital programs employ this model in their treatment programs. While there seems to be some overlap with substance abuse problems such as denial of problems, feeling out of control of one's behavior, and using food or drugs or alcohol to cope with problems, this is where the similarities end—obviously one needs food to live, which is not the case with drugs and alcohol.

Underweight and Undernourished

For some young adults, the lack of adequate body weight is a serious concern, particularly for those who have inherited a tendency to thinness. These people would likely fall into a BMI category (see page 144) of less than 18.5 and be from 10 percent to 20 percent below normal on a standard height-weight table. Males tend to be particularly concerned with too thin a body type, preferring a lean, muscular V-shape appearance.

Nutritionists believe that the healthiest way to gain weight is to increase the intake of calorie-dense food. These foods are characterized by high fat density resulting from high levels of vegetable fats (polyunsaturated fats). Foods that meet this requirement are dried fruits, bananas, nuts, granola, and cheeses made from low-fat milk. These foods should be consumed later in a meal so that the onset of satiety that quickly follows eating fat-rich foods does not occur. The current recommendation is to eat three calorie-dense meals of moderate size per day, interspersed with two or three substantial snacks. Using the

Food Guide Pyramid (see Chapter 5, page 109) as a guide, **underweight** people should eat the highest number of recommended servings for each group.

A second component of weight gain for those who are underweight is an exercise program that uses weight-training activities intended to increase muscle mass. As detailed in Chapter 4, the use of anabolic drugs without highly competent medical supervision has no role in healthful weight gain. In addition, carefully monitored aerobic activity should be undertaken in sessions that adequately maintain heart-lung health. At the same time, unnecessary activity that expends calories should be restricted. See Chapter 4 to review the female athlete triad and its relationship to underweight.

For those who cannot gain weight, even by using these approaches, a medical evaluation may offer an explanation. If no medical reason can be found, the person must begin to accept the reality of his or her unique body type.

When individuals fall below 80 percent of their desirable weight on standard height-weight tables and display BMI rates from 16 to 10, it is highly probable that they are not only underweight but, more important, *undernourished*.[44] This condition suggests clinically significant deficiencies in both the quantity of food being consumed and its nutritional value. Whether the undernourishment is associated with anorexia nervosa, other medical conditions characterized by weight loss (such as irritable bowel disease), or poverty or famine, affected people are in danger of death from starvation.

Key Terms

underweight a condition in which the body is below the desirable weight

---

Taking Charge of Your Health

- Investigate the resources available on your campus that you could use to determine your healthy weight and body composition profile.

- Evaluate your eating behaviors to find out if you are using food to cope with stress. If you are, develop a plan to use nonfood options, such as exercise or interaction with friends or family members, to deal with stress.

- Formulate a realistic set of goals for changing your weight and body composition in a time frame that allows you to do so in a healthful way.

- Establish a daily schedule that lets you make any necessary dietary and physical activity adjustments.

- Keep a daily journal of your weight-management efforts.

- Monitor your progress toward meeting your weight-management goals.

- Design a reward system for reaching each goal.

- Learn to accept your body, including the imperfections.

- Focus on other aspects of yourself besides your appearance.

SUMMARY

- Weight management has become an obsession in American culture as well as a significant health problem; an estimated 65 percent of U.S. adults are either overweight or obese.
- Doctors usually define "overweight" as a condition in which a person's weight is 1–19 percent higher than "normal," as defined by a standard height/weight chart. Obesity is usually defined as a condition in which a person's weight is 20 percent or more above normal weight. "Morbid obesity" refers to being 50–100 percent over normal weight, more than 100 pounds over normal weight, or sufficiently overweight to interfere with health or normal functioning.
- Some of the methods for assessing one's weight are Body Mass Index (BMI), current height and weight tables, waist to hip ratios, electrical impedance, BOD POD, skinfold measurements, hydrostatic weighing, and home scales.
- Basal Metabolic Rate (BMR) is a measure of resting energy expenditure that is taken upon awakening, 10–12 hours after eating, or 12–18 hours after significant physical activity.
- Thermic effect of food (TEF) refers to the amount of energy our bodies require for the digestion, absorption, and transportation of food.
- Four factors seem to play a significant role in the prevalence of obesity: sex, age, socioeconomic status, and race.
- The energy expenditure and energy storage centers of the body possess a genetically programmed awareness of the body's most physiologically desirable weight called *set point*.

- Environmental factors such as portion size, price, advertising, the availability of food, and the number of food choices presented can influence the amount the average person consumes.
- Psychological reasons for eating refer to eating not out of hunger but as a way of coping with feelings, as a way of socializing and celebrating with others, and by associating certain activities with eating.
- Weight loss occurs when the calories consumed are less than the energy the body needs for physiological maintenance and activity.
- The primary types of weight management techniques include dietary alterations, surgical interventions, medications, weight loss programs, and physical activity.
- A commitment to a lifestyle change of eating in healthy ways and engaging in regular aerobic exercise seems to be the most effective strategy for weight loss and weight maintenance.
- Anorexia nervosa is a psychological condition in which the individual weighs less than 85 percent of his/her expected weight for his/her age, gender, and height.
- People with bulimia nervosa use food and weight as a way of coping with stress, boredom, conflict in relationships, and low self-esteem. They engage in recurrent bingeing and purging to eliminate the food from their bodies.
- Binge eaters use food to cope in the same way that bulimics do and also feel out of control and unable to stop eating during binges but do not engage in purging behaviors.

REVIEW QUESTIONS

1. What percentage of U.S. adults are either overweight or obese?
2. How has the average caloric intake and physical activity level for Americans changed over the past two decades?
3. Define *overweight*, *obesity*, and *morbid obesity*.
4. List at least four of the methods used for assessing weight.
5. Define Basal Metabolic Rate (BMR).
6. Describe the thermic effect of food (TEF) and how it relates to the BMR.
7. What are four factors that seem to play a significant role in the prevalence of obesity?
8. Define *set point*.

9. The process of storing or burning more energy to maintain the body's "best" weight is called what?
10. What are two factors associated with a higher incidence of obesity?
11. Give four examples of how environmental factors can influence the amount the average person consumes.
12. Describe at least two psychological reasons for eating.
13. Give examples of four different types of weight-management techniques.
14. What is the most effective strategy for weight loss and weight maintenance?
15. Describe the symptoms of anorexia nervosa, bulimia nervosa, and binge eating disorder.

ENDNOTES

1. National Center for Chronic Disease Prevention and Health Promotion. *Defining Overweight and Obesity*, April 2005.
2. National Center for Health Statistics Center for Disease Control. *Obesity Still a Major Problem, New Data Show*, October 6, 2004.
3. Harvard Women's Health Watch: Panel issues new guidelines for healthy eating. *Harvard Medical School*, November 2002, Volume 10(3).
4. Sturm R, Wells KB. Does obesity contribute as much to morbidity as poverty or smoking? *Public Health* 115(3), 229–235, 2001.

5. Field AE, et al. Impact of overweight on the risk of developing common chronic disease during a 10-year period. *Arch Intern Med* 161(13), 1581–1586, 2001.

6. Poulton T. *No Fat Chicks.* Secaucus, NJ: Carol Publishing Group, 1997.

7. Maine M. *Body Wars.* Carlsbad, CA: Gurze Books, 2000.

8. Cash T, Henry P. Women's body images: The results of a national survey in the U.S.A. *Sex Role Res* 33(1), 19–29, 1995.

9. Pope H, Phillips K, Olivardia, R. *The Adonis Complex.* New York. Simon & Schuster Inc., 2000.

10. Brownell KD, Fairburn CG. *Eating Disorders and Obesity: A Comprehensive Handbook.* New York: Guilford Press, 1995.

11. National Institutes of Health, Body Mass Index Table, www.nhlbi.nih.gov/guidelines/obesity/bmi.tbl.htm.

12. Waist management, gauging your risk. *Consumer Reports,* p. 48, August 2003.

13. Roche AF. Anthropometric methods: New and old, what they tell us. *Int J Obess* 8(5), 509–523, 1984.

14. Dempster P, Aitkens S. A new air displacement method for the determination of human body composition. *Medical Science Sports Exercise* 27(2), 1692–1697, 1995.

15. International Health Racquet and Sportsclub Association. BOD POD Body Composition System to Descend on San Francisco's *IHRSA CONVENTION* as reported in the 29th Anniversary Exhibition in San Francisco's Moscone Convention Center, March 22–24, 2001.

16. Benardot, D. *Nutrition for Serious Athletes.* Atlanta, GA: Human Kinetics, 2000.

17. Thelen MH, Powell AL, Lawrence C, Kuhnent ME. Eating and body image concerns among children. *Journal of Consulting and Clinical Psychology* 21, 41, 46, 1992.

18. U.S. Department of Health and Human Services. *The Surgeon General's Call to Action to Prevent and Decrease Overweight and Obesity.* Rockville, MD: U.S. Department of Health and Human Service, Public Health Service, Office of the Surgeon General, 2001. Available from U.S. GPO, Washington, www.surgeongeneral.gov/topics/obesity/calltoaction/CalltoAction.pdf.

19. Sobal J. Obesity and socioeconomic status: A framework for examining relationships between physical and social variables. *Medical Anthropology* 13, 231–247, 1991.

20. Wadden TA, Stunkard AJ. *Handbook of Obesity Treatment.* New York: Guilford Press, 2002.

21. Halaas J, et al. Weight-reducing effects on the plasma protein encoded by the obese gene. *Science* 269(5223), 543–546, 1995.

22. Folsom AR, Jensen MD, Jacobs DR, Hilner JE, Tsai AW, Schreiner PJ. Serum leptin and weight gain over eight years in African American and Caucasian young adults. *Obesity Research* 7(1), 1–8, 1999.

23. Sakurai T, et al. Orexins and orexin receptors: A family of hypothalamic neuropeptides and G protein-coupled receptors that regulate feeding behavior. *Cell,* 92(4): 573–585, 1998.

24. LaLeche International. *The Womanly Art of Breast-Feeding,* 1997.

25. Set Point: What your body is trying to tell you. *National Eating Disorders Information Centre Bulletin* 7(2), June, 1992.

26. The truth about dieting. *Consumer Reports,* 26–31 June, 2002.

27. Saladin KS. *Anatomy & Physiology: The Unity of Form and Function.* Dubuque, IA: William C. Brown/McGraw-Hill, 1998.

28. Sorbara M, Geliebter A. Body image disturbance in obese outpatients before and after weight loss in relation to race, gender and age of onset of obesity. *Internal Journal of Eating Disorders,* 416–423, May, 2002.

29. Stunkard AJ, Wadden TA. *Obesity: Theory and Therapy.* New York: Raven Press, 1993.

30. Sobal J, Stunkard AJ. Socioeconomic status and obesity: A review of the literature. *Psychological Bulletin* 105, 260–275, 1989.

31. Sobal J, Rauschenbach B, Frongillo E. Marital status, fatness and obesity. *Social Science and Medicine* 35, 915–923, 1992.

32. Goode E. Obesity in America. *The New York Times,* August 19, 2003.

33. Weight Watchers. *Stop Stuffing Yourself: 7 Steps to Conquering Overeating.* New York: Wiley Publishing Inc., 1998.

34. Insel P, Turner RE, Ross D. *Nutrition.* Sudbury, MA: Jones and Bartlett Publishers, 2002.

35. Ganong WF. *Review of Medical Physiology* (18th ed.). Appleton & Lange, 1997.

36. Wardlaw GM. *Perspectives in Nutrition* (4th ed.). McGraw-Hill, 1999.

37. Ephedra ban puts herb industry on notice, *The New York Times,* December 31, 2003.

38. Center for Drug Evaluation and Research, U.S. Food and Drug Administration: FDA announces withdrawal of fenfluramine and dexfenfluramine. *News Release #97–32,* September 15, 1997.

39. Grazer FM, de Jong RH. Fatal outcomes from liposuction; census survey of cosmetic surgeons. *Plastic Reconstructive Surgery* 105 (1) 436–446, 2000.

40. *Diagnostic and Statistical Manual of Mental Disorders IV TR.* Washington, DC: American Psychiatric Association, 2000.

41. Gotthelf M. The new anorexia outrage. *Self Magazine,* 82–84. August 2001.

42. Lilenfeld L. Academy members debate over pro-anorexia websites. *Academy of Eating Disorders Newsletter,* June 2001.

43. Update: Chewing and spitting out food. *Eating Disorders Review,* July/August, 2002.

44. Ferro-Luzzi A, James WP. Adult malnutrition, simple assessment techniques for use in emergencies. *Br J Nutr* 75(1) 3–10, 1996.

Want to Lose Weight? Get More Sleep!

Research has recently discovered that not getting enough sleep doesn't just make you grumpy and sluggish—it can make you gain weight as well! People who sleep 2 to 4 hours a night have been found to be 73 percent more likely to be obese than those who sleep 7 to 9 hours. Sleeping 5 hours a night results in a 50 percent chance of being obese compared to those consistently sleeping 7 to 9 hours. Twenty-three percent of people who sleep 6 hours tend to be obese. In other words, the higher the BMI, the less sleep the person got.

Why does less sleep equal more weight? We used to think that sleeping too much made us gain weight and staying up meant we were more active and so burned calories, but this has been disproved. People tend to watch television, read, or be online late at night, and so they are not active. In addition, people tend to eat high-fat, high-sugar foods while they are engaging in these activities. Some people say that they eat sugary foods in order to give themselves more energy to stay up late to study or to get work done. Two hormones, ghrelin and leptin, have been found to regulate both sleep and hunger. A sleep study at the University of Chicago found that leptin levels were 18 percent lower and ghrelin levels 28 percent higher after subjects slept 4 hours. Sleep-deprived subjects reported feeling the most hungry and craved carbohydrates, the energy food. Ghrelin has been referred to as the accelerator for eating. When ghrelin levels are up, people feel hungrier. Leptin is the brake for eating; higher levels are associated with feeling full and decreased appetite.

These sleep studies seem to indicate that a hormonal relationship exists between sleep and hunger. The ghrelin level in people who routinely slept 5 hours a night was 15 percent higher, compared to 15 percent lower leptin levels in people who slept 8 hours a night. The first group also had higher BMIs than did individuals sleeping 8 hours at night. Studies have also found that children are not getting the 10 to 11 hours of sleep a night they require, which may also help explain the increase in childhood obesity.

So, one way for us to manage our weight is to manage our sleep better. This means managing our time better—prioritizing our commitments and activities and not overloading our schedules, so that we can get the rest we need.

Sources: "Sleep Loss May Equal Weight Gain," *USA Today,* December 7, 2004. "One More Reason to Get Enough Sleep," *Harvard Women's Health Watch,* May 2005.

personal assessment

How many calories do you need?

Resting Energy Requirement (RER)

Women

3–10 years 22.5 × weight (kg) + 499
10–18 years 12.2 × weight (kg) + 746
18–30 years 14.7 × weight (kg) + 496
30–60 years 08.7 × weight (kg) + 829
> 60 years 10.5 × weight (kg) + 596

Men

3–10 years 22.7 × weight (kg) + 495
10–18 years 17.5 × weight (kg) + 651
18–30 years 15.3 × weight (kg) + 679
30–60 years 11.6 × weight (kg) + 879
> 60 years 13.5 × weight (kg) + 487

Activity Energy Requirement (AER)

At bed rest: 1.20
Low activity (walking): 1.30
Average activity: 1.50–1.75
High activity: 2.0

Instructions: Calculate your resting energy requirement based on your sex, age, and weight. Then multiply your RER by your AER to determine how many calories you need each day to maintain your weight.

Example: Woman
24 years
120 lbs = 54.5 kg
High activity
(RER) × (AER) = Total Energy Requirement
14.7 × 54.5 (kg) + 496 × 2.0 = 2594 calories/day
Note: 1 kg = 2.2 lbs.

Data from *Energy and Protein Requirements: Report of a Joint FAO/WHO/UNU Expert Consultation.* Technical Report Series 724. World Health Organization, 1985; Zeam FJ: *Clinical Nutrition and Dietetics,* 1991, Macmillan.

personal assessment

Body love or body hate?

When you catch a glimpse of yourself in a mirror, do you smile at what you see or grimace? The following quiz will help you to assess your body self-esteem associated with your appearance. Please answer using the following rating scale:

1 = Rarely or never

2 = Sometimes

3 = Almost always or always

Add up your scores to determine your total score, and look at the summary below for an interpretation of your scores.

_____ 1. I worry about my weight and weighing "too much."

_____ 2. I prefer to eat by myself and not with other people.

_____ 3. My mood is determined by the scale and how I feel about my appearance.

_____ 4. I make negative comments about my appearance to myself and others.

_____ 5. I think I look less attractive on days that I haven't exercised.

_____ 6. I have a difficult time accepting compliments about my appearance from others.

_____ 7. I compare myself to other women and find myself lacking.

_____ 8. I ask other people how I look.

_____ 9. I avoid social situations, activities, and events involving food.

_____ 10. I feel more anxious about my body in the summertime because of the need to wear bathing suits and clothing suitable for warmer temperatures.

_____ **TOTAL SCORE**

Interpretation

If you scored between 10 and 15, you have positive body self-esteem and are accepting of yourself and your appearance.

If you scored between 16 and 23, you scored in the average range. While you are in good company, feeling about your body the way most people do, you may want to reframe your body image and develop more of an appreciation for your body and appearance.

If your score was between 24 and 30, you have poor or low body self-esteem. Your self-esteem in general is probably driven by how you see yourself, and you may be putting too much emphasis on your appearance and are too self-critical. You may feel as though you never are thin enough or look good enough and can always find a flaw when looking in the mirror. To improve your body self-esteem, focus on other aspects of yourself, focus on the positive aspects of your body, and be more accepting of yourself and less perfectionistic.

Chapter Seven

Making Decisions about Drug Use

Chapter Objectives

On completing this chapter, you will be able to:

- describe the effects of drugs on the central nervous system.
- discuss drug addiction and the three common aspects of the addiction.
- describe the physical and psychological dependence one develops when addicted to drugs.
- list the risks of combining drugs.
- list and describe the six classifications of psychoactive drugs, giving examples of each.
- list the serious side effects of non-prescription Ritalin use.
- list the short- and long-term effects of marijuana use.
- discuss the issue of drug testing.
- identify the important aspects of drug-treatment programs.

Eye on the Media

Do Media Scare Tactics Keep People from Using Drugs?

The media has tried to frighten people in many ways to keep them away from unhealthy behaviors. Bloody films showing the aftermath of a prom night car crash have been used to scare teenagers about dangerous drinking and driving behaviors. More recently, antidrug campaigns stated that buying illegal drugs helped finance anti-American terrorists. Television ads and public service announcements have featured celebrities speaking out against drug use.

Advertisements for drug and alcohol rehabilitation facilities have shown alcoholics drowning in a sea of alcohol, drug users being confronted by their families, and employees caught by a drug screening test. The message is that miserable life situations can be changed if people are willing to get help.

It's difficult to measure the effectiveness of these approaches to drug prevention. Many people recall these media presentations, so they do make an impression. But, given the many variables involved in drug-taking behavior—family influence, inherited predispositions, life events and situations, drug availability, and peer influence—it's impossible to pinpoint the influence of a single media event. These scare tactics seem to be especially effective among people who have already made the decision not to use drugs. They remind these people how dangerous it is to use drugs. For people who are thinking about starting drug use, these messages may be beneficial, since they portray drug use in a negative light.

For hard-core drug users, though, it's unlikely that scare tactics will be effective. These people tend to lead chaotic lives, may never see the ads, and often remain in denial about their addiction. Despite the fact that these ad campaigns are highly visible and costly, they seem to have only limited influence in drug prevention.

Effects of Drugs on the Central Nervous System

To better understand the disruption caused by the actions of psychoactive drugs, a general knowledge of the normal functioning of the nervous system's basic unit, the **neuron,** is required.

First, stimuli from the internal or external environment are received by the appropriate sensory receptor, perhaps an organ such as an eye or an ear. Once sensed, these stimuli are converted into electrical impulses. These impulses are then directed along the neuron's **dendrite,** through the cell body, and along the **axon** toward the *synaptic junction* near an adjacent neuron. On arrival at the **synapse,** the electrical impulses stimulate the production and release of chemical messengers called *neurotransmitters.*[1] These neurotransmitters transmit the electrical impulses from one neuron to the dendrites of adjoining neurons. Thus neurons function in a coordinated fashion to send information to the brain for interpretation and to relay appropriate response commands outward to the tissues of the body.

The role of neurotransmitters is critically important to the relay of information within the system. A substance that has the ability to alter some aspect of transmitter function has the potential to seriously disrupt the otherwise normally functioning system. Psychoactive drugs are capable of exerting these disruptive influences on the neurotransmitters. Drugs "work" by changing the way neurotransmitters work, often by blocking the production of a neurotransmitter or forcing the continued release of a neurotransmitter (see Figure 7-1).

Addictive Behavior

Experts in human behavior view drug use and abuse as just one of the many forms of addictive behavior. Such behavior includes addictions to shopping, eating, gambling, sex, television, video games, and work, as well as to alco-

---

Key Terms

neuron (**noor** on) a nerve cell

dendrite (**den** drite) the portion of a neuron that receives electrical stimuli from adjacent neurons; neurons typically have several such branches or extensions

axon the portion of a neuron that conducts electrical impulses to the dendrites of adjacent neurons; neurons typically have one axon

synapse (**sinn** aps) the location at which an electrical impulse from one neuron is transmitted to an adjacent neuron; also referred to as a *synaptic junction*

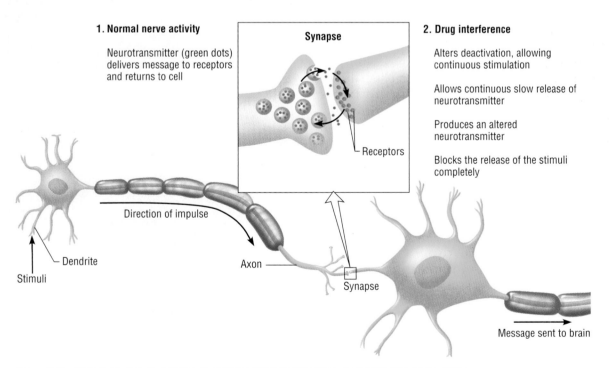

1. Normal nerve activity

Neurotransmitter (green dots) delivers message to receptors and returns to cell

Synapse

Receptors

2. Drug interference

Alters deactivation, allowing continuous stimulation

Allows continuous slow release of neurotransmitter

Produces an altered neurotransmitter

Blocks the release of the stimuli completely

Direction of impulse

Dendrite

Axon

Stimuli

Synapse

Message sent to brain

Figure 7-1 This illustration depicts the disruption caused by the action of psychoactive drugs on the central nervous system. Neurotransmitters are chemical messengers that transfer electrical impulses across the synapses between nerve cells. Psychoactive drugs interrupt this process, thus disrupting the coordinating functioning of the nervous system.

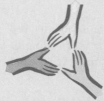

Learning from Our Diversity

Athletes Speak Out Against Drug Use

In the past decade, many public figures have been cautioning youth about the dangers of drug abuse. Politicians, rock stars, and actors have gone public with their antidrug messages. Some of them have admitted to having had drug-abuse problems in their own lives. Their personal accounts have probably influenced some drug abusers to curtail their drug-taking behaviors and seek professional help.

World-class athletes have also taken a public stance against drugs. In Washington, D.C., a group of former Olympians recently kicked off a campaign against the use of performance-enhancing drugs by young people. Gold medal winners Frank Shorter, Jim Ryan, Donna de Varona,

Edwin Moses, John Nabor, and Bruce Baumgartner gave their public support to this antisteroid campaign. The message to youth was that it's possible to achieve remarkable athletic success through hard work, personal sacrifice, and determination. The athletes headlining this campaign came from a variety of sports, so it's likely that their message reached a wide range of young people.

Not too long ago, the mother of basketball superstar Michael Jordan launched a campaign to discourage the use of inhalants by young people. Can you recall other antidrug messages delivered by famous athletes or their families?

---

hol or other drugs.

 TALKING POINTS How would you tell a friend that her video game playing is becoming an addiction that needs to be controlled?

The Process of Addiction

The process of developing an addiction has been a much-studied topic. Three common aspects of addictive behavior are exposure, compulsion, and loss of control.

Exposure

An addiction can begin after a person is exposed to a drug (such as alcohol) or a behavior (such as gambling) that he or she finds pleasurable. Perhaps this drug or behavior temporarily replaces an unpleasant feeling or sensation. This initial pleasure gradually, or in some cases quickly, becomes a focal point in the person's life.

Compulsion

Increasingly, the person spends more energy, time, and money pursuing the drug use or behavior. At this point in the addictive process, the person can be said to have a compulsion for the drug or behavior. Frequently, repeated exposure to the drug or behavior continues despite negative consequences, such as the gradual loss of family and friends, unpleasant physical symptoms resulting from taking a drug, or problems at work.

During the compulsion phase, a person's normal life often degenerates while she or he searches for increased pleasures from the drug or the behavior. An addicted person's family life, circle of friends, work, or study patterns become less important than does the search for more and better "highs." The development of tolerance and withdrawal are distinct possibilities. (These terms are dis-

cussed later in the chapter.)

Why some people develop compulsions and others do not is difficult to pinpoint, but addiction might be influenced by genetic makeup, family dynamics, physiological processes, personality type, peer groups, and available resources for help.

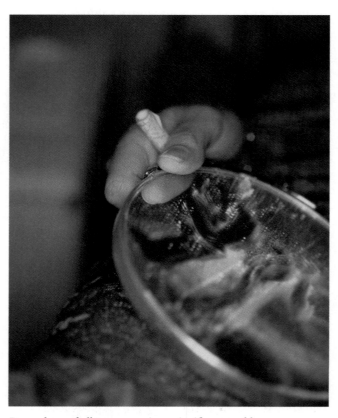

Drug abuse of all types remains a significant problem in our society.

Loss of Control

Over time, the search for highs changes to a desire to avoid the effects of withdrawal from the drug or behavior. Addicted people lose their ability to control their behavior. Despite overwhelming negative consequences (for example, deterioration of health, alienation of family and friends, or loss of all financial resources), addicted people continue to behave in ways that make their lives worse. The person addicted to alcohol continues to drink heavily, the person addicted to shopping continues to run up heavy debts, and the person addicted to food continues to eat indiscriminately. This behavior reflects a loss of control over one's life. Frequently, a person has addictions to more than one drug or behavior.

Intervention and Treatment

The good news for people with addictions is that help is available. Within the last two decades, much attention has been focused on intervention and treatment for addictive behavior. Many people with drug problems can be helped through programs such as those described in Changing for the Better above. These programs often include inpatient or outpatient treatment, family counseling, and long-term aftercare counseling.

It is common for people in aftercare treatment for addictive behavior to belong to a self-help support group, such as Alcoholics Anonymous, Gamblers Anonymous, or Sex Addicts Anonymous. These groups are often listed in the phone book or in the classified section of the newspaper.

Drug Terminology

Before discussing drug behavior, you must first be familiar with some basic terminology. Much of this terminology originates from the field of *pharmacology,* or the study of the interaction of chemical agents with living material.

What does the word *drug* mean? Each of us may have different ideas about what a drug is. Although a number of definitions are available, we will consider a drug to be "any substance, natural or artificial, other than food, that by its chemical or physical nature alters structure or function in the living organism."[1] Included in this broad definition is a variety of psychoactive drugs, medicines, and substances that many people do not usually consider to be drugs.

Psychoactive drugs alter the user's feelings, behavior, perceptions, or moods; they include stimulants, depressants, hallucinogens, opiates, and inhalants. (Changing for the Better above suggests ways to improve your mood without resorting to drug use.) Prescription medications function to heal unhealthy tissue as well as to ease pain, prevent illness, and diagnose health conditions. Although some psychoactive drugs are used for medical reasons, as in the case of tranquilizers and some narcotics, the most commonly prescribed medicines are antibiotics, hormone replacement drugs, sulfa drugs, diuretics, oral contraceptives, and cardiovascular drugs. Legal substances not usually considered to be drugs (but which certainly are drugs) include caffeine, tobacco, alcohol, aspirin, and other over-the-counter (OTC) preparations. These substances are used so commonly in our society that they are rarely perceived as true drugs.

For organizational reasons, this chapter primarily deals with psychoactive drugs. Alcohol is covered in Chapter 8. The effects of tobacco are discussed in Chapter 9. Prescription and OTC drugs and medicines are explored further in Chapter 15. Anabolic steroids, drugs used primarily for increasing muscle growth, are discussed in Chapter 4.

Routes of Administration

Drugs generally enter the body through one of four methods: ingestion, injection, inhalation, or absorption.

Ingestion, or oral administration, is the entry of drugs through the mouth and into the digestive tract. *Injection* refers to the use of a needle to insert a drug into the body. With *inhalation,* the drug enters the body through the lungs. *Absorption* refers to the administration of a drug through the skin or mucous membranes.

Dependence

Psychoactive drugs have a strong potential for the development of **dependence.** When users take a psychoactive drug, the patterns of nervous system function are altered. If these altered functions provide perceived benefits for the user, the drug use may continue, perhaps at increasingly larger dosages. If persistent use continues, the user can develop a dependence on the drug. Pharmacologists have identified two types of dependences: physical and psychological.

Key Terms

psychoactive drug any substance capable of altering feelings, moods, or perceptions

dependence general term that refers to the need to continue using a drug for psychological and/or physical reasons

---

A person can be said to have developed a *physical dependence* when the body cells have become reliant on a drug. Continued use of the drug is then required because body tissues have adapted to its presence.[2] The person's body needs the drug to maintain homeostasis, or dynamic balance. If the drug is not taken or is suddenly withdrawn, the user develops a characteristic **withdrawal illness.** The symptoms of withdrawal reflect the attempt by the body's cells to regain normality without the drug. Withdrawal symptoms are always unpleasant (ranging from mild to severe irritability, depression, nervousness, digestive difficulties, and abdominal pain) and can be life-threatening, as in the case of abrupt withdrawal from barbiturates or alcohol. In this chapter the term *addiction* is used interchangeably with physical dependence.

Continued use of most drugs can lead to **tolerance.** Tolerance is an acquired reaction to a drug in which continued intake of the same dose has diminishing effects.[2] The user needs larger doses of the drug to receive previously felt sensations. The continued use of depressants, including alcohol, and opiates can cause users to quickly develop a tolerance to the drug.

For example, college seniors who have engaged in four years of beer drinking usually recognize that their bodies have developed a degree of tolerance to alcohol. Many such students can vividly recall the initial and subsequent sensations they felt after drinking. For example, five beers consumed during a freshman social gathering might well have resulted in inebriation, but if these same students continued to drink beer regularly for four years, five beers would probably fail to produce the response they experienced as freshmen. Seven or eight beers might be needed to produce such a response. Clearly, these students have developed a tolerance to alcohol.

 TALKING POINTS Some of your friends have started making a contest of beer drinking. How would you tell them you think this is dangerous without sounding preachy?

Tolerance developed for one drug may carry over to another drug within the same general category. This phenomenon is known as **cross-tolerance.** The heavy abuser of alcohol, for example, might require a larger dose of a preoperative sedative to become relaxed before surgery than the average person would. The tolerance to alcohol "crosses over" to the other depressant drugs.

A person who possesses a strong desire to continue using a particular drug is said to have developed a *psychological dependence.* People who are psychologically dependent on a drug believe that they need to consume the drug to maintain a sense of well-being. They crave the drug for emotional reasons despite having persistent or recurrent physical, social, psychological, or occupational problems caused

or worsened by the drug use. Abrupt withdrawal from a drug by such a person would not trigger the fully expressed withdrawal illness, although some unpleasant symptoms of withdrawal might be felt. The term *habituation* is often used interchangeably with psychological dependence.

Drugs whose continued use can quickly lead to both physical and psychological dependence are depressants (barbiturates, tranquilizers, and alcohol), narcotics (the opiates, which are derivatives of the Oriental poppy: heroin, morphine, and codeine), and synthetic narcotics (Demerol and methadone). Drugs whose continued use can lead to various degrees of psychological dependence and occasionally to significant (but not life-threatening) physical dependence in some users are the stimulants (amphetamines, caffeine, and cocaine), hallucinogens (LSD, peyote, mescaline, and marijuana), and inhalants (glues, gases, and petroleum products).

Drug Misuse and Abuse

So far in this chapter we have used the term *use* (or *user*) in association with the taking of psychoactive drugs. At this point, however, it is important to define *use* and to introduce the terms **misuse** and **abuse.**[1] By doing so, we can more accurately describe the ways in which drugs are used.

The term *use* is all-encompassing and describes drug-taking in the most general way. For example, Americans use drugs of many types. The term *use* can also refer more narrowly to misuse and abuse.

Drug Classifications

Drugs can be categorized according to the nature of their physiological effects. Most psychoactive drugs fall into one of six general categories: stimulants, depressants, hallucinogens, cannabis, narcotics, and inhalants (Table 7.1).

Key Terms

withdrawal illness uncomfortable, perhaps toxic response of the body as it attempts to maintain homeostasis in the absence of a drug; also called *abstinence syndrome*

tolerance an acquired reaction to a drug; continued intake of the same dose has diminished effects

cross-tolerance transfer of tolerance from one drug to another within the same general category

misuse inappropriate use of legal drugs intended to be medications

abuse any use of a legal or illegal drug in a way that is detrimental to health

Table 7.1 Psychoactive Drug Categories

Drugs	Trade or Common Names	Medical Uses	Possible Effects
STIMULANTS			
Cocaine*	Coke, crack, gin, girlfriend, girl, double bubble, California cornflakes, caballo, bouncing powder, flake, snow	Local anesthetic	Increased alertness, excitation, euphoria, increased pulse rate and blood pressure, insomnia, loss of appetite
Amphetamines	Biphetamine, Delcobese, Desoxyn, Dexedrine, mediatric, black mollies, aimies, amps, bam, beans, benz	Hyperactivity, narcolepsy, weight control	
Methamphetamine	Speed, ice, chalk, meth, crystal, crank, fire, glass	Weight control	Memory loss, violence, psychotic behavior, cardiac and neurological damage
Phendimetrazine	Prelu-2		
Methylphenidate	Ritalin, Methidate		
Other stimulants	Adipex, Bacarate, Cylert, Didrex, Ionamin, Plegine, PreSate, Sanorex, Tenuate, ephedra		
DEPRESSANTS			
Chloral hydrate	Noctec, Somnos	Hypnotic	Slurred speech, disorientation, drunken behavior without odor of alcohol
Barbiturates	Amobarbital, Butisol, phenobarbital, phenoxbarbital, secobarbital, Tuinal, blockbusters, black bombers	Anesthetic, anticonvulsant, sedative, hypnotic	
Glutethimide	Doriden	Sedative, hypnotic	
Methaqualone	Optimil, Parest, Quaalude, Somnafec, Sopor	Sedative, hypnotic	
Benzodiazepines	Ativan, Azene, Clonopin, Dalmane, diazepam, Librium, Serax, Tranxene, Valium, Verstran	Antianxiety, anticonvulsant, sedative, hypnotic	
GHB	Gamma-hydroxybutyrate (G, liquid ecstasy, Georgia Home Boy)	None	Unconsciousness, seizures, amnesia, vomiting, coma
Other depressants	Equanil, Miltown, Noludar, Placidyl, Valmid	Antianxiety, sedative	
HALLUCINOGENS			
LSD	Acid, microdot, brown dot, cap, California sunshine, brown bomber	None	Delusions and hallucinations, poor perception of time and distance
Mescaline and peyote	Mesc, buttons, cactus, chief	None	
Amphetamine variants (designer drugs)	2,5-DMA, DOM, DOP, MDA, MDMA, PMA, STP, TMA, clarity, chocolate chips, booty juice	None	
Phencyclidine	Angel dust, hog, PCP, AD, boat, black whack, amoeba, angel hair, angel smoke	Veterinary anesthetic	
Phencyclidine analogs	PCE, PCPy, TCP	None	Euphoria, relaxed inhibitions, increased appetite, disorientation
Other hallucinogens	Bufotenin, DMT, DET, ibogaine, psilocybin	None	
CANNABIS			
Marijuana	Acapulco gold, black Bart, black mote, blue sage, bobo, butterflowers, cannabis-T, cess, cheeba, grass, pot, sinsemilla, Thai sticks	Under investigation	Euphoria, relaxed inhibitions, increased appetite, disoriented behavior
Tetrahydrocannabinol	THC	Under investigation	
Hashish	Hash	None	
Hashish oil	Hash oil	None	
NARCOTICS			
Opium	Dover's powder, paregoric, Parapectolin, cruz, Chinese tobacco, China	Analgesic, antidiarrheal	Euphoria, drowsiness, respiratory depression, constricted pupils, nausea
Morphine	Morphine, Pectoal syrup, emsel, first line	Analgesic, antitussive	
Codeine	Codeine, Empirin compound with codeine, Robitussin A-C	Analgesic, antitussive	
Heroin	Diacetylmorphine, horse, smack, courage pills, dead on arrival (DOA)	Under investigation	
Hydromorphone	Dilaudid	Analgesic	Intoxication, excitation, disorientation, aggression, hallucination
Meperidine (pethidine)	Demerol, Pethadol	Analgesic	
Methadone	Dolophine, Methadone, Methadose	Analgesic, heroin substitute	
Other narcotics	Darvon,† Dromoran, Fentanyl, LAAM, Leitine, Levo-Dromoran, Percodan, Tussionex, Talwin,† Lomotil	Analgesic, antidiarrheal, Antitussive	
INHALANTS			
Anesthetic gases	Aerosols, petroleum products, solvents	Surgical anesthetic	Intoxication, excitation, disorientation, aggression, hallucination, variable effects
Vasodilators (amyl nitrite, butyl nitrite)	Aerosols, petroleum products, solvents	None	

*Designated a narcotic under the Controlled Substances Act.
†Not designated a narcotic under the Controlled Substances Act.

Stimulants

In general, **stimulants** excite or increase the activity of the central nervous system (CNS). Also called "uppers," stimulants alert the CNS by increasing heart rate, blood pressure, and the rate of brain function. Users feel uplifted and less fatigued. Examples of stimulant drugs include caffeine, amphetamines, and cocaine. Most stimulants produce psychological dependence and tolerance relatively quickly, but they are unlikely to produce significant physical dependence when judged by life-threatening withdrawal symptoms. The important exception is cocaine, which seems to be capable of producing psychological dependence and withdrawal so powerful that continued use of the drug is inevitable in some users.

Caffeine

Caffeine, the tasteless drug found in chocolate, some soft drinks, energy drinks, coffee, tea, some aspirin products, and OTC "stay-awake" pills, is a relatively harmless stimulant when consumed in moderate amounts.[3] (Visit the Focus on Health Web site www.mhhe.com/hahn8e for a table listing the caffeine content in some products.) Many coffee drinkers believe that they cannot start the day successfully without the benefit of a cup or two of coffee in the morning.

For the average healthy adult, moderate consumption of caffeine is unlikely to pose any serious health threat. However, excessive consumption (equivalent to ten or more cups of coffee daily) could lead to anxiety, diarrhea, restlessness, delayed onset of sleep or frequent awakening, headache, and heart palpitations. Pregnant women are advised to avoid caffeine consumption.[4]

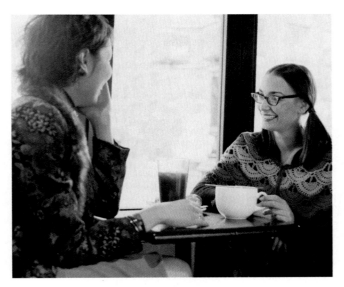

Coffeehouses have become popular places to relax, work, or spend time with friends.

Amphetamines

Amphetamines produce increased activity and mood elevation in almost all users. The amphetamines include several closely related compounds: amphetamine, dextroamphetamine, and methamphetamine. These compounds do not have any natural sources and are completely manufactured in the laboratory. Medical use of amphetamines is limited primarily to the treatment of obesity, **narcolepsy, and attention deficit hyperactivity disorder (ADHD).**

Amphetamines can be ingested, injected, or snorted (inhaled). At low-to-moderate doses, amphetamines elevate mood and increase alertness and feelings of energy by stimulating receptor sites for two naturally occurring neurotransmitters. They also slow the activity of the stomach and intestine and decrease hunger. In the 1960s and 1970s, in fact, amphetamines were commonly prescribed for dieters. Later, when it was discovered that the appetite suppression effect of amphetamines lasted only a few weeks, most physicians stopped prescribing them. At high doses, amphetamines can increase heart rate and blood pressure to dangerous levels. As amphetamines are eliminated from the body, the user becomes tired.

When chronically abused, amphetamines produce rapid tolerance and strong psychological dependence. Other effects of chronic use include impotence and episodes of psychosis. When use is discontinued, periods of depression may develop.

Methamphetamines

Today the abuse of amphetamines is a more pressing concern than it has been in the recent past because of the sharp increase in abuse of methamphetamine. Known by a variety of names and forms, including "crank," "ice," "crystal," "meth," "speed," "crystal meth," and "zip," methamphetamine is produced in illegal home laboratories.[5]

Crystal meth, or ice, is among the most dangerous forms of methamphetamine. Ice is a very pure form of methamphetamine that looks like rock candy.[6] When smoked or injected, the effects of ice are felt in about seven

---

Key Terms

stimulants psychoactive drugs that stimulate the function of the central nervous system

narcolepsy (nar co **lep** see) a sleep disorder in which a person has a recurrent, overwhelming, and uncontrollable desire to sleep

attention deficit hyperactivity disorder (ADHD) above-normal rate of physical movement; often accompanied by an inability to concentrate well on a specified task; also called *hyperactivity*

Meth Lab Warning Signs

- Strong chemical odors (ammonia, ether, cat urine)
- Blocked out windows in the residence
- Renters who pay rent in cash
- A high-traffic area, especially at night
- Significant amount of trash (containers, fuel cans, coffee filters, duct tape)
- Clear glass containers being brought into the residence
- Items including but not limited to batteries, house cleaners, gasoline, automobile chemicals, hot plates, alcohol, ether, rock salts, and diet aids

If you suspect a meth lab in your neighborhood, please contact your local police department (911).

[1] KCI The Anti-Meth Site. *Is There a Meth Lab Cookin' in Your Neighborhood?*, www.kci.org/meth_info/ neighborhood_lab.htm March 7, 2005.

seconds as a wave of intense physical and psychological exhilaration. This is due to the drug telling the brain to release large amounts of dopamine.[7] This effect lasts for several hours (much longer than the effects of *crack*) until the user becomes physically exhausted. When ingested orally or snorted, methamphetamine induces euphoria that may result in a quick addiction. Abuse can lead to memory loss, violence, and cardiac and neurological damage. Chronic use can result in Parkinson-like symptoms, rotten teeth ("meth mouth"), stroke, anorexia, increased heart rate and blood pressure, death,[5] nutritional difficulties, weight loss, reduced resistance to infection, and damage to the liver, lungs, and

kidneys. Psychological dependence is quickly established. Withdrawal causes acute depression and fatigue but not significant physical discomfort. (See the Star box on this page.)

Ephedra Health professionals are warning people about the dangers of using any over-the-counter herbal supplement containing ephedra. Also known as *ma huang*, ephedra is an amphetaminelike drug that can be especially dangerous for people with hypertension or other cardiovascular disease. Presently, ephedra is used in many over-the-counter decongestants and asthma drugs. However, in these products, warning labels indicate possible harmful side effects and drug interactions. Some herbal products that contain ephedra have been promoted as weight-control aids.[8] The FDA announced its ban on ephedra in dietary supplements in April 2004.

Ritalin A prescription stimulant drug that has surged in popularity in recent years is Ritalin. This drug is typically prescribed to children and adolescents (and increasing numbers of young adults) to help them focus attention if they are hyperactive or cannot concentrate. Ritalin can be abused when the drug is shared among friends. (See Star box on page 183.) Critics of Ritalin use argue that it is being overprescribed to treat a variety of problems, when a preferred course would be to identify and treat root causes of the problems. Supporters respond that Ritalin has enabled youth to succeed in school.

Cocaine

Cocaine, perhaps the strongest of the stimulant drugs, has received much media attention. It is the primary psychoactive substance found in the leaves of the South American coca plant.[9] The effects of cocaine are brief—from 5 to 30 minutes (Figure 7-2). Regardless of the form

Figure 7-2 Cocaine's effects on the body

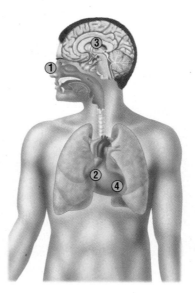

① **The nose:** as cocaine is snorted, nasal vessels immediately constrict and prohibit about 40% of the drug from entering the body. The remaining 60% enters the bloodstream.

② **The heart:** electrical impulses that regulate rhythmic pumping are impaired. Beating becomes irregular (arrhythmia). The heart can no longer supply itself with enough oxygenated blood.

③ **The brain:** dopamine and norepinephrine are released into the brain, producing a feeling of euphoria and confidence. Electrical signals to the heart are distorted, heart rate and pulse increase. A seizure may occur, causing coma and breathing stoppage.

④ **The heart:** blood circulation is out of control. The heart may simply flutter and stop, or it can be pumping so little oxygenated blood to the brain that the brain dies and the heart stops beating.

Ritalin and Adderall Abuse on College Campuses

Ritalin and Adderall abuse on college campuses continue to rise. Studies have shown that one in every five college students has used Ritalin illegally. Adderall is a fairly new drug similar to Ritalin, and it is being abused like Ritalin. Students who take Ritalin or Adderall without a prescription are using these drugs to help enhance concentration during late-night study sessions, to obtain a cocainelike high or to suppress their appetites. However, students may not realize the serious side effects they can experience from taking these drugs illegally.

Side effects of Ritalin can include nervousness, insomnia, loss of appetite, headaches, increased heart and respiratory rates, dilated pupils, dry mouth, perspiration, and feelings of superiority. Higher doses can result in tremors, convulsions, paranoia, and/or a sensation of bugs crawling under the skin. These health risks are considerably higher if Ritalin is snorted. Death can occur from abusing Ritalin.

Side effects of Adderall are similar to Ritalin. These effects include loss of appetite, weight loss, insomnia, headache, and dizziness. Owing to a longer-lasting dose, Adderall has been growing in popularity. In comparison to Ritalin users, Adderall patients have experienced softer side effects, withdrawal symptoms, stomach discomfort, and mood changes. Adderall abuse can also result in death.

Sources:
The Johns Hopkins News-Letter. *Ritalin Abuse Is Increasing*, www.jhunewsletter.com/vnews/display.v/ART/2002/11/22/3ddd766faebeb, February 21, 2005.
The Johns Hopkins News-Letter. *Hopkins Students Turning to Drugs to Keep Grades Up*, www.jhunewsletter.com/vnews/display.v/ART/2004/04/02/406cd1793dfb2?in_archive=1, February 21, 2005.
Attention Deficit Disorder Help Center. *Adderall Side Effects*, www.add-adhd-help-center.com/adderall_side_effects.htm, February 21, 2005.

---

in which it is consumed, cocaine produces an immediate, near-orgasmic "rush," or feeling of exhilaration. This euphoria is quickly followed by a period of marked depression. Used only occasionally as a topical anesthetic, cocaine is usually inhaled (snorted), injected, or smoked (as *freebase* or crack). There is overwhelming scientific evidence that users quickly develop a strong psychological dependence using cocaine. There is considerable evidence that physical dependence also rapidly develops. Cocaine users risk a weakened immune system making them "more susceptible to infections, including HIV."[10] However, physical dependence on cocaine does not lead to death upon withdrawal.

Freebasing Freebasing and the use of crack cocaine are the most recent techniques for maximizing the psychoactive effects of the drug. Freebasing first requires that the common form of powdered cocaine (cocaine hydrochloride) be chemically altered (alkalized). This altered form is then dissolved in a solvent, such as ether or benzene. This liquid solution is heated to evaporate the solvent. The heating process leaves the freebase cocaine in a powder form that can then be smoked, often through a water pipe. Because of the large surface area of the lungs, smoking cocaine facilitates fast absorption into the bloodstream.

One danger of freebasing cocaine is the risk related to the solvents used. Ether is a highly volatile solvent capable of exploding and causing serious burns. Benzene is a known carcinogen associated with the development of leukemia. Clearly, neither solvent can be used without increasing the level of risk normally associated with cocaine use. This method of making smokeable cocaine led to a new epidemic of cocaine use, smoking crack.

Crack In contrast to freebase cocaine, crack is made by combining cocaine hydrochloride with common baking soda. When this pastelike mixture is allowed to dry, a small rocklike crystalline material remains. This crack is heated in the bowl of a small pipe, and the vapors are inhaled into the lungs.[9] Some crack users spend hundreds of dollars a day to maintain their habit.

The effect of crack is almost instantaneous. Within 10 seconds after inhalation, cocaine reaches the CNS and influences the action of several neurotransmitters at specific sites in the brain. As with the use of other forms of cocaine, convulsions, seizures, respiratory distress, and cardiac failure have been reported with this sudden, extensive stimulation of the nervous system.

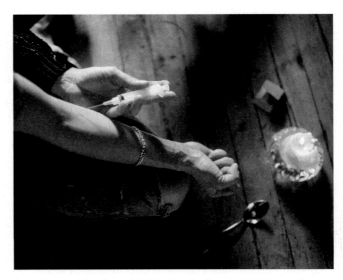

Intravenous injection of cocaine results in an almost immediate high for the user.

Within about 6 minutes, the stimulating effect of crack becomes completely expended, and users frequently become depressed. Dependence develops within a few weeks, since users consume more crack in response to the short duration of stimulation and rapid onset of depression.

Intravenous administration has been the preferred route for cocaine users who are also regular users of heroin and other injectable drugs. Intravenous injection results in an almost immediate high, which lasts about 10 minutes. A "smoother ride" is said to be obtained from a "speedball," the injectable mixture of heroin and cocaine (or methamphetamine). This type of mixture can be volatile and even fatal.[11]

Depressants

Depressants (or sedatives) sedate the user, slowing down CNS function. Drugs included in this category are alcohol (see Chapter 8), barbiturates, and tranquilizers. Depressants produce tolerance in abusers, as well as strong psychological and physical dependence.

Barbiturates

Barbiturates are the so-called sleeping compounds that function by enhancing the effect of inhibitory neurotransmitters. They depress the CNS to the point where the user drops off to sleep or, as is the case with surgical anesthetics, the patient becomes anesthetized. Medically, barbiturates are used in widely varied dosages as anesthetics and for treatment of anxiety, insomnia, and epilepsy.[2] Regular use of a barbiturate quickly produces tolerance—eventually such a high dose is required that the user still feels the effects of the drug throughout the next morning. Some abusers then begin to alternate barbiturates with stimulants, producing a vicious cycle of dependence. Other misusers combine alcohol and barbiturates or tranquilizers, inadvertently producing toxic or even lethal results. Abrupt withdrawal from barbiturate use frequently produces a withdrawal syndrome that can involve seizures, delusions, hallucinations, and even death.

Methaqualone (Quaalude, "ludes," Sopor) was developed as a sedative that would not have the dependence properties of other barbiturates.[1] Quaaludes were occasionally prescribed for anxious patients. Today, compounds resembling Quaaludes are manufactured in home laboratories and sold illegally so that they can be combined with small amounts of alcohol for an inexpensive, drunklike effect.

Tranquilizers

Tranquilizers are depressants that are intended to reduce anxiety and to relax people who are having problems managing stress. They are not specifically designed to produce sleep but rather to help people cope during their waking hours. Such tranquilizers are termed *minor* tranquilizers, of which alprazolam (Xanax) diazepam (Valium) and chlordiazepoxide (Librium) may be the most commonly prescribed examples. Unfortunately, some people become addicted to these and other prescription drugs.[12]

Some tranquilizers are further designed to control hospitalized psychotic patients who may be suicidal or who are potential threats to others. These *major tranquilizers* subdue people physically but permit them to remain conscious. Their use is generally limited to institutional settings. All tranquilizers can produce physical and psychological dependence and tolerance.

"Date Rape" Depressants "Date rape" drugs or club drugs are commonly used on college campuses. These drugs are usually slipped into the drink of an unsuspecting woman or man and can result in a coma or even death.

Common "date rape" drugs include GHB (gamma hydroxybutyrate), also known as G, liquid ecstasy, Easy-Lay, and Georgia Home Boy, and Rohypnol ("roophies"). When these drugs are consumed they cause a drunklike or sleepy state that can last for hours. During this time is when unsuspecting individuals are taken advantage of, against their will and sometimes against their knowledge.

High school and college students should not accept drinks from people they do not know. This recommendation extends to all parties where drinkers do not know what has been added to the punch or other drinks.[13]

Congress passed the 1996 Drug-Induced Rape Prevention and Punishment Act, and it is now a federal crime to give someone a drug, without the user's knowledge, to aid in sexual assault. The maximum penalty for this crime is 20 years in prison and a $250,000 fine.[2] GHB (G, liquid ecstasy) and ketamine (K, Special K, Cat) are additional depressants that are being used as date rape drugs.[14] These drugs should serve as a reminder to all partygoers to keep an extremely careful watch over their drinks. (See the Star box on page 185.)

Hallucinogens

As the name suggests, hallucinogenic drugs produce hallucinations—perceived distortions of reality. Also known as *psychedelic* drugs or *phantasticants*, **hallucinogens** reached their height of popularity during the 1960s. At that

---

Key Terms

hallucinogens psychoactive drugs capable of producing hallucinations (distortions of reality)

---

time, young people were encouraged to use hallucinogenic drugs to "expand the mind," "reach an altered state," or "discover reality." Not all the reality distortions, or "trips," were pleasant. Many users reported "bummers," or trips during which they perceived negative, frightening distortions.

Hallucinogenic drugs include laboratory-produced lysergic acid diethylamide (LSD), mescaline (from the peyote cactus plant), and psilocybin (from a particular genus of mushroom). Consumption of hallucinogens seems to produce not physical dependence but mild levels of psychological dependence. The development of tolerance is questionable. *Synesthesia,* a sensation in which users report hearing a color, smelling music, or touching a taste, is sometimes produced with hallucinogen use.

The long-term effects of hallucinogenic drug use are not fully understood. Questions about genetic abnormalities in offspring, fertility, sex drive and performance, and the development of personality disorders have not been fully answered. One phenomenon that has been identified and documented is the development of *flashbacks*—the unpredictable return to a psychedelic trip that occurred months or even years earlier. Flashbacks are thought to result from the accumulation of a drug within body cells.

LSD

The most well-known and powerful hallucinogen is lysergic acid diethylamide. LSD ("acid") is a drug that helped define the counterculture movement of the 1960s. During the 1970s and the 1980s, this drug lost considerable popularity. LSD use peaked in 1996, with an annual prevalence of 8.8 percent of high school seniors experimenting with LSD. The 2003 *Monitoring the Future* reported a sharp decrease in LSD use among high school seniors, at 1.9 percent. The researchers suggest that this sharp decline may be due to an increase in Ecstasy use or a drop in LSD availability.[15]

LSD is manufactured in home laboratories and frequently distributed in absorbent blotter paper decorated with cartoon characters.[16] Users place the paper on their tongue or chew the paper to ingest the drug. LSD can produce a psychedelic (mind-viewing) effect that includes altered perception of shapes, images, time, sound, and body form. Synesthesia is common to LSD users. Ingested in doses known as "hits," LSD produces a 6- to 9-hour experience.

Although the typical doses ("hits") today are about half as powerful as those in the 1960s, users still tend to develop high tolerance to LSD. Physical dependence does not occur. Not all LSD trips are pleasant. Hallucinations produced from LSD can be frightening and dangerous. Users can injure or kill themselves accidentally during a bad trip. Dangerous side effects include panic attacks, flashbacks, and occasional prolonged psychosis.

Designer Drugs

In recent years, chemists who produce many of the illicit drugs in home laboratories have designed versions of drugs listed on **FDA Schedule 1.** Under the Controlled Substances Act, substances regulated by the Food and Drug Administration are placed in one of five schedules. Schedule 1 contains the most dangerous drugs that have no medical use.[17] These *designer drugs* are similar to the controlled drugs on the FDA Schedule 1 but are sufficiently different so that they escape governmental control. The designer drugs are either newly synthesized products that are similar to already outlawed drugs but against which no law yet exists, or they are reconstituted or re-named illegal substances. Designer drugs are said to produce effects similar to their controlled drug counterparts.

People who use designer drugs do so at great risk because the manufacturing of these drugs is unregulated. The neurophysiological effect of these homemade drugs can be quite dangerous. So far, a synthetic heroin product (MPPP) and several amphetamine derivatives with hallucinogenic properties have been designed for the unwary drug consumer.

DOM (STP), MDA (the "love drug"), and ecstasy (MDMA or "XTC") are examples of amphetamine-derivative, hallucinogenic designer drugs. These drugs produce mild LSD-like hallucinogenic experiences, positive feelings, and enhanced alertness. They also have a number of potentially dangerous effects. Experts are particularly concerned that ecstasy can produce strong psychological dependence and can deplete serotonin, an important excitatory neurotransmitter associated with a state of alertness. Permanent brain damage is possible.[2] One recent major survey indicates that MDMA use is declining among teens.[13,18]

Phencyclidine

Phencyclidine (PCP, "angel dust") has been classified variously as a hallucinogen, a stimulant, a depressant, and an anesthetic. PCP was studied for years during the 1950s and 1960s and was found to be an unsuitable animal and human anesthetic.[19] PCP is an extremely unpredictable drug. Easily manufactured in home laboratories in tablet or powder form, PCP can be injected, inhaled, taken orally, or smoked. The effects vary. Some users report mild euphoria, although most report bizarre perceptions, paranoid feelings, and aggressive behavior. PCP overdose may cause convulsions, cardiovascular collapse, and damage to the brain's respiratory center.

In a number of cases the aggressive behavior caused by PCP has led users to commit brutal crimes against both friends and innocent strangers. PCP accumulates in cells and may stimulate bizarre behavior months after initial use.

Cannabis

Cannabis (marijuana) has been labeled a mild hallucinogen for a number of years. However, most experts now consider it to be a drug category in itself. Marijuana produces mild effects like those of stimulants and depressants. The implication of marijuana in a large number of traffic fatalities makes this drug one whose consumption should be carefully considered. Marijuana is actually a wild plant (*Cannabis sativa*) whose fibers were once used in the manufacture of hemp rope. When the leafy material and small stems are dried and crushed, users can smoke the mixture in rolled cigarettes ("joints"), cigars ("blunts"), or pipes. The resins collected from scraping the flowering tops of the plant yield a marijuana product called *hashish,* or *hash,* commonly smoked in a pipe.[20]

The potency of marijuana's hallucinogenic effect is determined by the percentage of the active ingredient tetrahydrocannabinol (THC) present in the product. The concentration of THC averages about 3.5 percent for marijuana, 7–9 percent for higher-quality marijuana (sinsemilla), 8–14 percent for hashish, and as high as 50 percent for hash oil.[2] Today's marijuana has THC levels that are higher than in past decades.

THC is a fat-soluble substance and thus is absorbed and retained in fat tissues within the body. Before being excreted, THC can remain in the body for up to a month. With the sophistication of today's drug tests, trace **metabolites** of THC can be detected for up to 30 days after consumption.[2] It is possible that the THC that comes from passive inhalation of high doses (for example, during an indoor rock concert) can also be detected for a short time after exposure.

Once marijuana is consumed, its effects vary from person to person (see Table 7.2 on page 187). Being "high" or "stoned" or "wrecked" means different things to different people. Many people report heightened sensitivity to music, cravings for particular foods, and a relaxed mood. There is consensus that marijuana's behavioral effects

---

Key Terms

FDA Schedule 1 a list of drugs that have a high potential for abuse but no medical use

metabolite a breakdown product of a drug

Table 7.2 Effects of Marijuana

Short-Term Effects	Long-Term Effects
• Increased heart rate and blood pressure • Feeling of elation • Drowsiness and sedation • Increased appetite • Red eyes • Food cravings • Slow reaction time • Feelings of depression, excitement, paranoia, panic, and euphoria • Problems with attention span, memory, learning, problem-solving, and coordination • Sleeplessness[1]	• Lung damage • Increased risk of bronchitis • Emphysema • Lung cancer • Heart attack[2] • Loss of motivation and short-term memory • Increased panic or anxiety • May become tolerant to marijuana • Damage to lungs, immune system, and reproductive organs • Can remain in the body for up to a month • Can cause birth defects • Five times more damaging to the lungs than tobacco products[1]

[1]National Institute on Drug Abuse. National Institutes of Health. *NIDA Research Report—Marijuana Abuse,* www.nida.nih.gov/ResearchReports/Marijuana/default.html, February 15, 2005.

[2]*Stronger Marijuana Is Major Health Risk. The Independent,* 1 February 2001.

include four probabilities: (1) users must learn to recognize what a marijuana high is like, (2) marijuana impairs short-term memory, (3) users overestimate the passage of time, and (4) users lose the ability to maintain attention to a task.

The long-term effects of marijuana use are still being studied. Chronic abuse may lead to an **amotivational syndrome** in some people. The irritating effects of marijuana smoke on lung tissue are more pronounced than those of cigarette smoke, and some of the over 400 chemicals in marijuana are now linked to lung cancer development. In fact, one of the most potent carcinogens, benzopyrene, is found in higher levels in marijuana smoke than in tobacco smoke. Marijuana smokers tend to inhale deeply and hold the smoke in the lungs for long periods. It is likely that at some point the lungs of chronic marijuana smokers will be damaged.

Long-term marijuana use is also associated with damage to the immune system and to the male and female reproductive systems and with an increase in birth defects in babies born to mothers who smoke marijuana. Chronic marijuana use lowers testosterone levels in men, but the effect of this change is not known. The effect of long-term marijuana use on a variety of types of sexual behavior is also not fully understood.

Because the drug can distort perceptions and thus perceptual ability (especially when combined with alcohol), its use by automobile drivers clearly jeopardizes the lives of many innocent people.

The only medical uses for marijuana are to relieve the nausea caused by chemotherapy, to improve the appetite in AIDS patients, and to ease the pressure that builds up in the eyes of glaucoma patients. However, a variety of other drugs, many of which are nearly as effective, are also used for these purposes. In May 2001, the U.S. Supreme Court ruled unanimously against the distribution of marijuana in medical clinics. In June 2005, the U.S. Supreme Court ruled in a 6–3 decision that the federal government can continue to ban the use of medicinal marijuana. Individuals who use marijuana for medicinal purposes risk federal legal action with state laws providing no defense.

Thai sticks are a potent form of marijuana.

Key Terms

amotivational syndrome behavioral pattern characterized by lack of interest in productive activities

Narcotics

The **narcotics** are among the most dependence-producing drugs. Medically, narcotics are used to relieve pain and induce sleep. On the basis of origin, narcotics can be subgrouped into the natural, quasisynthetic, and synthetic narcotics.

Natural Narcotics

Naturally occurring substances derived from the Oriental poppy plant include opium (the primary psychoactive substance extracted from the Oriental poppy), morphine (the primary active ingredient in opium), and thebaine (a compound not used as a drug). Morphine and related compounds have medical use as analgesics in the treatment of mild to severe pain.

Quasisynthetic Narcotics

Quasisynthetic narcotics are compounds created by chemically altering morphine. These laboratory-produced drugs are intended to be used as analgesics, but their benefits are largely outweighed by a high dependence rate and a great risk of toxicity. The best known of the quasisynthetic narcotics is heroin. Although heroin is a fast-acting and very effective analgesic, it is extremely addictive. Once injected into a vein or "skin-popped" (injected beneath the skin surface), heroin produces dreamlike euphoria and, like all narcotics, strong physical and psychological dependence and tolerance.

As with the use of all other injectable illegal drugs, the practice of sharing needles increases the likelihood of transmission of various communicable diseases, including Hepatitis C and HIV (see Chapter 12). Abrupt withdrawal from heroin use is rarely fatal, but the discomfort during **cold turkey** withdrawal is reported to be overwhelming. The use of heroin has increased during the last decade. The purity of heroin has improved while the price has dropped. Cocaine abusers may use heroin to "come down" from the high associated with cocaine.

Synthetic Narcotics

Meperidine (Demerol) and propoxyphene (Darvon), common postsurgical painkillers, and methadone, the drug prescribed during the rehabilitation of heroin addicts, are *synthetic narcotics*. These opiatelike drugs are manufactured in medical laboratories. They are not natural narcotics or quasisynthetic narcotics because they do not originate from the Oriental poppy plant. Like true narcotics, however, these drugs can rapidly induce physical dependence. One important criticism of methadone rehabilitation programs is that in some cases, they merely shift the addiction from heroin to methadone.

OxyContin   OxyContin, also known as hillybilly heroin, Oxy, Oxycotton, is a time-released legal prescription drug used to treat individuals with moderate to severe pain.[20] Illegal use of OxyContin brought national attention when individuals in rural areas of the country were found abusing this drug. Now abuse of OxyContin is continuing to spread across the country.[21] Classified as a narcotic drug, OxyContin is an addictive controlled substance with an addiction potential similar to morphine. This prescription drug is considered extremely dangerous as an illicit drug. Some methods of usage that increase the likelihood of dangerous effects, including death, are chewing the tablets, snorting crushed tablets, and dissolving the tablets in water and then injecting the drug. When OxyContin is not taken in tablet form, the controlled-release dosage is defeated and the user has a high potential of receiving a lethal dose due to the drug being released immediately into one's system.[22] Many other long-term consequences of OxyContin abuse are physical dependence and severe respiratory depression that may lead to death. Common withdrawal symptoms include restlessness, muscle and bone pain, insomnia, diarrhea, vomiting, cold flashes with goose bumps, and involuntary leg movements.[21] The FDA continues to monitor the abuse of OxyContin and has approved the strongest warning labels for this drug with the intent of changing prescription practices as well as increasing the physician's focus on the potential for abuse.[21]

Inhalants

Inhalants constitute a class of drugs that includes a variety of volatile (quickly evaporating) compounds that generally produce unpredictable, drunklike effects in users and feelings of euphoria.[23] Users of inhalants may also have some delusions and hallucinations. Some users may become quite aggressive. Drugs in this category include anesthetic gases (chloroform, nitrous oxide, and ether), vasodilators (amyl nitrite and butyl nitrite), petroleum products and commercial solvents (gasoline, kerosene, plastic cement, glue, typewriter correction fluid, paint, and paint thinner), and certain aerosols (found in some propelled spray products, fertilizers, and insecticides).

Key Terms

narcotics opiates; psychoactive drugs derived from the Oriental poppy plant; narcotics relieve pain and induce sleep

cold turkey immediate, total discontinuation of use of a drug; associated withdrawal discomfort

inhalants psychoactive drugs that enter the body through inhalation

Most of the danger in using inhalants lies in the damaging, sometimes fatal effects on the respiratory and cardiovascular systems. Furthermore, users may unknowingly place themselves in dangerous situations because of the drunklike hallucinogenic effects. Aggressive behavior might also make users a threat to themselves and others.

Combination Drug Effects

Drugs taken in various combinations and dosages can alter and perhaps intensify effects.

A **synergistic drug effect** is a dangerous consequence of taking different drugs in the same general category at the same time. The combination exaggerates each individual drug's effects. For example, the combined use of alcohol and tranquilizers produces a synergistic effect greater than the total effect of each of the two drugs taken separately. In this instance a much-amplified, perhaps fatal sedation will occur. In a simplistic sense, "one plus one equals four or five."

When taken at or near the same time, drug combinations produce a variety of effects. Drug combinations have additive, potentiating, or antagonistic effects. When two or more drugs are taken and the result is merely a combined total effect of each drug, the result is an **additive effect.** The sum of the effects is not exaggerated. In a sense, "one plus one plus one equals three."

When one drug intensifies the action of a second drug, the first drug is said to have a **potentiated effect** on the second drug. One popular drug-taking practice during the 1970s was the consumption of Quaaludes and beer. Quaaludes potentiated the inhibition-releasing, sedative effects of alcohol. This particular drug combination produced an inexpensive but potentially fatal drunklike euphoria in the user.

An **antagonistic effect** is an opposite effect one drug has on another drug. One drug may be able to reduce another drug's influence on the body. Knowledge of this principle has been useful in the medical treatment of certain drug overdoses, as in the use of tranquilizers to relieve the effects of LSD or other hallucinogenic drugs.

Society's Response to Drug Use

During the last 25 years, society has responded to illegal drug use with growing concern. Most adults see drug abuse as a clear danger to society. This position has been supported by the development of community, school, state, and national organizations directed toward the reduction of illegal drug use. These organizations have included such diverse groups as Parents Against Drugs, Partnership for a Drug-Free America, Mothers Against Drunk Driving (MADD), Narcotics Anonymous, and the U.S. Drug Enforcement Administration. Certain groups have concentrated their efforts on education, others on enforcement, and still others on the development of laws and public policy. Famous people, such as athletes, are also speaking out against drug use. (See Learning from Our Diversity on page 176.)

The personal and social issues related to drug abuse are very complex. Innovative solutions continue to be devised. Some believe that only through early childhood education will people learn alternatives to drug use. Starting drug education in the preschool years may have a more positive effect than waiting until the upper elementary or junior high school years. Recently, the focus on reducing young people's exposure to **gateway drugs** (especially tobacco, alcohol, and marijuana) may help slow down the move to other addictive drugs. Some people advocate harsher penalties for drug use and drug trafficking, including heavier fines and longer prison terms.

Others support legalizing all drugs and making governmental agencies responsible for drug regulation and control, as is the case with alcohol. Advocates of this position believe that drug-related crime and violence would virtually cease once the demand for illegal products is reduced. Sound arguments can be made on both sides of this issue. What's your opinion?

In comparison with other federally funded programs, the "war on drugs" is less expensive than farm support, food stamps, Medicare, and national defense. However, it remains to be seen whether any amount of money spent on enforcement, without adequate support for education, treatment, and poverty reduction, can reduce the illegal drug demand and supply. The United States now spends nearly $18 billion annually to fight the drug war.

Key Terms

synergistic drug effect (sin er **jist** ick) heightened, exaggerated effect produced by the concurrent use of two or more drugs

additive effect the combined (but not exaggerated) effect produced by the concurrent use of two or more drugs

potentiated effect (poe **ten** she ay ted) phenomenon whereby the use of one drug intensifies the effect of a second drug

antagonistic effect effect produced when one drug reduces or offsets the effects of a second drug

gateway drug an easily obtainable legal or illegal drug that represents a user's first experience with a mind-altering drug

About $11 billion is spent on law enforcement (supply reduction) and $6 billion on education, prevention, and treatment (demand reduction).[24]

Drug Testing

Society's response to concern over drug use includes the development and growing use of drug tests. Most of the specimens come from corporations that screen employees for commonly abused drugs. Among these are amphetamines, barbiturates, benzodiazepines (the chemical bases for prescription tranquilizers such as Valium and Librium), cannabinoids (THC, hashish, and marijuana), methaqualone, opiates (heroin, codeine, and morphine), and PCP. With the exception of marijuana, most traces of these drugs are eliminated by the body within a few days after use. Marijuana can remain detectable up to 30 days after use.

How accurate are the results of drug testing? At typical cutoff standards, drug tests will likely identify 90 percent of recent drug users. This means that about 10 percent of recent users will pass undetected. (These 10 percent are considered false negatives.) Nonusers whose drug tests indicate drug use (false positives) are quite rare. (Follow-up tests on these false positives would nearly always show negative results.) Human errors are probably more responsible than technical errors for inaccuracies in drug tests.

Recently, scientists have been refining procedures that use hair samples to detect the presence of drugs. These procedures seem to hold much promise, although certain technical obstacles remain. Watch for refinements in hair-sample drug testing in the near future.

Most Fortune 500 companies, the armed forces, various government agencies, and nearly all athletic organizations have already implemented mandatory drug testing. Corporate substance abuse policies are being developed, with careful attention to legal and ethical issues.

Do you think that the possibility of having to take a drug test would have any effect on college students' use of drugs?

College and Community Support Services for Drug Dependence

Students who have drug problems and realize they need help might select assistance based on the services available on campus or in the surrounding community and the costs they are willing to pay for treatment services.

One approach to convince drug-dependent people to enter treatment programs is the use of *confrontation*.

People who live or work with chemically dependent people are being encouraged to confront them directly about their addiction. Direct confrontation helps chemically dependent people realize the effect their behavior has on others. Once chemically dependent people realize that others will no longer tolerate their behavior, the likelihood of their entering treatment programs increases significantly. Although effective, this approach is very stressful for family members and friends and requires the assistance of professionals in the field of chemical dependence. These professionals can be contacted at a drug treatment center in your area.

Treatment

Comprehensive drug treatment programs are available in very few college or university health centers. College settings for drug dependence programs are more commonly found in the university counseling center. At such a center the emphasis will probably be not on the medical management of dependence but on the behavioral dimensions of drug abuse. Trained counselors and psychologists who specialize in chemical dependence counseling will work with students to (1) analyze their particular concerns, (2) establish constructive ways to cope with stress, and (3) search for alternative ways to achieve new "highs" (see the Personal Assessment on page 193).

 TALKING POINTS Do you think that confronting a friend about her cocaine use would prompt her to get help?

Medical treatment for the management of drug problems may need to be obtained through the services of a community treatment facility administered by a local health department, community mental health center, private clinic, or local hospital. Treatment may be on an inpatient or outpatient basis. Medical management might include detoxification, treatment of secondary health complications and nutritional deficiencies, and therapeutic counseling for chemical dependence.

Some communities have voluntary health agencies that deliver services and treatment programs for drug-dependent people. Check your telephone book for listings of drug-treatment facilities. Some communities have drug hot lines that offer advice for people with questions about drugs. (See the Changing for the Better box on page 177 for a list of anti–drug abuse organizations and hot line numbers.)

Costs of Treatment for Dependence

Drug-treatment programs that are administered by colleges and universities for faculty and students usually require no fees. Local agencies may provide either free services or services based on a **sliding scale.** Private hospitals, physicians, and clinics are the most expensive forms of treatment. Inpatient treatment at a private facility may cost as much as $1000 per day. Since the length of inpatient treatment averages 3 to 4 weeks, a patient can quickly accumulate a very large bill. However, with many types of health insurance policies now providing coverage for alcohol and other drug dependencies, even these services may not require additional out-of-pocket expenses.

Taking Charge of Your Health

- Assess your knowledge of drug use by completing the Personal Assessment on page 193.
- Calculate the amount of caffeine you consume daily. If you're drinking more than three cups of caffeinated beverages per day, develop a plan to reduce your overall intake.

- Prepare a plan of action to use if someone you know needs professional assistance with a drug problem.
- Identify five activities that can provide you with a drug-free high.
- Analyze your drug use patterns (if any), and assess the likelihood that you might fail a preemployment drug test.

- Assess your lifestyle for addictive behaviors that do not involve drugs, such as overexercising or watching too much TV. Develop a plan to moderate these activities and achieve more balance in your life.

SUMMARY

- A drug affects the CNS by altering neurotransmitter activity on the neuron.
- Drug use, drug abuse, tolerance, and dependence are important terms to understand.
- Drugs enter the body through ingestion, injection, inhalation, or absorption.
- Drugs can be placed into six categories: stimulants, depressants, hallucinogens, cannabis, narcotics, and inhalants.

- Combination drug effects include synergist, addictive, potentiated, and antagonistic effects.
- Drug testing is becoming increasingly common in our society.
- Drug abuse has a devastating effect on society.
- Society's response to drug abuse has been widely varied and has included education, enforcement, treatment, testing, and the search for drug-free ways to achieve highs.

REVIEW QUESTIONS

1. Describe how neurotransmitters work.
2. Identify and explain the three steps in the process of addiction.
3. How is the term *drug* defined in this chapter? What are psychoactive drugs? How do medicines differ from drugs?
4. Define the four routes of administration. Select a drug that reflects each of the ways drugs enter the body.
5. Explain what *dependence* means. Identify and explain the two types of dependence.
6. Define the word *tolerance*. What does *cross-tolerance* mean? Give an example of cross-tolerance.
7. Differentiate between drug misuse and drug abuse.

8. List the six general categories of drugs. For each category, give several examples of drugs and explain the effects they would have on the user. What are designer drugs?
9. Why do students without a prescription take Ritalin? What are the side effects and health risks of abusing Ritalin?
10. What is the active ingredient in marijuana? What are its common effects on the user? What are the short- and long-term effects of marijuana use?
11. Explain the terms *synergistic effect, additive effect, potentiated effect,* and *antagonistic effect.*
12. How accurate is drug testing?

ENDNOTES

1. Shier D, Butler J, Lewis R. *Hole's Essentials of Human Anatomy and Physiology* (9th ed.) New York: McGraw-Hill, 2002.

2. Ray O, Ksir C. *Drugs, Society, and Human Behavior* (10th ed.). New York: McGraw-Hill, 2004.

3. The Coffee Science Information Centre. *Caffeine*, http://www.cosic.org/, March 7, 2005.

4. *Caffeine*. Johns Hopkins online newsletter September 2002, www.intelihealth.com, March 7, 2005.

5. National Institute on Drug Abuse. National Institutes of Health. NIDA InfoFacts, *Methamphetamine*, www.nida.nih.gov/Infofax/methamphetamine.html, March 7, 2005.

6. U.S. Department of Justice. Drug Enforcement Administration, *Methemphetamine*, www.usdoj.gov/dea/concern/meth.htm, December 31, 2001.

7. Frackelmann, K. Breaking bonds of addiction: Compulsion traced to part of the brain, *USA Today*, April 18, 2002.

8. Ephedra Education Council. *Ephedra Supported by Science—A Ban Is Not, Industry Tells FDA*, April 8, 2003.

9. U.S. Department of Justice. Drug Enforcement Administration, *Drugs of Abuse*, www.dea.gov/pubs/abuse/5-stim.htm, 2005 Edition.

10. Cocaine weakens immune system. *Boston Herald*, March 7, 2003.

11. Pinger RR, Payne WA, Hahn DB, Hahn EJ. *Drugs: Issues for Today* (3rd ed.). New York: McGraw-Hill, 1998.

12. National Institute on Drug Abuse. National Institutes of Health, NIDA Research Report, *Prescription Drugs Abuse and Addiction*, www.drugabuse.gov/ResearchReports/Prescription/Prescription.html, NIH Publication No. 01-4881, July 2001.

13. National Institute on Drug Abuse. NIDA InfoFacts, *Rohypnol and GHB*, www.nida.nih.gov/Infofax/RohypnolGHB.html, February 14, 2004.

14. National Institute on Drug Abuse. National Institutes of Health, NIDA InfoFacts, *Club Drugs*, www.drugabuse.gov/Infofax/Clubdrugs.html, March 7, 2005.

15. Johnston LD, O'Malley PM, Bachman JG, Schulenberg, JE. *Monitoring the Future: National Survey Results on Drug Use: 1975–2003. Volume I: Secondary School Students*, www.monitoringthefuture.org/pubs/monographs/vol1_2003.pdf, NIH Publication No. 04-5507. Bethesda, MD: 2004.

16. National Institute on Drug Abuse. NIDA InfoFacts, *LSD*, www.nida.nih.gov/Infofax/lsd.html, February 15, 2005.

17. U.S. Drug Enforcement Administration. Controlled Substances Act, www.usdoj.gov/dea/agency/csa.htm, February 16, 2005.

18. Johnston LD, O'Malley PM, Bachman JG, Schulenberg, JE. National Press Release, *Overall Teen Drug Use Continues Gradual Decline; but Use of Inhalants Rises.* University of Michigan News and Information Services, Ann Arbor, MI: 2004.

19. National Institute on Drug Abuse. National Institutes of Health, NIDA InfoFacts, *Marijuana*, www.nida.nih.gov/Infofax/marijuana.html, February 16, 2005.

20. OxyContin Questions and Answers. Drug Information, U.S. Food and Drug Administration, Center for Drug Evaluation and Research, www.fda.gov/cder/drug/infopage/oxycontin/oxycontin-qa.htm, March 7, 2005.

21. OxyContin. *OxyContin Addiction and Treatment and Rapid Detox Services*, www.oxycontin-detox.com/index-overture-kw-oxycontin.html, March 7, 2005.

22. U.S. Food and Drug Administration. *FDA Strengthens Warnings for OxyContin*, www.fda.gov/bbs/topics/ANSWERS/2001/ANS01091.html, March 7, 2005.

23. Frackelmann, K. Inhalants' hidden treat: Access makes huffing popular but kids can recover with help, *USA Today*, June 25, 2002.

24. www.whitehousedrugpolicy.gov/publications/policy/04budget/exec_sum.pdf, May 21, 2003.

As We Go to Press

An anti-methamphetamine bill has been advancing in Congress to restrict the sales of over-the-counter cold medicines that contain pseudoephedrine, such as Sudafed, NyQuil, and Tylenol Cold, which are used in home laboratories to make methamphetamine. This bill will require consumers to present a photo identification card, sign a log, and be limited to a particular number of grams of pseudoephedrine bought in a 30-day period. Computer tracking would also prevent consumers from purchasing pseudoephedrine in other stores. Walgreen Company announced they would move all pseudoephedrine products behind the pharmacy counter nationwide in October 2005. Other retailers are restricting sales of pseudoephedrine to help curb methamphetamine production.

personal assessment

Test your drug awareness

1. What is the most commonly used drug in the United States?
   a. heroin
   b. cocaine
   c. alcohol
   d. marijuana

2. Name the three drugs most commonly used by children.
   a. alcohol, tobacco, and marijuana
   b. cocaine, crack, alcohol
   c. heroin, inhalants, marijuana

3. Which drug is associated with the most teenage deaths?
   a. heroin
   b. cocaine
   c. alcohol
   d. marijuana

4. By the 8th grade, how many kids have tried at least one inhalant?
   a. 1 in 100
   b. 1 in 50
   c. 1 in 25
   d. 1 in 5
   e. 1 in 2

5. "Crack" is a particularly dangerous drug because it is
   a. cheap.
   b. readily available.
   c. highly addictive.
   d. all of the above.

6. Fumes from which of the following can be inhaled to produce a high?
   a. spray paint
   b. model glue
   c. nail polish remover
   d. whipped cream canisters
   e. all of the above

7. People who have not used alcohol and other drugs before their 20th birthday:
   a. have no risk of becoming chemically dependent.
   b. are less likely to develop a drinking problem or use illicit drugs.
   c. have an increased risk of becoming chemically dependent.

8. A speedball is a combination of which two drugs?
   a. cocaine and heroin
   b. PCP and LSD
   c. valium and alcohol
   d. amphetamines and barbiturates

9. Methamphetamines are dangerous because use can cause
   a. anxiety/nervousness/irritability.
   b. paranoia/psychosis.
   c. loss of appetite/malnutrition/anorexia.
   d. hallucinations.
   e. aggressive behavior.
   f. all of the above.

10. How is marijuana harmful?
    a. It hinders the user's short-term memory.
    b. Students may find it hard to study and learn while under the influence of marijuana.
    c. It affects timing and coordination.
    d. All of the above

Answers to Personal Assessment

1. c
2. a
3. c
4. d
5. d
6. e
7. b
8. a
9. f
10. d

Source: *A Parent's Guide to Prevention*, U.S. Department of Education.

personal assessment

Getting a drug free high

Experts agree that drug use provides only short-term, ineffective, and often destructive solutions to problems. We hope that you have found (or will find) innovative, invigorating drug-free experiences that make your life more exciting. Circle the number for each activity that reflects your intention to try that activity. Use the following guide:

1. No intention of trying this activity
2. Intend to try this within 2 years
3. Intend to try this within 6 months
4. Already tried this activity
5. Regularly engage in this activity

1. Learn to juggle	1	2	3	4	5
2. Go backpacking	1	2	3	4	5
3. Complete a marathon race	1	2	3	4	5
4. Start a vegetable garden	1	2	3	4	5
5. Ride in a hot air balloon	1	2	3	4	5
6. Snow ski or water ski	1	2	3	4	5
7. Donate blood	1	2	3	4	5
8. Go river rafting	1	2	3	4	5
9. Learn to play a musical instrument	1	2	3	4	5
10. Cycle 100 miles	1	2	3	4	5
11. Go skydiving	1	2	3	4	5
12. Go rockclimbing	1	2	3	4	5
13. Play a role in a theater production	1	2	3	4	5
14. Build a piece of furniture	1	2	3	4	5
15. Solicit funds for a worthy cause	1	2	3	4	5
16. Learn to swim	1	2	3	4	5
17. Overhaul a car engine	1	2	3	4	5
18. Compose a song	1	2	3	4	5
19. Travel to a foreign country	1	2	3	4	5
20. Write the first chapter of a book	1	2	3	4	5

TOTAL POINTS _____

Interpretation

61–100	You participate in many challenging experiences
41–60	You are willing to try some challenging new experiences
20–40	You take few of the challenging risks described here

To Carry This Further . . .

Looking at your point total, were you surprised at the degree to which you are aware of alternative activities? What are the top five activities, and can you understand their importance? What activities would you add to this list?

chapter eight

Taking Control of Alcohol use

Chapter Objectives

On completing this chapter, you will be able to:

▌ describe the prevalence of drinking on college campuses.

▌ describe the physiological effects of alcohol and how these effects differ by gender.

▌ list the symptoms and first aid procedures for acute alcohol intoxication.

▌ explain how alcohol use plays a role in accidents, crime, and suicide.

▌ list the major organizations that support responsible drinking.

▌ describe problem drinking and alcoholism.

▌ define codependence and describe how it damages the alcoholic and codependent.

▌ explain how denial and enabling can prolong problem drinking.

▌ list the common traits of adult children of alcoholics.

Eye on the Media

TV Ads Target Drunk Driving

The first successful national campaign against drunk driving, "Designated Driver," began in 1998. Besides targeting specific audiences and using well-timed and strategically placed public service announcements, its developers convinced TV producers and writers to work references to the designated driver into the dialogue of their shows. Gradually, the message got through to young people. It does make sense to plan to have someone else drive if you're not going to be up to it. The designated-driver approach is still considered a good idea on college campuses today.

In contrast, the "Campaign for Alcohol Free Kids," relied heavily on dramatic graphics, such as grisly photos of car crash scenes on prom night. Although the overall visual impact was powerful, the campaign lacked a practical element. Worse, the ads seemed to be preaching.

The Ad Council's "Friends Don't Let Friends Drive Drunk" is based on the idea that we all have responsibility for one another. If someone is your friend, you want to take care of that person. So don't let your friend do something dangerous. Here the message is practical, not preachy.

The "You Drink & Drive, You Lose" campaign, a part of the National Public Education Campaign, targets two high-risk groups, 21- to 34-year-olds and repeat offenders. The message is simple: Make the right choice—don't drink and drive. The "Don't Lose It!" TV spot focuses on the fact that it's inconvenient to be stopped but the time spent at the checkpoint is for your own safety. It seems to be saying: "Sure, you're in a hurry, but this is important. So be patient." The graphics range from a serious-looking police officer talking to a motorist to hands locked in handcuffs.

What the successful campaigns have in common is a message that is simple, believable, and acceptable. Rather than scolding or preaching, the ads emphasize the fact that you have a choice and ask you to make the right choice.

"Road Predators," an American Public Television special that aired in December 1999, touched off strong contoversy. Funded by the Century Council, a corporation backed by a group of U.S. distillers, the program used tragic accounts of alcohol-related accidents to dramatize the fact that innocent people lose their lives, families are shattered, and billions of dollars are spent because of drunk drivers.

What is the motivation for an alcohol industry group to fund a campaign to discourage drunk driving? How do such campaigns compare with the tobacco industry's efforts to discourage smoking among teenagers? How effective do you think each kind of ad campaign is?

Campaign for Alcohol Free Kids: Who We Are, www.alcoholfreekids.com/au_who_ we_are.html, March 8, 2005.
Web Site Information: Ad Council, www.adcouncil. org/, March 8, 2005.

The push for zero tolerance laws, the tightening of standards for determining legal intoxication, and the growing influence of national groups concerned with alcohol misuse show that our society is more sensitive than ever to the growing misuse of alcohol.

People are concerned about the consequences of drunk driving, alcohol-related crime, and lowered job productivity. National data indicate that per capita alcohol consumption has gradually dropped in the United States since the early 1980s.[1] Alcohol use remains the preferred form of drug use for most adults (including college students), but as a society, we are increasingly uncomfortable with the ease with which alcohol can be misused.

Choosing to Drink

Clearly, people drink alcoholic beverages for many different reasons. Most people drink alcohol because it is an effective, affordable, and legal substance for altering the brain's chemistry. As **inhibitions** are removed by the influence of alcohol, behavior that is generally held in check is expressed (Figure 8-1). At least temporarily, drinkers become a different version of themselves—more outgoing, relaxed, and adventuresome.

> **TALKING POINTS** If alcohol did not make people more outgoing, relaxed, and adventuresome, then do you think they would consume as much?

Alcohol Use Patterns

From magazines to billboards to television, alcohol is one of the most heavily advertised consumer products in the country.[2] You cannot watch television, listen to the radio, or read a newspaper without being encouraged to buy a particular brand of beer, wine, or liquor. The advertisements create a warm aura about the nature of alcohol use. The implications are clear: alcohol use will bring you good times, handsome men or seductive women, exotic settings, and a chance to forget the hassles of hard work and study.

Given the many pressures to drink, it's not surprising that most adults drink alcoholic beverages. Two-thirds of all American adults are classified as drinkers. Yet one in three adults does not drink. In the college environment, where surveys indicate that 85–90 percent of all students drink, it's difficult for many students to imagine that every third adult is an abstainer. Although many college students assume that drinking is a natural part of their social life, others are making alternative choices. (See Discovering Your Spirituality on page 199.)

Alcohol consumption figures are reported in many different ways, depending on the researchers' criteria. Various sources support the contention that about one-third of adults 18 years of age and older are abstainers, about one-

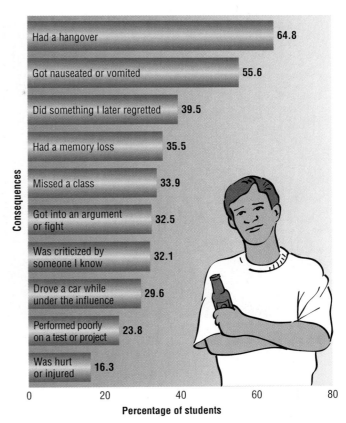

Figure 8-1 Negative consequences of alcohol use as reported by college students. (Occurred at least once in past year; year 2003 statistics from national sample of over 38,857 undergraduates from 89 colleges in U.S.)

Source: Core Institute. 2003. *The Core Alcohol and Drug Survey,* www.siu.edu/departments/coreinst/public_html/, February 27, 2005.

third are light drinkers, and one-third are moderate-to-heavy drinkers. As a single category, heavy drinkers make up about 10 percent of the adult drinking population. Students who drink in college tend to classify themselves as light-to-moderate drinkers. It comes as a shock to students, though, when they read the criteria for each drinking classification. According to the combination of quantity of alcohol consumed per occasion and the frequency of drinking, these criteria are established as shown in Table 8.1.

Moderate Drinking Redefined

Alcohol Research and Health defines moderate drinking as no more than two drinks each day for most men and

---

Key Terms

inhibitions inner controls that prevent a person from engaging in certain types of behavior

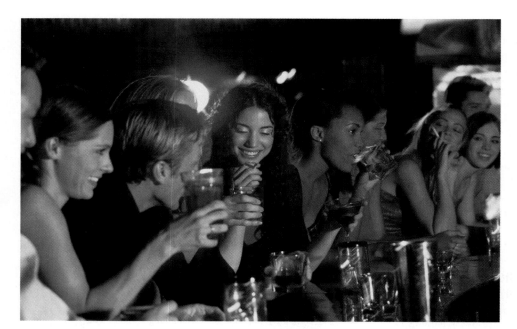

Two-thirds of American adults are classified as drinkers. Only one-third choose to abstain from alcohol.

Table 8.1 Criteria for Drinking Classifications

Classification	Alcohol-Related Behavior
Abstainers	Do not drink or drink less often than once a year
Infrequent drinkers	Drink once a month at most and drink small amounts per typical drinking occasion
Light drinkers	Drink once a month at most and drink medium amounts per typical drinking occasion, or drink no more than three to four times a month and drink small amounts per typical drinking occasion
Moderate drinkers	Drink at least once a week and small amounts per typical drinking occasion or three to four times a month and medium amounts per typical drinking occasion or no more than once a month and large amounts per typical drinking occasion
Moderate/heavy drinkers	Drink at least once a week and medium amounts per typical drinking occasion or three to four times a month and large amounts per typical drinking occasion
Heavy drinkers	Drink at least once a week and large amounts per typical drinking occasion[1]

Note: Small amounts = One drink or less per drinking occasion
Medium amounts = Two to four drinks per drinking occasion
Large amounts = Five or more drinks per drinking occasion (binge drinking)
Drink = 12 fluid oz of beer, 5 fluid oz of wine, or 1.5 fluid oz of 80 proof distilled spirits
U.S. Department of Health and Human Services: *Fourth Special Report to the U.S. Congress,* Washington, D.C., 1981, DHHS Pub No. ADM 81-1080.
Dufour M (1999). "What Is Moderate Drinking? Defining "Drinks" and Drinking Levels," *Alcohol Research and Health,* 23(1), 5–14.

one drink each day for women. A drink is defined as one 12-ounce regular beer, a 5-ounce glass of wine, or 1½ ounces of 80 proof distilled spirits.[3] These cutoff levels are based on the amount of alcohol that can be consumed without causing problems, either for the drinker or society. (The gender difference is due primarily to the higher percentage of body fat in women and to the lower amount of an essential stomach enzyme in women.) Elderly people are limited to no more than one drink each day, again because of a higher percentage of body fat.

These consumption levels are applicable to most people. Indeed, people who plan to drive, women who are pregnant, people recovering from alcohol addiction, people under age 21, people taking medications, and those with existing medical concerns should not consume alcohol. Additionally, although some studies have shown that low levels of alcohol consumption may have minor psychological and cardiovascular benefits, nondrinkers are not advised to start drinking.

Binge Drinking

Alcohol abuse by college students usually takes place through *binge drinking.* This practice refers to the consumption of five drinks in one sitting, at least once during the previous 2-week period. College students who fit the category of "heavy drinkers" rarely consume small amounts of alcohol each day but instead binge on alcohol 1 or 2 nights a week. Some students openly admit that they plan to "get really drunk" on the weekend. They plan to binge drink.

What's a Social Life without Alcohol?

When was the last time you went to a get-together where alcoholic drinks weren't served? It's probably been years. Socializing and drinking are connected in our consciousness in many ways. For instance, it's Friday night after a hard week and your friends ask you to join them for a beer. Why not? It'll be fun. Or you're invited to a party and want to bring something. How about a bottle of wine? That's easy and always appreciated.

Associating drinking with fun is something that many people, including college students, do. For various reasons, though, some college students are choosing to plan their fun around activities that don't involve drinking. Instead of going to a bar for a beer, they find a coffee shop and have a latte. Or they order soda with their pizza (not bad!). Others have discovered that they can get something that tastes great and is actually healthy at a juice bar.

What happens, though, when you go to a party and everyone else seems to be drinking? Choose something nonalcoholic—club soda, juice, soda, or water. (You probably won't be the only one doing this.) If someone gives you trouble about your choice, be firm. Just say that's what you want. You don't need to explain. And you don't have to say "yes" to be nice.

But maybe you want to drink at a party because it loosens you up and makes it easier to talk to people. How will you start a conversation without a drink to relax you? Think about how you talk easily and naturally with the people in your drama group or one of your favorite classes. You've got things in common, so it's easier to do. When you meet someone new at a party, look for common interests. You may feel self-conscious at first. But soon you'll forget about the fact that he or she is a stranger because you'll be involved in what you're talking about. Without that drink, you'll actually be more yourself.

Some students are making the commitment to be active instead of sitting around and drinking. They're going backpacking, joining a cycling group, taking an exercise class, or playing a team sport. What they're discovering is that it feels good—physically and mentally. They're socializing, doing something they enjoy, and getting in better shape. Think about something you've always wanted to try, and get going on it.

Making the choice to have fun without alcohol doesn't mean cutting yourself off from your friends. (If they're real friends, they'll respect your choice.) It's all about deciding what's right for you and making a commitment to that choice.

Individuals may experience peer pressure to participate in a drinking game. Drinking games are a form of binge drinking in which individuals consume large amounts of alcohol in a small period of time.

 TALKING POINTS How do you tell a friend that you think he has a drinking problem?

Binge drinking can be dangerous. Drunk driving, physical violence, property destruction, date rape, police arrest, and lowered academic performance are all closely associated with binge drinking. The direct correlation between the amount of alcohol consumed and lowered academic performance results in impaired memory, verbal skill deficiencies, and altered perceptions.[4] Frequently, the social costs of binge drinking are very high, especially when intoxicated people demonstrate their level of immaturity. How common is binge drinking on your campus?

In response to the personal dangers and campus trauma associated with binge drinking, colleges and universities are fighting back. Some colleges are conducting local alcohol education campaigns that feature innovative posters and materials displayed on campus. In the future, expect to see increasing efforts to reduce binge drinking on your campus to make it a safer environment.

For many students who drink, the college years are a time when they drink more heavily than at any other time in their life (Figure 8-2). Some will suffer serious consequences as a result (Figure 8-1). These years will also mark the entry into a lifetime of problem drinking for some.

The Nature of Alcoholic Beverages

Alcohol (also known as *ethyl alcohol* or *ethanol*) is the principal product of **fermentation.** In this process, yeast cells act on the sugar content of fruits and grains to produce alcohol and carbon dioxide.[5]

The alcohol concentration in beverages such as whiskey, gin, rum, and vodka is determined through a process called **distillation.** These distilled beverages are

Key Terms
fermentation a chemical process whereby plant products are converted into alcohol by the action of yeast cells on carbohydrate materials
distillation the process of heating an alcohol solution and collecting its vapors into a more concentrated solution

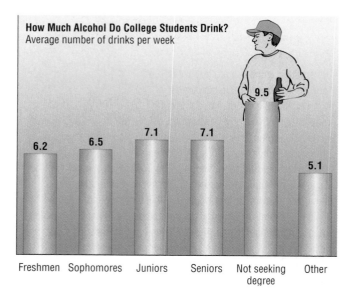

How Much Alcohol Do College Students Drink?
Average number of drinks per week

Freshmen 6.2 | Sophomores 6.5 | Juniors 7.1 | Seniors 7.1 | Not seeking degree 9.5 | Other 5.1

Figure 8-2 Average number of alcoholic drinks consumed by college drinkers (year 2003 statistics from national sample of over 38,857 undergraduates from 89 colleges in U.S.).

Source: Core Institute. 2003 *The Core Alcohol and Drug Survey,* www.siu.edu/departments/coreinst/ public _html/, March 8, 2005.

expressed by the term *proof,* a number that is twice the percentage of alcohol by volume in a beverage. Thus 70 percent of the fluid in a bottle of 140 proof gin is pure alcohol. Most proofs in distilled beverages range from 80 to 160. The familiar pure *grain alcohol* that is often added to fruit punches and similar beverages has a proof of almost 200.

The nutritional value of alcohol is extremely limited. Alcoholic beverages produced today through modern processing methods contain nothing but empty calories—about 100 calories per fluid ounce of 100-proof distilled spirits and about 150 calories for each 12-ounce bottle or can of beer.[6] Clearly, alcohol consumption is a significant contributor to the additional pounds that many college students accumulate. Pure alcohol contains only simple carbohydrates; it has no vitamins and minerals and no fats or protein.

"Lite" beer and low-calorie wines have been introduced in response to concerns about the number of calories that alcoholic beverages provide. They are not low-alcohol beverages but merely low-calorie beverages. Only beverages marked "low alcohol" contain a lower concentration of alcohol than the usual beverages of that type. Recently, manufacturers have introduced a new form of beer called low carbohydrate beer. For the diet-conscious consumer, low-carb beer contains a lower carbohydrate content but the same alcohol and calorie content that other beers have.

The popular new ice beers actually contain a higher percentage of alcohol than other types of beer. This is due to a production process that chills the fermented mixture sufficiently to allow ice crystals to form. When the ice crystals are removed, the beer contains a higher percentage of alcohol.

The Physiological Effects of Alcohol

First and foremost, alcohol is classified as a drug—a very strong CNS depressant. The primary depressant effect of alcohol occurs in the brain and spinal cord. Many people think of alcohol as a stimulant because of the way most users feel after consuming a serving or two of their favorite drink. Any temporary sensations of jubilation, boldness, or relief are attributable to alcohol's ability as a depressant drug to release personal inhibitions and provide temporary relief from tension.

Factors That Influence the Absorption of Alcohol

The **absorption** of alcohol is influenced by several factors, most of which can be controlled by the individual. These factors include the following:

- *Strength of the beverage.* The stronger the beverage, the greater the amount of alcohol that accumulates within the digestive tract.

- *Number of drinks consumed.* As more drinks are consumed, more alcohol is absorbed.

- *Speed of consumption.* If consumed rapidly, even relatively few drinks will result in a large concentration gradient that leads to high blood alcohol concentration.

- *Presence of food.* Food can compete with alcohol for absorption into the bloodstream, slowing the absorption of alcohol. When alcohol absorption is slowed, the alcohol already in the bloodstream can be removed. Slow absorption favors better control of blood alcohol concentration.

- *Body chemistry.* Each person has an individual pattern of physiological functioning that may affect the ability to process alcohol. For example, in some conditions, such as that marked by "dumping syndrome," the stomach empties more rapidly than is normal, and alcohol seems to be absorbed more quickly. The

Key Terms

absorption the passage of nutrients or alcohol through the walls of the stomach or the intestinal tract into the bloodstream

emptying time may be either slowed or quickened by anger, fear, stress, nausea, and the condition of the stomach tissues.

- *Race/Ethnicity.* Research suggests that alcohol tolerance levels may range from weak to strong based on an individual's race/ethnic origin.
- *Gender.* Women produce much less alcohol dehydrogenase than men do.[7] This enzyme is responsible for breaking down alcohol in the stomach. As a result, women absorb about 30 percent more alcohol into the bloodstream than men, despite an identical number of drinks and equal body weight.

Three other reasons help explain why women tend to absorb alcohol more quickly than men of the same body weight: (1) Women have proportionately more body fat than men. Since alcohol is not stored easily in fat, it enters the bloodstream relatively quickly. (2) Women's bodies have proportionately less water than do men's bodies of equal weight. Thus alcohol consumed does not become as diluted as in men. (3) Alcohol absorption is influenced by a woman's menstrual cycle. Alcohol is more quickly absorbed during the premenstrual phase of a woman's cycle. Also, there is evidence that women using birth control pills absorb alcohol faster than usual.[7]

With the exception of a person's body chemistry, race/ethnicity, and gender, all factors that influence absorption can be moderated by the alcohol user.

Blood Alcohol Concentration

A person's **blood alcohol concentration (BAC)** rises when alcohol is consumed faster than it can be removed (oxidized) by the liver.[8] As outlined in Figure 8-3, a fairly predictable sequence of events takes place when a person drinks alcohol at a rate faster than one drink every hour. When the BAC reaches 0.05 percent, initial measurable changes in mood and behavior take place. Inhibitions and everyday tensions appear to be released, while judgment and critical thinking are somewhat impaired. This BAC would be achieved by a 160-pound person consuming about two drinks in an hour.

At a level of 0.10 percent (one part alcohol to 1,000 parts blood), the drinker typically loses significant motor coordination. Voluntary motor function becomes quite clumsy. At this BAC, most states consider a drinker legally intoxicated and thus incapable of safely operating a vehicle. Although physiological changes associated with this BAC do occur, certain users do not feel intoxicated or do not outwardly appear to be impaired.

As the BAC rises from 0.20–0.50 percent, the health risk of acute alcohol intoxication increases rapidly. A BAC of 0.20 percent is characterized by the loud, boisterous, obnoxious drunk person who staggers. A 0.30 percent BAC produces further depression and stuporous behavior, and the drinker becomes so confused that he or she may not be capable of understanding anything. The 0.40 percent or 0.50 percent BAC produces unconsciousness. At this level, a person can die, since the brain centers that control body temperature, heartbeat, and breathing may be virtually shut down.

An important factor influencing the BAC is the individual's blood volume. The larger the person, the greater the amount of blood into which alcohol can be distributed. Conversely, the smaller person has less blood into which alcohol can be distributed, and as a result, a higher BAC will develop.

Sobering Up

Alcohol is removed from the bloodstream principally through the process of **oxidation.** Oxidation occurs at a constant rate (about $1/4$ to $1/3$ ounce of pure alcohol per hour) that cannot be appreciably altered. Since each typical drink of beer, wine, or distilled spirits contains about $1/2$ ounce of pure alcohol, it takes about 2 hours for the body to fully oxidize one typical alcoholic drink.[9]

Although people may try to sober up by drinking hot coffee, taking cold showers, or exercising, the oxidation rate of alcohol is unaffected by these measures. Thus far the FDA has not approved any commercial product that can help people achieve sobriety. Since alcohol causes dehydration, rehydration and the passage of time remains the only effective remedy for diminishing alcohol's effects.

First Aid for Acute Alcohol Intoxication

Not everyone who goes to sleep, passes out, or becomes unconscious after drinking has a high BAC. People who are already sleepy, have not eaten well, are sick, or are bored may drink a little alcohol and quickly fall asleep. However, people who drink heavily in a rather short time

> **Key Terms**
>
> **blood alcohol concentration (BAC)** the percentage of alcohol in a measured quantity of blood; BACs can be determined directly through the analysis of a blood sample or indirectly through the analysis of exhaled air
>
> **oxidation** the process that removes alcohol from the bloodstream

Figure 8-3 Effects of alcohol by number of drinks

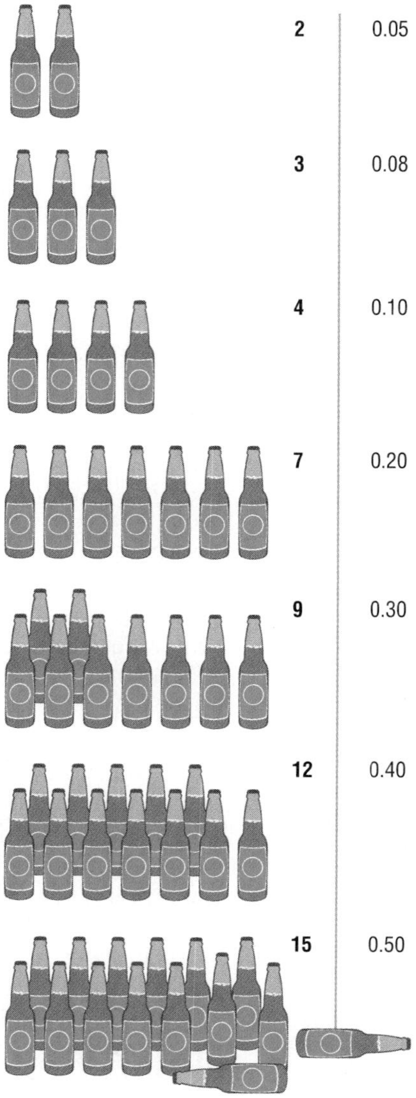

Number of drinks consumed in two hours	Alcohol in blood (percentage)	Typical effects
2	0.05	Judgment, thought, and restraint weakened; tension released, giving carefree sensation
3	0.08	Tensions of everyday life lessened; cheerfulness
4	0.10	Voluntary motor action affected, making hand and arm movements, walk, and speech clumsy
7	0.20	Severe impairment—staggering, loud, incoherent, emotionally unstable, 100 times greater traffic risk; exuberance and aggressive inclinations magnified
9	0.30	Deeper areas of brain affected, with stimulus-response and understanding confused; stuporous; blurred vision
12	0.40	Incapable of voluntary action; sleepy, difficult to arouse; equivalent of surgical anesthesia
15	0.50	Comatose; centers controlling breathing and heartbeat anesthetized; death increasingly probable

Note: A drink refers to a typical 12-ounce bottle of beer, a 1.5-ounce shot of hard liquor, or a 5-ounce glass of wine.

may be setting themselves up for an extremely unpleasant, toxic, potentially life-threatening experience because of their high BAC.

Although responsible drinking would prevent **acute alcohol intoxication** (poisoning), it will never be a reality for everyone. As a caring adult, what should you know about this health emergency that may help you save a life—perhaps even a friend's life?

The first real danger signs to recognize are the typical signs of **shock.** By the time these signs are evident, a drinker will already be unconscious. He or she will not be able to be aroused from a deep stupor. The person will probably have a weak, rapid pulse (over 100 beats per minute). The skin will be cool and damp, and breathing will be increased to once every 3 or 4 seconds. These breaths may be shallow or deep but will certainly occur in an irregular pattern. Skin will be pale or bluish. (In the case of a person with dark skin, these color changes will be

---

Key Terms

acute alcohol intoxication a potentially fatal elevation of the BAC, often resulting from heavy, rapid consumption of alcohol

shock profound collapse of many vital body functions; evident during acute alcohol intoxication and other health emergencies

more evident in the fingernail beds or in the mucous membranes inside the mouth or under the eyelids.) Whenever any of these signs are present, seek emergency medical help immediately. (See Changing for the Better above for a summary of these signs.)

Involuntary regurgitation (vomiting) can be another potentially life-threatening emergency for a person who has drunk too much alcohol. When a drinker has consumed more alcohol than the liver can oxidize, the pyloric valve at the base of the stomach tends to close. Additional alcohol remains in the stomach. This alcohol irritates the lining of the stomach so much that involuntary muscle contractions force the stomach contents to flow back through the esophagus. By removing alcohol from the stomach, vomiting may be a life-saving mechanism for conscious drinkers.

An unconscious drinker who vomits may be lying in such a position that the airway becomes obstructed by the vomitus. This person is at great risk of dying from **asphyxiation.** As a first-aid measure, unconscious drinkers should always be rolled onto their sides to minimize the chance of airway obstruction. If you are with someone who is vomiting, make certain that his or her head is positioned lower than the rest of the body. This position minimizes the chance that vomitus will obstruct the air passages.

Also keep a close watch on anyone who passes out from heavy drinking. Partygoers sometimes make the mistake of carrying these people to bed and then forgetting about them. Monitoring the physical condition of anyone who becomes unconscious from heavy drinking is crucial because of the risk of death. Observe the person at regular intervals until he or she appears to be clearly out of danger. This may mean an evening of interrupted sleep for you, but you could save a friend's life. Are you aware of any recent alcohol-related deaths among U.S. college students?

Alcohol-Related Health Problems

The relationship of chronic alcohol use to the structure and function of the body is reasonably well understood. Heavy alcohol use causes a variety of changes to the body that lead to an increase in morbidity and mortality. Figure 8-4 on page 204 describes these changes.

Research shows that chronic alcohol use also damages the immune system and the nervous system. Thus chronic users are at high risk for a variety of infections and neurological complications.[1] Additionally, many alcoholics suffer from malnutrition, in part because they do not consume a variety of foods. With the deterioration of the liver, stomach, and pancreas, chronic heavy drinkers also have poor absorption and metabolism of many nutrients.

Fetal Alcohol Syndrome and Fetal Alcohol Effects

A growing body of scientific evidence indicates that alcohol use by pregnant women can result in birth defects in unborn children. When alcohol crosses the **placenta,** it enters the fetal bloodstream in a concentration equal to that in the mother's bloodstream. Because of the underdeveloped nature of the fetal liver, this alcohol is oxidized much more slowly than the alcohol in the mother. During this time of slow detoxification, the developing fetus is certain to be overexposed to the toxic effects of alcohol. Mental retardation frequently develops.

This exposure has additional disastrous consequences for the developing fetus. Low birth weight, facial abnormalities (for example, small head, widely spaced eyes), and heart problems are often seen in such infants (Figure 8-5). This combination of effects is called

Key Terms

asphyxiation death resulting from lack of oxygen to the brain

placenta the structure through which nutrients, metabolic wastes, and drugs (including alcohol) pass from the bloodstream of the mother into the bloodstream of the developing fetus

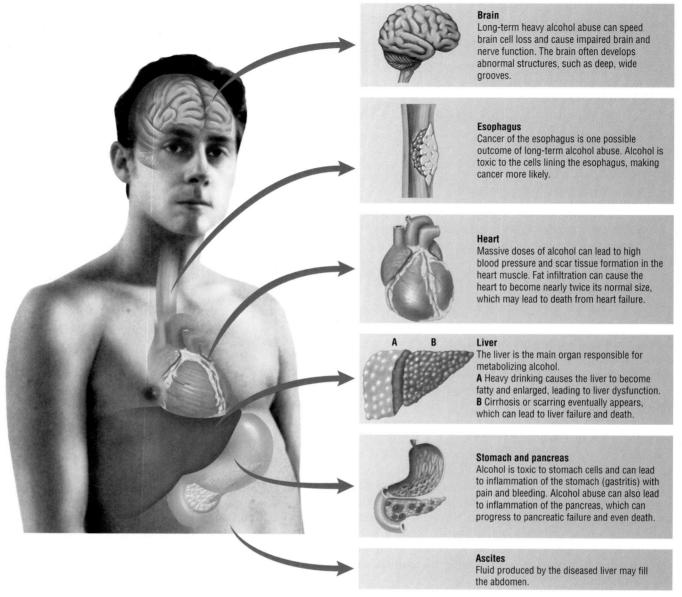

Figure 8-4 **Effects of Alcohol Use on the Body.** The mind-altering effects of alcohol begin soon after it enters the bloodstream. Within minutes, alcohol numbs nerve cells in the brain. The heart muscle strains to cope with alcohol's depressive action. If drinking continues, the rising BAC causes impaired speech, vision, balance, and judgment. With an extremely high BAC, respiratory failure is possible. Over time, alcohol abuse increases the risk for certain forms of heart disease and cancer and makes liver and pancreas failure more likely.

fetal alcohol syndrome. Recent estimates indicate that the full expression of this syndrome occurs at a rate of between 1 and 3 per 1,000 births. Partial expression (fetal alcohol effects [FAE]) can be seen in 3 to 9 per 1,000 live births. In addition, it is likely that many cases of FAE go undetected.[10]

Is there a safe limit to the number of drinks a woman can consume during pregnancy? Since no one can accurately predict the effect of drinking even small amounts of alcohol during pregnancy, the wisest plan is to avoid alcohol altogether.

Because of the critical growth and development that occur during the first months of fetal life, women who have any reason to suspect they are pregnant

---

Key Terms

fetal alcohol syndrome characteristic birth defects noted in the children of some women who consume alcohol during their pregnancies

---

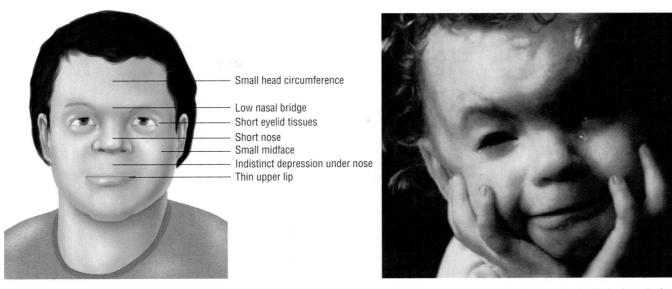

Small head circumference
Low nasal bridge
Short eyelid tissues
Short nose
Small midface
Indistinct depression under nose
Thin upper lip

Figure 8-5   Fetal Alcohol Syndrome. The facial features shown are characteristic of affected children. Additional abnormalities in the brain and other internal organs accompany fetal alcohol syndrome but are not obvious in the child's appearance.

should stop all alcohol consumption. Furthermore, women who are planning to become pregnant and women who are not practicing effective contraception must also consider keeping their alcohol use to a minimum.

Alcohol-Related Social Problems

Alcohol abuse is related to a variety of social problems. These problems affect the quality of interpersonal relationships, employment stability, and the financial security of both the individual and the family. Clearly, alcohol's negative social consequences lower our quality of life. In financial terms the annual cost of alcohol abuse and dependence has been estimated at more than $185 billion.[11]

Accidents

The four leading causes of accidental deaths in the United States (motor vehicle collisions, falls, drownings, and fires and burns) have significant statistical connections to alcohol use.

Motor Vehicle Collisions

Data from the National Highway Traffic Safety Administration (NHTSA) indicate that in 2004 over 17,000 alcohol-related vehicular crash deaths occurred. This figure represented 40 percent of the total traffic fatalities for 2003. Although 17,000 remains an unacceptably high figure, this total represented a 12 percent reduction from the nearly 20,000 alcohol-related fatalities reported in 1991.[12]

Presently in the United States, an alcohol-related car crash fatality occurs every 31 minutes. Every 2 minutes, an alcohol-related car crash injury happens. An estimated

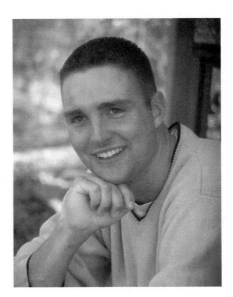

On August 4, 2000, 23-year-old Casey Ray Beaver was driving with two friends along U.S. Highway 71 near Goodman, Missouri, when an oncoming vehicle crossed the center line and collided with his car. Casey, a recent graduate of the University of Kansas, was pronounced dead at the scene, as was the driver of the other vehicle. The offender, who had seven prior convictions of driving under the influence and whose driver's license had been revoked seven years earlier, had a BAC above .10 percent, Casey was due to begin classes at the Illinois College of Optometry 10 days after the accident occurred.

Figure 8-6 A BAC of .08% constitutes legal intoxication. However, lower BACs can impair functioning enough to cause a serious accident.

Number of drinks in a 2-hour period
(1½ oz 86-proof liquor or 12 oz beer)

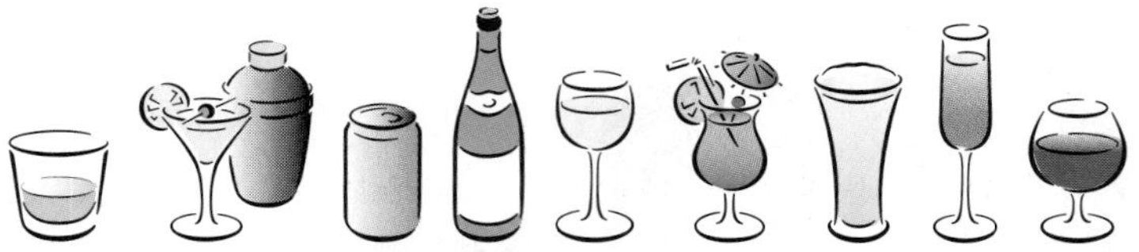

Body weight (lbs.)									
100	1	2	3	4	5	6	7	8	9
120	1	2	3	4	5	6	7	8	9
140	1	2	3	4	5	6	7	8	9
160	1	2	3	4	5	6	7	8	9
180	1	2	3	4	5	6	7	8	9
200	1	2	3	4	5	6	7	8	9

Could impair driving (BAC to .05%)

Driving significantly impaired (BAC .05% to .09%)

Driving seriously impaired (BAC .10% and up)

275,000 people were injured in such crashes in 2001. In 2002, the NHTSA reported that approximately 1.5 million drivers were arrested for drunk driving, reflecting an arrest rate of 1 for every 130 licensed drivers in the United States.[12]

One response to drunk driving has been for all states to raise the minimum legal drinking age to 21 years. This was accomplished in the mid-1980s. Another response was a federal law that President Clinton signed in October 2000. This law required all states to lower their drunk driving standard to .08 percent BAC by October 1, 2003 or the states would risk losing federal highway funds. All states have lowered the driving standard to .08 percent BAC. You can search the MADD Web site at www.madd.org to find out current .08 percent BAC law information (see Figure 8-6).[13]

Other programs and policies are being implemented that are designed to prevent intoxicated people from driving. Many states have enacted **zero-tolerance laws** to help prevent underage drinking and driving. Also included have been efforts to educate bartenders to recognize intoxicated customers, to use off-duty police officers as observers in bars, to place police roadblocks, to develop mechanical devices that prevent intoxicated drivers from starting their cars, and to encourage people to use designated drivers.

The use of designated drivers has received some of the credit for the significant reduction in drunk-driving deaths mentioned earlier. However, there may be a down side to this solution. Some health professionals are concerned that the use of designated drivers allows the nondrivers to drink more heavily than they might otherwise. In effect, designated drivers "enable" drinkers to be less responsible for their own behavior. The concern is that this freedom from responsibility might eventually lead to further problems for the drinkers. What do you think?

Falls

Many people are surprised to learn that falls are the second leading cause of accidental death in the United States. Alcohol use increases the risk for falls. Various studies suggest that alcohol is involved in between 21–77 percent of deadly falls and 18–53 percent of nonfatal falls.[14]

Drownings

Drownings are the third leading cause of accidental death in the United States. Studies have shown that alcohol use is implicated in 21–47 percent of these deaths.[14] High percentages of recreational boaters have been found to drink alcohol while boating.[15]

Fires and Burns

Fires and burns are responsible for an estimated 5,000 deaths each year in the United States, the fourth leading cause of accidental death. This cause is also connected to alcohol use: studies indicate that half of burn victims have BACs above the legal limit. Alcohol can impair judgment and swimming ability and reduce body temperature.[14]

Crime and Violence

Have you noticed that most of the violent behavior and vandalism on your campus is related to alcohol use? The

Key Terms

zero-tolerance laws laws that severely restrict the right to operate motor vehicles for underage drinkers who have been convicted of driving under any influence

connection of alcohol to crime has a long history. Prison populations have large percentages of alcohol abusers and alcoholics: people who commit crimes are more likely to have alcohol problems than are people in the general population. This is especially true for young criminals. Furthermore, alcohol use has been reported in 53–66 percent of all homicides, with the victim, the perpetrator, or both found to have been drinking. In rape situations, rapists are intoxicated 50 percent of the time and victims 30 percent of the time.[6]

Because of research methodological problems, pinpointing alcohol's connection to family violence is difficult.[16] However, it seems clear that among a large number of families, alcohol is associated with violence and other harmful behavior, including physical abuse, child abuse, psychological abuse, and abandonment.[6]

Suicide

Alcohol use has been related to large percentages of suicides. Alcoholism plays a large role in 30 percent of completed suicides.[17] Also, alcohol use is associated with impulsive suicides rather than with premeditated ones. Drinking is also connected with more violent and lethal means of suicide, such as the use of firearms.[6]

For many of these social problems, alcohol use impairs critical judgment and allows a person's behavior to quickly become reckless, antisocial, and deadly. Because most of us wish to minimize problems associated with alcohol use, acting responsibly when we host a party is a first step in this direction.

Hosting a Responsible Party

Some people might say that no party is totally safe when alcohol is served. These people are probably right, considering the possibility of unexpected **drug synergism,** overconsumption, and the consequences of released inhibitions. Fortunately, an awareness of the value of responsible party hosting seems to be growing among college communities. The impetus for this awareness has come from various sources, including respect for an

---

Key Terms

drug synergism (**sin** er jism) enhancement of a drug's effect as a result of the presence of additional drugs within the system

individual's right to choose not to drink alcohol, the growing recognition that many automobile accidents are alcohol-related, and the legal threats posed by **host negligence.**

Responsibly hosting parties at which alcohol is served is becoming a trend, especially among college-educated young adults. The Education Commission of the States' Task Force on Responsible Decisions about Alcohol has generated a list of guidelines for hosting a social event at which alcoholic beverages are served. The list includes the recommendations shown in Changing for the Better on page 207.

In addition, using a **designated driver** is an important component of responsible alcohol use. By planning to abstain from alcohol or to carefully limit their own alcohol consumption, designated drivers are able to safely transport friends who have been drinking.

 TALKING POINTS Have you noticed an increased use of designated drivers in your community? Would you be willing to be a designated driver?

Organizations That Support Responsible Drinking

The serious consequences of the irresponsible use of alcohol have led to the formation of a number of concerned-citizen groups. Although each organization has a unique approach, all attempt to deal objectively with two indisputable facts: Alcohol use is part of our society, and irresponsible alcohol use can be deadly.

Mothers Against Drunk Driving

Mothers Against Drunk Driving (MADD) is a national network of over 600 local chapters in the United States and Canada. This organization attempts to educate people about alcohol's effects on driving and to influence legislation and enforcement of laws related to drunk drivers. For more information about MADD, visit its Web site at www.madd.org.[13]

Students Against Destructive Decisions

Many students have known the acronym *SADD* to stand for the youth group Students Against Driving Drunk or Students Against Destructive Decisions. Recently, the group has restructured itself to expand beyond drunk driving to include other high-risk activities that are detrimental to youth, such as underage drinking, drug use, drugged driving, and failure to use seat belts.

Founded in 1981, this organization now has millions of members in thousands of chapters throughout the country. Remaining central to the drunk driving aspect of SADD is the "Contract for Life," a pact that encourages students and parents to provide safe transportation for each other if either is unable to drive safely after consuming alcohol. This contract also stipulates that no discussions about the incident are to be started until both can talk in a calm and caring manner. For more information about SADD, visit its Web site at www.saddonline.com.[18]

 TALKING POINTS How would you approach asking your parents or friends to join you in signing a "Contract for Life"?

BACCHUS and GAMMA Peer Education Network

BACCHUS (Boost Alcohol Consciousness Concerning the Health of University Students) began in 1975 as an alcohol-awareness organization at the University of Florida. Run by student volunteers, this organization promoted responsible drinking among college students who chose to drink. It was not an anti-alcohol group, but a "harm reduction" group. Over the years, hundreds of chapters were formed on campuses across the country.

When supporters of BACCHUS realized that many students interested in alcohol awareness were from fraternities and sororities, they developed GAMMA (Greeks Advocating Mature Management of Alcohol) to join BACCHUS to form a peer education network. Campuses are now able to choose BACCHUS, GAMMA, or any other acronym or name for their groups.

With the broadening of the original BACCHUS organization has come an expansion of the health issues this group addresses. Originally, the focus was on alcohol abuse and prevention. Now the BACCHUS and GAMMA Peer Education Network confronts a variety of student health and safety issues. For additional information

Key Terms
host negligence a legal term that reflects the failure of a host to provide reasonable care and safety for people visiting the host's residence or business
designated driver a person who abstains from or carefully limits alcohol consumption to be able to safely transport other people who have been drinking

about this organization, check out its Web site at www. bacchusgamma.org.[19]

Other Approaches

Other responsible approaches to alcohol use are surfacing nearly every day. Even among college fraternity organizations, attitudes toward the indiscriminate use of alcohol are changing. Many fraternity rush functions are now conducted without the use of alcohol, and growing numbers of fraternities are alcohol-free.

Another encouraging sign on college campuses is the increasing number of alcohol use task forces. Although each of these groups has its own focus and title, many are meeting to discuss alcohol-related concerns on their particular campus. These task forces often try to formulate detailed, comprehensive policies for alcohol use across the entire campus community. Membership on these committees often includes students (on-campus and off-campus, graduate and undergraduate), faculty and staff members, academic administrators, residence hall advisors, university police, health center personnel, alumni, and local citizens. Does your college have such a committee?

Problem Drinking and Alcoholism

Problem Drinking

At times the line separating **problem drinking** from alcoholism is difficult to distinguish (see the accompanying Star box). There may be no true line, with the exception that an alcoholic is unable to stop drinking. Problem drinking is a pattern of alcohol use in which a drinker's behavior creates personal difficulties or difficulties for other people. What are some of these behaviors? Examples might be drinking to avoid life stressors, going to work intoxicated, drinking and driving, becoming injured or injuring others while drinking, solitary drinking, morning drinking, an occasional **blackout,** high-risk sexual activity, and being told by others that you drink too much. For college students, two clear indications of

---

Progressive Stages of Alcohol Dependence

Early

- Escape drinking
- Binge drinking
- Guilt feelings
- Sneaking drinks
- Difficulty stopping once drinking has begun
- Increased tolerance
- Preoccupation with drinking
- Occasional blackouts

Middle

- Loss of control
- Self-hate
- Impaired social relationships
- Changes in drinking patterns (more frequent binge drinking)
- Temporary sobriety
- Morning drinking
- Dietary neglect
- Increased blackouts

Late

- Prolonged binges
- Alcohol used to control withdrawal symptoms
- Alcohol psychosis
- Nutritional disease
- Frequent blackouts

---

problem drinking are missing classes and lowered academic performance caused by alcohol involvement.

Problem drinkers are not always heavy drinkers; they might not be daily or even weekly drinkers. Unlike alcoholics, problem drinkers do not need to drink to maintain "normal" body functions. However, when they do drink, they (and others around them) experience problems—sometimes with tragic consequences. It's not surprising that problem drinkers are more likely than other drinkers to eventually develop alcoholism.

 TALKING POINTS Are there people around you who show signs of problem drinking?

Key Terms

problem drinking an alcohol use pattern in which a drinker's behavior creates personal difficulties or difficulties for other people

blackout a temporary state of amnesia experienced by a drinker; an inability to remember events that occurred during a period of alcohol use

---

Alcoholism

In the early 1990s a revised definition of **alcoholism** was established by a joint committee of experts on alcohol dependence.[20] This committee defined alcoholism as follows:

> Alcoholism is a primary, chronic disease with genetic, psychosocial, and environmental factors influencing its development and manifestations. The disease is often progressive and fatal. It is characterized by impaired control over drinking, preoccupation with the drug alcohol, use of alcohol despite adverse consequences, and distortions in thinking, most notably denial. Each of these symptoms may be continuous or periodic.

This definition incorporates much of the knowledge gained from addiction research during the last two decades. It is well recognized that alcoholics do not drink for the pleasurable effects of alcohol but to escape being sober. For alcoholics, being sober is stressful.

Unlike problem drinking, alcoholism involves a physical addiction to alcohol. For the true alcoholic, when the body is deprived of alcohol, physical and mental withdrawal symptoms become evident. These withdrawal symptoms can be life threatening.

Uncontrollable shaking can progress to nausea, vomiting, hallucinations, shock, and cardiac and pulmonary arrest. Uncontrollable shaking combined with irrational hallucinations is called *delirium tremens (DTs)*, an occasional manifestation of alcohol withdrawal.[21]

The complex reasons for the physical and emotional dependence of alcoholism have not been fully explained. Why, when more than 100 million adults use alcohol without becoming dependent on it, are 10 million or more others unable to control its use?

Could alcoholism be an inherited disease? Studies in humans and animals have provided strong evidence that genetics plays a role in some cases of alcoholism. Two forms of alcoholism are thought to be inherited: type 1 and type 2. Type 1 is thought to take years to develop and may not surface until midlife. Type 2 is a more severe form and appears to be passed primarily from fathers to sons. This form of alcoholism frequently begins earlier in a person's life and may even start in adolescence.

Genetics may also help protect some Asians from developing alcoholism. About half of all Far East Asians produce low levels of an important enzyme that helps metabolize alcohol. These people cannot tolerate even small amounts of alcohol. Genetic factors pertaining to the absorption rates of alcohol in the intestinal tract have been hypothesized to predispose some Native Americans to alcoholism. It is likely that more research will be undertaken concerning the role of genetic factors in all forms of chemical dependence.

The role of personality traits as conditioning factors in the development of alcoholism has received considerable attention. Factors ranging from unusually low self-esteem to an antisocial personality have been implicated. Additional factors making people susceptible to alcoholism may include excessive reliance on denial, hypervigilance, compulsiveness, and chronic levels of anxiety. Always complicating the study of personality traits is the uncertainty of whether the personality profile is a predisposing factor (perhaps from inheritance) or is caused by alcoholism.

Codependence

Not too long ago, a new term was coined to describe the relationship between drug-dependent people and those around them—**codependence.** This term implies a kind of dual addiction. The alcoholic and the person close to the alcoholic are both addicted, one to alcohol and the other to the alcoholic. People who are codependent often find themselves denying the addiction and enabling the alcohol-dependent person.

Unfortunately, this kind of behavior damages both the alcoholic and the codependent. The alcoholic's intervention and treatment may be delayed for a considerable time. Codependent people often pay a heavy price as well. They often become drug- or alcohol-dependent themselves, or they may suffer a variety of psychological consequences related to guilt, loss of self-esteem, depression, and anxiety. Codependents may be at increased risk for physical and sexual abuse.

Researchers continue to explore this dimension of alcoholism. Many students have found some of the resources identified in this chapter to be especially helpful.

Denial and Enabling

Problem drinkers and alcoholics frequently use the psychological defense mechanism of *denial* to maintain their drinking behavior. By convincing themselves that their lives are not affected by their drinking, problem drinkers and alcoholics are able to maintain their drinking patterns. A person's denial is an unconscious process that is apparent only to rational observers.

Key Terms

alcoholism a primary, chronic disease with genetic, psychosocial, and environmental factors influencing its development and manifestations

codependence an unhealthy relationship in which one person is addicted to alcohol or another drug and a person close to him or her is "addicted" to the alcoholic or drug user

Formerly, it was up to alcoholics to admit that their denial was no longer effective before they could be admitted to a treatment program. This is not the case today. Currently, family members, friends, or coworkers of alcohol-dependent people are encouraged to intervene and force an alcohol-dependent person into treatment.

 TALKING POINTS One of your professors is a known alcoholic. You wonder why no one has persuaded her to seek treatment. Would you intervene in any way to make that happen? If so, how?

During treatment, chemically dependent people must break through the security of denial and admit that alcohol controls their lives. This process is demanding and often time-consuming, but it is necessary for recovery.

For family and friends of chemically dependent people, denial is part of a process known as **enabling.** In this process, people close to the problem drinker or alcoholic inadvertently support drinking behavior by denying that a problem really exists. Enablers unconsciously make excuses for the drinker, try to keep the drinker's work and family life intact, and in effect make the continued abuse of alcohol possible. For example, college students enable problem drinkers when they clean up a drinker's messy room, lie to professors about a student's class absences, and provide class notes or other assistance to a drinker who can't keep up academically.

Alcohol counselors contend that enablers are an alcoholic's worst enemy because they can significantly delay the onset of effective therapy. Do you know of a situation in which you or others have enabled a person with an alcohol problem?

Alcoholism and the Family

Considerable disruption occurs in the families of alcoholics, not only from the consequences of the drinking behavior (such as violence, illness, and unemployment) but also because of the uncertainty of the family's role in causing and prolonging the situation. Family members often begin to adopt a variety of new roles that allow them to cope with the presence of the alcoholic in the family. Among the more commonly seen roles are the family hero, the lost child, the family mascot, and the scapegoat.[6] Unless family members receive appropriate counseling, these roles may remain intact for a lifetime.

Once an alcoholic's therapy has begun, family members are encouraged to participate in many aspects of the recovery. This participation will also help them understand how they are affected by alcoholism. If therapy and aftercare include participation in Alcoholics Anonymous (AA), family members will be encouraged to become affiliated with related support groups.

Helping the Alcoholic: Rehabilitation and Recovery

Once an alcoholic realizes that alcoholism is not a form of moral weakness but rather a clearly defined illness, the chances for recovery are remarkably good. It is estimated that as many as two-thirds of alcoholics can recover. Recovery is especially enhanced when the addicted person has a good emotional support system, including concerned family members, friends, and employer. When this support system is not well established, the alcoholic's chances for recovery are considerably lower.

AA is a voluntary support group of recovering alcoholics who meet regularly to help one another get and stay sober. Over 100,000 groups exist in 150 countries worldwide.[22] AA encourages alcoholics to admit their lack of power over alcohol and to turn their lives over to a higher power (although the organization is nonsectarian). Members of AA are encouraged not to be judgmental about the behavior of other members. They support anyone with a problem caused by alcohol.

Al-Anon and Alateen are parallel organizations that give support to people who live with alcoholics. Al-Anon is geared toward spouses and other relatives, and Alateen focuses on children of alcoholics. There are 28,000 Al-Anon groups and 3,000 Alateen groups worldwide. Both organizations help members realize that they are not alone and that successful adjustments can be made to nearly every alcoholic-related situation. AA, Al-Anon, and Alateen chapter organizations are usually listed in the telephone book or in the classified sections of local newspapers. You can locate Al-Anon and Alateen on the Web at www.al-anon.alateen.org.[23]

For people who feel uncomfortable with the concept that their lives are controlled by a higher power, *secular recovery programs* are becoming popular. These programs maintain that sobriety comes from within the alcoholic. Secular programs strongly emphasize self-reliance, self-determination, and rational thinking about one's drinking. Secular Organizations for Sobriety (SOS) and Rational Recovery are examples of secular recovery programs.

Drugs to Treat Alcoholism

Could there be a medical cure for alcoholism? For nearly 50 years, the only prescription drug physicians could use to help drinkers stop drinking was disulfiram (Antabuse).

Key Terms

enabling inadvertently supporting a drinker's behavior by denying that a problem exists

Antabuse would cause drinkers to become extremely nauseated whenever they used alcohol.

In 1995 the Food and Drug Administration approved the drug naltrexone (ReVia) that works by reducing the craving for alcohol and the pleasurable sensations felt when drinking. Combining naltrexone with conventional behavior modification has shown promising results. Additionally, the use of antidepressants by some alcoholics has been especially helpful during treatment.[1]

Current Alcohol Concerns

Adult Children of Alcoholic Parents

In recent years a new dimension of alcoholism has been identified—the unusually high prevalence of alcoholism among adult children of alcoholics (ACOAs). It is estimated that these children are about four times more likely to develop alcoholism than children whose parents are not alcoholics. Even the ACOAs who do not become alcoholics may have a difficult time adjusting to everyday living. Janet Geringer Woititz, author of the bestselling book *Adult Children of Alcoholics,*[24] describes 13 traits that most ACOAs exhibit to some degree (see the Star box).

In response to this concern, support groups have been formed to help prevent the adult sons and daughters of alcoholics from developing the condition that afflicted their parents (see the Star box). If a stronger link for an inherited genetic predisposition to alcoholism is found, these groups may play an even greater role in the prevention of alcoholism.

Common Traits of Adult Children of Alcoholics

Adult children of alcoholics may:

- Have difficulty identifying normal behavior
- Have difficulty following a project from beginning to end
- Lie when it would be just as easy to tell the truth
- Judge themselves without mercy
- Have difficulty having fun
- Take themselves very seriously
- Have difficulty with intimate relationships
- Overreact to changes over which they have no control
- Constantly seek approval and affirmation
- Feel that they are different from other people
- Be super-responsible or super-irresponsible
- Be extremely loyal, even in the face of evidence that the loyalty is undeserved
- Tend to lock themselves into a course of action without considering the consequences

Experts agree that adult children of alcoholics who believe they have come to terms with their feelings can sometimes face lingering problems. Support groups to contact include Al-Anon (www.al-anon.alateen.org), Adult Children of Alcohollics (www.adultchildren.org), and Children of Alcoholics Foundation (www.coaf.org).

Woititz JG. *Adult Children of Alcoholics.* Health Communications, Inc., 1990.

Women and Alcohol

For decades, women have consumed less alcohol and had fewer alcohol-related problems than men. At present, evidence is mounting that a greater percentage of women are choosing to drink and that some subgroups of women, especially young women, are drinking more heavily. An increased number of admissions of women to treatment centers may also reflect that alcohol consumption among women is on the rise.[6] Special approaches for women to use for staying sober are discussed in Learning from Our Diversity on page 213.

Studies indicate that currently there are almost as many female as male alcoholics. However, there appear to be differences between men and women when it comes to alcohol abuse: (1) More women than men can point to a specific triggering event (such as a divorce, death of a spouse, a career change, or children leaving home) that started them drinking heavily. (2) Alcoholism among women often starts later and progresses more quickly than alcoholism among men. (3) Women tend to be prescribed more mood-altering drugs than men are. So women face greater risk of drug interaction or cross-tolerance. (4) Nonalcoholic men tend to divorce their alcoholic spouses nine times more often than nonalcoholic women divorce their alcoholic spouses. Thus alcoholic women are not as likely to have a family support system to aid them in their recovery attempts. (5) Female alcoholics do not tend to receive as much social support as men in their treatment and recovery. (6) Unmarried, divorced, or single-parent women tend to have significant economic problems that may make entry into a treatment program especially difficult. (7) Women seem to be more susceptible than men are to having medical complications resulting from heavy drinking.[7] In light of the generally recognized educational, occupational, and social gains made by women during the last two decades, it will be interesting to see whether these male-female differences continue. What's your best guess?

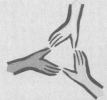

Learning from Our Diversity

Staying Sober: New Pathways for Women

Since 1935, when it was founded by two white American male alcoholics, Alcoholics Anonymous has expanded to encompass millions of members in virtually every region of the world who strive to achieve and maintain sobriety by adhering to AA's well-known 12-step program of recovery. With its strong spiritual orientation emphasizing the acknowledgment of a "higher power," AA offers safety, comfort, and structure to people of all ages and backgrounds, and both sexes. For decades, women as well as men have made AA the cornerstone of their efforts to get sober and stay sober.

Not all women, however, are comfortable with AA's focus on Christian spirituality and the perceived masculine orientation of its chief text, Alcoholics Anonymous (familiarly known as the "Big Book"), and other program literature. These women place an equally high value on sober living as do AA adherents, but they prefer to pursue that goal in other settings. In recent years, alternatives to AA have emerged that offer peer group acceptance and support for recovering alcoholic women but do so in a nonspiritual, nonsexist context.

One such group, Women for Sobriety, is a mutual aid organization for women with alcohol problems that was founded in 1975 by Dr. Jean Kirkpatrick. The WFS program focuses on improving self-esteem; members achieve sobriety by taking responsibility for their actions and by learning not to dwell on negative thoughts. Another alternative, Rational Recovery, is open to both men and women. RR, which is based on the theories of psychologist Albert Ellis's Rational Emotive Therapy, also uses a cognitive, nonspiritual approach that fosters cohesiveness and provides the emotional support sought by people who seek to gain and maintain sobriety.

Particularly for "marginalized" alcoholic women such as lesbians, racial and ethnic minorities, and those of non-Christian religious backgrounds, alcoholism treatment professionals increasingly are being encouraged to present the full range of support-group options, including but not emphasizing the approach of Alcoholics Anonymous.

If you were seeking help to achieve and maintain sobriety, would you be more inclined to attend a program based on spirituality, or one that offers a rational, cognitive approach? Why?

Sources:
Galanter M, et al. Rational recovery: Alternative to AA for addiction? *American Journal of Drug and Alcohol Abuse,* 1993, vol. 19, p. 499.

Hall J: Lesbians' participation in Alcoholics Anonymous: Experience of social, personal, and political tensions. *Contemporary Drug Problems,* Spring 1996, vol. 23, no. 1, p. 113.

Kaskutas L: A road less traveled: Choosing the "Women for Sobriety" program. *Journal of Drug Issues,* Winter 1996, vol. 26, no. 1, p. 77.

Women for Sobriety, Inc. www.womenforsobriety.org/, March 10, 2005.

Alcohol Advertising

Every few years, careful observers can see subtle changes in the ways the alcoholic beverage industry markets its products. Recently, the marketing push appears to be directed toward minorities (through advertisements for malt liquor and fortified wines), women (through wine and wine cooler ads), and youth (through trendy, young adult-oriented commercials), and spiffy Web sites.

On the college campus, aggressive alcohol campaigns have used rock stars, beach party scenes, athletic event sponsorships, and colorful newspaper supplements as vehicles to encourage the purchase of alcohol. Critics claim that most of the collegiate advertising is directed at the "below age 21" crowd and that the prevention messages are not strong enough to offset the potential health damage to this population. How do you feel about alcohol advertising on your campus? If you're a nontraditional-age student, do you find the advertising campaigns amusing or potentially dangerous?

Taking Charge of Your Health

- Determine whether you are affected by someone's drinking by doing the Personal Assessment on page 217.

- Prepare for a possible alcohol-related emergency by reviewing the signs listed in the Changing for the Better box on page 203.

- Assess your level of social responsibility by using the Changing for the Better box on page 207.

- If you think that you are a problem drinker or an alcoholic, join a support group to get help.

- Enter into a "Contract for Life" with your parents or closest friends, a pact that says that you will provide safe transportation for one another if any of you are unable to drive safely after consuming alcohol.

- Make a commitment to responsible alcohol use by joining a campus group that works toward this goal.

SUMMARY

- Alcohol is the drug of choice among college students and the rest of American society.
- Many factors affect the rate of absorption of alcohol into the bloodstream.
- As BAC rises, predictable depressant effects take place.
- People with acute alcohol intoxication must receive first-aid care immediately.
- The health effects of chronic alcohol abuse are serious.
- Problem drinking reflects an alcohol use pattern in which a drinker's behavior creates personal difficulties or problems for others.

- Alcoholism is a primary, chronic disease with a variety of possible causes and characteristics.
- Denial, enabling, codependence, ACOAs, and alcohol advertising are current issues related to alcohol abuse in the United States.
- Recovery and rehabilitation programs can be effective in helping alcoholics become sober.
- Antabuse, naltrexone, and antidepressants are drugs prescribed by physicians to help alcoholics in treatment.
- Federal legislation has pushed all states to lower the legal BAC standard to .08%.

REVIEW QUESTIONS

1. What percentage of American adults consume alcohol? Approximately what percentage of adults are classified as abstainers? What percentage of college students drink?
2. What is binge drinking?
3. What is meant by the term *proof*?
4. What is the nutritional value of alcohol? How do "lite" and low-alcohol beverages compare?
5. Identify and explain the various factors that influence the absorption of alcohol. Why is it important to be aware of these factors?
6. What is BAC? Describe the general sequence of physiological events that takes place when a person drinks alcohol at a rate faster than the liver can oxidize it.
7. What are the signs and symptoms of acute alcohol intoxication? What are the first-aid steps you should take to help a person with this problem?
8. Describe the characteristics of fetal alcohol syndrome and fetal alcohol effects.
9. Explain the differences between problem drinking and alcoholism.
10. What is codependence? What roles do denial and enabling play in alcoholism?
11. What are some common traits of ACOAs?
12. What unique alcohol-related problems exist for women?
13. Describe the activities undertaken by SADD, MADD, BACCHUS, and GAMMA and by AA, Al-Anon, and Alateen.

ENDNOTES

1. U.S. Department of Health and Human Services. *Alcohol and Health: Tenth Special Report to the U.S. Congress*, NIH Publication No 00-1583, 2000. Washington, DC: U.S. Government Printing Office.
2. U.S. Bureau of the Census: *Statistical Abstract of the United States, 1999* (199th ed.). Washington, DC: U.S. Government Printing Office, 1999.
3. Defour, M. What is moderate drinking? Defining "drinks" and drinking levels. *Alcohol Research and Health*, 23(1), 5–14, 1999.
4. Brown SA, Tapert SF, Granholm E, et al. Neurocognitive functioning of adolescents: Effects of protracted alcohol use. *Alcoholism, Clinical and Experimental Research*, 24(2), 164–171, 2000.
5. Zest for Life. Alcohol and ethanol information page, www.anyvitamins.com/alcohol-ethanol-info.htm, March 9, 2005.
6. Kinney J. *Loosening the Grip: A Handbook of Alcohol Information* (7th ed.). New York: McGraw-Hill, 2003.
7. Be Responsible About Drinking. Women and Alcohol, www.brad21.org/alcohol_ and_women.html, March 9, 2005.
8. Pinger RR, et al. *Drugs: Issues for Today* (3rd ed.). New York: McGraw-Hill, 1998.
9. Ray O, Ksir C. *Drugs, Society and Human Behavior* (8th ed.). New York: McGraw-Hill, 1999.
10. ADA: Division of Drug and Alcohol Abuse. As a Matter of Fact . . . Fetal Alcohol Syndrome, www.well.com/user/woa/fsfas.htm, March 9, 2005.
11. National Institute on Alcohol Abuse and Alcoholism. *Tenth Special Report to the U.S. Congress on Alcohol and Health*. Chapter 6. NIH Publication No. 00-1583. Rockville, MD: U.S. Department of Health and Human Services, 2000.
12. *Traffic Safety Facts 2003: Alcohol*. U.S. Department of Transportation, National Highway Traffic Safety Administration.
13. About Us. Mothers Against Drunk Driving, www.madd.org, March 9, 2005.
14. *Alcohol and Unintentional Injury: A Brief Review of the Literature*. The Trauma Foundation, www.tf.org/tf/alcohol/ariv/reviews/injurev5.html, June 16, 2003.
15. Training Guide for USLA Safety Tips: General Information on Drowning. USLA Lifeguards for Life, www.usla.org/PublicInfo/Safety_guide.shtml, June 16, 2003.
16. Vaughn, C. *Children of Alcoholics: At Risk for Family Violence*. U.S. Department of Health and Human Services and SAMHSA's National Clearinghouse for Alcohol and Drug Information, February 10, 2003.
17. *Facts about Suicide*. CDC Prevention, National Center for Health Statistics, 1998.
18. SADD History. Students Against Drunk Driving, www.saddonline.com, March 1, 2005.

19. Organization History and Mission. The Bacchus and Gamma Peer Education Network, www.bacchusgamma.org/, March 1, 2005.

20. Morse RM, et al. The definition of alcoholism. *JAMA* 1992; 268(8): 1012–1014.

21. Burns, M. *Delirium Tremens,* emedicine.com, November 8, 2004.

22. AA at a Glance. Alcoholics Anonymous, www.alcoholics-anonymous.org, March 1, 2005.

23. Web Site information, Al-Anon/Alateen, www.al-anon.alateen.org/, March 1, 2005.

24. Woititz JG. *Adult Children of Alcoholics.* Health Communications, Inc., 1990.

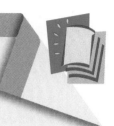

As We Go to Press

To help enforce underage drinking laws, the Justice Department announced in August 2005 that all 50 states and the District of Columbia would each be awarded $350,000. This $20 million federal initiative consists of block grants to be used for media outreach programs stressing the dangers of binge drinking, underage drinking, drinking and driving, and a zero-tolerance policy for offenders. This funding would also support alcohol-free programming for minors.

personal assessment

Are you troubled by someone's drinking?

The following questions are designed to help you decide whether you are affected by someone's drinking and could benefit from a program such as Al-Anon. Record your number of yes and no responses in the boxes at the end of the questionnaire.

	Yes	No
1. Do you worry about how much someone else drinks?	____	____
2. Do you have money problems because of someone else's drinking?	____	____
3. Do you tell lies to cover up for someone else's drinking?	____	____
4. Do you feel that if the drinker loved you, he or she would stop drinking to please you?	____	____
5. Do you blame the drinker's behavior on his or her companions?	____	____
6. Are plans frequently upset or meals delayed because of the drinker?	____	____
7. Do you make threats, such as: "If you don't stop drinking, I'll leave you"?	____	____
8. Do you secretly try to smell the drinker's breath?	____	____
9. Are you afraid to upset someone for fear it will set off a drinking bout?	____	____
10. Have you been hurt or embarrassed by a drinker's behavior?	____	____
11. Are holidays and gatherings spoiled because of the drinking?	____	____
12. Have you considered calling the police for help in fear of abuse?	____	____
13. Do you search for hidden alcohol?	____	____
14. Do you often ride in a car with a driver who has been drinking?	____	____
15. Have you refused social invitations out of fear or anxiety that the drinker will cause a scene?	____	____

	Yes	No
16. Do you sometimes feel like a failure when you think of the lengths to which you have gone to control the drinker?	____	____
17. Do you think that if the drinker stopped drinking, your other problems would be solved?	____	____
18. Do you ever threaten to hurt yourself to scare the drinker?	____	____
19. Do you feel angry, confused, or depressed most of the time?	____	____
20. Do you feel there is no one who understands your problems?	____	____
TOTAL	____	____

Interpretation

If you answered yes to three or more of these questions, Al-Anon or Alateen may be able to help. You can contact Al-Anon or Alateen by looking in your local telephone directory or by writing to Al-Anon Family Group Headquarters, Inc., 1600 Corporate Landing Parkway, Virginia Beach, VA 23454-5617, or you may call (888) 4AL-ANON.

To Carry This Further . . .

Sometimes the decision to seek help from a support group is a difficult one. If you answered yes to any of the preceding questions, spend a few moments reflecting on your responses. How long have you been experiencing problems because of someone else's drinking? How would sharing your feelings with others—people who have dealt with very similar problems—help you cope with your own situation? Knowing you're not alone can often be a great relief; it's up to you to take the first step.

chapter nine

Rejecting Tobacco Use

Chapter Objectives

On completing this chapter, you will be able to:

- examine smoking rates among demographic groups, student groups on your campus, and groups in different states, and speculate on the underlying reasons for these trends.

- identify techniques used by the tobacco industry to encourage people to smoke.

- critically evaluate tobacco advertisements to determine what audience particular ads target, and what messages they send to consumers.

- administer the 10-item Hooked on Nicotine Checklist (HONC) to friends who smoke to determine the existence and depth of dependence.

- explain the bolus theory, the adrenocorticotropic hormone (ACTH) theory, and the self-medication theory of nicotine addiction.

- explain the particulate phase and the gaseous phase of tobacco smoke and identify the primary components of each.

- describe the relationship between smoking and cardiovascular disease.

- trace the role of smoking in the development of respiratory-tract cancer.

- identify smoking-cessation aids, including various nicotine-delivery techniques, and describe steps that smokers can take to reduce or eliminate their use of tobacco.

- explain the dangers of secondhand smoke and develop steps to reduce your exposure to it.

Eye on the Media

Tobacco Industry Denies Ads Target Kids

On various occasions during the past 8 years, the tobacco industry has run television commercials intended to "educate" the public about the fundamental changes that the tobacco industry has undertaken in terms of marketing, particularly in light of charges that the industry previously targeted children in an attempt to develop a new generation of smokers. In these commercials several changes were described, all of which were attributed to the 1998 settlement (formally signed in 1999) reached between the tobacco industry and the states' attorneys general stemming from a massive class action suit to recoup Medicaid money. There was no mention in the commercials that the original agreement reached between the states and the tobacco industry in June of 1997 was much more restrictive and closely reflective of the intent of the court in curbing the marketing activities of the tobacco industry. The more permissive 1998 settlement, known as the Master Settlement Agreement (MSA), arose when the tobacco industry promised to vigorously fight the 1997 agreement in court. Thus, compromises favoring the tobacco industry were made by the states to save time and resources that would otherwise be lost to additional litigation.

The accompanying chart shows selected examples of the differences between the 1997 agreement and the final 1999 settlement. Because of the tobacco industry's ability to afford media exposure, the American public will continue to be led to believe that the tobacco industry complied completely with the intent of the courts.

In yet a more current example of the tobacco industry's relationship to media exposure, RJR withdrew its corporate sponsorship of NASCAR's premier racing series, the Winston Cup Series. By finally complying with the 1999 Master Settlement Agreement RJR can redirect hundreds of millions of dollars once spent on NASCAR into other areas of media exposure, such as advertisements in magazines popular with teens (such as *Sports Illustrated* and *Hot Rod*) and point-of-purchase displays in convenience stores and drug stores.[1]

[1]Wakefield, MA, et al. "Tobacco Industry Marketing of Point of Purchase after the 1999 MSA Billboard Ban," *AJPH* 9, No. 6, June 2002.

Master Settlement Agreement (MSA)

Restriction	1997 Agreement	1999 (MSA)
Outdoor and Transit Ads	Bans all outdoor and transit ads	Allows signs of up to 14 sq feet on any building or property where tobacco products are sold, including those near schools and playgrounds. Bans other billboards and transit ads.
Cartoons and Human Images	Banned	Allows human images, such as the Marlboro man. Bans cartoons.
Brand Name Sponsorships	Banned	Each company allowed one brand name sponsorship of an event or series of events. Prohibits events in which contestants are under 18 years of age.
Free Samples	Banned	Free samples allowed in adult-only facilities.

Tobacco Use in American Society

If you were to visit certain businesses, entertainment spots, or sporting events in your community, you might leave convinced that virtually every adult is a tobacco user. Certainly, for some segments of society, tobacco use is the rule rather than the exception. You may be quite surprised to find out that the great majority of adults do not use tobacco products. Table 9.1 displays current cigarette smoking by males and females for each state.[2] Note that Kentucky, a major tobacco-producing state, has the highest percentage of smokers (32.6 percent), whereas Utah, a state in which nearly three-fourths of the residents are Mormons and thus refrain from tobacco and alcohol use, reports the smallest percentage of tobacco uses (12.7 percent). How does your home state compare?

Following the Surgeon General's 1964 report (the first official statement of concern by the federal government regarding the dangers of smoking),[3] the prevalence of smoking began a decline that lasted until 1991, when a

Table 9.1 Current Cigarette Smoking by Sex and State: 2002

In percent. Current cigarette smoking is defined as persons who reported having smoked 100 or more cigarettes during their lifetime and who currently smoke every day or some days. Based on the Behavioral Risk Factor Surveillance System, a telephone survey of health behaviors of the civilian, noninstitutionalized U.S. population, 18 years old and over; for details, see source.

State	Total	Male	Female	State	Total	Male	Female	State	Total	Male	Female
U.S.	23.1	25.9	20.9	KS	22.1	23.2	20.9	ND	21.5	23.1	20.0
				KY	32.6	34.8	30.5	OH	26.6	28.4	25.0
AL	24.4	27.5	21.6	LA	23.9	26.6	21.5	OK	26.7	29.7	23.8
AK	29.4	31.9	26.7	ME	23.6	26.4	21.1	OR	22.4	24.6	20.2
AZ	23.5	27.0	20.1	MD	22.0	25.7	18.6	PA	24.6	26.1	23.2
AR	26.3	28.7	24.1	MA	19.0	20.2	18.0	RI	22.5	24.3	20.9
CA	16.4	19.7	13.3	MI	24.2	25.1	23.5	SC	26.6	29.1	24.4
CO	20.4	21.4	19.4	MN	21.7	24.3	19.4	SD	22.6	25.6	19.7
CT	19.5	20.6	18.4	MS	27.4	33.2	22.2	TN	27.8	31.0	24.9
DE	24.7	25.4	24.1	MO	26.6	29.6	23.9	TX	22.9	26.8	19.1
DC	20.4	23.8	17.5	MT	21.3	21.3	21.4	UT	12.7	14.2	11.3
FL	22.1	23.6	20.7	NE	22.8	26.3	19.4	VT	21.2	21.5	20.9
GA	23.3	26.8	20.0	NV	26.0	28.5	23.5	VA	24.6	28.5	20.9
HI	21.1	26.2	16.0	NH	23.2	23.9	22.6	WA	21.5	23.6	19.4
ID	20.6	21.6	19.7	NJ	19.1	20.4	17.9	WV	28.4	29.8	27.2
IL	22.9	26.1	19.8	NM	21.2	23.3	19.3	WI	23.4	25.4	21.4
IN	27.7	29.8	25.8	NY	22.4	25.9	19.3	WY	23.7	25.3	22.0
IA	23.1	26.3	20.2	NC	26.4	30.7	22.3				

Source: U.S. Centers for Disease Control and Prevention, Atlanta, GA, *Morbidity and Mortality Weekly Report,* Vol. 52, No. 53, January 9, 2004.

Table 9.2 Patterns of Cigarette Smoking

Prevalence by Sex

Total	Men	Women
22.5	25.2	20.0

Note: Subjects have smoked more than 100 cigarettes and reported smoking every day or some days.

Percentage by Ethnicity and Race

Total	White	Black	Hispanic	American Indian or Alaska Native	Asian or Pacific Islander
22.5	23.6	22.4	16.7	40.8	13.3

Note: Subjects have smoked more than 100 cigarettes and smoked at the time of the survey.

Cigarette smoking among adults—United States, 2002. *MMWR*, Vol. 53, No. 20, May 28, 2004.

leveling off was noted that lasted for the next three years. Since 1994 the percentage of the population who smoke has declined slowly but progressively. Current statistics reveal that 22.5% of American adults smoke cigarettes on a daily or near-daily basis. Men are more likely to smoke (25.9 percent) than are women (20.9 percent).[2] When subsegments of the population, based on race and ethnicity, were studied it was found that whites and blacks were essentially smoking with the same prevalence (23.6 percent and 22.4 percent).[6] At the same time, Hispanics were considerably less likely to smoke, while American Indians and Alaska Natives (40.3 percent) were more likely to smoke. Persons of Asian or Pacific Island descent were the Americans least likely to smoke (13.3 percent) (see Table 9.2).[4]

Cigarette Smoking among College Students

Until very recently, the rate of cigarette smoking among college graduates was lower than that reported for the population as a whole, and it was significantly lower than the rate for persons with very little formal education. In fact, the prevalence of smoking among college students decreased progressively from 21 percent in 1964 to 14 percent in 1995.[5] However, an upward trend in cigarette use by college students has been noted, with a recent study indicating that 31.4 percent had smoked within the past month.[6] In contrast, a downward trend in smoking by 12-graders has been reported for five out of the last six consecutive years (1998–2004), with 25.0 percent smoking during the past month in the most recent year.[7] Because the majority of today's college students have matriculated

from high school during these years, we could have expected a progressive decline in college student smoking. Such was not the case, however, suggesting that factors encountered after matriculation are fostering smoking among college students. This is, in fact, possible since among the 2002 twelfth graders with college aspirations, only 21.6 percent were cigarette smokers.[7]

When a college community is viewed as a whole regarding which segments of the student body are most likely to smoke, there appears to be a direct relationship between the level of alcohol consumption and cigarette smoking. Additional direct relationships appear between smoking and other drug use and in housing where smoking is permitted. Similar, although perhaps less influential, relationships are seen among tobacco use and coping style, depression, and perceptions of life satisfaction.[8]

The historically predictable relationship between higher levels of completed education and the lessened likelihood of smoking remains clearly evident even today. For example, when comparing the percentage of heavy smokers (a pack or more per day) on the basis of education completed, the influence of education is evident—less than high school (37.5m/31.3f percent), high school graduate (22.0m/26.2f percent), some college (25.4m/21.9f percent), and college graduate (11.0m/10.7f percent).[9] Unfortunately, the more recently reported incidence of smoking among college students (2004) seems to indicate that today's college students are smoking at a level more characteristic of high school dropouts from a decade ago.

The most disturbing aspect of the increase in reported smoking among college students, beyond the eventual influence it will have on health and life expectancy, is its negation of the traditional belief that the college and university experience "protected" this segment of the society from making some ill-informed choices. As recently as the mid-1990s it was still possible to believe that the college population was "too well informed" and "too future oriented" to engage widely in an addictive behavior that fosters dependence, compromises health, and eventually shortens life. Today that proposition seems to lack some of its former validity, but one hopes that the corner is being turned.

Other Demographic Factors Influencing Tobacco Use

In addition to gender, race, ethnicity, and education level, other demographic facts appear to influence the extent to which smoking occurs. Included among these factors are the age groups into which persons fall, the region of the country in which they live, the size of their communities, and their employment status.

If age grouping is begun with 18- to 25-year-olds and progresses to 65 years of age and older, the general trend is

A Simple Dependency Test Regarding Your Relationships with Cigarettes

To nonsmokers it must seem that smokers would realize the existence of their dependency on cigarettes; however, such might not be the case. The Hooked On Nicotine Checklist (HONC) appearing below is a simple way to determine whether a cigarette-based dependency exists. If you are a smoker, answer each question asked by the HONC in an honest manner; then give careful consideration to your findings. If you are a nonsmoker, ask a smoker to complete the HONC and share responses to each item with you—a good discussion could ensue.

Nicotine Addiction's 10 Warning Signs
HONC—Hooked On Nicotine Checklist

1. Have you ever tried to quit but couldn't?
2. Do you smoke now because it is really hard to quit?
3. Have you ever felt like you were addicted to tobacco?
4. Do you ever have strong cravings to smoke?
5. Have you ever felt like you really needed a cigarette?
6. Is it hard to keep from smoking in places where you are not supposed to, like school?

In answering the last four questions, when you tried to stop smoking, or when you have not used tobacco for a while . . .

7. Did you find it hard to concentrate?
8. Did you feel more irritable?
9. Did you feel a strong need or urge to smoke?
10. Did you feel nervous, restless or anxious because you couldn't smoke?

Answering "yes" to any one of these 10 questions indicates that you may already be hooked on nicotine and are chemically dependent. Think about it! Your "yes" answer is your own honest self-assessment that you have already lost the freedom and ability to simply and effortlessly walk away. Two-thirds of all teens whom you see smoking regularly will spend their entire life as slaves to nicotine.

Source: HONC—(Hooked on Nicotine Checklist), Tobacco Control, Sept. 2002
Dr. JR Difranza, Development of Symptoms of Tobacco Dependency in Youths.
Reliability Study of HONC Factors—July 2002.
Created by www.WhyQuit.com. Join us for motivation, education, and support!

---

for the percentage of persons smoking (during the past month) within each group to go down. For example, among the younger age group, 18- to 24-year-olds, 32.4 percent of males and 24.6 percent of females reported having smoked during the preceding month, whereas among the 25- to 34-year-olds, 27.5 percent of males and 21.6 percent of females smoked during the preceding month, and in the 45- to 64-year-old group, 24.5 percent of males and 21.1 percent of females smoked during the preceding month. In comparison, in the oldest age group, the 65-year-olds and older, only 10.1 percent of males and 8.6 percent of females smoked cigarettes within the preceding 30 days. Most likely over the course of time, both quitting and premature death serve to reduce the percentage of smokers.

Comparing smoking during the preceding month among people in different regions of the country reveals that persons living in the north central portion of the country are the most likely to smoke (26 percent). In contrast, persons living in the West are least likely to have smoked during the preceding month (20.0 percent). People in the South (25.4 percent) and the Northeast (23.9 percent) fall in between.[9] In terms of population density, one might be surprised to learn that persons living outside metropolitan areas are more likely to have smoked during the preceding month (30.5 percent), whereas persons living in small metropolitan areas (27.2 percent) and large metropolitan areas (26.5 percent) are less likely to have smoked during the same period.[10]

Employment status also affects the likelihood of regular smoking. Persons who are employed part-time are more likely to have smoked during the past month (31.2 percent) than are people who are employed full-time (25.5 percent)—most likely reflecting the greater opportunity of the former group to smoke, since today's work place is increasingly a smoke-free environment. In stark contrast to those who have some degree of employment, the unemployed are by far the most likely to have smoked during the preceding month (48.2 percent).[11] This fact may reflect not only the lower level of education found among this group but also the immediate gratification that smoking brings to persons who may have little opportunity to seriously pursue long-range goals and the postponed gratification that striving for such goals can often require.

Marketing of Tobacco Products

Shredded plant material, wrapped in paper or leaf, ignited with a flame, and then placed on or near the delicate tissues of the mouth . . . what other human behavior does this resemble? If you answered *None!* to this question, then you appreciate that smoking is unique, and, therefore, that it must be learned. How it is learned is currently a less than fully understood process that most likely requires a variety of stimuli ranging from modeling to actual experimentation. The role of advertising as a source of models has long been suspected and intensely debated. Today, as in the past, controversy surrounds the intent of the tobacco industry's advertising. Are the familiar logos seen in a variety of media intended to challenge the brand loyalty of those who have already decided to smoke, as the industry claims? Or are the ads intended to entice new smokers, older children and young adolescents, in sufficient numbers to replace the 3,000 smokers who die each day from the consequences of tobacco use? This latter objective is now known, by admission of the tobacco industry, to have been pursued for decades. Its effectiveness has also been documented. The cartoon character Joe Camel was an especially successful tool for enticing children and teens to begin smoking.

Over the years the tobacco industry has used all aspects of mass media advertising, including radio, television, print, billboards, and sponsorship of televised athletic events and concerts, to sell its products. In addition, it has often distributed free samples and sold merchandise bearing the company or product logo.

Today the tobacco industry has been denied access to television and radio, and it can no longer distribute free samples to minors, but the industry continues to be active and innovative in other aspects of the media to which it has access. For example, Philip Morris contemplated the introduction of an upscale lifestyle magazine to be provided free to over 1 million smokers. Interestingly, the magazine would feature articles about healthful activities that many long-time smokers would be unable to engage in because of the effects of smoking.

In the 9 months following the 1999 Master Settlement Agreement, the tobacco industry increased their magazine advertising budget by 30 percent over presettlement levels in magazines with 15 percent or more youth (under 18 years of age) readership, even though they had agreed to discontinue advertising in youth-oriented publications. Most recently, increased tobacco advertising has been noted in magazines that appeal specifically to younger women, working women, fans of hip-hop music, and women of color.

The development of nonmarket brands of cigarettes for free distribution to patrons of bars and restaurants who are attempting to "bum" cigarettes represents a second form of "advertising." This "premarketing" introduction of a prototype brand technically does not violate the law regarding the distribution of samples. To date, several hundred establishments in several major cities have participated.

A final current example of the tobacco industry's subtle but effective presence in the mind of the public is that of tobacco use in motion pictures. In spite of a 1990 tobacco industry policy and the 1999 Master Settlement Agreement, both of which prohibit "brand placement" of tobacco products in films, cigarette and cigar smoking continue to be disproportionately represented in current films. Unfortunately, children and adolescents can easily identify with these characters (and their smoking), since they are generally depicted in a positive light. As an example, in a 2001 survey, two-thirds of the 43 movie stars most frequently named by 10- to 19-year-olds were seen smoking in their most recent films.[12] Perhaps even younger children were exposed to tobacco placement when Philip Morris was able to place its products in *Who Framed Roger Rabbit* and *The Muppet Movie*.[13]

Pipe and Cigar Smoking

Many people believe that pipe or cigar smoking is a safe alternative to cigarette smoking. Unfortunately, this is not the case. All forms of tobacco present users with a series of health threats (see the Star box on page 223 and Table 9.4 on page 231).

When compared with cigarette smokers, pipe and cigar smokers have cancer of the mouth, throat, larynx (voice box), and esophagus at the same frequency. Cigarette smokers are more likely than pipe and cigar smokers to have lung cancer, cancer of the larynx, chronic obstructive lung disease (COLD), also called chronic obstructive pulmonary disease (COPD), and heart disease. The cancer risk of death to smokers is four times greater from lung cancer and ten times greater from laryngeal cancer than it is for nonsmokers.

In comparison to cigarette smokers, pipe and cigar smokers are considerably fewer in number. Interestingly, cigar smoking enjoyed a resurgence through much of the 1990s. However, during 1998–1999 a substantial decline in sales of premium cigars occurred. Whether this downturn represents an emerging dissatisfaction with cigars as an enjoyable use of tobacco or simply reflects adjustments in the import market remains uncertain. In 1995 cigars generated sales of $1 billion, mainly to younger adults, including a very small but growing percentage of women.

Perhaps because of the increase in cigar smoking noted above, the National Cancer Institute commissioned the first extensive study of regular cigar smoking. That report confirmed and expanded on the health risks identified in earlier smaller studies.[14] In a study conducted in England, 7,735 middle-aged male cigar and pipe smokers were followed for nearly 22 years. Evaluation of the morbidity and mortality data collected determined that cigar and pipe smokers showed an increased risk for major coronary heart disease events and stroke events and an increased mortality rate for cardiovascular disease and for overall mortality.[15]

In response to the recognition of these risks, the FTC now requires that cigar manufacturers disclose the tobacco content and additives in their products. Most recently the FTC announced its intention of requiring five rotating health warnings to appear on cigars, including two that have been currently agreed on by the FTC and major cigar manufacturers: *Cigars Are Not a Safe Alternative to Cigarettes* and *Cigar Smoking Can Cause Cancer of the Mouth and Throat, Even If You Don't Inhale.*

The use of smokeless tobacco, a third alternative to cigarette smoking, is discussed later in the chapter.

If one were to judge on the basis of the number of newly opened cigar stores and clubs catering to cigar smokers, as well as the highly visible magazine *Cigar Aficionado,* one could conclude that cigar smoking was the hottest trend in tobacco use. To a degree this contention is true when one considers that in 1991 only 2.2 percent of the adult population smoked cigars on a regular basis, whereas by 1998 the size of the cigar-smoking population had risen to 5.2 percent. However, the most recent data available (2002) suggest only a slight increase, to 5.4 percent. We can hope that this very small increase suggests a possible leveling off of the cigar craze of the 1990s. Cigar smokers who continue to smoke and those of you who might be interested in this form of tobacco use should consider the following information from the American Lung Association:

- *Secondhand (sidestream) cigar smoke is more poisonous than secondhand cigarette smoke is.* The smoke from one cigar equals that of three cigarettes. Carbon monoxide emissions from one cigar are 30 times higher than those for one cigarette.

- *Cigar smoking can cause cancer of the larynx (voice box), mouth, esophagus, and lungs.* Cancer death rates for cigar smokers are 34% higher than those for nonsmokers.

- *Ninety-nine percent of cigar smokers have atypical cells found in the larynx.* These cells are the first step toward malignancy (cancer).

- *Cigar smokers are three to five times more likely to die of lung cancer than are nonsmokers.*

- *Cigar smokers have five times the risk of emphysema compared to nonsmokers.*

- *Nicotine does not have to be inhaled to damage the heart and blood vessels.* It is absorbed into the bloodstream through the mucous membranes of the mouth. Nicotine increases the heart rate and constricts the blood vessels, which reduces blood flow to the heart.

Tobacco Use and the Development of Dependence

Although not true for every tobacco user (see the discussion of "chippers" later in this section), the vast majority of users, particularly cigarette smokers, will develop a dependency relationship with the nicotine contained in tobacco. This state of **dependence** causes users to consume greater quantities of nicotine over extended periods of time, further endangering their health.

Dependence can imply both a physical and psychological relationship. Particularly with cigarettes, *physical dependence* or *addiction,* with its associated *tolerance, withdrawal,* and **titration,** is strongly developed by 40 percent of all smokers. The development of addiction reflects a strong genetic predisposition to physical dependence.[16] Most of the remaining population of smokers will experience lesser degrees of physical dependence. Psychological *dependence* or *habituation,* with its accompanying psychological components of *compulsion* and *indulgence,* is almost universally seen.

Compulsion is a strong emotional desire to continue tobacco use despite restrictions on smoking and the awareness of health risks. Very likely, users are "compelled" to engage in continual tobacco use in fear of the unpleasant physical, emotional, and social effects that result from discontinuing use. In comparison to compulsion, indulgence is seen as "rewarding" oneself for aligning with a particular behavior pattern—in this case, smoking. Indulgence is made possible by the existence of various reward systems built around the use of tobacco, including a perceived image, group affiliation, and even appetite suppression intended to foster weight control.

Much to the benefit of the tobacco industry, dependence on tobacco is easily established. Many experts believe that physical dependence on tobacco is far more easily established than is physical dependence on alcohol, cocaine (other than crack), or heroin. Of all people who experiment with cigarettes, 85 percent develop various aspects of a dependence relationship.

A small percentage of smokers, known as "chippers," can smoke on occasion without becoming dependent. Most likely, chippers respond differently to environmental cues than do more dependent smokers,[17] thus smoking less frequently. They may be truly "social smokers" in that they smoke only with a few selected friends or in a very limited number of places. Unfortunately,

---

Key Terms

dependence a physical and/or psychological need to continue the use of a drug

titration (tie **tray** shun) the particular level of a drug within the body; adjusting the level of nicotine by adjusting the rate of smoking

many inexperienced smokers feel that they too are only social smokers; however, a few months, or even a few days, of this type of occasional smoking could be a transitional period into a dependence pattern of tobacco use.

Sandwiched between regular smokers and chippers is a newly emerging group of smokers—part-time smokers. Today these smokers constitute about 20 percent of all smokers.[18] The practice most likely reflects the reality of the high cost of cigarettes and restrictions in the workplace. The health effects of this form of smoking appear to be the same as for regular smokers.

Theories of Nicotine Addiction

The establishment and maintenance of physical dependence or addiction is less than fully understood. Most experts, however, believe that for a specific individual, addiction has a multifaceted etiology, or cause, with increasing attention being directed toward a genetic basis for addiction. Accordingly, several theories have been proposed to explain the development of dependence. We present a brief account of some of these theories. Readers are reminded that many of these theories are technically sophisticated and only a most basic description can be provided in a personal health textbook. The more emotional aspects of dependence formation are discussed later in the chapter.

Genetic Influences

Although the specific genetic pathways that influence both the initiation and maintenance of smoking (or other forms of tobacco use) are less than fully understood, a role for genetic influence is evident. Applying new statistical techniques to earlier studies of smoking patterns in families and between identical twins, it is now believed that initiation and maintenance of initial smoking is 60 percent driven by genetic influences.[19] Of course, the smoking of the first few cigarettes is a choice made by beginning smokers. In a yet-to-be-determined percentage of beginning smokers, the *initiation* of smoking, or the desire to continue with this new behavior, is underlined by a genetic predisposition to neurohormonally "appreciate" the stimulating effects of nicotine. Once smoking has been so easily and successfully initiated, the continuation of smoking is then *maintained* by the same, or closely related, genetic predisposition for neurohormonal excitation of the central nervous system. The "hook" for a lifetime of smoking is, thus, set in large part by a genetic susceptibility.[20] The remaining influence needed for initiation and maintenance of initial smoking is 20 percent environmental and 20 percent the unique needs of individuals.[19]

Once the relatively brief period of initial exposure (initiation) and early maintenance is passed, the role of

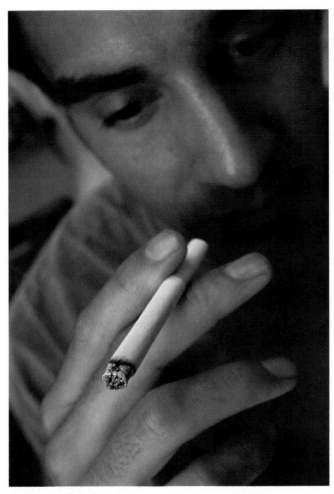

A smoker inhales about 70,000 times during the first year of smoking, resulting in a nicotine addiction that often lasts a lifetime.

genetic influences may be even more powerful—providing 70 percent of the maintenance stimulus required over decades of smoking. Environmental and personality factors subside accordingly.[19]

Bolus Theory

In the **bolus theory** of nicotine addiction, one of the oldest and most general theories of addiction, each inhalation of smoke releases into the blood a concentrated

---

Key Terms

bolus theory a theory of nicotine addiction based on the body's response to the bolus (ball) of nicotine delivered to the brain with each inhalation of cigarette smoke

quantity of nicotine (a ball or bolus) that reaches the brain and results in a period of neurohormonal excitement. The smoker perceives this period of stimulation as pleasurable but, unfortunately, short-lived. Accordingly, the smoker attempts to reestablish this pleasurable feeling by again inhaling and sending another bolus of nicotine on its way to the brain. The 70,000 or more inhalations during the first year of smoking serve to condition the novice smoker, resulting in a lifelong pattern of cigarette dependence. The level needed for arousal is different for each individual smoker, depending on the length of addiction, the level of tolerance, genetic predisposition, and environmental and personal stimuli.

Recognition of two types of smokers emerges from an understanding of the bolus theory of smoking. *Peak smokers* are those smokers who become dependent on the arousal of pleasure centers in the brain that are stimulated by the rapid increase of nicotine levels following inhalation and distribution of nicotine within the CNS. In contrast, the *trough maintenance smokers* maintain an even consistently higher level of nicotine titration in order to avoid the negative consequences of withdrawal. These feelings are experienced as unpleasant and thus are to be avoided.

Adrenocorticotropic Hormone (ACTH) Theory

Yet another theory of dependence suggests that nicotine stimulates the release of adrenocorticotropic hormone (ACTH) from the anterior pituitary, or "master gland" of the endocrine system (see Chapter 3) causing the release of **beta endorphins** (naturally occurring opiatelike chemicals) that produce mild feelings of euphoria. Perhaps this stresslike response mechanism involving ACTH accounts for the increased energy expenditure seen in smokers and thus their tendency to maintain a lower body weight. Others, however, have questioned the ability of nicotine to stimulate endorphin release.[21]

When these physiological responses are viewed collectively, nicotine may be seen as biochemically influencing brain activity by enhancing the extent and strength of various forms of "communication" between different brain areas and even glands of the endocrine system. If this is the case, it is apparent why, once addicted, the functioning of the smoker's control systems is much altered in comparison with that of nonsmokers.

Self-Medication Theory

Another explanation of the addiction to smoking, called *self-medication,* suggests that nicotine, through the effects of mood-enhancing dopamine, may allow smokers to "treat" feelings of tiredness, lack of motivation, or even depression.[22] In other words, a smoke lifts the spirits, if only briefly. Eventually, however, smokers become dependent on tobacco as a "medication" to make themselves feel better. Thus, because tobacco is a legal drug that is readily available, it becomes preferred to prescription medications and illegal drugs, such as cocaine and the stimulants, that elevate mood.

Regardless of the mechanism involved, as tolerance to nicotine develops, smoking behavior is adjusted to either maintain arousal or prevent the occurrence of withdrawal symptoms. At some point, however, the desire for constant arousal is probably superseded by the smoker's desire not to experience withdrawal.

The importance of nicotine as the primary factor in establishing dependence on tobacco is supported by research that demonstrates that smokers will not select a nontobacco cigarette if a tobacco cigarette is available. Even tobacco cigarettes with a very low level of nicotine seem to be unacceptable to most smokers, as do cigarettes with very low nicotine but with high tar content. Interestingly, users of low-nicotine cigarettes tend to inhale more frequently and deeply to obtain as much nicotine as possible.

Even more impressive (and alarming) regarding nicotine's dependency-producing power is seen in conjunction with the small amount of time needed to become dependent. Using the HONC instruments described in the Star box on page 221, it is now established that beginning smokers (recall that most smokers begin during adolescence) become dependent on cigarettes within 3 weeks to 3 months of smoking on as little as two cigarettes per day. Males are more likely to be a bit more resistant to dependency, taking a month or two, whereas females can become dependent in a matter of a very few days of initial experimentation.[23]

 TALKING POINTS A smoker says that she does not consider smoking to be a form of drug use. She becomes angry at the suggestion that cigarettes are part of a drug-delivery system. How would you respond to her position?

Acute Effects of Nicotine on Nervous System Function

In comparison with the more chronic effects of nicotine on the central nervous system (CNS) that may eventually result in physical dependence or addiction, nicotine also

---

Key Terms

beta endorphins mood-enhancing, pain-reducing, opiatelike chemicals produced within the smoker's body in response to the presence of nicotine

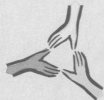

produces changes of short duration. In the CNS, nicotine activates receptors within the nucleus accumbens (a reward center) and the locus caeruleus (a cortical activating center) of the brain. Stimulation of the brain is seen by changes in electroencephalogram (EEG) patterns, reflecting an increase in the frequency of electrical activity. This is part of a general arousal pattern signaled by the release of the neurotransmitters **norepinephrine,** dopamine, acetylcholine, and serotonin. Heavy use of tobacco products, resulting in high levels of nicotine in the bloodstream, eventually produces a blocking effect as more and more receptor sites for these neurotransmitters are filled. The result is a generalized depression of the CNS.

The level of plasma nicotine associated with normal levels of heavy smoking (one to two packs per day) would not likely produce the depressive effect just described. However, in chain smokers (four to eight packs per day), plasma nicotine levels would be sufficient to have a depressive influence on nervous system function. In fact, it has been suggested that chain smoking is driven by the fruitless effort to counter the depressive influence of chronically excessively high levels of nicotine.

In carefully controlled studies involving both animals and humans, nicotine increased the ability of subjects to concentrate on a task. However, the duration of this improvement was limited. Most people would agree that this brief benefit is not enough to justify the health risks associated with chronic tobacco use.

Non–Nervous-System Acute Effects of Nicotine

Outside the CNS, nicotine affects the transmission of nerve signals at the point where nerves innervate muscle tissue (called the *neuromuscular junction*) by mimicking the action of the neurotransmitter acetylcholine. Nicotine occupies receptor sites at the junction and prevents the transmission of nerve impulses from nerve cell to muscle cell.

Nicotine also causes the release of epinephrine from the adrenal medulla (see Chapter 3), which results in an increase in respiration rate, heart rate, blood pressure, and

---

Key Terms

norepinephrine (nor epp in **eff** rin) an adrenalinlike chemical produced within the nervous system

coronary blood flow. These changes are accompanied by the constriction of the blood vessels beneath the skin, a reduction in the motility in the bowel, loss of appetite, and changes in sleep patterns.

Although a lethal dose of nicotine could be obtained through the ingestion of a nicotine-containing insecticide, to "smoke oneself to death" in a single intense period of cigarette use would be highly improbable. In humans, 40 to 60 mg (.06–.09 mg/kg) is a lethal dose. A typical cigarette supplies .05–2.5 mg of nicotine, and that nicotine is relatively quickly broken down for removal from the body.

Psychosocial Factors Related to Dependence

Recall that a psychological aspect of dependence (habituation) exists and is important in maintaining the smoker's need for nicotine. Both research and general observation support many of the powerful influences this aspect of dependence possesses, especially for beginning smokers, before the onset of physical addiction. Consequently, in the remainder of this section, we will explore nonphysiological factors that may contribute to the development of this aspect of dependence.

Modeling

Because tobacco use is a learned behavior, it is reasonable to accept that modeling acts as a stimulus to experimental smoking. **Modeling** suggests that susceptible people smoke to emulate, or model their behavior after, smokers whom they admire or with whom they share other types of social or emotional bonds. Particularly for young adolescents (ages 14 to 17), smoking behavior correlates with the smoking behavior of slightly older peers and very young adults (ages 18 to 22), older siblings, and, most important, parents. Negative parental influences on cigarette smoking by their children include their own smoking status, and/or their failure to clearly state their disapproval of smoking.[24] Further, for parents who smoke, it is important that they cease smoking before their children turn 8 years of age if they wish to maximize an anti-smoking message.

Modeling is particularly evident when smoking is a central factor in peer group formation and peer group association and can lead to a shared behavioral pattern that differentiates the group from others and from adults. Further, when risk-taking behavior and disregard for authority are common to the group, smoking becomes the behavioral pattern that most consistently identifies and bonds the group. Particularly for those young people who lack self-directedness or the ability to resist peer pressure, initial membership in a tobacco-using peer group may become inescapable. The ability to counter peer pressure is a salient component of successful anti-smoking programs for use with older children and younger adolescents.

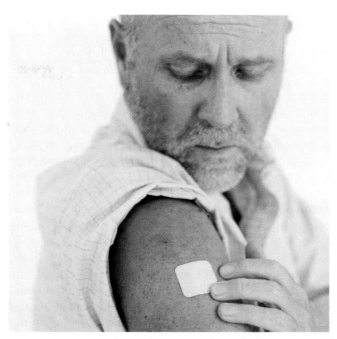

Smoker with arm patch

In addition, when adolescents have lower levels of self-esteem and are searching for an avenue to improve self-image, a role model who smokes is often seen as tough, sociable, and sexually attractive. These three traits have been played up by the tobacco industry in their carefully crafted advertisements. In fact, teens from any background may see the very young and attractive models used in tobacco (and beer) advertisements as being more peerlike in age than they really are. FCC regulations require that models for both products be 21 years of age or older, regardless of how youthful they might (and the advertisers hope they do) appear to older children and young adolescents. (See the Learning from Our Diversity box on page 226 for a counterapproach to the acceptance of tobacco.)

Manipulation

In addition to modeling as a psychosocial link with tobacco use, cigarette use may meet the beginning smoker's need to manipulate something and at the same time provide the manipulative "tool" necessary to offset boredom, feelings of depression, or social immaturity. Clearly the availability of affordable smoking paraphernalia

> **Key Terms**
>
> **modeling** the process of adopting the admired behavioral patterns of another person

provides smokers with ways to reward themselves. A new cigarette lighter, a status brand of tobacco, or a beach towel with a cigarette's logo are all reinforcements to some smokers. Fortunately, the last item will become increasingly harder to find since logos can no longer be placed on items such as beach towels. For others, the ability to take out a cigarette or fill a pipe adds a measure of structure and control to situations in which they might otherwise feel somewhat ill at ease. The cigarette becomes a readily available and dependable "friend" to turn to during stressful moments.

Susceptibility to Advertising

The images of the smoker's world portrayed by the media can be particularly attractive. For adolescents, women, minorities, and other carefully targeted groups of adults, the tobacco industry has paired suggestions of a better life with the use of its products. To these users and potential users, the self-reward of power, liberation, affluence, sophistication, or adult status is achieved by using the products that they are told are associated with these desired states. Thus the self-rewarding use of tobacco products becomes a means of hoped-for achievement.

With this multiplicity of forces at work, we can understand why so many who experiment with tobacco use find that they quickly, in combination with genetic predisposition, become emotionally dependent on tobacco. Human needs, both physiological and psychosocial, are many and complex. Tobacco use meets the needs on a short-term basis, whereas dependence, once established, replaces these needs with a different, more immediate set of needs.

Despite the satisfaction of the dependency that continued smoking brings, approximately 80 percent of adult smokers have, on at least one occasion, expressed a desire to quit, and the majority of these have actually attempted to become nonsmokers. Today, with the over-the-counter availability of transdermal nicotine patches, nicotine-containing gum, prescription medications such as antidepressants, and nicotine inhalers, the number of smokers making concerted and repeated attempts to stop smoking is up considerably over that seen in the past. It therefore seems apparent that tobacco use is a source of **dissonance.** This dissonance stems from the need to deal emotionally with a behavior that is both highly enjoyable and highly dangerous but known to be difficult to stop. The degree to which this dissonance exists probably varies from user to user.

Preventing Teen Smoking

Even before the 1997 release of tobacco industry documents confirming the targeting of young adolescents, the federal government stated its intention to curb these cigarette advertisements. In August 1995 the FDA described the specific actions that it hoped it would be given authority to implement. These policies were, in large part, incorporated into *Healthy People 2000* and retained in *Healthy People 2010*. If these policies, in combination with other initiatives, are effective, the adolescent smoking rate will be lowered to no more than 16 percent by 2010.

1. Limit tobacco advertising in publications that appeal to teens and restrict billboards with tobacco-related content to no closer than 1,000 feet of schools and playgrounds. (An August 1995 study in California found that stores near schools displayed significantly more tobacco-related advertisements than those farther from schools.)
2. Restrict the use of logo and other tobacco-related images on nontobacco-related products, such as towels, T-shirts, and caps.
3. Bar certain sources of access to tobacco products, such as mail order sales, the distribution of free samples, and vending machines.
4. Halt sponsorship of high-visibility events, such as auto racing and athletic contests in which brand names appear on highly televised surfaces, including hoods, fenders, uniforms, and arena sign boards. (It is estimated that the Marlboro logo is seen 5,933 times during the course of a 90-minute televised Nextel Cup auto race.)
5. Require merchants to obtain proof of age when selling tobacco products to adolescents. (This particular component of the initial plan became law in 1997. Merchants are required to validate the age of people whom they suspect to be younger than 27 years of age before selling cigarettes to those 18 years of age and older. If found in violation, both the salesperson and the store owner will be fined $500.)

By mid-1998 the federal government's desire to reduce youth smoking through implementation of the steps just described was mired in a larger package of tobacco-related policies being debated in Congress. This undertaking was related to the class action suit filed by all 50 (46 as a single large class and 4 as a smaller class) states against the tobacco industry in an attempt to recoup Medicaid expenditures for treating tobacco-related illnesses. As Congress attempted to construct a settlement that would be acceptable to all parties, the impasse fragmented attempts to reduce youth smoking. Unfortunately, this outcome diluted some restrictions on tobacco advertisements, as well as the FDA's

---

Key Terms

dissonance (**dis** son ince) a feeling of uncertainty that occurs when a person believes two equally attractive but opposite ideas

ability to reduce smoking by defining cigarettes as drug delivery systems. In fact, in 2000 the United States Supreme Court ruled that the FDA lacked the regulatory authority to bring tobacco products under its control, unless Congress was willing to rescind laws that currently define tobacco as an agricultural product that can be freely marketed to persons 18 years of age or older. (If defined as a drug delivery system, cigarettes would be obtainable only with a physician's prescription, which would essentially prevent, or greatly limit, children's access to them.)

As noted earlier in the chapter, the Master Settlement Agreement of 1999, which required the tobacco industry to pay the states 246 billion dollars, was able to restrict some forms of youth-oriented advertising and funds anti-smoking education, which may accomplish some of the changes initially proposed. Unfortunately, during the economic downturn many states have used these funds to meet taxation shortfalls.

Tobacco: The Source of Physiologically Active Compounds

When burned, the tobacco in cigarettes, cigars, and pipe mixtures is the source of an array of physiologically active chemicals, many of which are closely linked to significant changes in normal body structure and function. At the burning tip of the cigarette, the 900°C (1,652°F) heat oxidizes tobacco (as well as paper, wrapper, filter, and additives). With each puff of smoke, the body is exposed to approximately 4,700 chemical compounds, hundreds of which are known to be physiologically active, toxic, and carcinogenic. These chemicals have their origin in the tobacco or the over 1,450 additives, including pesticides and other agricultural chemicals. An annual 70,000 puffs taken in by the one-pack-a-day cigarette smoker results in an environment that makes the most polluted urban environment seem clean by comparison.

Table 9.3 presents a partial list of toxic and carcinogenic compounds of tobacco smoking. In addition to tobacco smoke, these materials, and hundreds of others

not listed, are routinely found within many materials used in industrial and residential settings.

Particulate Phase

Cigarette, cigar, and pipe smoke can be described on the basis of two phases. These phases include a particulate phase and a gaseous phase. The **particulate phase** includes **nicotine,** water, and a variety of powerful chemicals known collectively as tar. **Tar** includes phenol, cresol, pyrene, DDT, and a benzene-ring group of compounds that includes benzo[a]pyrene. Most of the carcinogenic

---

Table 9.3 A Partial Listing of Toxic and Carcinogenic Components of Cigarette Smoke

Agent

Carbon Monoxide   (1)
Nitrogen Oxides (NO$_x$)   (2)
Hydrogen Cyanide   (3)
Formaldehyde   (4)
Acrolein   (5)
Acetaldehyde   (6)
Ammonia   (7)
Hydrazine   (8)
Vinyl Chloride   (9)
Benzo[a]pyrene   (10)
Aromatic Amines   (11)
Aromatic Nitrohydrocarbons   (12)
Polonium-210   (13)
Nickel   (14)
Arsenic   (15)
Cadmium   (16)

Nontobacco Sources of Selected Chemical Compounds Found in Tobacco Smoke

(1) released by internal combustion engines (cars, trucks, buses, etc.)
(2) released by internal combustion engines
(3) burning of polyurethane form (insulating material)
(4) released by internal combustions and the burning of many forms of building material
(5) burning of fat (e.g., barbecuing of meats)
(6) released by internal combustion engines
(7) found in fertilizers, many cleaning agents, and released during decomposition of organic material
(8) rocket fuel exhaust
(9) released by burning plastics
(10) produced when grilling meats and found in wood smoke and soot
(11) released during the decomposition of organic material
(12) found in fumes produced by the incineration of municipal wastes
(13) released into air during radioactive decay
(14) leakage from or burning of nickel-cadmium batteries
(15) found in localized ground-water areas
(16) found in pesticides and batteries, and released by municipal waste incineration

Source: Mulcahy S. *The Toxicology of Cigarette Smoke and Environmental Tobacco Smoke,* A Review of Cigarette Smoke and Its Toxicological Effects, www.csn.ul.ie/-stephen/reports/bc4927.html.

---

compounds are found within the tar. A person who smokes one pack of cigarettes per day collects four ounces of tar in his or her lungs in a year. Only the gases and the smallest particles reach the small sacs of the lungs, called the *alveoli*, where oxygen exchange occurs. The carcinogen-rich particles from the particulate phase are deposited somewhere along the air passage leading to the lungs.

Gaseous Phase

The **gaseous phase** of tobacco smoke, like the particulate phase, is composed of a variety of physiologically active compounds, including carbon monoxide, carbon dioxide, ammonia, hydrogen cyanide, isopyrene, acetaldehyde, and acetone. At least 60 of these compounds have been determined to be **carcinogens** or co-carcinogenic promoters, thus capable of stimulating the development of cancer. Carbon monoxide is, however, the most damaging compound found in this component of tobacco smoke. Its effect is discussed next.

Carbon Monoxide

Like every inefficient engine, a cigarette, cigar, or pipe burns (oxidizes) its fuel with less than complete conversion into carbon dioxide, water, and heat. As a result of this incomplete oxidation, burning tobacco forms **carbon monoxide (CO)** gas. Carbon monoxide is one of the most harmful components of tobacco smoke.

Carbon monoxide is a colorless, odorless, tasteless gas that possesses a very strong physiological attraction for hemoglobin, the oxygen-carrying pigment on each red blood cell. When CO is inhaled, it quickly bonds with hemoglobin and forms a new compound, carboxyhemoglobin. In this form, hemoglobin is unable to transport oxygen to the tissues and cells where it is needed.

Although it is true that normal body metabolism always keeps an irreducible minimum of CO in our blood (0.5–1 percent), the blood of smokers may have levels of 5–10 percent CO saturation.[25] We are exposed to additional CO from environmental sources such as automobiles and buses and other combustion of fossil fuels. When we consider the combination of a smoker's CO with environmental CO, we are not surprised that smokers more easily become out of breath than nonsmokers do. The half-life of CO combined with hemoglobin is approximately 4 to 6 hours. Most smokers replenish their level of CO saturation at far shorter intervals than this.

As mentioned, the presence of excessive levels of carboxyhemoglobin in the blood of smokers leads to shortness of breath and lowered endurance. Because an adequate oxygen supply to all body tissues is critical for normal functioning, any oxygen reduction can have a serious impact on health. Brain function may be eventually reduced, reactions and judgment are dulled, and of course, cardiovascular function is impaired. Fetuses are especially at risk for this oxygen deprivation (hypoxia) because fetal development is so critically dependent on a sufficient oxygen supply from the mother.

Illness, Premature Death, and Tobacco Use

For people who begin tobacco use as adolescents or young adults, smoke heavily, and continue to smoke, the likelihood of premature death is virtually ensured. Two-pack-a-day cigarette smokers can expect to die 7 to 8 years earlier than their nonsmoking counterparts will. (Only nonsmoking-related deaths that can afflict smokers and nonsmokers alike keep the difference at this level rather than much higher.) Not only will these people die sooner, but they will also probably be plagued with painful, debilitating illnesses for an extended time. Smoking is responsible for nearly 440,000 premature deaths each year.[26] Table 9.4 presents an overview of illnesses known to be caused or worsened by tobacco use.

Cardiovascular Disease

Although cancer is now the leading cause of death for Americans under 80 years of age, cardiovascular disease is the leading cause of death among all adults, accounting for 927,448 deaths in the United States in 2004.[27] Tobacco use, and cigarette smoking in particular, is clearly one of the major factors contributing to this cause of death. Although overall progress is being made in reducing the incidence of cardiovascular-related deaths, tobacco use impedes these efforts. So important is tobacco use as a contributing factor in deaths from cardiovascular disease that the cigarette smoker more than doubles the risk of experiencing a **myocardial infarction,** the leading cause

---

Key Terms

gaseous phase portion of the tobacco smoke containing carbon monoxide and many other physiologically active gaseous compounds

carcinogens environmental agents, including chemical compounds within cigarette smoke, that stimulate the development of cancerous changes within cells

carbon monoxide (CO) chemical compound that can "inactivate" red blood cells

myocardial infarction heart attack; the death of heart muscle as a result of a blockage in one of the coronary arteries

Table 9.4 Selected Established and Suspected Health Effects of Cigarette Smoking

Category of Condition	Established and Suspected Effects
1. Lung Disease	lung cancer, chronic obstructive lung disease; increased severity of asthma; increased risk of developing various respiratory infections
2. Cancer Risk	esophageal, laryngeal, oral, bladder, kidney, stomach, pancreatic, vulvar, cervical, and colorectal cancers
3. Heart Disease	coronary heart disease; angina pectoris; heart attack; repeat heart attack; arrhythmia; aortic aneurysm; cardiomyopathy
4. Peripheral Vascular Disease	pain and discomfort in the legs and feet resulting from restricted blood flow into the extremities
5. Skin Changes	wrinkling; fingernail discoloration; psoriasis; palmoplantar pustulosis
6. Surgical Risk	need for more anesthesia; increased risk of postsurgical respiratory infection; increased need for supplemental oxygen following surgery; delayed wound healing
7. Orthopedic Problems	disc degeneration; less successful back surgery; musculoskeletal injury; delayed fracture healing
8. Rheumatologic Conditions	osteoporosis and osteoarthritis
9. Environmental Tobacco Smoke and Pediatric Illnesses	infections of the lower respiratory tract; more severe asthma; middle ear infections; Crohn's disease and ulcerative colitis; sudden infant death syndrome; impaired delivery of oxygen to body tissues
10. Complications in Obstetrics and Gynecology	infertility; miscarriage; fetal growth retardation; prematurity; stillbirth; transmission of HIV to the fetus from the infected biological mother; birth defects; intellectual impairment of offspring; sudden infant death syndrome; earlier menopause
11. Male Infertility and Sexuality Dysfunctions	decreased sperm motility; decreased sperm density; impotence
12. Neurological Disorders	transient ischemic attack; stroke; worsened multiple sclerosis
13. Brain and Behavior	depression
14. Abnormalities of the Ears, Nose, and Throat	snoring and hearing loss
15. Eyes	cataracts; complications from Graves' disease; macular degeneration; optic neuropathy
16. Oral Health	periodontal disease
17. Endocrine System	increased metabolic rate; blood-sugar abnormalities; increased waist-to-hip ratio; redistribution of body fat
18. Gastrointestinal Diseases	stomach and duodenal ulcers; Crohn's disease
19. Immune System	impaired humoral and cell-mediated immunity
20. Emergency Medicine	injuries from fires; occupational injuries

Source: Kapier KN, et al. *Cigarettes: What the Warning Label Doesn't Tell You.* American Council on Science and Health, 1997.
Note: Recently *The 2004 United States Surgeon General's Report: The Health Consequences of Smoking* added abdominal aneurysms, periodontal disease, and myeloid leukemia to the list of illnesses and diseases attributed to smoking and listed in Table 9.4.

of death from cardiovascular disease. Smokers also increase their risk of **sudden cardiac death** by two to four times. Fully one-third of all cardiovascular disease can be traced to cigarette smoking.

The relationship between tobacco use and cardiovascular disease is centered on two major components of tobacco smoke: nicotine and carbon monoxide.

Nicotine and Cardiovascular Disease
The influence of nicotine on the cardiovascular system occurs when it stimulates the nervous system to release norepinephrine. This powerful stimulant increases the

heart rate. In turn, an elevated heart rate increases cardiac output, thus increasing blood pressure. The extent to which this is dangerous depends in part on the coronary circulation's ability to supply blood to the rapidly

> **Key Terms**
>
> **sudden cardiac death** immediate death resulting from a sudden change in the rhythm of the heart

A healthy lung (right) vs. the lung of a smoker (left).

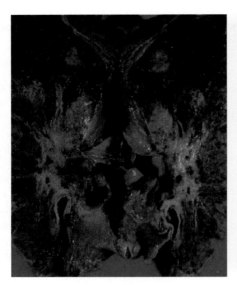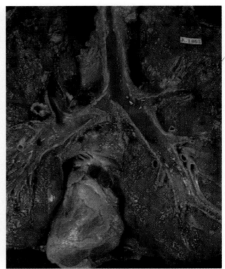

contracting heart muscle. The development of **angina pectoris** and the possibility of sudden heart attack are heightened by this sustained elevation of heart rate, particularly in those individuals with existing coronary artery disease (see Chapter 10).

Nicotine is also a powerful vasoconstrictor of the peripheral blood vessels. As these vessels are constricted by the influence of nicotine, the pressure against their walls increases. Research shows that irreversible atherosclerotic damage to major arteries also occurs with smoking.

For over a decade it has been known that nicotine also increases blood **platelet adhesiveness.** As the platelets become more and more likely to "clump," a person is more likely to develop a blood clot. In people already prone to cardiovascular disease, more rapidly clotting blood is an unwelcome liability. Heart attacks occur when clots form within the coronary arteries or are transported to the heart from other areas of the body.

In addition to other influences on the cardiovascular system, nicotine possesses the ability to decrease the proportion of high-density lipoproteins (HDLs) and to increase the proportion of low-density lipoproteins (LDLs) and very-low-density lipoproteins that constitute the body's serum cholesterol. Low-density lipoproteins appear to support the development of atherosclerosis and are clearly increased in the bloodstreams of smokers. (See Chapter 10 for further information about cholesterol's role in cardiovascular disease.)

Carbon Monoxide and Cardiovascular Disease

A second substance contributed by tobacco influences the type and extent of cardiovascular disease found among tobacco users. Carbon monoxide interferes with oxygen transport within the circulatory system.

As described earlier in the chapter, carbon monoxide is a component of the gaseous phase of tobacco smoke and readily joins with the hemoglobin of the red blood cells. Carbon monoxide has an affinity for hemoglobin 206 times that of oxygen. Once the hemoglobin of a red cell has accepted carbon monoxide molecules, the hemoglobin is transformed into carboxyhemoglobin. Thereafter, the carboxyhemoglobin permanently weakens the red blood cell's ability to transport oxygen. So long as smoking continues, these red blood cells remain relatively useless during the remainder of their 120-day lives. Levels of carboxyhemoglobin in heavy smokers are associated with significant increases in the incidence of myocardial infarction.

When a person has impaired oxygen-transporting abilities, physical exertion becomes increasingly demanding on both the heart and the lungs. The cardiovascular system will attempt to respond to the body's demand for oxygen, but these responses are themselves impaired as a result of the influence of nicotine on the cardiovascular system. If tobacco does create the good life, as advertisers claim, it also unfortunately lessens the ability to participate actively in that life.

Cancer

Over the past 60 years, research from the most reputable institutions in this country and abroad has consistently concluded that tobacco use is a significant factor in the development of virtually all forms of cancer and the most significant factor in cancers involving the respiratory system.

> **Key Terms**
>
> **angina pectoris** (an **jie** nuh **peck** tor is) chest pain that results from impaired blood supply to the heart muscle
>
> **platelet adhesiveness** tendency of platelets to clump together, thus enhancing the speed at which the blood clots

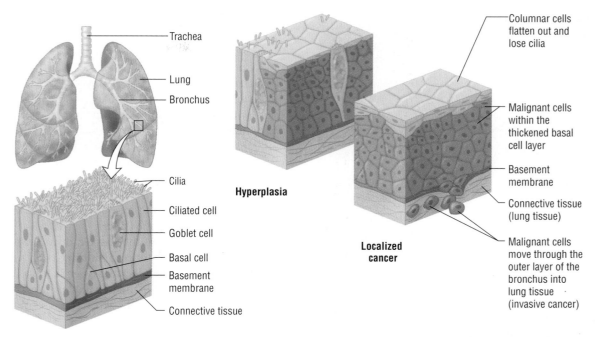

Figure 9–1 Tissue changes associated with bronchogenic carcinoma (lung cancer)

In describing cancer development, the currently used reference is 20 pack-years, or an amount of smoking equal to smoking one pack of cigarettes a day for 20 years. Thus the two-pack-a-day smoker can anticipate cancer-related tissue changes in as few as 10 years, while the half-pack-a-day smoker may have 40 years to wait. Regardless, the opportunity is there for all smokers to confirm these data by developing cancer as predicted. It is hoped that most people will think twice before disregarding this evidence.

Data supplied by the American Cancer Society (ACS) indicate that during 2004 an estimated 1,372,910 Americans developed cancer.* These cases were nearly equally divided between the sexes and resulted in approximately 570,280 deaths. In the opinion of the ACS, 30 percent of all cancer cases are heavily influenced by tobacco use. Lung cancer alone accounted for about 172,570 of the new cancer cases and 163,510 deaths in 2004. Fully 87 percent of men with lung cancer were cigarette smokers.[26] A genetic "missing link" between smoking and lung cancer was established, when mutations to an important tumor suppressor gene were identified. If it was necessary to have a final "proof" that smoking causes lung cancer, that proof appears to be in hand.

Cancer of the entire respiratory system, including lung cancer and cancers of the mouth and throat, accounted for about 184,800 new cases of cancer and 168,140 deaths.[26] Despite these high figures, not all smokers develop cancer.

---

*Excluding cases of nonmelanoma skin cancer.

Respiratory Tract Cancer

Recall that tobacco smoke produces both a gaseous and a particulate phase. As noted, the particulate phase contains the tar fragment of tobacco smoke. This rich chemical environment contains more than four thousand known chemical compounds, hundreds of which are known to be carcinogens.

In the normally functioning respiratory system, particulate matter suspended in the inhaled air settles on the tissues lining the airways and is trapped in **mucus** produced by specialized *goblet cells*. This mucus, with its trapped impurities, is continuously swept upward by the beating action of hairlike **cilia** of the ciliated columnar epithelial cells lining the air passages (Figure 9-1). On reaching the throat, this mucus is swallowed and eventually removed through the digestive system.

When tobacco smoke is drawn into the respiratory system, however, its rapidly dropping temperature allows the particulate matter to accumulate. This brown, sticky

Key Terms

mucus clear, sticky material produced by specialized cells within the mucous membranes of the body; mucus traps much of the suspended particulate matter within tobacco smoke

cilia (**sill** ee uh) small, hairlike structures that extend from cells that line the air passages

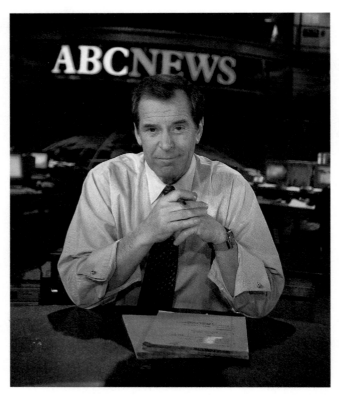

Peter Jennings, who died from lung cancer in 2005.

tar contains compounds known to harm the ciliated cells, goblet cells, and the basal cells of the respiratory lining. As the damage from smoking increases, the cilia become less effective in sweeping mucus upward to the throat. When cilia can no longer clean the airway, tar accumulates on the surfaces and brings carcinogenic compounds into direct contact with the tissues of the airway.

At the same time that the sweeping action of the lining cells is being slowed, substances in the tar are stimulating the goblet cells to increase the amount of mucus they normally produce. The "smoker's cough" is the body's attempt to remove this excess mucus.

With prolonged exposure to the carcinogenic materials in tar, predictable changes will begin to occur within the respiratory system's basal cell layer (Figure 9-1). The basal cells begin to display changes characteristic of all cancer cells. In addition, an abnormal accumulation of cells occurs. When a person stops smoking, preinvasive lesions do not repair themselves as quickly as once thought.[28]

By the time lung cancer is usually diagnosed, its development is so advanced that the chance for recovery is very poor. Still today, only 15 percent of all lung cancer victims survive for 5 years or more after diagnosis.[26] Most die in a very uncomfortable, painful way.

Cancerous activity in other areas of the respiratory system, including the larynx, and within the oral cavity (mouth) follows a similar course. In the case of oral cavity cancer, carcinogens found within the smoke and within the saliva are involved in the cancerous changes. Tobacco users, such as pipe smokers, cigar smokers, and users of smokeless tobacco, have a higher (4 to 10 times) rate of cancer of the mouth, tongue, and voice box.

In addition to drawing smoke into the lungs, tobacco users swallow saliva that contains an array of chemical compounds from tobacco. As this saliva is swallowed, carcinogens are absorbed into the circulatory system and transported to all areas of the body. The filtering of the blood by the liver, kidneys, and bladder may account for the higher-than-normal levels of cancer in these organs among smokers. Smoking may also accelerate the rate of development of pancreatic cancer.

As reported earlier in the chapter, documents released in 1997 from within the tobacco industry clearly show that the major tobacco companies were aware of tobacco's role in the development of cancer and had made a concerted effort to deprive the American public access to such knowledge.

Chronic Obstructive Lung Disease

Chronic obstructive lung disease (COLD), also known as chronic obstructive pulmonary disease (COPD), is a disorder in which the amount of air that flows in and out of the lungs becomes progressively limited. COLD is a disease state that is made up of two separate but related diseases: **chronic bronchitis** and **pulmonary emphysema.**

With chronic bronchitis, excess mucus is produced in response to the effects of smoking on airway tissue, and the walls of the bronchi become inflamed and infected. This produces a characteristic narrowing of the air passages. Breathing becomes difficult, and activity can be severely restricted. With cessation of smoking, chronic bronchitis is reversible.

Emphysema causes irreversible damage to the tiny air sacs of the lungs, the **alveoli.** Chest pressure builds when air becomes trapped by narrowed air passages (chronic bronchitis) and the thin-walled sacs rupture. Emphysema patients lose the ability to ventilate fully. They feel as though they are suffocating. You may have seen people with

---

Key Terms

chronic bronchitis persistent inflammation and infection of the smaller airways within the lungs

pulmonary emphysema an irreversible disease process in which the alveoli are destroyed

alveoli (al **vee** oh lie) thin, saclike terminal ends of the airways; the site at which gases are exchanged between the blood and inhaled air

this condition in malls and other locations as they walk slowly by, carrying or pulling their portable oxygen tanks.

More than 10 million Americans suffer from COLD. It is responsible for a greater limitation of physical activity than any other disease, including heart disease. COLD patients tend to die a very unpleasant, prolonged death, often from a general collapse of normal cardiorespiratory function that results in congestive heart failure (see Chapter 10).

Additional Health Concerns

In addition to the serious health problems stemming from tobacco use already described, other health-related changes are routinely seen. These include a generally poor state of nutrition, a decline in insulin sensitivity, a decline in short-term memory, the gradual loss of the sense of smell, and premature wrinkling of the skin. Tobacco users are also more likely to experience strokes (a potentially fatal condition), lose bone mass leading to osteoporosis, experience more back pain and muscle injury, and find that fractures heal more slowly. Further, smokers who have surgery spend more time in the recovery room. Although not perceived as a health problem by people who continue smoking to control weight, smoking does appear to minimize weight gain. In studies using identical twins, twins who smoked were six to eight pounds lighter than their nonsmoking siblings. Current understanding about why smoking results in lower body weight is less than complete. One factor may be an increase in Basal Metabolic Rate (BMR) (see Chapter 6) brought about by the influence of nicotine on sympathetic nervous system function. Additionally, smokers have a four-fold greater risk of developing serious gum (periodontal) disease, now thought to be a risk factor for cardiovascular disease. Also, smokers may need supplementation for two important water-soluble vitamins, vitamin C and vitamin B.

Smoking and Reproduction

In all its dimensions, the reproductive process is impaired by the use of tobacco, particularly cigarette smoking and environmental tobacco smoke in close proximity to pregnant women.[29] Problems can be found in association with infertility, problem pregnancy, breast-feeding, and the health of the newborn. So broadly based are reproductive problems and smoking that the term *fetal tobacco syndrome* or *fetal smoking syndrome*[30] is regularly used in clinical medicine. Some physicians even define a fetus being carried by a smoker as a "smoker" and, upon birth, as a "former smoker."

Infertility

Recent research indicates that cigarette smoking by both men and women can reduce levels of fertility. Among men, smoking adversely affects blood flow to erectile tissue, reduces sperm motility, and alters sperm shape, and it causes an overall decrease in the number of viable sperm. Among women, the effects of smoking are seen in terms of abnormal ovum formation, including a lessened ability on the part of the egg to prevent polyspermia, or the fertilization by multiple sperm. Smoking also negatively influences estrogen levels, resulting in underdevelopment of the uterine wall and ineffective implantation of the fertilized ovum. Lower levels of estrogen may also influence the rate of transit of the fertilized egg through the fallopian tube, making it arrive in the uterus too early for successful implantation or, in some cases, restricting movement to the point that an **ectopic, or tubal, pregnancy** may develop. Also, the early onset of menopause is associated with smoking.

Although causative pathways remain somewhat unclear, the influences of smoking are noted in two aspects of male infertility, sperm degradation and erectile dysfunction. In the former cases, several chemicals in tobacco smoke are able to cross the blood-testis barrier and structurally alter the DNA of the genetic material within the sperm. The presence of abnormal sperm in the male compromises the chances of fertilization. In erectile dysfunction, smoking, most likely through the effects of nicotine on blood-flow dynamics, decreases blood flow into the erectile tissues of the penile shaft, resulting in the inability to obtain or sustain an erection.[31,32]

Problem Pregnancy

The harmful effects of tobacco smoke on the course of pregnancy are principally the result of the carbon monoxide and nicotine to which the mother and her fetus are exposed. Carbon monoxide from the incomplete oxidation of tobacco is carried in the maternal blood to the placenta, where it diffuses across the placental barrier and enters the fetal circulation. Once in the fetal blood, the carbon monoxide bonds with the fetal hemoglobin to form fetal carboxyhemoglobin. As a result of this exposure to carbon monoxide, the fetus is progressively deprived of normal oxygen transport and eventually becomes compromised by chronic **hypoxia.**

Nicotine also exerts its influence on the developing fetus. Thermographs of the placenta and fetus show signs of marked vasoconstriction within a few seconds after inhalation by the mother. This constriction further reduces the oxygen supply, resulting in hypoxia. In addition, nicotine stimulates the mother's stress response, placing the mother and fetus under the potentially harmful influence

---

Key Terms

ectopic (tubal) pregnancy pregnancy resulting from the implantation of the fertilized ovum within the inner wall of the fallopian tube

hypoxia oxygenation deprivation at the cellular level

of elevated epinephrine and corticoid levels (see Chapter 3). Any fetus exposed to all of these agents is more likely to be miscarried, stillborn, or born prematurely. Even when carried to term, children born to mothers who smoked during pregnancy have lower birth weights and may show other signs of a stressful intrauterine life.

Breast-Feeding

Women who decide to breast-feed their infants and continue to smoke continue to expose their children to the harmful effects of tobacco smoke. It is well recognized that nicotine appears in breast milk and thus is capable of exerting its vasoconstricting and stress-response influences on nursing infants. Mothers who stop smoking during pregnancy should be encouraged to continue to refrain from smoking while they are breast-feeding.

Neonatal Health Problems

Babies born to women who smoked during pregnancy are, on average, shorter and have a lower birth weight than do children born to nonsmoking mothers. During the earliest months of life, babies born to mothers who smoke experience an elevated rate of death caused by sudden infant death syndrome. Statistics also show that infants are more likely to develop chronic respiratory problems, more frequent colic, be hospitalized, and have poorer overall health during their early years of life. Problems such as those just mentioned may also be seen in children of nonsmoking mothers, when they were exposed prenatally to environmental tobacco smoke. In addition, environmental tobacco smoke exposure extending beyond the home and into the workplace may increase the probability of problem pregnancies and neonatal health problems. Most recently, the interest in the effects of tobacco smoke on pregnancy has been extended to include behavioral differences seen in infants born to women who smoked during pregnancy.[33]

Parenting, in the sense of assuming responsibility for the well-being of children, does not begin at birth, but during the prenatal period. In the case of smoking, this is especially true. Pregnant women who continue smoking are disregarding the well-being of the children they are carrying. Other family members, friends, and coworkers who subject pregnant women to cigarette, pipe, or cigar smoke are, in a sense, exhibiting their own disregard for the health of the next generation.

Oral Contraceptives and Tobacco Use

Women who smoke and use oral contraceptives, particularly after age 35, are placing themselves at a much greater risk of experiencing a fatal cardiovascular accident (heart attack, stroke, or **embolism**) than are oral contraceptive users who

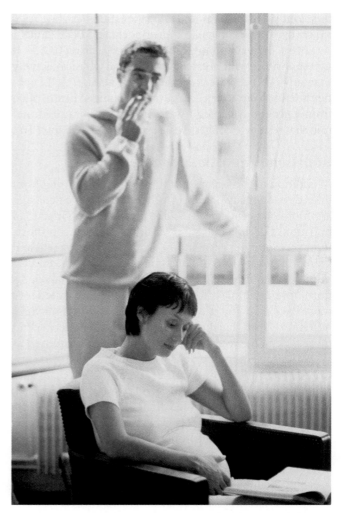

Pregnant women and those around them should refrain from smoking to protect the health of the developing fetus.

do not smoke. This risk of cardiovascular complications increases further for oral contraceptive users 40 years of age or older. Women who both smoke and use oral contraceptives are four times more likely to die from myocardial infarction (heart attack) than are women who only smoke. Because of this adverse relationship, *it is strongly recommended that women who use oral contraceptives not smoke.*

Smokeless Tobacco Use

As the term implies, smokeless tobacco, such as Skoal and Copenhagen, is not burned; rather, it is placed into the mouth. Once in place, the physiologically active nicotine

---

Key Terms

embolism a potentially fatal condition in which a circulating blood clot lodges in a smaller vessel

---

and other soluble compounds are absorbed through the mucous membranes and into the blood. Within a few minutes, chewing tobacco and snuff generate blood levels of nicotine in amounts equivalent to those seen in cigarette smokers.

Chewing tobacco is taken from its foil pouch, formed into a small ball (called a "wad," "chaw," or "chew"), and placed into the mouth. Once in place, the bolus of tobacco is sucked and occasionally chewed, but not swallowed.

Snuff, a more finely shredded smokeless tobacco product, is marketed in small round cans. Snuff is formed into a small mass (or "quid") for dipping or used in prepackaged pouches. The quid or pouch is placed between the jaw and the cheek; the user sucks the quid or pouch, then spits out the brown liquid. Snuff, as once used, was actually a powdered form of tobacco that was inhaled through the nose.

Although smokeless tobacco would seem to free the tobacco user from many of the risks associated with smoking, chewing and dipping are not without their own substantial risks. The presence of *leukoplakia* (white spots) and *erythroplakia* (red spots) on the tissues of the mouth indicate precancerous changes. In addition, an increase in **periodontal disease** (with the pulling away of the gums from the teeth, resulting in later tooth loss), the abrasive damage to the enamel of the teeth, and the high concentration of sugar in processed tobacco all contribute to dental problems among users of smokeless tobacco. In those who develop oral cancer, the risk is dramatically heightened if the cancer metastasizes from the site of origin in the mouth to the brain. Clearly, users should be aware of any signs of damage being done by their use of smokeless tobacco. (See the Changing for the Better box on this page.) The validity of this warning was made clear in 1998 when about half of smokeless tobacco-using major league baseball players were found to have tobacco-related lesions when oral examinations were performed by team dentists on the first day of spring training.

In addition to the damage done to the tissues of the mouth, the need to process the inadvertently swallowed saliva that contains dissolved carcinogens places both the digestive and urinary systems at risk of cancer.

In the opinion of health experts, the use of smokeless tobacco and its potential for life-threatening disease is very real and should not be disregarded. Consequently, television advertisements have been banned, and the following warnings have been placed in rotation on all smokeless tobacco products:

> WARNING: THIS PRODUCT MAY CAUSE MOUTH CANCER
>
> WARNING: THIS PRODUCT MAY CAUSE GUM DISEASE AND TOOTH LOSS
>
> WARNING: THIS PRODUCT IS NOT A SAFE ALTERNATIVE TO CIGARETTE SMOKING

Changing for the Better

Early Detection of Oral Cancer

I started using smokeless tobacco a few years ago, thinking it was safe. Recently, I read an article about it that was frightening. What are the real danger signs?

If you have any of the following signs, see your dentist or physician immediately:

- Lumps in the jaw or neck area
- Color changes or lumps inside the lips
- White, smooth, or scaly patches in the mouth or on the neck, lips, or tongue
- A red spot or sore on the lips or gums or inside the mouth that does not heal in 2 weeks
- Repeated bleeding in the mouth
- Difficulty or abnormality in speaking or swallowing

Clearly, smokeless tobacco is a dangerous product, and little doubt exists that continued use of tobacco in this form is a serious problem to health in all its dimensions.

The Risks of Involuntary (Passive) Smoking

The smoke generated by the burning of tobacco can be classified as either **mainstream smoke** (the smoke inhaled and then exhaled by the smoker) or **sidestream smoke** (the smoke that comes from the burning end of the cigarette, pipe, or cigar that simply disperses into the air without being inhaled by the smoker). When either form of tobacco smoke is diluted and stays within a common source of air, it can eventually be referred to as **environmental tobacco smoke.** All three forms of tobacco smoke lead to

Key Terms

periodontal disease destruction of soft tissue and bone that surround the teeth

mainstream smoke smoke inhaled and then exhaled by a smoker

sidestream smoke smoke that comes from the burning end of a cigarette, pipe, or cigar

environmental tobacco smoke tobacco smoke, regardless of its source, that stays within a common source of air

The Hidden Price Tag of Smoking

"I started to hug him but felt myself drawing back. It was almost like a reflex action." Those are the words of a young woman after greeting her brother when he returned home from his first semester at college. The young man had recently become a smoker, and his sister was reacting to the strong smell of smoke on his clothes and hair.

Dramatic as it may sound, smoking does set up barriers between people. First, there's the health issue. Some nonsmokers are adamant about not wanting people they care about to smoke. They also want to protect their children from this danger. And they certainly don't want to breathe in smoke themselves. So, at a family gathering, a smoker may want to have a cigarette after dinner, in the living room with everyone else. But the nonsmokers say no—go outside if you want to smoke. In the process, a birthday dinner or a special holiday is marred by this disagreement.

Whether the person is a family member or a friend, it's difficult to feel close to someone who's doing something you disapprove of—such as smoking. But, from the smoker's point of view, it's hard to feel good about someone who acts superior and doesn't accept you as you are. What do children think about all this? Does a "good" aunt or uncle smoke? If smoking is bad, as a little girl constantly hears at school and at home, why does her favorite uncle smoke?

On the job, smoking has gone the way of the three-martini lunch. It's just not politically correct. In fact, many companies have a no-smoking policy, or smoking is allowed in designated areas only. Ever drive by a big factory or office building and see a group of people standing outside, perhaps huddled under umbrellas? They're not organizing a strike—they're having a smoke. Once again, the smoker feels isolated.

Just as in the family group, the smoker feels the judgment of others—only now it's her boss or secretary who's frowning.

In addition to the more modest work-site restrictions just described, today the hammer has fallen even harder on the heads of smokers—companies are beginning to reject job applications from smokers. (It's hard to hide the telltale signs of smoking and relatively easy to learn from references whether an applicant is a smoker.) Additionally, companies have begun terminating employees who smoke, even when they don't smoke at work. Some companies will pay for smoking-cessation assistance, so long as the employees remain active participants in the program and eventually quit smoking. Countersuits brought by rejected applicants and terminated employees will certainly begin filtering through the court system, but until final rulings are made, smokers should be prepared for increasing discrimination.

The price of smoking is hard to measure. The damage to the smoker's health is beyond dispute. But the spiritual and psychological costs are also real. How does it feel to always be the outsider? The unaccepted? Why does the smoker have to take the chance of missing an exciting play in the stadium to go smoke a cigarette? Or feel the resentment of others at work because he leaves to take a smoking break every hour? Many who have stopped smoking—often after several attempts—say that they thought about more than their health in deciding to quit. They thought about many situations—involving family, outdoor activities, and work—before they threw away the pack and said: "That was my last cigarette."

involuntary or passive smoking and can present health problems for both nonsmokers and smokers. (See Discovering Your Spirituality above.)

Surprisingly, mainstream smoke makes up only 15 percent of our exposure to the harmful substances associated with involuntary smoking. Sidestream smoke is responsible for 85 percent of the harmful substances associated with secondhand smoke exposure. Because it is not filtered by the tobacco, the filter, or the smoker's body, sidestream smoke contains more free nicotine and produces higher yields of carbon dioxide and carbon monoxide. Much to the detriment of nonsmokers, sidestream smoke has a much higher quantity of highly carcinogenic compounds, called *N-nitrosamines*, than mainstream smoke has.

Current scientific opinion suggests that smokers and nonsmokers are exposed to very much the same smoke when tobacco is used within a common airspace. The important difference is the quantity of smoke inhaled by smokers and nonsmokers. It is likely that for each pack of cigarettes smoked by a smoker, nonsmokers who must share a common air supply with the smokers involuntarily smoke the equivalent of three to five cigarettes per day. Even today, because of the small size of the particles produced by burning tobacco, environmental tobacco smoke cannot be completely removed from a workplace, restaurant, or shopping mall by the most effective ventilation system.

Recently reported research indicates that involuntary smoke exposure may be responsible for 35,000 to 40,000 premature deaths per year from heart disease among nonsmokers in the United States.[26] Other estimates range upward to 53,000 premature deaths when lung cancer and COPD are included. In addition, large numbers of people exposed to involuntary smoke develop eye irritation, nasal symptoms, headaches, and a cough. Furthermore, most nonsmokers dislike the odor of tobacco smoke.

For these reasons, state, local, and private-sector initiatives to restrict smoking have been introduced. Most buildings in which people work, study, play, reside, eat, or shop now have some smoking restrictions. Some have complete smoking bans. Nowhere is smoking more noticeably prohibited than in the U.S. airline industry. Currently, smoking is banned on all domestic plane flights of less than 6 hours, and major American airlines have extended the ban on smoking to international flights as well.

Involuntary smoking poses major threats to nonsmokers within residential settings. Spouses and children of smokers are at greatest risk for involuntary smoking. Scientific studies suggest that nonsmokers married to smokers are three times more likely to experience heart attacks than nonsmoking spouses of nonsmokers, and the former have a 30 percent greater risk of lung cancer than do the latter. It should be noted, however, that a recent study of 35,561 nonsmoking spouses of smoking partners failed to show significantly higher death rates from heart disease, lung cancer, and COPD than did nonsmoking spouses in nonsmoking relationships.[34] Between the time of publication of the study and October of 2004, however, dozens of letters to the editor were sent to the *British Medical Journal,* publisher of the original study. A substantial number of these letters called attention to flaws in the design of the study, faulty statistical interpretation, and a potential conflict of interest between the authors and the tobacco industry.

In spite of what may or may not be the effects of passive smoking on the nonsmoking partners of smokers, the effects of environmental tobacco smoke on the health of children seems well established. The children of parents who smoke are twice as likely as children of nonsmoking parents to experience bronchitis or pneumonia during the first year of life. In addition, throughout childhood these children will experience more wheezing, coughing, and sputum production than will children whose parents do not smoke. Otitis media (middle ear infection), one of the most frequently seen conditions in pediatric medicine, is also significantly more common in children under age 3 who reside with one or more adults who smoke.

In July 1998, the tobacco industry challenged in court the salient 1993 EPA report that was the basis for restricting smoking in a wide array of public places and work sites. The federal judge who heard the case concluded that the principal study used in the report was flawed in its methodology and that its conclusions therefore were of questionable validity. Since this decision, the scientific community has documented to a very substantial degree the inherent dangers of passive or environmental tobacco smoke to the health of nonsmokers and smokers alike. Accordingly, restrictions on public smoking have been large

scale and continue to be imposed. These restrictions include statewide bans on smoking in public places in California, Connecticut, Delaware, Florida, Idaho, Maine, Massachusetts, New York, Rhode Island, South Dakota, and Utah. Additionally, many cities and towns have enacted their own bans, particularly in states that have no statewide bans. Examples are Anchorage, Tempe, Boulder, Honolulu, Fort Wayne (IN), Albuquerque, Columbus (OH), Eugene, and Austin.[35]

Although the United States does not have a single encompassing ban on smoking in public places, several countries have enacted such bans. Among them are Australia, Italy, Scotland, England, Cuba, Ireland, Uganda, Greece, Sweden, and Romania.

Many colleges and universities are instituting bans on smoking near the entrances to classroom buildings and residence halls. At Ball State University, cigarettes must be extinguished within 30 feet of an entrance. This restriction on smoking reflects the fact that environmental tobacco smoke accumulates under overhangs and in alcoves.

Nontobacco Sources of Nicotine

Regardless of whether they are intended as aids to smoking cessation or only supplemental forms of nicotine for use when smoking is not permitted, numerous new forms of nicotine delivery systems have appeared in the marketplace in recent years. An area of growing concerns is, of course, that these nontobacco delivery sources of nicotine could provide introductory exposure to nicotine, at a tragically early age, for the next generation of nicotine-dependent youth. Included among these nontobacco sources of nicotine are multiple flavors of nicotine suckers, nicotine-flavored gum, nicotine straws, nicotine-enhanced water (Nico Water), inhalers, sprays, drops, lozenges, and transdermal patches. To date, only Nico Water has been formally addressed by the Food and Drug Administration (and their request for control was rejected by the courts), other than those that came into the marketplace as prescription-only or approved OTC products.

Stopping What You Started

Experts in health behavior contend that before people will discontinue harmful health behaviors, such as tobacco use, they must appreciate fully what they are expecting of themselves. This understanding grows in relationship to the following:

1. *Knowledge* about the health risks associated with tobacco use
2. *Recognition* that these health risks are applicable to all tobacco users

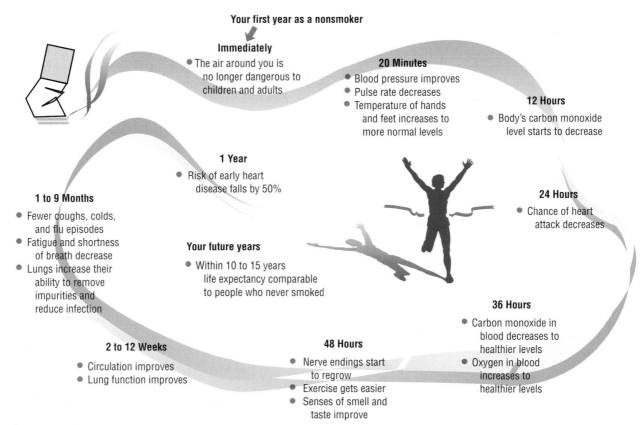

Your first year as a nonsmoker

Immediately
- The air around you is no longer dangerous to children and adults

20 Minutes
- Blood pressure improves
- Pulse rate decreases
- Temperature of hands and feet increases to more normal levels

12 Hours
- Body's carbon monoxide level starts to decrease

1 Year
- Risk of early heart disease falls by 50%

1 to 9 Months
- Fewer coughs, colds, and flu episodes
- Fatigue and shortness of breath decrease
- Lungs increase their ability to remove impurities and reduce infection

Your future years
- Within 10 to 15 years life expectancy comparable to people who never smoked

24 Hours
- Chance of heart attack decreases

36 Hours
- Carbon monoxide in blood decreases to healthier levels
- Oxygen in blood increases to healthier levels

2 to 12 Weeks
- Circulation improves
- Lung function improves

48 Hours
- Nerve endings start to regrow
- Exercise gets easier
- Senses of smell and taste improve

Figure 9–2 The health benefits of quitting smoking begin immediately and become more significant the longer you stay smoke-free.

3. *Familiarity* with steps that can be taken to eliminate or reduce these risks
4. *Belief* that the benefits to be gained by no longer using tobacco will outweigh the pleasures gained through the use of tobacco
5. *Certainty* that one can start and maintain the behaviors required to stop or reduce the use of tobacco

These steps combine both knowledge and desire (or motivation). Being knowledgeable about risks, however, will not always stop behaviors that involve varying degrees of psychological and physical dependence. The 75 percent failure rate thought to be common among tobacco-cessation programs suggests that the motivation is not easy to achieve or maintain. In fact, on the basis of information reported by the Hazelden Foundation, for persons who are successful in quitting, approximately 18.6 years elapse between the first attempt to stop and the actual time of quitting. The many health benefits of quitting smoking are shown in Figure 9-2.

A variety of smoking-cessation programs exist, including those using highly organized formats, with or without the use of prescription or OTC nicotine replace-

ment systems. In past years, most of the 1.3 million people who managed to quit smoking each year did so by throwing away their cigarettes (going cold turkey) and paying the physical and emotional price of waiting for their bodies to adjust to life without nicotine. Today, however, the use of nicotine replacement products in combination with external smoking cessation approaches, such as those described later in this chapter, or the use of prescription medication, such as antidepressants, is more common. Changing for the Better on page 241 provides a plan for smoking cessation that incorporates nicotine replacement products.

Programs to help people stop their tobacco use are available in a variety of formats, including educational programs, behavior modification, aversive conditioning, hypnosis, acupuncture, and various combinations of these approaches. Programs are offered in both individual and group settings and are operated by hospitals, universities, health departments, voluntary health agencies, churches, and private practitioners. The better programs will have limited success rates—20–50 percent as measured over one year (with self-reporting), whereas the remainder will have even poorer results. If results are monitored using the assessment of nicotine breakdown products in the blood, the effectiveness rate of these programs falls even lower, as some "successful" self-reporters are not completely honest in their reporting of cessation.

Two methods for weaning smokers from cigarettes to a nontobacco source of nicotine are nicotine-containing chewing gum (Nicorette) and transdermal patches, in either prescription or OTC versions (Nicoderm, Nicotrol, Habitrol, Prostep, and others), using either single-strength or step-down formulas. A brief description of both gum and the transdermal patch is provided next, although subtle variations exist between prescription and OTC formulations and between brands.

Nicotine-Containing Chewing Gum Correct use of nicotine-containing chewing gum requires an immediate cessation of smoking, an initial determination of dosage (4 mg or 2 mg of nicotine per piece), knowledge of the appropriate manner of chewing each piece of gum, the appropriate time to chew each piece, the maximum number of pieces to be chewed each day, and time to begin withdrawal from the therapy. When used in combination with physician guidance or program support provided by the manufacturer, cessation using nicotine-containing gum may have a success rate of 40 percent or more, based on blood evaluation. Nicotine-containing chewing gum therapy ranges in cost from an initial $60 kit to weekly refills of approximately $30.

Table 9.5 How Methods of Smoking Cessation Stack Up

Of the nation's estimated 48 million smokers, 70% want to quit, and 46% try each year. Only 1 in 40 succeeds. Federal guidelines, based on published studies, estimate varied success rates for a number of medications designed to help smokers quit.

Medications	Nicotine gum	Nicotine inhaler	Buproprion SR (Zyban)	Nicotine spray	Nicotine patch	Combination
Number of studies	13	4	2	3	27	3
Five-month quit rate	23.7%	22.8%	30.5%	30.5%	17.7%	28.6%
Advantage	Can be used to offset cravings	Mimics smoking	Nonnicotine, an antidepressant	Higher nicotine levels	Private, one/day	Combines benefits
Disadvantage	Poor taste	Low nicotine levels	Must screen for seizures	Irritation, sneezing	Skin irritation	Not FDA-approved
Over the counter (OTC) or prescription (Rx)	OTC	Rx	Rx	Rx	Both	Both

Source: *Treating Tobacco Use and Dependence.* U.S Public Health Service: John Hughes, University of Vermont, November 2000.

Transdermal Nicotine Patches The more recently developed transdermal (through the skin) nicotine patches appear to be less effective (25 percent) than does the gum just described, but in many ways the patches are more easily used. If a step-down version (21 mg, 14 mg, 7 mg) is employed, determinations must be made as to the appropriate initial dosage (based on number of cigarettes smoked per day and body weight), the length of time at the initial dosage before stepping down, and the manner of withdrawal after a usual 8- to 12-week treatment period. The single-dose (15 mg) version, of course, eliminates the step-down component. Costs associated with transdermal nicotine replacement therapy are similar to those for the gum-based program.

In addition to the nicotine-replacement products already described, a nicotine inhaler and spray has been approved by the FDA. Because of the large surface area of the lungs and rapid absorption into the blood, inhalation-based delivery of nicotine has become a very attractive alternative to transdermal and oral routes of replacement.

In all delivery forms and formulations, nicotine replacement therapy can be associated with contraindications and adverse reactions, including skin irritation, redness, and irregular heart rates. People who are concerned that nicotine-replacement therapies are simply a "trade-off" of addictions (from cigarettes to gum, patches, or a nasal spray) should remember that while using the therapy the former smoker is no longer being exposed to carbon monoxide and carcinogens, and the step-down feature allows for a gradual return to a totally nicotine-free lifestyle. Therefore, a short period of cross-addiction should be viewed simply as the cost of recovery.

Recently developed prescription medications, used in combination with other cessation methods improve the latter's effectiveness rate to somewhat above the 40 percent (perhaps approaching 50 percent) level reported for nicotine-containing chewing gum, according to a blood-based assessment. These drugs affect receptors in the CNS, reducing the pleasurable effects of nicotine and thus decreasing dependency. Among the more recently "discovered" prescription medications for smoking cessation is methoxsalen. Although intended for the treatment of psoriasis, a skin condition, this medication has been found to constructively alter the breakdown of nicotine in persons who have a particular genetic mutation that lessens their need for frequent cigarettes. Another recently approved drug for use in smoking cessation is varenicline. On the basis of clinical trials, it is reported that nearly one-half of all persons receiving the drug were able to cease smoking. Should this efficacy carry over into long-term trials, this medication would equal or most likely exceed the most effective approaches now available.

Several additional nicotine-free prescription medications to aid smoking cessation have now been approved or are nearing approval. These agents can be used alone or with nicotine replacement therapy. Zyban and Wellbutrin are antidepressant drugs that increase the production of dopamine, a neurotransmitter. Production of dopamine declines when a smoker quits, creating the craving to smoke. Prozac, the serotonin-reuptake inhibitor antidepressant approved for the treatment of depression, bulimia nervosa, PMS, and obsessive-compulsive disorder, has also shown promise as an adjunct to smoking cessation. See Table 9.5 for a comparison of various cessation approaches.

In a recent meta-analysis of smoking cessation program success involving African Americans, it was found that there is no statistically significant difference between the success of this racial group and others. Of interest, however, was a finding that church-based programs might be more successful for smoking cessation than previously recognized.

Taking Charge of Your Health

- Commit yourself to establishing a smoke-free environment in the places where you live, work, study, and recreate.

- Support friends and acquaintances who are trying to become smoke-free.

- Support legislative efforts, at all levels of government, to reduce your exposure to environmental tobacco smoke.

- Be civil toward tobacco users in public spaces, but respond assertively if they infringe on smoke-free spaces.

- Support agencies and organizations committed to reducing tobacco use among young people through education and intervention.

SUMMARY

- The percentage of American adults who smoke is continuing to decline.
- In spite of a reversal on the part of more recent college graduates, cigarette smoking has traditionally been inversely related to the level of formal education.
- A number of demographical variables influence the incidence of tobacco use.
- The tobacco industry continues to aggressively market its products to potential smokers.
- Multiple theories regarding nicotine's role in dependence have been advanced, including a better understanding of the proportional influences of genetics, environment, and personality.
- Nicotine exerts acute effects both within the central nervous system and on a variety of other tissues and organs.
- Tobacco smoke can be divided into gaseous and particulate phases. Each phase has its unique chemical composition.
- Thousands of chemical components and hundreds of carcinogenic agents are found in tobacco smoke.
- Nicotine and carbon monoxide have predictable effects on the function of the cardiovascular system.
- The development of nearly one-third of all cancers can be attributed to tobacco use, and virtually every form of cancer is found more frequently in smokers than in nonsmokers.

- Chronic obstructive lung disease (COLD), also called chronic obstructive pulmonary disease (COPD), is a likely consequence of long-term cigarette smoking, with early symptoms appearing shortly after beginning regular smoking.
- Smoking alters normal structure and function of the body, as seen in a wide variety of noncardiovascular and noncancerous conditions, such as infertility, problem pregnancy, and neonatal health concerns. Additional health concerns include the diminished ability to smell, periodontal disease, vitamin inadequacies, and bone loss leading to osteoporosis.
- The use of smokeless tobacco carries its own health risks, including oral cancer.
- The presence of secondhand smoke results in involuntary (or passive) smoking by those who must share a common air source with smokers. This secondhand smoke threatens the health of the spouse, children, and coworkers of the smoker.
- Stopping smoking can be undertaken in any one of several ways, including the use of nicotine-replacement products, such as nicotine-containing gum, transdermal nicotine patches, and nicotine inhalers, as well as medications that influence the recognition of neurotransmitters that bring pleasure to smokers.

REVIEW QUESTIONS

1. What percentage of the American adult population smoke? In what direction has change been occurring?
2. What is the current direction that adolescent smoking is taking?
3. What was the outcome of the class action suit brought by the forty-six states, and what was the effect of the Master Settlement Agreement (1999) on the ability of the tobacco industry to market its products?
4. In comparison to cigarettes, what health risks are associated with pipe and cigar smoking?
5. What are the two principal dimensions of nicotine dependence? What are specific aspects seen within physical dependence?
6. Identify each of the theories of nicotine dependence discussed in the chapter.
7. How do modeling and manipulation explain the development of emotional dependence on tobacco?

8. In the amount consumed by the typical smoker, what is the effect of nicotine on central nervous system function? How does this differ in chain smokers?
9. What effects does nicotine have on the body outside of the central nervous system? How does the influence of nicotine resemble that associated with the stress response?
10. What is the principal effect of carbon monoxide on cardiac function?
11. What influences does passive smoking have on nonsmoking adult partners of smokers? On their children?
12. How is the federal government attempting to limit the exposure that children and adolescents currently have to tobacco products and tobacco advertisements?
13. What prescription and OTC products are now available to assist smokers in quitting?
14. What percentage of smokers are able to quit, and what is the best way to confirm that quitting has actually occurred?

Sold only online by its developer, a new smokeless cigarette contains tobacco but is neither lighted nor heated in any manner. In the absence of any burning or heating, there is no smoke, tar, and carbon monoxide. This product is the Aeros Smokeless Cigarette, and it was developed by Woodleaf Corporation of Newport Beach, California. Online promotional material suggests that Aeros was developed over 8 years in conjunction with FDA criteria for a smokeless cigarette.

The Aeros cigarette is described as being a sealed plastic tube containing a tightly packed carefully formulated tobacco mixture. "Smoking" the Aeros involves cutting both ends of the plastic tube and inhaling through the appropriate opened end. Over the course of about 8 inhalations the user enjoys the aroma, taste, and nicotine of the tobacco, without the health-detracting particulate and gaseous components of normal cigarettes. The developer assures the "smoker" that no tobacco touches the lips. Data provided by an independent laboratory reports that 0 milligrams of tar and .05 milligrams of nicotine are delivered by each cigarette. The FDA appears to concur with the developer's contention that the Aeros Smokeless Cigarette could be legally used in all traditional nonsmoking environments.

ENDNOTES

1. Wakefield MA, et al. Tobacco industry marketing of point of purchase after the 1999 MSA billboard ban. *AJPH 9,* No. 6, June 2002.
2. U.S. Centers for Disease Control and Prevention. *MMWR,* Vol 52, No. 53. January 9, 2004.
3. *Smoking and Health: Report of the Advisory Committee to the Surgeon General of the Public Health Service.* U.S. Department of Health and Human Services. Public Health Service. 1964.
4. Cigarette smoking among adults—United States, 2002. *MMWR,* Vol. 53, No. 20. May 28, 2004.
5. National Center for Health Statistics, United States, *Health, 1998, with Socioeconomic Status and Health Chartbook.* NCHS, 1998.
6. Substance Abuse and Mental Health Service Administration. *Results from the 2003 National Survey on Drug Use and Health: National Findings.* NSDUH Series H-25, DHHS Publication No. SMA 04-3964, 2004.
7. Johnston LD, et al. *Monitoring the future national results on adolescent drug use: Overview and key findings, 2004.* NIH Publication No. 05-5726. National Institute on Drug Abuse, 2005.
8. Patterson F, et al. Cigarette smoking practices among American college students: Review and future directions. *J Am Coll Health.* 2004 Mar–Apr; 52(5):203–210.
9. Schoenborn CA, Jackline VL, Barnes PM. *Cigarette Smoking Behavior of Adults: United States, 1998.* Advanced Data from Vital and Health Statistics, No. 331. Division of Interview Statistics, National Center for Vital Statistics, February 2003.
10. *National Household Survey on Drug Abuse—Main Findings 1998* (H-11) Substance Abuse and Mental Health Services. Department of Health and Human Services, 2000.
11. *National Survey on Drug Use and Health 2000–2003* (formerly called the *National Survey On Drug Abuse*) (G-30), Substance Abuse and Mental Health Services, Department of Health and Human Services, 2004.
12. Tickle JJ, et al. Favorite movie stars, their tobacco use in contemporary movies, and its association with adolescent smoking. *Tob Control.* 2001 Mar 10(1):16–22.
13. *More Antismoking Issues in Movies and TV.* TobaccoFree.org. The Foundation for a Smokefree America, www.tobaccofree.org/films.htm, 2005.
14. Burns DM, et al. *Cigars: Health Effects and Trends.* Cancer Monograph Series (No. 9) National Cancer Institute, 1998.
15. Shaper AG, Wannamethee SG, Walker M. Pipe and cigar smoking and major cardiovascular events, cancer incidence, and all-cause mortality in middle-aged British men. *In J Epidemiol.* 2003 Oct; 32(5):802–808.
16. Zickler P. Evidence builds that genes influence cigarette smoking. *NIDA Notes.* 2000; 15(3):1–15.
17. Sasyette MA, et al. A multi-dimensional analysis of cue-elicited craving in heavy smokers and tobacco chippers. *Addiction.* 2001; 96(10):1419–1432.
18. Hassmiller KM, et al. Nondaily smokers: Who are they? *Am J Public Health.* 2003 Aug; 93(8):1321–1327.
19. Sullivan PF, Kendler KS. The genetic epidemiology of smoking. *Nicotine Tob Res, Suppl.* 2:51–57, 1999.
20. Sullivan PF, et al. Candidate genes for nicotine dependence via linkage, epistasis, bioinformatics. *Am J Med Genet B Neuropsychiatr Genet.* 2004. Apr 1; 126(1):23–36.
21. Pomerleau OF. Endogenous opioids and smoking: A review of progress and problems. *Psychoneuroendocrinology.* 1998 Feb; 23(2):115–130.
22. Balfour DJ, Ridkey DL. The effects of nicotine on neural pathways implicated in depression. *Pharmacol Biochem Behav.* 2000; 66(1):79–85.
23. DiFranza JR, et al. Development of symptoms of tobacco dependency in youth: 30-month follow-up from the DANDY study. *Tob Control.* 2002; 11(3):228–235.
24. Bricker JB, et al. Nine-year prospective relationship between parental smoking cessation and children's daily smoking. *Addiction.* 2003; 98(5):585–593.

25. Saladin KS. *Anatomy and Physiology: The Unit of Form and Function* (4th ed.). New York: McGraw-Hill, 2007.

26. American Cancer Society. *Cancer Facts and Figures—2005.* Atlanta: Cancer Society, 2005.

27. American Heart Association: *Heart Disease and Stroke Statistics*—2005 Update, 2004.

28. Lam S, et al. Sex-related differences in bronchial epithelial changes associated with tobacco smoking. *L Natl Cnacer Inst.* 91(8):691–696, April 1999.

29. DiFranza JR, Aligne CA, Weitzman M. Prenatal and postnatal environmental tobacco smoke exposure: children's health. *Pediatrics.* 2004 Apr; 113(4 Suppl): 1007–1015.

30. Habek D, et al. Fetal tobacco syndrome and perinatal outcome. *Fetal Diagn Ther.* 2002 November–December; 17(6):367–371.

31. Sepaniak S, et al. Negative impact of cigarette smoking on male fertility: From spermatozoa to the offspring. *J Obstet Biol Reprod.* 2004 Sept; 33(5):384–390.

32. Gades NM, et al. Association between smoking and erectile dysfunction: A population-based study. *AM J Epidemiol.* 2005 Feb 15; 16(4):341–351.

33. Maughan B, et al. Prenatal smoking and early childhood conduct problems: Testing genetic and environmental explanations of the association. *Arch Gen Psychiatr.* 2004 Aug; 61(8):836–843.

34. Enstrom JE, Kabat GC. Environmental tobacco smoke and tobacco-related mortality in a prospective study of Californians, 1990–1998. *BMJ.* 2003 May; 326(7398):1048–1057.

35. Smoke Free USA. March 2005. www.smokefreeworld.com/usa.sjtml.

personal assessment

How much do you know about cigarette smoking?

Are the following assumptions about smoking true or false?
Take your best guess, and then read the answer to the right
of each statement.

Assumption

1. There are now safe cigarettes on the market.

2. A small number of cigarettes can be smoked without risk.
3. Most early changes in the body resulting from cigarette smoking are temporary.
4. Filters provide a measure of safety to cigarette smokers.
5. Low-tar, low-nicotine cigarettes are safer than high-tar, high-nicotine brands.

6. Mentholated cigarettes are better for the smoker than are nonmentholated brands.

7. It has been scientifically proven that cigarette smoking causes cancer.
8. No specific agent capable of causing cancer has ever been identified in the tobacco used in smokeless tobacco.
9. The cure rate for lung cancer is so good that no one should fear developing this form of cancer.

10. Smoking is not harmful as long as the smoke is not inhaled.

11. The "smoker's cough" reflects underlying damage to the tissue of the airways.

12. Cigarette smoking does not appear to be associated with damage to the heart and blood vessels.
13. Because of the design of the placenta, smoking does not present a major risk to the developing fetus.

14. Women who smoke cigarettes and use an oral contraceptive should decide which they wish to continue, because there is a risk in using both.
15. Air pollution is a greater risk to our respiratory health than is cigarette smoking.

16. Addiction, in the sense of physical addiction, is found in conjunction with cigarette smoking.

Discussion

F Depending on the brand, some cigarettes contain less tar and nicotine; none are safe, however.
F Even a low level of smoking exposes the body to harmful substances in tobacco smoke.
T Some changes, however, cannot be reversed—particularly changes associated with emphysema.
T However, the protection is far from adequate.
T Many people, however, smoke low-tar, low-nicotine cigarettes in a manner that makes them just as dangerous as stronger cigarettes.
F Menthol simply makes cigarette smoke feel cooler. The smoke contains all the harmful agents found in the smoke from regular cigarettes.
T Particularly lung cancer and cancers of the larynx, esophagus, oral cavity, and urinary bladder.
F Unfortunately, smokeless tobacco is no safer than the tobacco that is burned. The user of smokeless tobacco swallows much of what the smoker inhales.
F Approximately 15% of people who have lung cancer will live the 5 years required to meet the medical definition of "cured."
F Because of the toxic material in smoke, even its contact with the tissue of the oral cavity introduces a measure of risk in this form of cigarette use.
T The cough occurs in response to an inability to clear the airway of mucus as a result of changes in the cells that normally keep the air passages clear.
F Cigarette smoking is in fact the single most important risk factor in the development of cardiovascular disease.
F Children born to women who smoked during pregnancy show a variety of health impairments, including smaller birth size, premature birth, and more illnesses during the first year of life. Smoking women also have more stillbirths than do nonsmokers.
T Women over 35 years of age, in particular, are at risk of experiencing serious heart disease should they continue using both cigarettes and an oral contraceptive.
F Although air pollution does expose the body to potentially serious problems, the risk is considerably less than that associated with smoking.
T Dependence, including true physical addiction, is widely recognized in cigarette smokers.

chapter ten

Reducing Your Risk of Cardiovascular Disease

Chapter Objectives

On completing this chapter, you will be able to:

- describe the prevalence of cardiovascular disease compared to other diseases.
- list the cardiovascular disease risk factors and distinguish between those that can and cannot be modified.
- explain how each of the modifiable cardiovascular disease risk factors can be changed.
- explain the signs of a heart attack and the recommended action that should be taken.
- explain how coronary heart disease is diagnosed and treated.
- explain the recommendations for prevention and treatment of hypertension.
- distinguish between the different types of stroke.

Eye on the Media

The Pressure Is Building

A recent *Time* magazine cover story, "The Stealth Killer," discussed the growing problem of hypertension in the United States. Current estimates suggest that 65,000,000 Americans have this condition, and the rates are projected to keep increasing. One of the issues discussed in the article was the concept that hypertension is a "silent" process. In other words, people cannot feel high blood pressure; rather, it has to be measured to be detected. One of the principal reasons for the projected increased prevalence of hypertension is that obesity is strongly related to hypertension. Obesity rates have reached epidemic proportions in our country, including increased levels in children. One of the most alarming aspects of this is that children are now being diagnosed with type 2 diabetes and hypertension, which typically was first observed in adults aged 40 years and older. The long-term consequences of hypertension—both financial and health-related—will be tremendously magnified if hypertension occurs 20 years earlier than usual.

Source: "Blowing a Gasket," *Time,* December 6, 2004. Volume 164, Number 23.

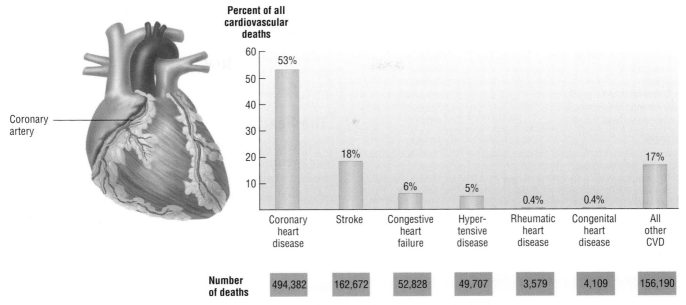

Percent of all cardiovascular deaths

	Coronary heart disease	Stroke	Congestive heart failure	Hypertensive disease	Rheumatic heart disease	Congenital heart disease	All other CVD
Percent	53%	18%	6%	5%	0.4%	0.4%	17%
Number of deaths	494,382	162,672	52,828	49,707	3,579	4,109	156,190

Figure 10-1 Of the 923,467 deaths in the United States in 2002* resulting from cardiovascular diseases, half were attributable to heart attack.[2]

(*The most recent year for which statistics are available.)

If you're a traditional-age college student, you may find it difficult to understand the importance of **cardiovascular** health. Unless you were born with a heart problem, you may think that cardiovascular damage will not occur until you reach your 50s or 60s. During your young adult years, you're much more likely to be concerned about cancer and sexually transmitted diseases.

Yet autopsy reports on teenagers and young adults who have died in accidents are now showing that relatively high percentages of young people have developed changes consistent with coronary artery disease; that is, fatty deposits have already formed in their coronary arteries. (See Learning from Our Diversity on page 251.) Since the foundation for future heart problems starts early in life, cardiovascular health is a very important topic for all college students.

Heart disease continues to be the number one killer of Americans; between 1990 and 2000 the death rates from cardiovascular disease (CVD) declined 17 percent.[2] The American Heart Association, in its 2004 *Heart and Stroke Statistical Update,* credits this reduction to a combination of changing American lifestyles and medical advances in the diagnosis and treatment of CVD.[2]

This chapter explains how the heart works. It also will help you identify your CVD risk factors and suggest ways you can alter certain lifestyle behaviors to reduce your risk of developing heart disease.

Prevalence of Cardiovascular Disease

Cardiovascular diseases were directly related to 38 percent of deaths in the United States in 2002 and indirectly related to a large percentage of additional deaths.[2] Heart disease, stroke, and related blood vessel disorders combined to kill nearly 1 million Americans in 2002 (Figure 10-1).[2] This figure represents more deaths than were caused by cancer, accidents, pneumonia, influenza, lung diseases, diabetes, and AIDS combined. CVD causes one out of every 2.6 deaths in the United States.[2] Indeed, cardiovascular disease is our nation's number one "killer" (see Table 10.1).

Key Terms

cardiovascular pertaining to the heart (cardio) and blood vessels (vascular)

Table 10.1 Estimated Prevalence of Major Cardiovascular Diseases*

Coronary heart disease	13,000,000
Hypertension	65,000,000
Stroke	5,400,000
Congenital heart disease	1,000,000
Rheumatic heart disease	1,800,000
Congestive heart failure	4,900,000
TOTAL[†]	91,100,000

*70,100,000 people total.

[†]The sum of the individual estimates exceeds 70,100,000 because many people have more than one cardiovascular disorder. For example, many people with coronary heart disease also have hypertension.

Normal Cardiovascular Function

The cardiovascular or circulatory system uses a muscular pump to send a complex fluid on a continuous trip through a closed system of tubes. The pump is the heart, the fluid is blood, and the closed system of tubes is the network of blood vessels.

The Vascular System

The term *vascular system* refers to the body's blood vessels. Although we might be familiar with the arteries (vessels that carry blood away from the heart) and the veins (vessels that carry blood toward the heart), arterioles, capillaries, and venules are also included in the vascular system. Arterioles are the farther, small-diameter extensions of arteries. These arterioles lead eventually to capillaries, the smallest extensions of the vascular system. At the capillary level, exchanges of oxygen, food, and waste occur between cells and the blood.

Once the blood leaves the capillaries and begins its return to the heart, it drains into small veins, or venules. The blood in the venules flows into increasingly larger vessels called *veins.* Blood pressure is highest in arteries and lowest in veins, especially the largest veins, which empty into the right atrium of the heart.

The Heart

The heart is a four-chambered pump designed to create the pressure required to circulate blood throughout the body. Usually considered to be about the size of a person's clenched fist, this organ lies slightly tilted between the lungs in the central portion of the **thorax.** The heart does not lie completely in the center of the chest. Approximately two-thirds of the heart is to the left of the body midline, and one third is to the right.

Two upper chambers, called *atria,* and two lower chambers, called *ventricles,* form the heart.[3] The thin-walled atrial chambers are considered collecting chambers, and the thick-walled muscular ventricles are considered the pumping chambers. The right and left sides of the heart are divided by a partition called the *septum.* Use Figure 10-2 to follow the flow of blood through the heart's four chambers.

For the heart muscle to function well, it must be supplied with adequate amounts of oxygen. The two main **coronary arteries** (and their numerous branches)

> **Key Terms**
>
> **thorax** the chest; portion of the torso above the diaphragm and within the rib cage
>
> **coronary arteries** vessels that supply oxygenated blood to heart muscle tissues

Regular exercise helps strengthen the heart muscle and increase HDL cholesterol.

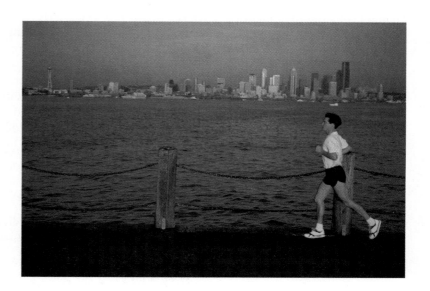

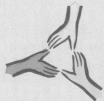

Learning from Our Diversity

Prevention of Heart Disease Begins in Childhood

Youth is one aspect of diversity that is sometimes overlooked. Yet age is important, especially when adults have influence over children's health behavior. Many adults never seriously consider that their health behaviors are imitated by the children around them. When adults care little about their own health, they can also be contributing to serious health consequences in young people. Nowhere is this age diversity issue more pronounced than in the area of cardiovascular health.

For many aspects of wellness, preventive behaviors are often best learned in childhood, when they can be repeated and reinforced by family members and caregivers. This is especially true for preventive actions concerning heart disease. Although many problems related to heart disease appear at midlife and later, the roots of heart disease start early in life.

The most serious childhood health behaviors associated with heart disease are poor dietary practices, lack of physical activity, and cigarette smoking. Unfortunately, the current state of health for America's youth shows severe deficiencies in all three areas. Children's diets lack nutrient density and remain far too high in overall fat. Teenage children are becoming increasingly overweight and obese. Studies consistently show a decline in the amount of physical activity by today's youth, since television and video games have become the after-school companions for many children. In addition, cigarette smoking continues to rise among schoolchildren, especially teenagers.

These unhealthy behaviors are laying the foundation for coronary artery disease, hypertension, stroke, and other diseases in the future. The focus should be on health measures in childhood that prevent cardiovascular problems rather than treatment of older, already affected people. Parents must make efforts to encourage children to eat more nutritiously and be physically active. Adults should discourage cigarette use by young people. Perhaps the best approach for adults is to set a good example by adopting heart-healthy behaviors themselves. Following the Food Guide Pyramid (page 143) and exercising regularly are excellent strategies that can be started early in life.

---

accomplish this. These arteries are located outside the heart (see Figure 10-1). If the coronary arteries are diseased, a heart attack (myocardial infarction) is possible.

Heart Stimulation

The heart contracts and relaxes through the delicate interplay of **cardiac muscle** tissue and cardiac electrical centers called *nodes*. Nodal tissue generates the electrical impulses necessary to contract heart muscle.[4] The heart's electrical activity is measured by an instrument called an *electrocardiograph* (ECG or EKG), which provides a print-out called an electrocardiogram, which can be evaluated to determine cardiac electrical functioning.

> **Key Terms**
>
> **cardiac muscle** specialized muscle tissue that forms the middle (muscular) layer of the heart wall

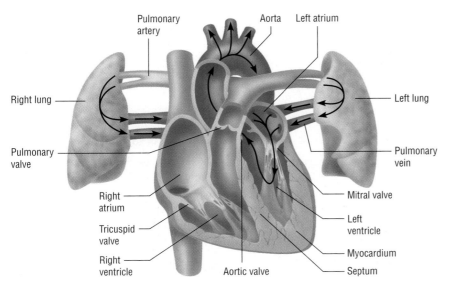

Figure 10-2 The heart functions like a complex double pump. The right side of the heart pumps deoxygenated blood to the lungs. The left side of the heart pumps oxygenated blood through the aorta to all parts of the body. Note the thickness of the walls of the ventricles. These are the primary pumping chambers.

Blood

The average-sized adult has approximately 5 quarts of blood in his or her circulatory system. The functions of blood, which are performed continuously, are similar to the overall functions of the circulatory system and include the following:

- Transportation of nutrients, oxygen, wastes, hormones, and enzymes
- Regulation of water content of body cells and fluids
- Buffering to help maintain appropriate pH balance of body fluids
- Regulation of body temperature; the water component in the blood absorbs heat and transfers it
- Prevention of blood loss; by coagulating or clotting, the blood can alter its form to prevent blood loss through injured vessels
- Protection against toxins and microorganisms, accomplished by chemical substances called *antibodies* and specialized cellular elements circulating in the bloodstream

Cardiovascular Disease Risk Factors

As you have just read, the heart and blood vessels are among the most important structures in the human body. By protecting your cardiovascular system, you lay the groundwork for an exciting, productive, and energetic life. The best time to start protecting and improving your cardiovascular system is early in life, when lifestyle patterns are developed and reinforced. (See Learning from Our Diversity, page 251.) Of course, it's difficult to move backward through time, so the second best time to start protecting your heart is today. Improvements in certain lifestyle activities can pay significant dividends as your life unfolds. (Complete the Personal Assessment on page 267 to determine your risk for heart disease.)

The American Heart Association encourages people to protect and enhance their heart health by examining the ten cardiovascular risk factors related to various forms of heart disease.[5] A *cardiovascular risk factor* is an attribute that a person has or is exposed to that increases the likelihood that he or she will develop some form of heart disease. The first three risk factors are ones you will be unable to change. An additional six risk factors are ones you can change. One final risk factor is one that is thought to be a contributing factor to heart disease.

Risk Factors That Cannot Be Changed

The three risk factors that you cannot change are increasing age, male gender, and heredity.[5] However, your knowledge that they might be an influence in your life should encourage you to make a more serious commitment to the risk factors you can change.

Increasing Age

Heart diseases tend to develop gradually over the course of one's life. Although we may know of a few people who experienced a heart attack in their 20s or 30s, most of the serious consequences of heart disease are evident in older ages. For example, approximately 84 percent of people who die from heart diseases are age 65 and older.[2]

Male Gender

Before age 55, women have lower rates of heart disease than men do. Yet when women move through menopause (typically in their 50s), their rates of heart disease are similar to those of men (see the Star box on page 253). It is thought that women are somewhat more protected from heart disease than men because of their natural production of the hormone estrogen during their fertile years.

Heredity

Like increasing age and male gender, heredity cannot be changed. By the luck of the draw, some people are born into families in which heart disease has never been a serious problem; others are born into families in which heart disease is quite prevalent. In this latter case, children are said to have a genetic predisposition (tendency) to develop heart disease as they grow and develop throughout their lives. These people have every reason to be highly motivated to reduce the risk factors they can control.

Race is also a consideration related to heart disease. African Americans have moderately high blood pressure at rates twice that of whites and severe hypertension at rates three times higher than whites. Hypertension significantly increases the risk of both heart disease and stroke; however, it can be controlled through a variety of methods. It is especially important for African Americans to take advantage of every opportunity to have their blood pressure measured so that preventive actions can be started immediately if necessary.

Risk Factors That Can Be Changed

Six cardiovascular risk factors are influenced largely by our lifestyle choices. These risk factors are cigarette and tobacco smoke, physical inactivity, high blood cholesterol level, high blood pressure, diabetes mellitus, and obesity and overweight.[4] Healthful behavior changes you make for these "big six" risk factors can help you protect and enhance your cardiovascular system.

Women and Heart Disease

Is heart disease mainly a problem for men? According to the American Heart Association, the answer is a resounding NO. In fact, data indicate that 53 percent of all cardiovascular disease deaths occur in women. Cardiovascular disease is the leading cause of death for American women and kills nearly twice as many women as do all forms of cancer combined. Presently, one in five women has some sort of heart or blood vessel disease. Over 60 percent of stroke deaths occur in women. Also 38 percent of women who have heart attacks will die within a year, compared with 25 percent of men. From age 55, higher percentages of women than men have high blood pressure.[1]

For many years, it was thought that men were at much greater risk than women were for the development of cardiovascular problems. Today it is known that young men are more prone to heart disease than young women are, but once women reach menopause (usually in their early to middle 50s), their rates of heart-related problems quickly equal those of men.

The protective mechanism for young women seems to be the female hormone estrogen. Estrogen appears to help women maintain a beneficial profile of blood fats. When the production of estrogen is severely reduced at menopause, this protective factor no longer exists. Prescribing postmenopausal hormone replacement therapy (PHT) was a common practice by many physicians in treating a number of factors in postmenopausal women. One of the benefits of PHT was considered to be prevention of cardiovascular diseases. However, in 2002 a major clinical research trial was stopped owing to the finding that more women on PHT were experiencing heart attacks and strokes. Thus, the American Heart Association now recommends that PHT should not be used for the purpose of preventing cardiovascular diseases. Certainly, PHT may still be utilized for other purposes (i.e., relief of menopausal symptoms or osteoporosis prevention).[2] Women who are prescribed PHT need to be aware of the increased risk for cardiovascular disease in evaluating its value. Certainly, much more research is underway that may influence the use of PHT in the future. Women should discuss the risks and benefits of PHT with their physicians.

Young women should not rely solely on naturally produced estrogen to prevent heart disease. The general recommendations for maintaining heart health—good diet, adequate physical activity, monitoring blood pressure and cholesterol levels, controlling weight, avoiding smoking, and managing stress—will benefit women at every stage of life.

[1]American Heart Association: www.americanheart.org/Heart and Stroke_A_Z_Guide/womens/, September 1, 2001.
[2]American Heart Association: www.americanheart.org/presenter.jhtml?identifier=4536, July 21, 2003.

Tobacco Smoke

Smokers have a heart attack risk that is 2–4 times that of nonsmokers. Smoking cigarettes is the major risk factor associated with sudden cardiac death. In fact, smokers have two to four times the risk of dying from sudden cardiac arrest than nonsmokers do.

Cigarette or tobacco smoke also adversely affects nonsmokers who are exposed to environmental tobacco smoke. Studies suggest that the risk of death caused by heart disease is increased about 30 percent in people exposed to secondhand smoke in the home. Because of the health threat to nonsmokers, restrictions on indoor smoking in public areas and business settings are increasing tremendously in every part of the country.

For years, it was believed that if you had smoked for many years, it was pointless to try to quit; the damage to one's health could never be reversed. However, the American Heart Association now indicates that by quitting smoking, regardless of how long or how much you have smoked, your risk of heart disease declines rapidly. For people who have smoked a pack or less of cigarettes per day, within 3 years after quitting smoking, their heart disease risk is virtually the same as those who never smoked.

This news is exciting and should encourage people to quit smoking, regardless of how long they have smoked.

Of course, if you have started to smoke recently, the healthy approach would be to quit now—before the nicotine controls your life and leads to heart disease or damages your lungs or causes lung cancer. (For additional information about the health effects of tobacco, see Chapter 9.)

 TALKING POINTS A friend complains of not being able to quit smoking after several serious attempts. How could you direct this person toward a new approach?

Physical Inactivity

Lack of regular physical activity is a significant risk factor for heart disease. Regular aerobic exercise (discussed in Chapter 4) helps strengthen the heart muscle, maintain healthy blood vessels, and improve the ability of the vascular system to transfer blood and oxygen to all parts of the body. Additionally, physical activity helps lower overall blood cholesterol levels for most people, encourages weight loss and retention of lean muscle mass, and allows people to moderate the stress in their lives.

With all the benefits of physical activity, it amazes health professionals that so many Americans refuse to become regularly active. Some people feel that they don't have enough time or that they must work out strenuously. However, you'll recall from Chapter 4 that only 20 to 60 minutes of moderate aerobic activity three to five times each week can decrease your risk of heart disease. This is not a large price to pay for a lifetime of cardiovascular health. Find a partner and get started! (Discovering Your Spirituality on page 255 discusses how the benefits of physical activity extend into the spiritual dimension of your life.)

If you are middle-aged or older and have been inactive, consult with a physician before starting an exercise program. Also, if you have any known health condition that could be aggravated by physical activity, check with a physician first.

 TALKING POINTS You've started exercising many times by yourself, but you can't seem to stick to it. How would you convince a new friend that you can help each other get started on regular physical activity and keep it up?

High Blood Cholesterol Level

The third controllable risk factor for heart disease is high blood cholesterol level. Generally speaking, the higher the blood cholesterol level, the greater the risk for heart disease. When high blood cholesterol levels are combined with other important risk factors, the risks become much greater.

Fortunately, blood cholesterol levels are relatively easy to measure. Many campus health, fitness, and wellness centers provide cholesterol screenings for employees and students. These screenings help identify people whose cholesterol levels (or profiles) may be potentially dangerous. Medical professionals have been able to determine the link between a person's diet and his or her cholesterol levels. People with high blood cholesterol levels are encouraged to consume a heart-healthy diet (see Chapter 5) and to become physically active. In recent years a variety of cholesterol-lowering drugs have also been developed that are very effective. Cholesterol will be discussed further later in this chapter.

High Blood Pressure

The fourth of the "big six" cardiovascular risk factors is high blood pressure, or *hypertension*. You will soon be reading more about hypertension, but for now, suffice it to say that high blood pressure can seriously damage a person's heart and blood vessels. High blood pressure causes the heart to work much harder, eventually causing the heart to enlarge and weaken. It increases the chances for stroke, heart attack, congestive heart failure, and kidney disease.

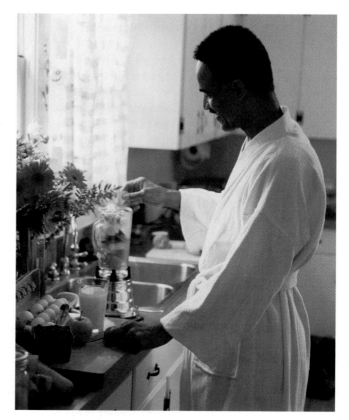

People who have high cholesterol should follow a heart-healthy diet based on the Food Guide Pyramid (see Chapter 5).

When high blood pressure is present along with other risk factors, the risk for stroke or heart attack is increased tremendously. Yet this "silent killer" is easy to monitor and can be effectively controlled using a variety of approaches. This is the positive message about high blood pressure.

Diabetes Mellitus

Diabetes mellitus (discussed in detail on page 292) is a debilitating chronic disease that has a significant effect on the human body. In addition to increasing the risk of developing kidney disease, blindness, and nerve damage, diabetes increases the likelihood of developing heart and blood vessel diseases. Over 65 percent of people with diabetes die of some type of heart or blood vessel disease. The cardiovascular damage is thought to occur because of the abnormal levels of cholesterol and blood fat found in individuals with diabetes. With weight management, exercise, dietary changes, and drug therapy, diabetes can be relatively well controlled in most people. Even with careful management of this disease, diabetic patients are susceptible to eventual heart and blood vessel damage.

Yoga: Creating Peaceful Time

In a typical college day that includes academic, social, and financial pressures, you can lose the sense of who you really are. Do you ever find yourself wondering why you're making certain choices and what's really important to you? Meditative practices such as yoga offer you the chance to slow down and recapture a sense of yourself.

The word *yoga* comes from a Sanskrit root meaning "union" or "joining," referring to the integration of body, mind, and spirit. Yoga has evolved from ancient beginnings in the Himalayan mountains of India. Accounts of its origin differ, and some suggest that it reaches back 6,000 years. Yoga is practiced by people of all social, economic, and religious backgrounds. Many past yoga masters have been Hindus, but there is no need to embrace or even understand Hinduism if you want to practice yoga.

Yoga is a structured physical and mental discipline, designed to ease tension, improve concentration, and increase mental clarity. Like other meditative disciplines, it emphasizes the benefits of consistent, daily practice. A typical workout, as recommended by the American Yoga Association, lasts 20 minutes: two minutes of breathing exercises, two minutes of warming up, eight minutes of stretching, and eight minutes of meditation. After working out, you can expect to feel relaxed and energized, rather than exhausted.

Each exercise, called an *asan* or *ansana,* has specific effects. The "diamond pose," for example, limbers the lower back, hips, and groin muscles. Specialized workouts—to address pregnancy, sports, weight-loss programs, and other needs—can be created by including carefully selected exercises.

Yoga requires no special equipment and can be practiced in a small space such as a bedroom. Instructors in the United States have worked to make yoga accessible to the American lifestyle by developing special routines that can be pursued during travel, business, or the academic day. Classes are frequently offered on college campuses or in community centers, but any large bookstore stocks books that offer guidance to the beginner who wants to practice alone.

You'll find that most yoga practices offer ethical advice to help you reduce mental and emotional disturbances. Principles include nonviolence, truthfulness, and tolerance, but, again, you don't need to embrace these principles to practice yoga.

Clinical research has not conclusively demonstrated yoga's health benefits, but anecdotal evidence strongly suggests that disciplined practice can offer insight into the self and improve balance in your life.

 TALKING POINTS How would you show support for a friend who is struggling with the dietary requirements of diabetes?

Obesity and Overweight

Even if they have no other risk factors, obese people are more likely than nonobese people to develop heart disease and stroke. Obesity, particularly if located primarily around the abdomen, places considerable strain on the heart, and it tends to influence both blood pressure and blood cholesterol levels. Also, obesity tends to trigger diabetes in predisposed people. The importance of maintaining body weight within a desirable range minimizes the chance of obesity ever happening. To accomplish this, maintain an active lifestyle and follow the dietary guidelines in Chapter 5.

 TALKING POINTS How could you tactfully bring up a friend's weight problem to show concern for his or her health?

Contributing Risk Factors

The American Heart Association identifies other risk factors that may contribute to CVD. These include *individual response to stress, sex hormones, birth control pills,* and *drinking too much alcohol.* Unresolved stress can encourage negative health dependencies (for example, smoking, poor dietary practices, underactivity) that lead to changes in blood fat profiles, blood pressure, and heart workload. Female sex hormones tend to protect women from CVD until they reach menopause, but male hormones do the opposite. Birth control pills (see Chapter 14) can increase the risk of blood clots and heart attack, although the risk is small unless the woman also smokes and is over age 35. The consumption of too much alcohol can cause elevated blood pressure, heart failure, and lead to stroke, although moderate drinking (no more than one drink per day for women and two drinks per day for men) is associated with lower risk of heart disease.[2]

Forms of Cardiovascular Disease

The American Heart Association describes the six major forms of CVD as coronary heart disease, hypertension, stroke, congenital heart disease, rheumatic heart disease, and congestive heart failure. A person may have just one of these diseases or a combination of them at the same time. Each form exists in varying degrees of severity. All are capable of causing secondary damage to other body organs and systems.

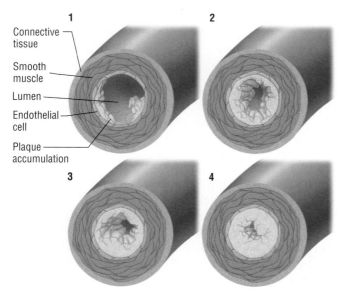

Figure 10-3 Progression of atherosclerosis. This diagram shows how plaque deposits gradually accumulate to narrow the lumen (interior space) of an artery. Although enlarged here, coronary arteries are only as wide as a pencil lead.

Labels on figure:
1
2
Connective tissue
Smooth muscle
Lumen
Endothelial cell
Plaque accumulation
3
4

Coronary Heart Disease

This form of CVD, also known as *coronary artery disease,* involves damage to the vessels that supply blood to the heart muscle. The bulk of this blood is supplied by the coronary arteries. Any damage to these important vessels can cause a reduction of blood (and its vital oxygen and nutrients) to specific areas of heart muscle. The ultimate result of inadequate blood supply is a heart attack.

Atherosclerosis

The principal cause for the development of coronary heart disease is atherosclerosis (Figure 10-3). **Atherosclerosis** produces a narrowing of the coronary arteries. This narrowing stems from the long-term buildup of fatty deposits, called *plaque,* on the inner walls of the arteries. This buildup reduces the blood supply to specific portions of the heart. Some arteries of the heart can become so blocked (occluded) that all blood supply is stopped. Heart muscle tissue begins to die when it is deprived of oxygen and nutrients. This damage is known as **myocardial infarction.** In lay terms, this event is called a *heart attack.* (Changing for the Better on page 257 explains how to recognize the signs of a heart attack and what to do next.)

Cholesterol and Lipoproteins For many years, scientists have known that atherosclerosis is a complicated disease that has many causes. Some of these causes are not well understood, but others are clearly understood. *Cholesterol,* a soft, fatlike material, is manufactured in the liver and small intestine and is necessary in the formation of sex hormones, cell membranes, bile salts, and nerve fibers. Elevated levels of serum cholesterol (200 mg/dl or more for adults age 20 and older, and 170 mg/dl or more for young people below age 20) are associated with an increased risk for developing atherosclerosis.[2]

About half of American adults age 20 and older exceed the "borderline high" 200 mg/dl cholesterol level. It is estimated that nearly 40 percent of American youth age 19 and below have "borderline high" cholesterol levels of 170 mg/dl and above. About one out of five American adults has a "high" blood cholesterol level, that is, 240 mg/dl or greater.

Initially, most people can help lower their serum cholesterol level by adopting three dietary changes: lowering their intake of saturated fats, lowering their intake of dietary cholesterol, and lowering their caloric intake to a level that does not exceed body requirements. The aim is to reduce excess fat, cholesterol, and calories in the diet while promoting sound nutrition. By carefully following such a diet plan, people with high serum cholesterol levels may be able to reduce their cholesterol levels by 30 to 55 mg/dl. However, dietary changes do not affect people equally; some will experience greater reductions than others. Some will not respond at all to dietary changes and may need to take cholesterol-lowering medications and increase their physical activity.

Cholesterol is attached to structures called lipoproteins. Lipoproteins are particles that circulate in the blood and transport lipids (including cholesterol).[5] Two major classes of lipoproteins exist: **low-density lipoproteins (LDLs)** and **high-density lipoproteins (HDLs).** A person's total cholesterol level is chiefly determined by the amount of the LDLs and HDLs in a measured sample of blood. For example, a person's total cholesterol level of 200 mg/dl could be represented by an LDL level of 130

Key Terms

atherosclerosis buildup of plaque on the inner walls of arteries

myocardial infarction heart attack; the death of part of the heart muscle as a result of a blockage in one of the coronary arteries

low-density lipoprotein (LDL) the type of lipoprotein that transports the largest amount of cholesterol in the bloodstream; high levels of LDL are related to heart disease

high-density lipoprotein (HDL) the type of lipoprotein that transports cholesterol from the bloodstream to the liver, where it is eventually removed from the body; high levels of HDL are related to a reduction in heart disease

and an HDL level of 40, or an LDL level of 120 and an HDL level of 60. (Note that other lipoproteins do exist and carry some of the cholesterol in the blood.)

After much scientific study, it has been determined that high levels of LDL are a significant promoter of atherosclerosis. This makes sense because LDLs carry the greatest percentage of cholesterol in the bloodstream. LDLs are more likely to deposit excess cholesterol into the artery walls. This contributes to plaque formation. For this reason, LDLs are often called the "bad cholesterol." High LDL levels are determined partially by inheritance, but they are also clearly associated with smoking, poor dietary patterns, obesity, and lack of exercise.

In contrast, high levels of HDLs are related to a decrease in the development of atherosclerosis. HDLs are thought to transport cholesterol out of the bloodstream. Thus HDLs have been called the "good cholesterol." Certain lifestyle alterations, such as quitting smoking, reducing obesity, increasing physical activity, and replacing saturated fats with monosaturated fats, help many people increase their level of HDLs.

Reducing total serum cholesterol levels is a significant step in reducing the risk of death from coronary heart disease. For people with elevated cholesterol levels, a 1 percent reduction in serum cholesterol level yields about a 2 percent reduction in the risk of death from heart disease. Thus a 10–15 percent cholesterol reduction can reduce risk by 20–30 percent.[6] See Table 10.2 for LDL classifications and current recommended follow-up and Table 10.3 for additional classifications.

Angina Pectoris When coronary arteries become narrowed, chest pain, or *angina pectoris,* is often felt. This

Table 10.2 Classification and Recommended Follow-up Based on LDL Cholesterol Level

LDL Cholesterol Level	Classification	Initiate Therapeutic Lifestyle Changes (TLC)
<100	Optimal	—
100–129	Near optimal/ Above optimal	If CHD or diabetes is present
130–159	Borderline high	If you have 2 or more risk factors
160–189	High	Yes, and see physician
≥190	Very high	Yes, and see physician

Note: The National Cholesterol Education Program (NCEP) now recommends that all adults have their LDL cholesterol measured. See http://nhlbi.nih.gov/about/ncep/index.htm.

Table 10.3 Classification of Total Cholesterol, Triglycerides, and HDL Cholesterol. All values expressed in mg/dL.

	Normal or Desirable	Borderline-High	High
Total cholesterol	< 200	200–239	≥ 240
Triglycerides	< 150	150–199	≥ 200
	Low	**Normal**	**High**
HDL cholesterol	< 40	40–59	≥ 60

pain results from a reduced supply of oxygen to heart muscle tissue. Usually, angina is felt when the coronary artery disease patient becomes stressed or exercises too strenuously. Angina reportedly can range from a feeling of mild indigestion to a severe viselike pressure in the chest. The pain may extend from the center of the chest to the arms and even up to the jaw. Generally, the more severe the blockage, the more pain is felt.

Some cardiac patients relieve angina with the drug *nitroglycerin,* a powerful blood vessel dilator. This prescription drug, available in slow-release transdermal (through the skin) patches or small pills that are placed under the patient's tongue, causes a major reduction in the workload of the heart muscle. Other cardiac patients may be prescribed drugs such as **calcium channel blockers** or **beta blockers.**

Arrhythmias Arrhythmias are disorders of the heart's normal sequence of electrical activity that are experienced by more than 2 million Americans. They result in an irregular beating pattern of the heart. Arrhythmias can be so brief that they do not affect the overall heart rate. Some arrhythmias, however, can last for long periods of time and cause the heart to beat either too slowly or too fast. A slow beating pattern is called *bradycardia* (fewer than 60 beats per minute), and a fast beating pattern is called *tachycardia* (more than 100 beats per minute).

Hearts that beat too slowly may be unable to pump a sufficient amount of blood throughout the body. The body becomes starved of oxygen, and loss of consciousness and even death can occur. Hearts that beat too rapidly do not allow the ventricles to fill sufficiently. When this happens, the heart cannot pump enough blood throughout the body. The heart becomes, in effect, a very inefficient machine. It beats rapidly but cannot pump much blood from its ventricles. This pattern may lead to fibrillation, which is the life-threatening, rapid uncoordinated contraction of the heart. Interestingly, whether the heart pumps too slowly or too rapidly, the result is the same: inadequate blood flow throughout the body.

The person most prone to arrhythmia is a person with some form of heart disease, including atherosclerosis, hypertension, or inflammatory or degenerative conditions. The prevalence of arrhythmia tends to increase with age. Certain congenital defects may make a person more likely to have an arrhythmia. Some chemical agents, including high or low levels of minerals (potassium, magnesium, and calcium) in the blood, addictive substances (caffeine, tobacco, other drugs), and various cardiac medications, can all provoke arrhythmias.

Arrhythmias are most frequently diagnosed through an ECG (electrocardiogram), which records electrical activity of the heart. After diagnosis, a range of therapeutic approaches can be used, including simple monitoring (if the problem is relatively minor), drug therapy, use of a pacemaker, or the use of implantable defibrillators.

Emergency Response to Heart Crises

Heart attacks need not be fatal. The consequences of any heart attack depend on the location of the damage to the heart, the extent to which heart muscle is damaged, and the speed with which adequate circulation is restored. Injury to the ventricles may very well prove fatal unless medical countermeasures are immediately undertaken. The recognition of a heart attack is critically important. (See Changing for the Better on page 257.)

Cardiopulmonary resuscitation (CPR) is one of the most important immediate countermeasures that trained people can use when confronted with a victim of heart attack. Programs sponsored by the American Red Cross and the American Heart Association teach people how to recognize, evaluate, and manage heart attack emergencies. CPR trainees are taught how to restore breathing and circulation in persons requiring emergency care. Frequently, colleges offer CPR training through courses in various departments. With revised CPR procedures in place in 2001, we encourage students to take a course and become certified. Additionally, members of the public are encouraged to obtain training in the use of automated external defibrillators (AED). These devices are now found in most public buildings and can markedly improve the chances of resuscitating a victim.

Key Terms

calcium channel blockers drugs that prevent arterial spasms; used in the control of blood pressure and the long-term management of angina pectoris

beta blockers drugs that prevent overactivity of the heart, which decreases occurrence of angina pectoris and helps control blood pressure

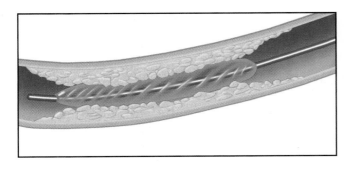

A

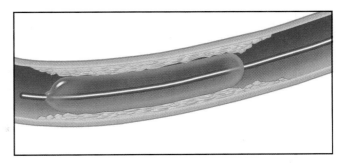

B

Figure 10-4   Angioplasty. A: A "balloon" is surgically inserted into the narrowed coronary artery.
B: The balloon is inflated, compressing plaque and fatty deposits against the artery walls.

Diagnosis and Coronary Repair

Once a person's vital signs have stabilized, further diagnostic examinations can reveal the type and extent of damage to heart muscle. Initially an ECG might be taken, which may be able to identify if areas of ischemia (insufficient blood flow) or damage has occurred to the heart muscle. Another test which may be used is echocardiography. This procedure can also detect ischemia. The diagnostic ability of both of these tests is improved if used in conjunction with exercise (that is, stress ECG or stress echocardiography). This test analyzes the electrical activity of the heart. *Heart catheterization,* also called *coronary arteriography,* is a minor surgical procedure that starts with placement of a thin plastic tube into an arm or leg artery. This tube, called a *catheter,* is guided through the artery until it reaches the coronary circulation, where a *radiopaque dye* is then released. X-ray films called *angiograms* record the progress of the dye through the coronary arteries so that areas of blockage can be easily identified.

Once the extent of damage is identified, a physician or team of physicians can decide on a medical course of action. Currently popular is an extensive form of surgery called **coronary artery bypass surgery.** An estimated 515,000 patients had bypass surgeries in 2002.[2] The purpose of such surgery is to detour (bypass) areas of coronary artery obstruction by usually using a section of an artery from the patient's chest (the internal mammary artery) and grafting it from the aorta to a location just beyond the area of obstruction. Multiple areas of obstruction result in double, triple, or quadruple bypasses.

Angioplasty   An alternative to bypass surgery, *angioplasty* involves the surgical insertion of a doughnut-shaped "balloon" directly into the narrowed coronary artery (Figure 10-4). When the balloon is inflated, plaque and fatty deposits are compressed against the artery walls, widening the space through which blood flows. The balloon usually remains in the artery for less than 1 minute.

Renarrowing of the artery will occur in about one quarter of angioplasty patients. Balloon angioplasty can be used for blockages in the heart, kidneys, arms, and legs. The decision whether to have angioplasty or bypass surgery can be a difficult one to make. Nearly 1,657,000 angioplasty procedures were performed in 2002.[2]

The FDA approved a device for clearing heart and leg arteries. This device is called a *motorized scraper.* Inserted through a leg artery and held in place by a tiny inflated balloon, this motor-driven cutter shaves off plaque deposits from inside the artery. A nose cone in the scraper unit stores the plaque until the device is removed.

The use of laser beams to dissolve plaque that blocks arteries has been slowly evolving. The FDA has approved three laser devices for use in clogged leg arteries. In 1992 the FDA approved the use of an excimer laser for use in coronary arteries.

Aspirin   Studies released a decade ago highlighted the role of aspirin in reducing the risk of heart attack in men with no history of previous attacks. Specifically, the studies concluded that for men with hypertension, elevated cholesterol levels, or both, taking one aspirin per day was a significant factor in reducing their risk of heart attack. Aspirin works by making the blood less able to clot. This reduces the likelihood of blood vessel blockages. Presently, opinions differ regarding the age at which this preventive action should begin. The safest advice is to check with your physician before starting aspirin therapy.

> **Key Terms**
>
> **coronary artery bypass surgery** surgical procedure designed to improve blood flow to the heart by providing new routes for blood to take around points of blockage

Recent research now indicates that aspirin therapy is also beneficial for women.[7]

Alcohol For years, scientists have been uncertain about the extent to which alcohol consumption is related to a reduced risk for heart disease. The current thinking is that moderate drinking (defined as no more than two drinks per day for men and one drink per day for women) is related to a lower heart disease risk. However, the benefit is much smaller than proven risk reduction behaviors such as stopping smoking, reducing cholesterol level, lowering blood pressure, and increasing physical activity. Experts caution that heavy drinking increases cardiovascular risks and that nondrinkers should not start to drink just to reduce heart disease risk.

Heart Transplants and Artificial Hearts For almost 40 years, surgeons have been able to surgically replace a person's damaged heart with that of another human being. Although very risky, these transplant operations have added years to the lives of a number of patients who otherwise would have lived only a short time. In 2002, 2,057 heart transplants were performed in the United States.[2]

Artificial hearts have also been developed and implanted in humans. These hearts have extended the lives of many patients, but they have kept them unpleasantly tethered with tubes and wires to large power source machines. However, a major medical breakthrough took place in July 2001, when the world's first self-contained artificial heart was successfully implanted into a 59-year-old patient.

Hypertension

Just as your car's water pump recirculates water and maintains water pressure, your heart recirculates blood and maintains blood pressure. When the heart contracts, blood is forced through your arteries and veins. Your blood pressure is a measure of the force that your circulating blood exerts against the interior walls of your arteries and veins.

Blood pressure is measured with a *sphygmomanometer*. This instrument is attached to an arm-cuff device that can be inflated to stop the flow of blood temporarily in the brachial artery. This artery is a major supplier of blood to the lower arm. It is located on the inside of the upper arm, between the biceps and triceps muscles.

A health professional using a stethoscope will listen for blood flow while the pressure in the cuff is released. Two pressure measurements will be recorded: the **systolic pressure** is the highest blood pressure against the vessel walls during the heart contraction, and the **diastolic pressure** is the lowest blood pressure against

the vessel walls when the heart relaxes (between heartbeats). Expressed in units of millimeters of mercury displaced on the sphygmomanometer, blood pressure is recorded as the systolic pressure over the diastolic pressure, for example, 115/82.

Although a blood pressure of less than 120/80 is considered "normal" for an adult, lower values do not necessarily indicate a medical problem. In fact, many young college women of average weight will indicate blood pressures that seem to be relatively low (100/60, for example), yet these lowered blood pressures are quite "normal" for them.

TALKING POINTS You're having a regular physical examination, and your doctor remarks that your blood pressure puts you in the category of "borderline hypertension." What questions would you ask about managing this condition?

Hypertension refers to a consistently elevated blood pressure. Generally, concern about blood pressure begins when a person has a systolic reading of 140 or above or a diastolic reading of 90 or above. People with prehypertension are advised to seek lifestyle measures to prevent any further elevation in their blood pressure. Approximately 65 million American adults and children have hypertension. The American Heart Association reports that African Americans, Hispanic Americans, and American Indians have higher rates of high blood pressure than white Americans.[2,5] In contrast, Asian/Pacific Islanders have significantly lower rates of hypertension.[2]

Although the causes of 90–95 percent of the cases of hypertension are not known, the health risks produced by uncontrolled hypertension are clearly understood. Throughout the body, long-term hypertension makes arteries and arterioles become less elastic and thus incapable of dilating under a heavy workload. Brittle, calcified blood vessels can burst unexpectedly and produce serious strokes (brain accidents), kidney failure (renal accidents), or eye damage **(retinal hemorrhage).** Furthermore, it

---

Key Terms

systolic pressure blood pressure against blood vessel walls when the heart contracts

diastolic pressure blood pressure against blood vessel walls when the heart relaxes

retinal hemorrhage uncontrolled bleeding from arteries within the eye's retina

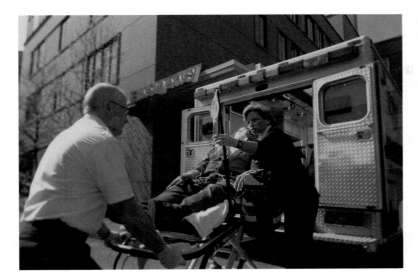

Emergency response teams help keep cardiac patients alive during transit to a medical facility.

appears that blood clots are more easily formed and dislodged in a vascular system affected by hypertension. Thus hypertension can be a cause of heart attacks. Clearly, hypertension is a potential killer.

Ironically, despite its deadly nature, hypertension is referred to as "the silent killer" because people with hypertension often are not aware that they have the condition. They cannot feel the sensation of high blood pressure. The condition does not produce dizziness, headaches, or memory loss unless one is experiencing a medical crisis. It is estimated that approximately 30 percent of the people who have hypertension do not realize they have it.[8] Many who are aware of their hypertension do little to control it. Only a small percentage (34 percent) of people who have hypertension control it adequately, generally through dietary control, regular exercise, relaxation training, and drug therapy.

Hypertension is not thought of as a curable disease; rather, it is a controllable disease. Once therapy is stopped, the condition returns. As a responsible adult, use every opportunity you can to measure your blood pressure on a regular basis.

Prevention and Treatment

Weight reduction, physical activity, moderation in alcohol use, and sodium restriction are often used to reduce hypertension. For overweight or obese people, a reduction in body weight may produce a significant drop in blood pressure. Physical activity helps lower blood pressure by expending calories (which may lead to weight loss in those who are overweight or obese) and through other physiological changes that affect the circulation. Moderation in alcohol consumption (no more than 1–2 drinks daily) helps reduce blood pressure in some people.

The restriction of sodium (salt) in the diet also helps some people reduce hypertension. Interestingly, this strategy is effective only for those who are **salt sensitive** — estimated to be about 25 percent of the population. Reducing salt intake would have little effect on the blood pressure of the rest of the population. Nevertheless, since our daily intake of salt vastly exceeds our need for salt, the general recommendation to curb salt intake still makes good sense.

Many of the stress reduction activities discussed in Chapter 3 are receiving increased attention in the struggle to reduce hypertension. In recent years, behavioral scientists have reported the success of meditation, biofeedback, controlled breathing, and muscle relaxation exercises in reducing hypertension. Look for further research findings in these areas in the years to come.

There are literally dozens of drugs available for use by people with hypertension. Unfortunately, many patients refuse to take their medication on a consistent basis, probably because of the mistaken notion that "you must feel sick to be sick." Nutritional supplements, such as calcium, magnesium, potassium, and fish oil, have not been proven to be effective in lowering blood pressure.

Stroke

Stroke is a general term for a wide variety of crises (sometimes called *cerebrovascular accidents* [*CVAs*] or brain

---

Key Terms

salt sensitive term used to describe people whose bodies overreact to the presence of sodium by retaining fluid and thus experience an increase in blood pressure

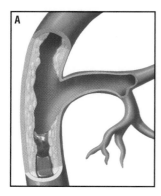

Thrombus
A clot that forms within a narrowed section of a blood vessel and remains at its place of origin.

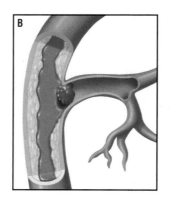

Embolus
A clot that moves through the circulatory system and becomes lodged at a narrowed point within a vessel.

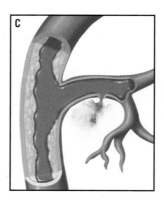

Hemorrhage
The sudden bursting of a blood vessel.

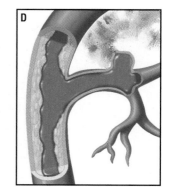

Aneurysm
A sac formed when a section of a blood vessel thins and balloons; the weakened wall of the sac can burst, or rupture, as shown here.

Figure 10-5 Causes of stroke

attacks) that result from blood vessel damage in the brain. African Americans have a much greater risk of stroke than white Americans do, probably because African Americans have a greater likelihood of having hypertension than do white Americans. Data for 2002 indicate that 162,672 deaths and half a million new cases of stroke occurred.[2] Just as the heart muscle needs an adequate blood supply, so does the brain. Any disturbance in the proper supply of oxygen and nutrients to the brain can pose a threat.

Perhaps the most common form of stroke results from the blockage of a cerebral (brain) artery. Similar to coronary occlusions, **cerebrovascular occlusions** can be started by a clot that forms within an artery, called a *thrombus,* or by a clot that travels from another part of the body to the brain, called an *embolus* (Figure 10-5, A and B). The resultant accidents (cerebral thrombosis or cerebral embolism) cause more than 85 percent of all strokes. The portion of the brain deprived of oxygen and nutrients can literally die.

A third type of stroke can result from an artery that bursts to produce a crisis called *cerebral hemorrhage* (Figure 10-5, C). Damaged, brittle arteries can be especially susceptible to bursting when a person has hypertension.

A fourth form of stroke is a *cerebral aneurysm.* An aneurysm is a ballooning or outpouching on a weakened area of an artery (Figure 10-5, D). Aneurysms may occur in various locations of the body and are not always life-threatening. The development of aneurysms is not fully understood, although there seems to be a relationship between aneurysms and hypertension. It is quite possible that many aneurysms are congenital defects. In any case, when a cerebral aneurysm bursts, a stroke results.

Table 10.4 Warning Signs of Stroke

The American Heart Association encourages everyone to be aware of the following signs:

- Sudden, temporary weakness or numbness of the face, arm, and leg on one side of the body
- Temporary loss of speech or trouble in speaking or understanding speech
- Temporary dimness or loss of vision, particularly in one eye
- Unexplained dizziness, unsteadiness, or sudden falls

Many severe strokes are preceded by "mini-strokes," warning signals such as the above, experienced days, weeks, or months before the more severe event. Prompt medical or surgical attention to these symptoms may prevent a fatal or disabling stroke from occurring.

A person who reports any warning signs of stroke (Table 10.4) or any mini stroke, called a **transient ischemic attack (TIA),** will undergo a battery of diagnostic tests, which could include a physical examination, a search for possible brain tumors, tests to identify areas of the brain affected, use of the electroencephalogram, cerebral

Key Terms

cerebrovascular occlusion blockages to arteries supplying blood to the cerebral cortex of the brain; strokes

transient ischemic attack (TIA) strokelike symptoms caused by temporary spasm of cerebral blood vessels

arteriography, and the use of the **CT** (computed tomography) **scan** or **MRI** (magnetic resonance imaging) **scan.** Many additional tests are also available.

Treatment of stroke patients depends on the nature and extent of the damage. Some patients require surgery (to repair vessels and relieve pressure) and acute care in the hospital. Others undergo drug treatment, especially the use of anticoagulant drugs, including aspirin and TPA (tissue plasminogen activators; the "clot buster" drug).

The advancements made in the rehabilitation of stroke patients are amazing. Although some severely affected patients have little hope of improvement, our increasing advancements in the application of computer technology to such disciplines as speech and physical therapy offer encouraging signs for stroke patients and their families.

Congenital Heart Disease

A congenital defect is one that is present at birth. The American Heart Association estimates that each year about 36,000 babies are born with a congenital heart defect. In 2001, 4,109 children (mostly infants) died of congenital heart disease.[2]

A variety of abnormalities may be produced by congenital heart disease, including valve damage, holes in the walls of the septum, blood vessel transposition, and an underdevelopment of the left side of the heart. All of these problems ultimately prevent a newborn from adequately oxygenating tissues throughout the body. A bluish skin color (cyanosis) is seen in some infants with such congenital heart defects. These infants are sometimes referred to as *blue babies.*

The cause of congenital heart defects is not clearly understood, although one cause, *rubella,* has been identified. The fetuses of mothers who contract the rubella virus during the first 3 months of pregnancy are at great risk of developing *congenital rubella syndrome (CRS),* a catch-all term for a wide variety of congenital defects, including heart defects, deafness, cataracts, and mental retardation. Other hypotheses about the development of congenital heart disease implicate environmental pollutants; maternal use of drugs, including alcohol, during pregnancy; and unknown genetic factors (see the Star box).

Treatment of congenital defects usually requires surgery, although some conditions may respond well to drug therapy. Defective blood vessels and certain malformations of the heart can be surgically repaired. This surgery is so successful that many children respond quite quickly to the increased circulation and oxygenation. Many are able to lead normal, active lives.

Rheumatic Heart Disease

Rheumatic heart disease is the final stage in a series of complications started by a streptococcal infection of the

Risk Factors for Congenital and Rheumatic Heart Disease

Risk Factors for Congenital Heart Disease
Fetal exposure to rubella, other viral infections, pollutants, alcohol, or tobacco smoke during pregnancy

Risk Factors for Rheumatic Heart Disease
Streptococcal infection

Common Symptoms of Strep Throat
Sudden onset of sore throat, particularly with pain when swallowing
Fever
Swollen, tender glands under the angle of the jaw
Headache
Nausea and vomiting
Tonsils covered with a yellow or white pus or discharge

throat (strep throat). The Star box lists symptoms of strep throat. This bacterial infection, if untreated, can result in an inflammatory disease called *rheumatic fever* (and a related condition, *scarlet fever*). Rheumatic fever is a whole-body (systemic) reaction that can produce fever, joint pain, skin rashes, and possible brain and heart damage. A person who has had rheumatic fever is more susceptible to subsequent attacks. Rheumatic fever tends to run in families. Over 3,500 Americans died from rheumatic fever and rheumatic heart disease in 2002.[2]

Damage from rheumatic fever centers on the heart's valves. For some reason the bacteria tend to proliferate in the heart valves. Defective heart valves may fail either to open fully (*stenosis*) or to close fully (*insufficiency*). Diagnosis of valve damage might initially come when a physician hears a backwashing or backflow of blood

Key Terms

CT scan computed tomography scan; an x-ray procedure that is designed to visualize structures within the body that would not normally be seen through conventional x-ray procedures

MRI scan magnetic resonance imaging scan; an imaging procedure that uses a giant magnet to generate images of body tissues

rheumatic heart disease chronic damage to the heart (especially heart valves) resulting from a streptococcal infection within the heart; a complication associated with rheumatic fever (a **murmur**). Further tests—including chest X rays, cardiac catheterization, and echocardiography—can reveal the extent of valve damage. Once identified, a faulty valve can be replaced surgically with a metal or plastic artificial valve or a valve taken from an animal's heart.

Congestive Heart Failure

Congestive heart failure is a condition in which the heart lacks the strength to continue to circulate blood normally throughout the body. In 2001, 52,828 people died from congestive heart failure. During congestive heart failure, the heart continues to work, but it cannot function well enough to maintain appropriate circulation. Venous blood flow starts to "back up." Swelling occurs, especially in the legs and ankles. Fluid can collect in the lungs and cause breathing difficulties and shortness of breath, and kidney function may be damaged.[2]

Congestive heart failure can result from heart damage caused by congenital heart defects, lung disease, rheumatic fever, heart attack, atherosclerosis, or high blood pressure. Generally, congestive heart failure is treatable through a combined program of rest, proper diet, modified daily activities, and the use of appropriate drugs. Without medical care, congestive heart failure can be fatal.

Additional Conditions

Besides the cardiovascular diseases already discussed, the heart and blood vessels are also subject to other pathological conditions. Tumors of the heart, although rare, occur. Infectious conditions involving the pericardial sac that surrounds the heart (*pericarditis*) and the innermost layer of the heart (*endocarditis*) are more commonly seen. In addition, inflammation of the veins (*phlebitis*) is troublesome to some people.

Peripheral Artery Disease **Peripheral artery disease (PAD),** also called *peripheral vascular disease (PVD)*, is a blood vessel disease characterized by pathological changes to the arteries and arterioles in the extremities (primarily the legs and feet but sometimes the hands). These changes result from years of damage to the peripheral blood vessels. Important causes of PAD are cigarette smoking, a high-fat diet, obesity, and sedentary occupations. In some cases, PAD is aggravated by blood vessel changes resulting from diabetes.

PAD severely restricts blood flow to the extremities. The reduction in blood flow is responsible for leg pain or cramping during exercise, numbness, tingling, coldness, and loss of hair in the affected limb. The most serious consequence of PAD is the increased likelihood of developing ulcerations and tissue death. These conditions can lead to gangrene and may eventually necessitate amputation.

The treatment of PAD consists of multiple approaches and may include efforts to improve blood lipid levels (through diet, exercise, or drug therapy), reduce hypertension, reduce body weight, and eliminate smoking. Blood vessel surgery is also a possible treatment approach.

Key Terms

murmur an atypical heart sound that suggests a back-washing of blood into a chamber of the heart from which it has just left

congestive heart failure inability of the heart to pump out all the blood that returns to it; can lead to dangerous fluid accumulations in veins, lungs, and kidneys

peripheral artery disease (PAD) damage resulting from restricted blood flow to the extremities, especially the legs and feet

---

Taking Charge of Your Health

- Complete the Personal Assessment on page 267 to determine your risk for heart attack and stroke.

- Review the Food Guide Pyramid in Chapter 5 (page 109), and make changes to your diet so that it is more "heart healthy."

- Begin or continue an aerobic exercise program that is appropriate for your current fitness level.

- If you are a smoker, resolve to quit smoking. Visit your physician to talk about safe and effective approaches. Begin putting your plan into action.

- Develop a plan to lower your dietary intake of fat to keep your blood cholesterol level low.

- Have your blood pressure checked, and review your weight, physical activity, alcohol intake, and salt intake to determine whether you can make changes in any of these areas.

- If you are overweight or obese, develop a plan to combine dietary changes and increased physical activity to lose weight gradually but steadily.

SUMMARY

- Cardiovascular disorders are responsible for more disabilities and deaths than any other disease.
- The cardiovascular system consists of the heart, blood, and blood vessels. This system performs many functions.
- Our overall health depends on the health of the cardiovascular system.
- A cardiovascular risk factor is an attribute that a person has or is exposed to that increases the likelihood of heart disease.
- The "big six" risk factors are tobacco smoke, physical inactivity, high blood cholesterol level, high blood pressure, diabetes mellitus, and obesity and overweight. These are controllable risk factors.
- Increasing age, male gender, and heredity are risk factors that cannot be controlled.

- Four contributing risk factors to heart disease are individual response to stress, sex hormones, birth control pills, and drinking too much alcohol.
- The major forms of cardiovascular disease include coronary artery disease, hypertension, stroke, congenital heart disease, rheumatic heart disease, and congestive heart failure. Each disease develops in a specific way and may require a highly specialized form of treatment.
- Atherosclerosis is the pathophysiological process that results in the narrowing of coronary arteries.
- It is important to recognize the warning signs of both heart attacks and strokes.

REVIEW QUESTIONS

1. Identify the principal components of the cardiovascular system. Trace the path of blood through the heart and cardiovascular system.
2. How much blood does the average adult have? What are some of the important functions of blood?
3. Define cardiovascular risk factor. What relationship do risk factors have to cardiovascular disease?
4. Identify those risk factors for cardiovascular disease that cannot be changed. Identify those risk factors that can be changed. Identify the risk factors that can be contributing factors.

5. What are the six major forms of cardiovascular disease? For each of these diseases, describe what the disease is, its cause (if known), and its treatment.
6. Describe how high-density lipoproteins differ from low-density lipoproteins.
7. What problems does atherosclerosis produce?
8. Why is hypertension referred to as "the silent killer"?
9. What are the warning signals of stroke?
10. What is peripheral artery disease?

ENDNOTES

1. American Heart Association. *2004 Heart and Stroke Statistical Update,* 2004.
2. Seeley RR, Stephens TD, Tate P. *Essentials of Anatomy and Physiology* (3rd ed.). New York: McGraw-Hill, 1999.
3. Brubaker PH, Kaminsky LA, Whaley MH. *Coronary Artery Disease.* Champaign, IL: Human Kinetics, 2002.
4. American Heart Association. Heart and Stroke Facts, 2003.

5. Cholesterol: Up with the good, *Harvard Heart Letter* 5:11, July 1995, 3–4.
6. Aspirin for coronary disease: Beneficial in women, too, *Harvard Heart Letter* 7:7, March 1997, 8.
7. National Heart Lung and Blood Institute. www.nhlbi.nih.gov/guidelines/hypertension/index.htm July 21, 2003.

As We Go to Press

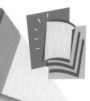

The American Heart Association Journal *Hypertension*[1] recently published a study that reported that women who use acetaminophen, ibuprofen, or naproxen (all frequently used analgesic medications) had a greater risk for developing hypertension. Use of aspirin was not associated with developing hypertension. Certainly, as with all early studies on a topic, more research is necessary to fully understand the issues. At this time, women who regularly use any of these medications should consult with their physicians.

[1] Forman, JP, Stampfer MJ, Curhan GC, in *Hypertension* (Journal of the American Heart Association) 46:1–8, 2005.

personal assessment

what is your risk for heart disease?

Cholesterol

Your serum cholesterol level is

   0 190 or below
+ 2 191 to 230
+ 6 231 to 289
+12 290 to 319
+16 Over 320

Your HDL cholesterol is

− 2 Over 60
   0 45 to 60
+ 2 35 to 44
+ 6 29 to 34
+12 23 to 28
+16 Below 23

Smoking

In the past, you

   0 Never smoked, or quit more than 5 years ago
+ 1 Quit 2 to 4 years ago
+ 3 Quit about 1 year ago
+ 6 Quit during the past year

You now smoke

+ 9 ½ to 1 pack a day
+12 1 to 2 packs a day
+15 More than 2 packs a day

The quality of the air you breathe is

   0 Unpolluted by smoke, exhaust, or industry at home and at work
+ 2 Live or work with smokers in unpolluted area
+ 4 Live and work with smokers in unpolluted area
+ 6 Live or work with smokers **and** live or work in air-polluted area
+ 8 Live **and** work with smokers **and** live and work in air-polluted area

Blood Pressure

Your blood pressure is

   0 120/75 or below
+ 2 120/75 to 140/85
+ 6 140/85 to 150/90
+ 8 150/90 to 175/100
+10 175/100 to 190/110
+12 190/110 or above

Exercise

Your exercise habits are

   0 Exercise vigorously 4 or 5 times a week
+ 2 Exercise moderately 4 or 5 times a week
+ 4 Exercise only on weekends
+ 6 Exercise occasionally
+ 8 Little or no exercise

Weight

Your weight is

   0 Always at or near ideal weight
+ 1 Now 10% overweight
+ 2 Now 20% overweight
+ 3 Now 30% or more overweight
+ 4 Now 20% or more overweight and have been since before age 30

Stress

You feel overstressed

   0 Rarely at work or at home
+ 3 Somewhat at home but not at work
+ 5 Somewhat at work but not at home
+ 7 Somewhat at work **and** at home
+ 9 Usually at work **or** at home
+12 Usually at work **and** at home

Diabetes

Your diabetic history is

   0 Blood sugar always normal
+ 2 Blood glucose slightly high (prediabetic) or slightly low (hypoglycemic)
+ 4 Diabetic beginning after age 40 requiring strict dietary or insulin control
+ 5 Diabetic beginning before age 30 requiring strict dietary or insulin control

Alcohol

You drink alcoholic beverages

   0 Never or only socially, about once or twice a month, or only one 5-ounce glass of wine or 12-ounce glass of beer or 1½ ounces of hard liquor about 5 times a week
+ 2 Two to three 5-ounces glasses of wine or 12-ounce glasses of beer or 1½ ounce cocktails about 5 times a week
+ 4 More than three 1½-ounce cocktails or more than three 5-ounce glasses of wine or 12-ounce glasses of beer almost every day

Interpretation

Add all sources and check next page.

0 to 20:   **Low risk.** Excellent family history and lifestyle habits.

21 to 50:   **Moderate risk.** Family history or lifestyle habits put you at some risk. You might lower your risks and minimize your genetic predisposition if you change any poor habits.

51 to 74:   **High risk.** Habits and family history indicate high risk of heart disease. Change your habits now.

Above 75:   **Very high risk.** Family history and a lifetime of poor habits put you at very high risk of heart disease. Eliminate as many of the risk factors as you can.

To Carry This Further . . .

Were you surprised with your score on this assessment? What were your most significant risk factors? Do you plan to make any changes in your lifestyle to reduce your cardiovascular risks? Why or why not?

Chapter eleven

Living with Cancer and Other Chronic Conditions

Chapter Objectives

On completing this chapter, you will be able to:

▌ describe cancer statistics and identify groups who are at high risk for developing particular forms of cancer.

▌ explain the role of cell regulation in the development of cancer, and discuss the relationship of genetic mutations, viral infections, and carcinogens to the loss of cell regulation.

▌ name specific steps that individuals can take to aid in early detection of specific cancers, including breast cancer, melanoma, and testicular cancer.

▌ discuss the importance of medical screening for specific cancers, and identify several procedures used to screen for particular forms of cancer.

▌ offer several lifestyle changes that effectively reduce your cancer risk.

▌ summarize the status of our current "War on Cancer."

▌ explain what an autoimmune disorder is.

▌ describe the genetic causes and the symptoms of several inherited conditions.

▌ discuss treatment options for a number of chronic conditions.

▌ explain the difference between type 1 and type 2 diabetes, and discuss the importance of physical activity and diet in remaining glucose tolerant as we get older.

Eye on the Media

Support Is Just a Click Away

Support groups are composed of people who come together to help one another through the demands of a chronic health condition. These groups have traditionally been organized by institutions in the local health care community, such as hospitals, by the local affiliates of national organizations, such as the American Cancer Society, or by citizens who have the same chronic condition. Today, however, more and more support group members are connected not by physical proximity but by the Internet.

Health self-help groups on the Internet develop in one of two ways. The first occurs when a brick-and-mortar organization, such as a national agency or health care institution, develops a support group for its homepage. The second way is for a person with the condition (or a family member of that person) to organize an online group.

You can find a health support group simply by surfing the net. Or you can be referred to a site by a health care professional, friend, family member, colleague, or someone with a similar condition. You can also go to the homepage of a medical institution or a national agency to find out if it provides a support group link.

For someone with a newly diagnosed chronic condition, the initial contact with a support group may be made to get information about the condition and its treatment. For others, it is a way of connecting with other people who have the condition. Web support groups provide windows to the outside world, particularly for those whose conditions limit their mobility and social contacts. The Internet support group transcends the restrictions of various diseases to make new connections possible.

Note that online support groups' members are rarely physicians or other highly trained health professionals, so you shouldn't rely on this source for specific technical information. Instead, your main sources of information about medical management of a chronic condition should be your health care providers. Seasoned members of support groups need to remind themselves that newly diagnosed members are inexperienced and vulnerable. It will take them time to adjust to the frankness and clinical sophistication demonstrated by some group members in addressing their health problems.

Some hospitals provide laptop computers to patients so they can maintain contact with their support groups. In this way, health care institutions are encouraging patients to support their efforts and, perhaps, helping them recover more quickly.

Most people can attest to the disruptive influence an illness can have on their ability to participate in day-to-day activities. When we are ill, school, employment, and leisure activities are replaced by periods of lessened activity and even periods of bed rest or hospitalization. When an illness is chronic, the effect of being ill may extend over long periods, perhaps even an entire lifetime. People with chronic illness must eventually find a balance between day-to-day function and the continuous presence of their condition. Cancer is usually a chronic illness.

In spite of our understanding of its relationship to human health and our ceaseless attempts to prevent and cure it, progress in the "war on cancer" has been relatively limited. In this regard, cancer is clearly an "expensive" condition, both in terms of its human consequences and its monetary costs. It is estimated that 1,372,910 people developed cancer in 2005. Once diagnosed, approximately 64 percent (adjusted for other causes of death) of this group will be alive 5 years later.[1] If one limits 2005's new cases to those forms of cancer for which early detection through screening is applicable (breast, colon, rectum, cervix, prostate, oral cavity, and skin), 85 percent will be alive after 5 years. This 5-year period, called *relative survivability,* includes "persons who are living 5 years after diagnosis, whether disease free, in remission, or under treatment with evidence of cancer."[1] Understandably, the term *cured* is used guardedly since an initially diagnosed case of cancer can affect survivability beyond the end of the 5-year time period. Regardless of survivability, for those who develop cancer, the physical, emotional, and social costs will be substantial.

No single explanation can be given for why progress in eliminating cancer has been so limited. It is a combination of factors, including the aging of the population, continued use of tobacco, the high-fat American diet, the continuing urbanization and pollution of our environment, the lack of health insurance for an estimated 45 million Americans to pay for early diagnosis and proper treatment,[2] or simply our delayed recognition of cancer's true role in deaths once ascribed to other causes. Regardless, we continue to be challenged to control this array of abnormal conditions that we collectively call cancer. There is, however, increasing optimism that with new pharmacological agents and the development of vaccines to prevent and treat cancers real progress will finally be made.

 TALKING POINTS A close friend justifies her high cancer-risk lifestyle by saying that "everyone will die of something." How would you counter this point?

Cancer: A Problem of Cell Regulation

Just as a corporation depends on individuals to staff its various departments, the body depends on its basic units of function, the cells. Cells band together as tissues, such as muscle tissue, to perform a prescribed function. Tissues in turn join to form organs, such as the heart, and organs are assembled into the body's several organ systems, such as the cardiovascular system. Such is the "corporate structure" of the body.

If individuals and cells are the basic units of function for their respective organizations, the failure of either to perform in a prescribed, dependable manner can erode the overall organization to the extent that it might not be able to continue. Cancer, the leading cause of death among adults under 80 years of age,[3] is a condition reflecting cell dysfunction in its most extreme form. In cancer, the normal behavior of cells ceases.

Cell Regulation

Most of the body's tissues lose cells over time. This continual loss requires that replacement cells come from areas of young and less specialized cells. The process of specialization required to turn the less specialized cells into mature cells is controlled by genes within the cells. On becoming specialized, these newest cells copy, or replicate, themselves. These two processes are carefully monitored by the cells' **regulatory genes.** Failure to regulate replication specialization results in abnormal, or potentially cancerous, cells.

In addition to genes that regulate replication and specialization, cells also have genes designed to repair mistakes in the copying of genetic material (the basis of replication) and genes to suppress the growth of abnormal cells should it occur. Thus, repair genes and tumor suppressor genes, such as the *p53* gene (altered or missing in half of all cancers), can also be considered regulatory genes in place to prevent the development of abnormal cells. Should these genes fail to function properly, resulting in the development of malignant (cancerous) cells, the immune system (see Chapter 12) will ideally recognize their presence and remove them before a clinical (diagnosable) case of cancer can develop.

> **Key Terms**
>
> **regulatory genes** genes that control cell specialization, replication, DNA repair, and tumor suppression

Because, when they are not working properly, replication, specialization, repair, and suppressor genes can become cancer-causing genes, or **oncogenes,** these four types of genes can also be referred to as **proto-oncogenes,** or potential oncogenes.[4] How proto-oncogenes become oncogenes is a question that cannot be completely answered at this time. Regardless, abnormal cells produce abnormal proteins, and the absence of normal proteins alters the body's ability to function appropriately, from the molecular to the organ system level.

Oncogene Formation

All cells have proto-oncogenes, so what events alter otherwise normal regulatory genes, causing them to become cancer-causing genes? Three mechanisms, genetic mutations, viral infections, and carcinogens, have received much attention.

Genetic mutations develop when dividing cells miscopy genetic information. If the gene that is miscopied is a gene that controls specialization, replication, repair, or tumor suppression (a proto-oncogene), the oncogene that results will allow the formation of cancerous cells. A variety of factors, including aging, free radical formation, and radiation, are associated with the miscopying of the complex genetic information that constitutes the genes found within the cell, including those intended to prevent cancer.

In both animals and humans, cancer-producing viruses, such as the feline leukemia virus in cats and the human immunodeficiency virus (HIV) and multiple forms of the human papilloma virus (HPV) in humans (see Chapter 12) have been identified. These viruses seek out cells of a particular type, such as cells of the immune system, or the lining of the cervix, and substitute some of their genetic material for some of the cells' thus converting them into virus-producing cells. In so doing, they convert proto-oncogenes into oncogenes. Once converted into oncogenes, the altered genes are passed on through cell division.

A third possible explanation for the conversion of proto-oncogenes into oncogenes involves the presence of environmental agents known as *carcinogens.* Over an extended period, carcinogens, such as chemicals found in tobacco smoke, polluted air and water, toxic wastes, and even high-fat foods, may convert proto-oncogenes into oncogenes. These carcinogens may work alone or in combination with co-carcinogenic promoters (see Chapter 9, Table 9.3) to alter the genetic material, including regulatory genes, within cells. Thus people might develop lung cancer only if they are exposed to the right combination of carcinogens over an extended period.

You may already see that some of the specific risk factors in each area—such as radiation in the development of mutations, sexually transmitted viruses in cancers of the reproductive tract, and smoking-introduced carcinogens in the development of lung cancer—can be moderated by adopting health-promoting behaviors.

In light of the complexity of cancer, some people in the scientific community believe that cancer can never be truly prevented. Rather, they feel that the ability to stop and then reverse cancerous changes at an early stage of development is more likely than is the prevention of this complex disease process. However, this text addresses the concepts of prevention in the belief that prevention-based practices reflect our personal contribution to the "war on cancer."

The Cancerous Cell

Compared with noncancerous cells, cancer cells function in similar and dissimilar ways. It is the dissimilar aspects that often make them unpredictable and difficult to manage.

Perhaps the most unusual aspect of cancerous cells is their infinite life expectancy. Specifically, it appears that cancerous cells can produce an enzyme, *telomerase,* that blocks the cellular biological clock that informs normal cells that it is time to die.[5] In spite of this ability to live forever, cancer cells do not necessarily divide more quickly than normal cells do. In fact, they can divide at the same rate or even on occasion at a slower rate.

In addition, cancerous cells do not possess the *contact inhibition*[6] (a mechanism that influences the number of cells that can occupy a particular space at a particular time) of normal cells. In the absence of this property, cancer cells accumulate, altering the functional capacity of the tissue or organ they occupy. Further, the absence of *cellular cohesiveness*[6] (a property seen in normal cells that "keeps them at home") allows cancer cells to spread through the circulatory or lymphatic system to distant points via **metastasis**

Key Terms

oncogenes faulty regulatory genes that are believed to activate the development of cancer

proto-oncogenes (pro toe **on** co genes) normal regulatory genes that may become oncogenes

metastasis (muh **tas** ta sis) the spread of cancerous cells from their site of origin to other areas of the body

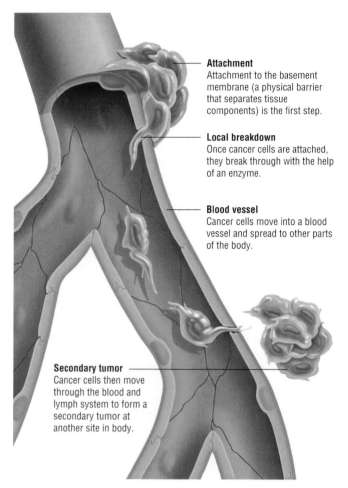

Attachment
Attachment to the basement membrane (a physical barrier that separates tissue components) is the first step.

Local breakdown
Once cancer cells are attached, they break through with the help of an enzyme.

Blood vessel
Cancer cells move into a blood vessel and spread to other parts of the body.

Secondary tumor
Cancer cells then move through the blood and lymph system to form a secondary tumor at another site in body.

Figure 11-1 How cancer spreads. Locomotion (movement) is essential to the process of metastasis (spread of cancer). Scientists have identified a protein that causes cancer cells to grow arms, or pseudopodia, enabling them to move to other parts of the body.

(Figure 11-1). Interestingly, once migrating cancer cells arrive at a new area of the body, they "rediscover" their cellular cohesive capabilities. A final unique characteristic of cancerous cells is their ability to command the circulatory system to send them additional blood supply to meet their metabolic needs and to provide additional routes for metastasis. This *angiogenesis*[6] capability of cancer cells makes them extremely hardy compared with noncancerous cells.

Benign Tumors

Noncancerous, or **benign,** tumors can also form in the body. These **tumors** are usually enclosed by a membrane and do not spread from their point of origin. Benign tumors can be dangerous when they crowd out normal tissue within a confined space.

Types of Cancer

Cancers are named according to the types of cells or tissues from which they originate. Although physicians routinely use these labels, another set, to be described later, is more familar to laypersons:

carcinoma—Found most frequently in the skin, nose, mouth, throat, stomach, intestinal tract, glands, nerves, breasts, urinary and genital structures, lungs, kidneys, and liver; approximately 85 percent of all malignant tumors are classified as carcinomas

sarcoma—Formed in the connective tissues of the body; bone, cartilage, and tendons are the sites of sarcoma development; only 2 percent of all malignancies are of this type

melanoma—Arises from the melanin-containing cells of skin; found most often in people who have had extensive sun exposure, particularly a deep, penetrating sunburn; although once rare, the amount of this cancer has increased markedly in recent years; remains among the most deadly forms of cancer

neuroblastoma—Originates in the immature cells found within the central nervous system; neuroblastomas are rare; usually found in children

adenocarcinoma—Derived from cells of the endocrine glands

hepatoma—Originates in cells of the liver; although not thought to be directly caused by alcohol use, seen more frequently in people who have experienced **sclerotic changes** in the liver

leukemia—Found in cells of the blood and blood-forming tissues; characterized by abnormal, immature white blood cell formation; several forms are found in children and adults

lymphoma—Arises in cells of the lymphatic tissues or other immune system tissues; includes lymphosarcomas and Hodgkin's disease; characterized by abnormal white cell production and decreased resistance

---

Key Terms

benign noncancerous; tumors that do not spread

tumor mass of cells; may be cancerous (malignant) or noncancerous (benign)

sclerotic changes (skluh **rot** ick) thickening or hardening of tissues

---

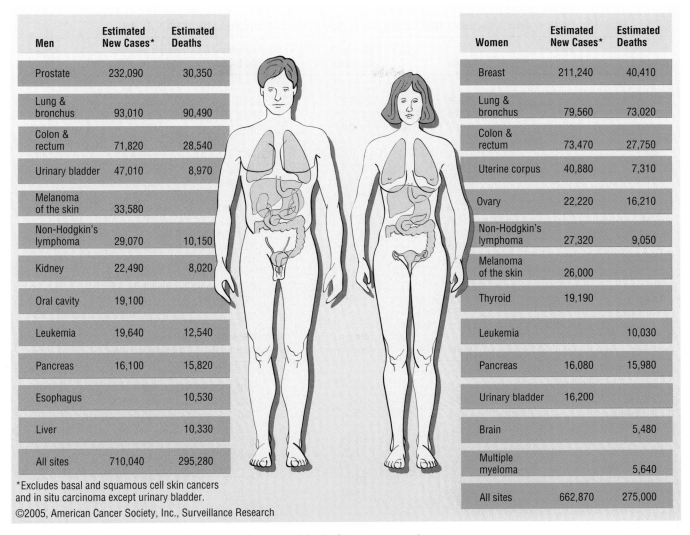

Men	Estimated New Cases*	Estimated Deaths
Prostate	232,090	30,350
Lung & bronchus	93,010	90,490
Colon & rectum	71,820	28,540
Urinary bladder	47,010	8,970
Melanoma of the skin	33,580	
Non-Hodgkin's lymphoma	29,070	10,150
Kidney	22,490	8,020
Oral cavity	19,100	
Leukemia	19,640	12,540
Pancreas	16,100	15,820
Esophagus		10,530
Liver		10,330
All sites	710,040	295,280

*Excludes basal and squamous cell skin cancers and in situ carcinoma except urinary bladder.

©2005, American Cancer Society, Inc., Surveillance Research

Women	Estimated New Cases*	Estimated Deaths
Breast	211,240	40,410
Lung & bronchus	79,560	73,020
Colon & rectum	73,470	27,750
Uterine corpus	40,880	7,310
Ovary	22,220	16,210
Non-Hodgkin's lymphoma	27,320	9,050
Melanoma of the skin	26,000	
Thyroid	19,190	
Leukemia		10,030
Pancreas	16,080	15,980
Urinary bladder	16,200	
Brain		5,480
Multiple myeloma		5,640
All sites	662,870	275,000

Figure 11-2 These 2005 estimates of new cases of cancer and deaths from cancer reveal some significant similarities between men and women. Note that lung cancer is the leading cause of cancer deaths for both genders.

Figure 11-2 presents information about the estimated new cases of cancer and deaths from cancer at various sites in both men and women.[1] Table 11.1 shows that cancer incidence and mortality rates vary among different racial and ethnic groups.

Cancer at Selected Sites in the Body

A second and more familiar way to describe cancer is on the basis of the organ site at which it occurs. The following discussion relates to some of these more familiar sites. A lack of space, in combination with the wide array of human cancers, limits the number of specific malignancies that can be described. Remember, also, that regular screening procedures can lead to early identification of cancer at these sites. (See Table 11.2 on page 279.)

Lung Cancer

Lung cancer is one of the most lethal and frequently diagnosed forms of cancer. Primarily because of the advanced stage of the disease at the time symptoms first appear, only 15 percent of all people with lung cancer (all stages) survive 5 years beyond diagnosis.[1] By the time a person is sufficiently concerned about having a persistent cough, blood-streaked sputum, and chest pain, it is often too late for treatment to be effective. This failure to be able to diagnose lung cancer in its earlier stages could, however, begin to change. Currently the National Cancer Institute is studying the efficacy of *spiral CT scans* in

Table 11.1 Incidence and Mortality Rates* by Site, Race, and Ethnicity, US, 1997–2001

Incidence	White	African American	Asian American and Pacific Islander	American Indian and Alaska Native	Hispanic/ Latino[†]
All sites					
Males	556.5	689.2	385.9	263.2	419.8
Females	429.8	400.1	302.8	222.5	309.9
Breast (female)	141.7	119.9	96.8	54.2	89.6
Colon & rectum					
Males	63.1	72.9	56.3	38.3	49.6
Females	45.9	56.5	38.6	32.7	32.5
Lung & bronchus					
Males	77.9	117.2	60.5	46.0	45.2
Females	51.3	54.5	28.5	23.4	23.9
Prostate	167.4	271.3	100.7	51.2	140.0
Stomach					
Males	10.8	18.8	21.9	15.7	17.8
Females	5.0	9.9	12.4	8.9	10.0
Liver & intrahepatic bile duct					
Males	7.2	11.8	21.1	8.3	13.5
Females	2.9	3.9	7.7	4.8	5.8
Uterine cervix	8.9	11.8	9.5	6.0	16.2

Mortality	White	African American	Asian American and Pacific Islander	American Indian and Alaska Native	Hispanic/ Latino[†]
All sites					
Males	245.5	347.3	151.2	167.0	174.0
Females	165.5	196.5	100.5	113.4	111.6
Breast (female)	26.4	35.4	12.6	13.6	17.3
Colon & rectum					
Males	24.8	34.3	15.8	17.1	18.0
Females	17.1	24.5	10.8	11.7	11.6
Lung & bronchus					
Males	76.6	104.1	40.2	49.8	39.6
Females	41.6	39.9	19.2	26.6	14.9
Prostate	28.8	70.4	13.0	20.2	23.5
Stomach					
Males	5.8	13.3	11.9	7.3	9.7
Females	2.8	6.3	7.0	4.1	5.3
Liver & intrahepatic bile duct					
Males	6.1	9.3	15.6	8.3	10.6
Females	2.7	3.8	6.6	4.3	5.1
Uterine cervix	2.6	5.6	2.8	2.8	3.6

*Per 100,000, age-adjusted to the 2000 US standard population.

[†]Hispanic/Latinos are not mutually exclusive from whites, African Americans, Asian Americans, and Pacific Islanders, and American Indians and Alaska Natives.

Source: Ries LAG, Eisner MP, Kosary CL, Hankey BF, Miller BA, Clegg L, Mariotto A, Fay MP, Feuer EJ, Edwards BK (eds). *SEER Cancer Statistics Review, 1975–2001.* National Cancer Institute, Bethesda, MD: http://seer.cancer.gov/csr/1975_2001, 2004. American Cancer Society, Surveillance Research, 2005.

detecting lung tumors earlier than can be done by conventional chest x-rays. However, an initial assessment of the technology questions its cost-effectiveness and potential for excessive false-positive findings.

Risk Factors

Today it is known that genetic predisposition is important in the development of lung cancer. Perhaps, in fact, the majority of people who develop this form of cancer have an inherited "head start." When people who are genetically at risk also smoke, their level of risk for developing lung cancer is significantly greater than it is for nonsmokers. Of particular interest at this time are multiple genes on chromosome 3. Damage to three tumor suppressors on this chromosome is found in virtually every case of small-cell lung cancer and 90 percent of nonsmall-cell lung cancer. Most of the remaining lung cancer cases appear in people who smoke but are not genetically predisposed.

Cigarette smoking is unquestionably the single most important behavioral factor in the development of lung cancer. For men who smoke, the rate of lung cancer is 22 times higher than it is for men who do not smoke. For women who smoke, the rate is 12 times higher than for women who do not smoke. Smokers account for 87 percent of all reported cases of lung cancer, and lung cancer itself produces at least 30 percent of all cancer-caused deaths.[1]

Since 1987, lung cancer has exceeded breast cancer as the leading cause of cancer death in women, although more new cases of breast cancer than lung cancer are diagnosed each year. The incidence of lung cancer in men has shown a gradual decline over the last several years that parallels their declining use of tobacco products. In comparing 2003 estimated new cases of lung cancer in women with 2005 data, it appears for the first time that the incidence of lung cancer has also begun declining in women.[1] One hopes that this decline in new cases of lung cancer in women reflects a continuing decline in tobacco use.

Environmental agents, such as radon, asbestos, and air pollutants, make a smaller contribution to the development of lung cancer. Radon alone may be the principal causative agent in most lung cancer found in nonsmokers.

Prevention

The preceding information clearly suggests that not smoking or quitting smoking (see page 239) and avoidance of second-hand tobacco smoke (see page 237) are the most important factors in the prevention of lung cancer. In addition, place of residence, particularly as it relates to air pollution, is a long-suspected risk factor for lung cancer.[7] Nonsmokers who are considering living with a smoker or working in a confined area where second-hand tobacco smoke is prevalent should carefully consider the risk of developing lung cancer. A recent study does, however, lessen concern over moderate alcohol use and the risk of developing lung cancer.[8]

Treatment

The prognosis for surviving lung cancer remains extremely guarded. Depending on the type of lung cancer, its extent, and factors related to the patient's overall health, various combinations of surgery, radiation, and chemotherapy remain the physicians' primary approach to treatment. Today, for persons with early stage lung cancer, chemotherapy, following surgery, has increased survivability slightly. Additionally, new medications that primarily shrink tumors are also available. An experimental vaccine (GVAX) now in the early stages of testing has shown extremely encouraging results in patients with non-small-cell lung cancer, the most common form of the disease.[9] Also, a once-promising drug, *Iressa*, used as a last-resort drug by terminally ill lung cancer patients, now seems far less promising after subsequent study, thus is basically ineffective against the lethality of advanced lung cancer.

Breast Cancer

Surpassed only by lung cancer, breast cancer is the second leading cause of death from cancer in women. It is the third leading cause of cancer deaths overall. Nearly one in eight women will develop breast cancer in her lifetime, resulting in an estimated 211,240 new invasive cases and 40,410 deaths in 2005.[1] In men, an estimated 1,690 new cases and 460 deaths occurred in 2005[1] (See Learning from Our Diversity on page 277.) As women age, their risk of developing breast cancer increases. Early detection is the key to complete recovery. Ninety-seven percent of women who discover their breast cancer before it has spread (metastasized) will survive more than 5 years.[1]

Risk Factors

Although all women and men are at some risk of developing breast cancer, the following groups of women have a higher risk.

- Women whose menstrual periods began at an early age, or whose menopause occurred late (although the former may be more important than the latter is)
- Women who had no children, had their first child later in life, or did not nurse[10]
- Women who have used hormone replacement therapy (HRT), particularly combined estrogen and progestin[11]
- Women who have a high degree of breast density (high level of glandular tissues relative to fat) or biopsy-established hyperplasia[1]
- Women whose diets are high in saturated fats, who are sedentary, or who are obese after menopause[12] (particularly central body cavity obesity; see Chapter 6)
- Women who carry the *BRAC1* and/or *BRAC2* mutated tumor suppressor genes, or those women with a strong family history of breast cancer

As mentioned above, significant concern exists regarding the long-term use of hormone replacement therapy and the development of breast cancer in postmenopausal women. In fact, in a government-sponsored study (Women's Health Initiative Study) the link appeared so strongly and early that the study was terminated much earlier than had been planned. Researchers found that tumor development in women taking HRT versus those on a placebo was more common, that tumors were larger at diagnosis, and that tumors were more often invasive.[11] Many physicians are now advising that HRT be used only on a very short-term basis to relieve the symptoms of menopause, rather than the much longer period of time previously deemed appropriate.

The effects of environmental pollutants and regional influences have also been investigated as causative factors in the development of breast cancer. Environmental pollutants

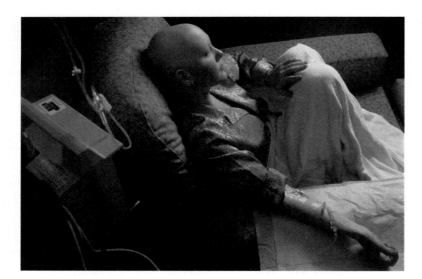

Chemotherapy is a treatment for many types of cancer.

vary from region to region and are influenced by a number of factors, including the type of industrial and agricultural activity in a particular area. A wide array of regional factors may be involved, including genetic background of people in a given area and lifestyle differences involving diet, alcohol consumption, and exercise patterns.

The role of genetic predisposition in the development of breast cancer has also received considerable attention. For example, a small percentage (perhaps 5 percent) of women with breast cancer have inherited or developed mutations in one or both of two tumor suppressor genes (proto-oncogenes), *BRCA1* and *BRCA2*. Discovered in 1994 and 1995, respectively, and currently the focus of extensive research, more than 200 mutations in these genes have been identified. In a recent study involving 5,000 Ashkenazi Jews (Jews of Central and Eastern European descent) living in the Washington, D.C., area, mutation in the *BRCA1* gene resulted in a 56 percent greater chance of developing breast cancer by age 70 (versus a 13 percent greater risk for people without a mutated version of the gene).[13] In the years since these genes' identification, studies have been ongoing in an attempt to more accurately define the level of risk for developing breast cancer among women who carry one or both *BRCA1* or *2* mutations. The desirability of fine-tuning the level of risk holds important implications in establishing recommendations for screening and in the development of public education programs.[14] Both of these genes are also associated with increased risk of developing ovarian cancer (see page 282) and, perhaps, prostate cancer in men.

Other genetic links to breast cancer have been identified. For example, one involves an increased risk for breast cancer development in black women. The gene in question is *BPI*, a gene that, if shut off, allows cancer cells to establish cellular immortality. Factors that influence this gene to become dysfunctional have not been identified.

The Personal Assessment on page 301 may be helpful in determining your relative level of risk of developing breast cancer.

Prevention

As already discussed, a variety of risk factors are thought to be important in the development of most cases of breast cancer. Accordingly, some degree of prevention is possible when factors such as diet; alcohol use; physical activity level; decisions about contraception, pregnancy, and breastfeeding; occupational exposure to toxins; and even place of residence are considered.

For women who have a primary family history of breast cancer (sisters, mother, or grandmothers with the disease) and who have been found to carry one or both of the *BRCA* genes discussed, an extreme form of prevention is also possible—**prophylactic mastectomy.** In this surgical procedure, both noncancerous breasts are removed, in an attempt to eliminate the possibility of future cancer development. When carefully planned, breast reconstruction surgery can be undertaken immediately, with satisfactory results. A high level of satisfaction (70 percent) was found among women who had undergone this procedure.[15]

At the present time pharmacological prevention represents the newest approach to reducing the incidence

---

Key Terms

prophylactic mastectomy surgical removal of the breasts to prevent breast cancer in women who are at high risk of developing the disease

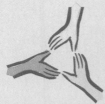
of breast cancer. Two medications, Evista, or raloxifene (a drug developed for use in osteoporosis prevention), and tamoxifen (an estrogen-receptor blocker developed for use in the treatment of cancer) have been found to be effective in lowering the risk of cancer in high-risk women. However, a warning (August 2000) from the FDA reminds physicians that tamoxifen can have serious side effects, including the development of uterine cancer and potentially fatal blood clots.

Early Detection: Breast Self-Examination

For several decades a fundamental component of early detection of breast cancer has been breast self-examination (BSE). Generally recommended for women 20 years of age and older, the procedure was to be performed during the menstrual period or during the day immediately following the end of the menstrual period, when estrogen levels are at their lowest and cystic activity in breast tissue is minimal (or on the same day of each month by postmenopausal women). The proper technique is illustrated in the Changing for the Better box on page 278. Although breast self-examination is an easily learned technique, today its value is being strongly challenged by researchers in both this country and in China. It has, in fact, become the contention of some that teaching BSE to another generation of women is a misuse of time and money that could be better spent on other screening techniques. Others, however, feel that women who know

the technique should not be discouraged from using BSE, but they also should be regularly reminded of its significant limitations in finding tumors. In 2003, the American Cancer Society (ACS) revised its recommendation for breast cancer screening to better address the doubts regarding BSE's limitations. Specific to BSE the following statement summarizes the ACS's position.

> Previously, the guidelines (for BSE) recommended women perform breast self-exam every month. Now, (we) recommend that, beginning in their 20s, women should be told about the benefits and limitations of BSE, and that it is acceptable for women to choose not to do BSE, or to do it occasionally. The importance of promptly reporting changes to a physician is emphasized.
>
> The reason for this change is that research has shown that BSE plays a very small role in detecting breast cancer compared with self-awareness.

In any case, monthly BSE can be viewed as an adjunct to regularly scheduled breast examinations conducted by a physician (CBE) and to the routine use of mammography.

In light of the concern regarding the role of BSE in early cancer detection, the second rung of early detection, Clinical Breast Examination (CBE), is also being critically reviewed because of the lack of standard procedures for conducting the examination. Steps are being taken to develop standardized protocols. Currently, the ACS appears to remain totally committed to the importance of CBE.[16]

Breast Self-Examination

I've never felt confident about doing a breast self-exam. What is the proper technique?

The following explains how to do a breast self-examination:

1. In the shower: Examine your breasts during a bath or shower; hands glide more easily over wet skin. With your fingers flat, move gently over every part of each breast. Use right hand to examine left breast, left hand for right breast. Check for any lump, hard knot, or thickening. This self-examination should be done monthly, preferably a day or two after the end of the menstrual period.
2. Before a mirror: Inspect your breasts with arms at your sides. Next, raise your arms high overhead. Look for any changes in contour of each breast, a swelling, dimpling of skin, changes in the nipple. Then rest palms on hips, and press down firmly to flex your chest muscles. Left and right breast will not exactly match— few women's breasts do.
3. Lying down: To examine your right breast, put a pillow or folded towel under your right shoulder. Place right hand behind your head—this distributes breast tissue more evenly on the chest. With left hand, fingers flat, press gently in small circular motions around an imaginary clock face. Begin at outermost top of your right breast for 12 o'clock, then move to 1 o'clock, and so on around the circle back to 12 o'clock. A ridge of firm tissue in the lower curve of each breast is normal. Then move in an inch toward the nipple; keep circling to examine every part of your breast, including the nipple. This requires at least three more circles. Now slowly repeat the procedure on your left breast with a pillow under your left shoulder and left hand behind head. Notice how your breast structure feels. Finally, squeeze the nipple of each breast gently between thumb and index finger. Any discharge, clear or bloody, should be reported to your doctor immediately.

Breast cancer can occur in men, too, and they should perform this examination monthly. Regular examination will teach you what is normal for you and will give you confidence in your examination.

InfoLinks

www.mskcc.org

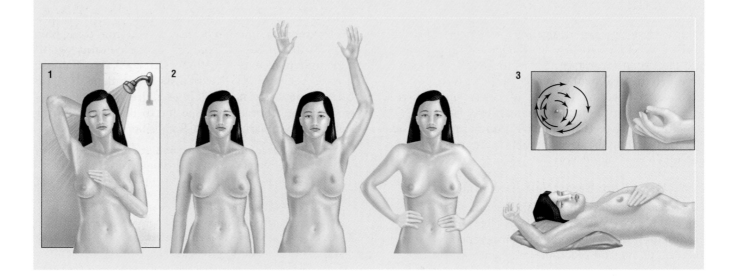

Early Detection: Mammography

Although researchers once disagreed about the age at which women should begin routine mammography and the extent to which mammography is effective in finding masses in dense breast tissue, today mammograms are physicians' best tool for the early detection of breast cancer. Accordingly, the American Cancer Society recommends that mammography begin at age 40.

Whether women begin routine mammography at 40, as advised by the ACS, or as early as 35 years of age, particularly women with previous symptoms or a family history of breast disease, women should continue these examinations on an annual basis. Recommendations regarding mammography for older women (65+) are, however, a bit more individually determined and should be discussed annually with physicians. For older women,

Table 11.2 Most Recent American Cancer Society Screening Guidelines, 2005, for the Early Detection of Cancer in Asymptomatic People

Site	Recommendation
Breast	• Yearly mammograms are recommended starting at age 40. The age at which screening should be stopped should be individualized by considering the potential risks and benefits of screening in the context of overall health status and longevity. • Clinical breast exam should be part of a periodic health exam, about every 3 years for women in their 20s and 30s, and every year for women 40 and older. • Women should know how their breasts normally feel and report any breast change promptly to their health care providers. Breast self-exam is an option for women starting in their 20s. • Women at increased risk (e.g., family history, genetic tendency, past breast cancer) should talk with their doctors about the benefits and limitations of starting mammography screening earlier, having additional tests (i.e., breast ultrasound and MRI), or having more frequent exams.
Colon & rectum	Beginning at age 50, men and women should begin screening with 1 of the examination schedules below: • A fecal occult blood test (FOBT) or fecal immunochemical test (FIT) every year • A flexible sigmoidoscopy (FSIG) every 5 years • Annual FOBT or FIT and flexible sigmoidoscopy every 5 years* • A double-contrast barium enema every 5 years • A colonoscopy every 10 years *Combined testing is preferred over either annual FOBT or FIT, or FSIG every 5 years, alone. People who are at moderate or high risk for colorectal cancer should talk with a doctor about a different testing schedule.*
Prostate	The PSA test and the digital rectal examination should be offered annually, beginning at age 50, to men who have a life expectancy of at least 10 years. Men at high risk (African American men and men with a strong family history of 1 or more first-degree relatives diagnosed with prostate cancer at an early age) should begin testing at age 45. For both men at average risk and high risk, information should be provided about what is known and what is uncertain about the benefits and limitations of early detection and treatment of prostate cancer so that they can make an informed decision about testing.
Uterus	**Cervix:** Screening should begin approximately 3 years after a woman begins having vaginal intercourse, but no later than 21 years of age. Screening should be done every year with regular Pap tests or every 2 years using liquid-based tests. At or after age 30, women who have had 3 normal test results in a row may get screened every 2 to 3 years. Alternatively, cervical cancer screening with HPV DNA testing and conventional or liquid-based cytology could be performed every 3 years. However, doctors may suggest a woman get screened more often if she has certain risk factors, such as HIV infection or a weak immune system. Women 70 years and older who have had 3 or more consecutive normal Pap tests in the last 10 years may choose to stop cervical cancer screening. Screening after total hysterectomy (with removal of the cervix) is not necessary unless the surgery was done as a treatment for cervical cancer. **Endometrium:** The American Cancer Society recommends that at the time of menopause all women should be informed about the risks and symptoms of endometrial cancer, and strongly encouraged to report any unexpected bleeding or spotting to their physicians. Annual screening for endometrial cancer with endometrial biopsy beginning at age 35 should be offered to women with or at risk for hereditary nonpolyposis colon cancer (HNPCC).
Cancer-related checkup	For individuals undergoing periodic health examinations, a cancer-related checkup should include health counseling, and, depending on a person's age and gender, might include examinations for cancers of the thyroid, oral cavity, skin, lymph nodes, testes, and ovaries, as well as for some nonmalignant diseases.

American Cancer Society guidelines for early cancer detection are assessed annually in order to identify whether there is new scientific evidence sufficient to warrant a reevaluation of current recommendations. If evidence is sufficiently compelling to consider a change or clarification in a current guideline or the development of a new guideline, a formal procedure is initiated. Guidelines are formally evaluated every 5 years regardless of whether new evidence suggests a change in the existing recommendations. There are 9 steps in this procedure, and these "guidelines for guideline development" were formally established to provide a specific methodology for science and expert judgment to form the underpinnings of specific statements and recommendations from the Society. These procedures constitute a deliberate process to ensure that all Society recommendations have the same methodological and evidence-based process at their core. This process also employs a system for rating strength and consistency of evidence that is similar to that employed by the Agency for Health Care Research and Quality (AHCRQ) and the US Preventive Services Task Force (USPSTF).©2005, American Cancer Society, Inc.

overall health status and expectations for reaching a normal life expectancy are weighed relative to the lessening cost-effectiveness of mammography.

Because of the important role routine mammography plays in the early identification of breast lesions, the Mammography Quality Standards Act (MQSA), formulated by the FDA (April 1998), is a valuable step toward ensuring that mammography is performed by experienced technicians, using correctly calibrated equipment, and interpreted by skilled radiologists. Every woman should be certain that her mammography is being performed in a MQSA-certified facility. Table 11.2

provides screening guidelines for breast and other cancers.

Treatment

Regardless of the method of detection, if a lump is found, a breast biopsy can determine whether the lump is cancerous. If the lump is cancerous but localized, treatment is highly effective, with cure rates at nearly 100 percent. The most frequently used treatments are **lumpectomy** combined with radiation, lumpectomy without radiation, and mastectomy. The use of chemotherapy following surgery is strongly advocated as well.

When drug therapy is deemed desirable in treating breast cancer, oncologists may consider two drugs that have recently become available or whose earlier protocols have been redefined. The first, tamoxifen, discussed earlier in terms of breast cancer prevention, is a hormonelike drug that prevents estrogen from stimulating cancer cell growth. The use of tamoxifen has proven highly effective in women who have the type of breast cancer stimulated by the presence of estrogen.

The second drug, herceptin, is an antibodylike agent used in combination with other chemotherapeutic drugs in highly advanced breast cancer. This newly approved drug interferes with the activity of a protein produced by the *HER-2* oncogene that normally fosters tumor cell division.

As we would expect, additional cancer treatment and prevention drugs are becoming available. Two such drugs, Fermara and Arimidex, which belong to a class of drugs called *aromatase inhibitors,* reduce or stop the production of estrogen. Currently researchers are determining the manner in which these drugs will join (or replace) tamoxifen in the treatment of breast cancer.[17]

Cervical Cancer

In 2005 an estimated 10,370 new cases of cancer of the cervix (the anatomical neck of the uterus) occurred in the United States.[1] Fortunately, the death rate from cervical cancer has dropped greatly since 1950, largely because of the **Pap test.** This test screens for precancerous cellular changes (called *cervical intraepithelial neoplasia,* or *CIN*) and malignant cells. If malignant cells are found, it is hoped that they represent only cancer in situ (at the site of origin), rather than a more advanced invasive stage of the disease. Unfortunately, this simple and relatively inexpensive screening test is still underused, particularly in women over age 60, the group in which cervical cancer is most frequently found.

Risk Factors

Because of the clear association between sexually transmitted infections and cervical cancer, risk factors for this form of cancer include early age of first intercourse, large number of sexual partners, history of infertility (which may indicate chronic pelvic inflammatory disease), and clinical evidence of *human papillomavirus* infections (see page 327 in Chapter 12). For patients with previous HPV infections or whose sexual history suggests a higher risk for HPV, a ThinPrep Pap test has been shown effective in detecting the DNA from four HPVs that are known to be cancer causing, while being as easy to use as the more widely used Pap smear. Today the test is approved only for identifying HPV infection, but it is also capable of detecting both chlamydia and gonorrhea. At the time of writing, clinical trials are underway on a vaccine designed to protect against some HPV infections. Initial human studies have been highly effective in preventing infections from the most virulent of the HPVs. On the basis of these trials it has been shown that the vaccines are approximately 93 percent effective against HPVs 16 and 18 (the most virulent of the 15 human cancer-causing HPVs), are well tolerated, and remain effective for at least 5 years.[18] In addition to sexual history, cigarette smoking and socioeconomic factors are also risk factors for cervical cancer. The latter most likely relates to less frequent medical assessment, including infrequent Pap tests. (The Personal Assessment on page 301 will help women evaluate their risk of developing cervical cancer.)

 TALKING POINTS Three risk factors are associated with HPV-induced cervical cancer: early age of first sexual intercourse, higher-than-average number of partners, and lack of protection against sexually transmitted diseases (for example, condoms). How would you introduce this topic to a teenage daughter, sister, or niece?

Prevention

Sexual abstinence is the most effective way of reducing the risk of developing cervical cancer (for example, Catholic nuns have extremely low rates of cervical cancer). However, abstinence is unlikely to be the choice for most women; other alternatives include fewer sexual partners, more careful selection of partners to minimize contact with those at

---

Key Terms

lumpectomy a surgical treatment for breast cancer in which a minimal amount of breast tissue is removed; when appropriate, this procedure is an alternative to mastectomy, in which the entire breast and underlying tissue are removed

Pap test a cancer screening procedure in which cells are removed from the cervix and examined for precancerous changes

high risk, the use of condoms, and the use of spermicides. In addition, of course, regular medical assessment, including annual Pap tests (and the ThinPrep Pap test), represents prevention through early detection. When widely available, the HPV vaccine will further increase prevention.

Early Detection

At this time, the importance of women having Pap tests for cervical cancer performed on a regular basis cannot be overemphasized. However, the specific scheduling of cervical screening is undergoing adjustment. For young sexually active women, initial screening using the Pap smear (preferably in combination with the ThinPrep) should be undertaken within 3 years of first exposure. For young women not sexually at risk, or for women who have had a hysterectomy, the initial screening with the Pap smear can be determined in consultation with health care providers. Once initiated, however, following three consecutive annual negative tests, the interval between tests may be increased upon discussion with health care providers. The American Cancer Society estimates that cervical cancer claimed the lives of 3,710 women in 2005.

The Pap test is not perfect, however. When tests are read in laboratories highly experienced in interpreting Pap slides, about 7 percent will be false negatives, resulting in a 93 percent accuracy rate. In less-experienced laboratories, false negatives may be as high as 20 percent. In addition, not all women whose test results are accurately assessed as abnormal receive adequate follow-up care, nor do they have subsequent Pap tests regularly enough. Table 11.3 discusses Pap smear results.

Table 11.3 What Pap Smear Results Mean

Pap smear results and their meanings can include:
- **Normal.** The cervical cells are healthy.
- **Unsatisfactory for evaluation.** The slide can't be read. Causes include douching, bleeding, infection, or not enough cells on the slide. The test should probably be repeated in 2–3 months.
- **Benign.** The Pap smear showed infection, irritation, or normal cell repair. If you have an infection, you might need medication.
- **Ascus.** The Pap smear showed some abnormal changes in the cells, but the cause is not clear. Infection is a common cause.
- **Low-grade changes.** You might have been infected with the human papilloma virus (HPV). Some types of the virus are associated with an increased risk for cancer of the cervix. Your health care provider will recommend specific follow-up. This might include another Pap smear or a colposcopy—a look at the cervix with a high-power microscope.
- **High-grade changes.** The cells of the cervix can progress toward cancer, but they aren't cancer yet. Fewer than half of the women with this test will develop cancer. Colposcopy is needed. Biopsy and treatment might be necessary.

In addition to changes discovered by a Pap test, symptoms that suggest potential cervical cancer include abnormal vaginal bleeding between periods and frequent spotting.

Treatment

Should precancerous cellular changes (CIN) be identified, treatment can include one of several alternatives. Physicians can destroy areas of abnormal cellular change using cryotherapy (freezing), electrocoagulation, laser destruction, or surgical removal of abnormal tissue. More advanced (invasive) cancer of the cervix can be treated with a hysterectomy combined with other established cancer therapies. A combination of radiation and chemotherapy is the most effective treatment for cervical cancer.

Uterine (Endometrial) Cancer

The American Cancer Society estimates that in 2005, 40,880 cases of uterine cancer (cancer within the inner wall of the body of the uterus, rather than within the cervix or neck of the uterus) were diagnosed in American women. In addition, 7,310 women died of the disease.[1] Although African Americans have a lower incidence of uterine cancer than white women do, their death rate is nearly twice as high.[19]

Risk Factors

Unlike cervical cancer, in which a strong viral link has been identified, the principal risk factor related to the development of endometrial cancer is a high estrogen level. Accordingly, the following factors are related to higher levels of estrogen and, thus, to the development of endometrial cancer:

- Early menarche (early onset of menstruation)
- Late menopause
- Lack of ovulation (infertility)
- Never having given birth
- Estrogen replacement therapy (ERT not moderated with progesterone)
- Use of tamoxifen (a drug used in breast cancer therapy)
- History of polycystic ovary syndrome
- Hereditary nonpolyposis colon cancer

To some degree, endometrial cancer is seen more frequently in people who are diabetic, obese, hypertensive or who have gallbladder disease.

Prevention

The risk factors associated with high levels of estrogen are areas in which prevention might be targeted. In addition, the need for regular gynecological care that includes pelvic examination is a principal factor in minimizing the risk of uterine cancer. Pregnancy and the use of oral contraceptives both provide some protection from endometrial cancer.[1]

Early Detection

Compared with cervical cancer, which is routinely identified through Pap tests, endometrial cancer is much more likely to be suspected on the basis of symptoms (irregular or postmenopausal bleeding) and confirmed by biopsy. Although more invasive, biopsy is a more effective method than ultrasound to diagnose uterine cancer.

Treatment

The treatment for early or localized endometrial cancer is generally surgical removal of the uterus (hysterectomy). Other therapies, such as radiation, chemotherapy, and hormonal therapy, may then be added to the treatment regimen. However, in terms of hormone replacement therapy (HRT), in which estrogen is combined with a synthetic progesterone, the FDA, The National Institute on Aging, and various medical associations now advise that no women 65 or older with an intact uterus should take HRT owing to several concerns, including an increased risk for endometrial cancer. For women who are undergoing menopause and experiencing troublesome symptoms such as night sweats and hot flashes, HRT should be used in the smallest doses that provide relief and for the shortest duration of time possible.

Ovarian Cancer

Since the death in 1989 of actress Gilda Radner, a star in the early years of *Saturday Night Live,* public awareness of ovarian cancer has increased in the United States. The American Cancer Society estimates that in 2005 there were 22,200 new cases diagnosed, and 16,210 women died of the disease.[1] Most cases develop in women over age 40 who have not had children or began menstruation at an early age. The highest rate is in women over age 60. Today ovarian cancer causes more deaths than does any other form of female reproductive system cancer.

For a relatively small percentage of all women (10 percent), the inheritance of either the *BRCA1* or *BRCA2* suppressor gene mutation (see page 276) significantly increases the risk of developing both breast and ovarian cancer. Today it is estimated that about 20 percent of all cases of ovarian cancer stem from these genetic mutations.

Beyond the 20 percent of cases attributed to genetic mutations, what might account for the majority of ovarian cancers? A number of studies, with varying degrees of assurance, suggest that decades of estrogen replacement therapy (ERT) used to counter symptoms of menopause,

maintain bone mass, and provide hormonal protection from heart disease could be responsible for the majority of ovarian cancer.[20] As mentioned in conjunction with endometrial cancer, today hormone replacement therapy is used, and then for only the briefest period of time.

Prevention

Methods of preventing or lowering the risk of developing ovarian cancer are very similar to those recommended for breast cancer. These include using oral contraceptives, giving birth and breast-feeding (for at least 3 months), reducing dietary fat intake, abstaining from alcohol use, and performing regular physical activity.

For the small group of women with a strong family history of ovarian cancer, a **prophylactic oophorectomy** should be seriously considered. In this surgical procedure, both ovaries are removed. Carefully monitored hormone replacement therapy is then used to provide the protective advantages of estrogen in maintaining cardiovascular health and bone density.

Early Detection

Because of its vague symptoms, ovarian cancer has been referred to as a *silent cancer.* Women in whom ovarian cancer has been diagnosed often report that the only symptoms of their cancer's presence were digestive disturbances, gas, urinary incontinence, stomach distention, and a crampy abdominal pain over a few short weeks. The latter should be medically evaluated immediately.[21]

For women with a strong family history of ovarian cancer (four primary family members who have had breast or ovarian cancer, with two or more cases occurring before age 50) or women of Ashkenazi Jewish descent (see page 276), genetic screening and transvaginal ultrasound screening are likely to be recommended. These women may also be referred for participation in one of several prevention trials now under way.

Treatment

At this time, treatment of ovarian cancer requires surgical removal of the ovary, followed by aggressive use of chemotherapy. Use of the chemotherapeutic drug Taxol, obtained from the bark and needles of the Pacific yew tree, results in a 50 percent survival rate 19 months after the completion of therapy. Most recently, use of an experimental

---

Key Terms

prophylactic oophorectomy surgical removal of the ovaries to prevent ovarian cancer in women at high risk of developing the disease

three-drug combination has resulted in a 70 percent survival rate 22 months after chemotherapy.

Prostate Cancer

If the names Bob Dole, General Norman Schwarzkopf, Colin Powell, and Rudy Giuliani are familiar, then you know four older men who have been diagnosed with and treated for prostate cancer. In fact, prostate cancer is so common that in 2005 an estimated 232,090 new cases were diagnosed and 30,500 men died of the disease.[1] Prostate cancer is the second leading cause of cancer deaths in American men, exceeded only by lung cancer deaths. Cancer of the prostate is the most common form of cancer in men and a leading cause of death from cancer in older men.

The prostate gland is a walnut-size gland located near the base of the penis. It surrounds the neck of the bladder and the urethra. The prostate secretes a number of components of semen, such as nutrients used to fuel sperm motility.

Risk Factors

Compared with other cancers, the risk factors for prostate cancer are less clearly defined. The most predictable risk factor is age. Nearly 80 percent of all prostate cancer cases are diagnosed in men over 65 years of age; however, cases in men under age 50 are infrequent. African American men and men with a family history of prostate cancer are at greater risk of developing this form of cancer [167.4/100,000 (W) versus 271.3/100,000 (AA)].[1] A link between prostate cancer and dietary fat intake, including excessive red meat and dairy product consumption, has also been suggested. With the discovery of the *BRCA1* and *BRCA2* genes related to breast and ovarian cancer, a genetic link with prostate cancer was also established. Men with one of these genetic mutations have an increased risk of developing prostate cancer.

Prevention

Although the American Cancer Society does not specifically address prevention of prostate cancer, prevention is not an unrealistic goal. Clearly, moderation of dietary fat intake is a preventive step. Increased dietary intake levels of vitamin E and the micronutrient selenium have been shown to play a preventive role in prostate cancer. In addition, effective treatment of benign prostatic hyperplasia (BPH) (prostate enlargement) with the drug Proscar (finasteride) has proven effective in preventing low-grade tumors in clinical trials.[22]

Early Detection

The symptoms of prostate disease, including prostate cancer, include difficulty in urinating, frequent urination, continued wetness following urination, blood in urine, low-back pain, and aches in upper thighs. A physician should be consulted if any of these symptoms appear, particularly in men aged 50 or older. Screening for prostate cancer should begin by age 40. This screening consists of an annual rectal examination performed by a physician and a blood test, the **prostate-specific antigen (PSA) test,** administered every 2 years. Another version of the PSA test has also been developed. This test can identify the "free" antigen most closely associated with the more aggressive forms of prostate cancer, thus cutting down on the false positives and extensive use of biopsies. In addition, an ultrasound rectal examination is used in men whose PSA scores are abnormally high. Currently debate is occurring within the medical community regarding the need to increase rigor of PSA levels and the need to look more closely at the suddenness at which levels increase.

Treatment

Today prostate cancer is treated surgically, or through the use of external radiation or the implantation of radioactive seeds (brachytherapy) into the gland, in combination with short-term use of hormonal therapy. Of course, each form of treatment carries the potential for side effects, including an 80 percent chance of impotence over a 10-year period; incontinence with surgery; diarrhea and tiredness with external radiation; some anal discomfort in association with the implantation of radioactive seeds into the prostate with internal radiation, and thinning of the bones with long-term hormone therapy.

One form of prostate cancer grows so slowly that men whose cancer is of this type, whose tumors are very localized, and whose life expectancy is less than 10 years at the time of diagnosis, do not receive treatment but rather are closely monitored for any progression of the cancer. For men who have the more aggressive form of the cancer, or whose tumor is no longer localized, physicians can employ a range of therapies, including surgery, radiation, chemotherapy, and hormonal therapy. In addition, an experimental vaccine has recently been tested on humans with promising results.[23]

Testicular Cancer

Cancer of the testicle is among the least common forms of cancer; however, it is the most common solid tumor

---

Key Terms

prostate-specific antigen (PSA) test a blood test used to identify prostate-specific antigen, an early indicator that the immune system has recognized and mounted a defense against prostate cancer

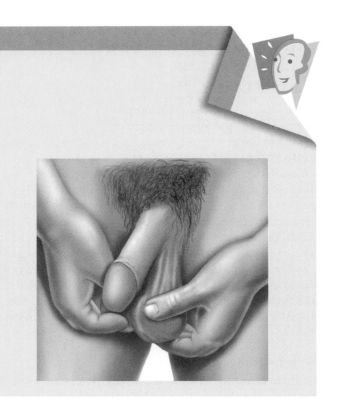
in men ages 15 to 34. Awareness of this type of cancer was raised in 1996 and 1997, when seven-time winner of the tour de France Lance Armstrong and champion figure skater Scott Hamilton were diagnosed with testicular cancer. In both men, chronic fatigue and abdominal discomfort were the first symptoms of the disease. The American Cancer Society estimates that in 2005 testicular cancer was diagnosed in 8,010 men and caused the deaths of 390.[1]

Risk Factors

Risk factors for testicular cancer are variable, ranging from family history to environmental factors. The disease is more frequently seen in White Americans and in men whose testicles were undescended during childhood. Additional risk factors, such as difficulty during the mother's pregnancy, elevated temperature in the groin, and mumps during childhood, have been reported. The incidence of this cancer has been increasing in recent decades, while a corresponding drop in sperm levels has also been observed. Although no single explanation can be given for these changes, environmental factors such as agricultural pesticide toxicity may be involved. Once pesticides are concentrated in the tissues of the human body, during pregnancy they mimic estrogen. This, in turn, may lead to testicular dysgenesis syndrome, or the failure of the testicles to develop normally.[24]

Testicular cancer is more frequently seen among white-collar workers than among people in blue-collar occupations. The suspicion that testicular cancer is linked to vasectomies appears to be unfounded.

Prevention

Because risk factors for testicular cancer are so variable, prevention is limited to regular self-examination of the testicles. Symptoms such as fatigue, abdominal discomfort, and enlargement of the testicle should be reported to a physician, since these can be associated with other disease processes. A male infant with one or both testicles in the undescended position (resulting in an empty scrotum) should be seen promptly by a physician so that corrective procedures can be undertaken.

Early Detection

In addition to the fatigue and abdominal distress reported by both Armstrong and Hamilton, other symptoms of testicular cancer include a small, painless lump on the side or near the front of the testicle, a swollen or enlarged testicle, and a heaviness or dragging sensation in the groin or scrotum. The importance of testicular self-examination, as well as early diagnosis and prompt treatment, cannot be overemphasized for men in the at-risk age group of 15 to 34 years. Changing for the Better above explains how to perform a testicular self-examination.

Treatment

Depending on the type, stage, and degree of localization of the tumor, surgical intervention generally includes removal of the testicle, spermatic cord, and regional lymph nodes. Chemotherapy and radiation might also be used. Today, treatment is very effective, with 96 percent of all testicular cancer patients surviving 5 years and 99.4 percent surviving 5 years when the cancer was localized at the time of diagnosis. It should be noted, however, that concern exists regarding the development of other forms of cancer, such as leukemia, later in life.

Colorectal Cancer

Cancer of the colon and rectum (colorectal cancer) cause the second greatest number of cancer deaths, 56,290 in 2005, second only to lung cancer. In the most general sense, two types of tumors, carcinoma and lymphoma, can be found in both the colon and rectum. However, even within the most common form of colorectal cancer, there may subtle difference in type of tumors (or their origins) which influence the degree of potential spread and, thus, the nature of treatment itself. Fortunately, when diagnosed in a localized state, colorectal cancer has a relatively high survival rate (90 percent when localized and 63.4 percent for all stages).[1]

Risk Factors

Underlying the development of colorectal cancer are at least two potentially important areas of risk: genetic susceptibility and dietary patterns. Genes have recently been discovered that lead to familial colon cancer and familial polyposis (abnormal tissue growth that occurs before the formation of cancer) and are believed to be responsible for the tendency of colorectal cancer to run in families. Dietary risk factors include diets that are high in saturated fat from red meat and low in fruits and vegetables, which contain antioxidant vitamins and fiber. In regard to fiber's ability to prevent colorectal cancer, however, the ability of dietary fiber, when taken in supplement form, is in question.

Prevention

Small outpouchings in the lower intestinal tract wall, called *polyps,* are frequently important in the eventual development of colorectal cancer. Prompt removal of polyps has been shown to lower the risk of colorectal cancer. Further, some evidence indicates that the development of colorectal cancer may be prevented or slowed through regular exercise, the regular use of low-dose (81 mg) aspirin (consistently for at least two decades), an increase in dietary calcium intake, and long-term folic acid supplementation. Additionally, oral contraceptive use may be protective for women.

Again, routine screening for colorectal cancer should be considered a form of prevention, much as PSA testing is for prostate cancer and mammography is for breast cancer.

Early Detection

Symptoms of colorectal cancer include bleeding from the rectum, blood in the stool, and a change in bowel habits. In addition, a family history of inflammatory bowel disease, polyp formation, or colorectal cancer should make one more alert to symptoms.[1] In people over age 50, any sudden change in bowel habits that lasts 10 days or longer should be evaluated by a physician. The American Cancer Society recommends preventive health care that includes digital (manual) rectal examination after age 40, a stool blood test after age 50, and sigmoidoscopy every 3 to 5 years and **colonoscopy** every 10 years after age 50. Some experts question the advisability of using **sigmoidoscopy** as the routine screening procedure for colorectal cancer in comparison to using colonoscopy, which can more effectively find distal (higher up in the colon) cancerous changes.

Although colonoscopy is currently the "gold standard" in the screening for colorectal cancer, new technologies are on the horizon. Four alternatives include the PreGen-Plus test that identifies cancer-indicating DNA mutations appearing in stool samples; a yet-named blood test capable of identifying "loss of imprinting" (LOI) factor associated with a high risk for colorectal cancer; virtual colonoscopy using a miniaturized camera that can, after being swallowed, be followed as it moves through the lower intestinal tract, generating digitized pictures of the entire colon; and the CT colonography (CTC) that uses serial tomography (type of CAT scan) to visualize the colon, thus eliminating the need to scope the colon.

It should be noted that the digital stool-sample test, used as the only stool-sample test by most doctors and taken during physical examinations,[25] as well as the newer test to find traces of cancer cell DNA in the stool, have both been found to be less effective than previously believed.[26]

Treatment

When one or more of these screening procedures suggests the possibility of disease within the lower intestinal tract, a careful visual evaluation of the entire length of the colon will be undertaken. During colonoscopy, areas of concern can be biopsied and the presence of a malignancy

---

Key Terms

colonoscopy (co lun **os** ko py) examination of the entire length of the colon, using a flexible fiberoptic scope to inspect the structure's inner lining

sigmoidoscopy examination of the sigmoid colon (lowest section of the large intestine) using a short, flexible fiberoptic scope

confirmed. Upon diagnosis, a localized and noninvasive malignancy will be removed surgically. When an invasive tumor is identified, supportive treatment with radiation or chemotherapy is necessary. Metastatic cancer requires chemotherapy.

Pancreatic Cancer

Pancreatic cancer is one of the most lethal forms of cancer, with a survival rate of only 4 percent 5 years after diagnosis.[1] Because of this gland's important functions in both digestion and metabolic processes related to glucose utilization (see the discussion of diabetes mellitus), its destruction by a malignancy leaves the body in a state incompatible with living.

In 2005 an estimated 32,180 new cases of pancreatic cancer were diagnosed and 31,800 deaths occurred.[1]

Risk Factors

Pancreatic cancer is more common in men than women, occurs more frequently with age, and develops most often in African American men. Smoking is clearly a risk factor for this form of cancer, with smokers more than twice as likely to develop the disease. Other risk factors have been tentatively suggested, such as chronic inflammation of the pancreas (pancreatitis), diabetes mellitus, alcohol-induced liver deterioration (cirrhosis), obesity, and high-fat diets.[1] Relatively little else is known about risk factors and, thus, prevention.

Prevention

Not smoking and abstaining from alcohol use are the most effective steps toward preventing this form of cancer. Further, reducing the risk of type 2 diabetes mellitus, through weight loss and exercise, (see page 292) would also make an important contribution to prevention. Annual medical examinations are, of course, associated with overall cancer prevention.

Early Detection

Early detection of this cancer is difficult because of the absence of symptoms until late in its course. Perhaps for people with a history of chronic pancreatitis, physicians might consider routine ultrasound assessment or computerized axial tomography scans (CAT scans). Once symptoms appear, a biopsy is performed.

Treatment

At this time there is no effective treatment for pancreatic cancer. Surgical removal of malignant sites within the gland, in addition to radiation and chemotherapy, is usually tried. Certainly, if a particular patient with pancreatic cancer qualifies, enrollment in a clinical trial would be worth consideration.

Lymphatic Cancer

An estimated 63,740 new cases of lymphoma (7,350 cases of Hodgkin's disease and 56,390 cases of non-Hodgkin's lymphoma) were diagnosed in 2005. The number of deaths from both forms of lymphoma was near 20,610. The incidence of Hodgkin's disease has declined over the last 30 years, while the incidence of non-Hodgkin's disease has nearly doubled, but is now holding steady.

Risk Factors

Risk factors for lymphoma are difficult to determine. Some possible factors are a general reduction in immune protection, exposure to toxic environmental chemicals such as pesticides and herbicides, and viral infections.[1] As you will learn in Chapter 12, the virus that causes AIDS (HIV) is a leukemia/lymphoma virus that was initially called HTLV-III (human T-cell leukemia/lymphoma virus-type III). A related leukemia/lymphoma virus, HTLV-I, is also suspected in the development of lymphatic cancer. The Epstein-Barr virus (EBV) may also play a role in lymphatic cancer development.

Prevention

Beyond limiting exposure to toxic chemicals and sexually transmitted viruses, few recommendations can be made about prevention. Again, early detection and diagnosis can serve as a form of prevention, since early-stage cancer is more survivable than advanced disease.

Early Detection

Unlike other cancers, the early symptoms of lymphoma are diverse and similar to symptoms of other illnesses, most of which are not serious. These symptoms include enlarged lymph nodes (frequently a sign of any infection that the immune system is fighting), fever, itching, weight loss, and anemia.

Treatment

Although surgery (beyond a biopsy) is usually not associated with the treatment of lymphoma, a variety of other therapies are employed. Depending on the stage and type of lymphoma, therapy may involve only radiation treatment of localized lymph nodes, as is seen in non-Hodgkin's lymphoma. Radiation combined with chemotherapy is generally used in the treatment late-stage non-Hodgkin's lymphoma. More recently, other therapies, including more aggressive chemotherapy, monoclonal antibody therapy, and bone marrow and stem cell transplantation, have been employed.

After completion of therapy, 1-year survival rates for Hodgkin's disease are near 95 percent and near 77 percent for non-Hodgkin's lymphoma. By the end of 5 years, these rates have dropped to 84 percent and 55 percent, respectively.[1] Lower rates of survival are seen at 10 years and beyond.

Skin Cancer

Thanks largely to our desire for a fashionable tan, many teens and adults have spent more time in the sun (and in tanning booths) than their skin can tolerate. As a result, skin cancer, once common only among people who had to work in the sun, is occurring with alarming frequency. In 2005, more than a million Americans developed basal or squamous cell skin cancer and 59,580 cases of highly dangerous malignant melanoma were diagnosed.[1]

Deaths from skin cancer do occur, with 10,590 estimated in 2005. More than 80 percent of these deaths were the result of malignant melanoma.

Risk Factors

Severe sunburning during childhood and chronic sun exposure during adolescence and younger adulthood are largely responsible for the "epidemic" of skin cancer being reported. The current emphasis on screening for skin cancer may also be increasing the incidence of early-stage cancer being reported. Occupational exposure to some hydrocarbon compounds can also cause skin cancer.

In spite of the progress reported by the American Academy of Dermatology, Americans continue to seek natural sources of sun or tanning salons for cosmetically related tanning, or they find that their exposure cannot be avoided owing to the nature of their jobs. In regard to "purposeful tanning" either outdoors or indoors, recent research has given some credibility to the contention that tanning is emotionally "addictive."[27] Researchers are now beginning to see this factor as a detrimental player in ongoing efforts to persuade the public to increase their avoidance of ultraviolet radiation exposure.

Prevention

Prevention of skin cancer should be a high priority for people who enjoy the sun or must work outdoors. The use of sunscreen with an a sun protection factor (SPF) of 15 or greater is very important. In addition, parents can help their children prevent skin cancer later in life by restricting their outdoor play from 11:00 A.M. to 2:00 P.M., requiring them to wear hats that shade their faces, and applying a sunscreen with an SPF of 15 on them regardless of skin tone. An evaluation of sunscreen effectiveness studies by Sloan-Kettering Cancer Center, however, suggests that sunscreens provide little protection against the deeply penetrating UV-A rays associated with the development of melanoma in susceptible people, and less protection than once thought against the UV-B rays associated with burning and wrinkling of the skin. Practicing dermatologists nonetheless continue to recommend their use. Regardless of the extent to which sunscreens provide protection, users are reminded that the level of protection provided is not doubled by simply doubling the SPF—for example, a sunscreen carrying an SPF of 30 does not provide twice the protection provided by a product with an SPF of 15.

The Personal Assessment on page 301 will help you determine your risk of developing this kind of cancer.

Early Detection

Although many doctors do not emphasize this point enough, the key to the successful treatment of skin cancer is early detection. For basal cell or squamous cell cancer, a pale, waxlike, pearly nodule or red, scaly patch may be the first symptom. Other types of skin cancer may be indicated by a gradual change in the appearance of an existing mole. A physician should be consulted if such a change is noted. Melanoma usually begins as a small, molelike growth that increases progressively in size, changes color, ulcerates, and bleeds easily. To help detect melanoma, the American Cancer Society recommends using the guidelines below:

A is for asymmetry.

B is for border irregularity.

C is for color (change).

D is for a diameter greater than 6 mm.

E is for elevation (raised margins).

Figure 11-3 shows a mole that would be considered harmless and one that clearly demonstrates the ABCDE characteristics just described. (Changing for the Better on page 288 shows how to make a regular inspection of the skin.)

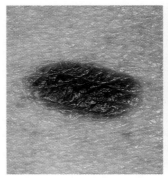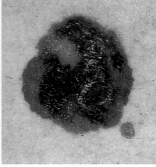

A   B

Figure 11-3 A: Normal mole. This type of lesion is often seen in large numbers on the skin of young adults and can affect any body site. Note its symmetrical shape, regular borders, uniform color, and relatively small size (about 6 millimeters). **B:** Malignant melanoma. Note its asymmetrical shape, irregular borders, uneven color, and relatively large size (about 2 centimeters).

Self-Examination for Melanoma

Through a routine physical exam, my brother found out he has melanoma. How should I check myself for this condition?

How to look for melanoma

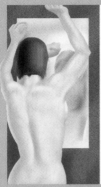 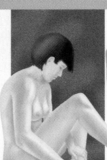 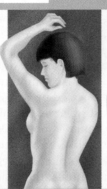 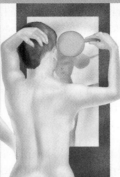 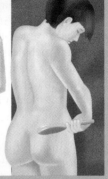

1. Examine your body front and back in the mirror, then right and left sides with arms raised.

2. Bend your elbows and carefully look at your palms, forearms, and under your upper arms.

3. Look at the backs of your legs and feet, the spaces between your toes, and the soles of your feet.

4. Examine the back of your neck and scalp with a hand mirror. Part your hair for a closer look.

5. Finally, check your back and buttocks with a mirror.

What to look for
Potential signs of malignancy in moles or pigmented spots:

Asymmetry	**Irregularity**	**Color**	**Size**
One half unlike the other half	Border irregular or poorly defined	Color varies from one area to another; shades of tan, brown, or black	Diameter larger than 6 mm, as a rule (diameter of a pencil eraser)

Most recently, a relationship between the presence of abnormal moles, called *dysplastic nevi* (flat, irregularly shaped, mottled in color, with irregular edges), and the risk of developing malignant melanoma has been established. By counting these "indicator moles," physicians can judge the relative risk of developing this serious form of skin cancer before it first appears.

Table 11.4 lists cancer's seven warning signs.

Treatment

When nonmelanoma skin cancer is found, an almost 100 percent cure rate can be expected. Treatment of these skin cancers can involve surgical removal by traditional excising or laser vaporization, destruction by burning or freezing, or destruction using x-ray therapy. When the more serious melanomas are found at an early stage, a high cure rate (95 percent) is accomplished using the same techniques. However, when malignant melanomas are more advanced, extensive surgery and chemotherapy are necessary. The 5-year survival rate for regionalized forms of the

Table 11.4 Cancer's Seven Warning Signals

Listed below are the 7 warning signs of cancer, which the acronym **CAUTION** will help you remember.

1. **C**hange in bowel or bladder habits
2. **A** sore that does not heal
3. **U**nusual bleeding or discharge
4. **T**hickening or lump in the breast or elsewhere
5. **I**ndigestion or difficulty in swallowing
6. **O**bvious change in a wart or mole
7. **N**agging cough or hoarseness

If you have a warning signal for more than 5 days, see your doctor!

disease drops to 60 percent, and, unfortunately, long-term disease recovery is uncommon (16 percent).[1]

Status of the "War on Cancer"

It has been over 35 years since President Nixon (1971) declared a national "War On Cancer," and today the results are both encouraging and discouraging. On the positive side impressive technological advances have been and continue to be made in the diagnosis and treatment of cancer. As mentioned throughout the chapter, new screening procedures as well as treatment protocols seem to appear at a consistent rate. Additionally, the death rates from a variety of cancers have fallen, including a 70 percent decrease in the rate for Hodgkin's disease and a 14 percent decline in the death rate for breast cancer. Death rates for cervical, stomach, uterine, colon, bladder, and thyroid cancers have also fallen. Particularly important is a general increase in the public's awareness of cancer prevention and early detection.

On the negative side is the reality that cancer is not only a biological disease but also a disease (or more than 100 diseases) with strong sociopolitical implications. Central to this area are factors such as the inability of the majority of Americans to make needed changes in lifestyle in regard to smoking, alcohol use, exercise, weight management, and dietary practices. Also impeding progress is the absence of health care insurance for 45 million Americans, which prevents early diagnosis and treatment of cancer. In fact, virtually every cancer in adults is impacted negatively by one or more of these largely modifiable complicating factors.

In addition to factors such as the lack of health insurance for millions of Americans and the inability (or unwillingness) of large segments of the American population to modify current lifestyles, a third force, the federal government, is also potentially negatively affecting the war against cancer. In letter dated January 25, 2005, a coalition of 40 organizations working to win the cancer war (including the American Cancer Society, the American College of Surgeons, and the Cancer Research and Prevention Foundation) called on the president to reconsider his planned overall cut in the Fiscal Year 2006 budget of the National Cancer Institute (NCI). The coalition, *One Voice Against Cancer,* reminded the administration that the NCI's goal of eliminating death and suffering from cancer by 2015 will incur egregious damage from a yearly parade of budget reductions.[28]

Prevention Through Risk Reduction

Because cancer will probably continue to be the leading cause of death among adults under the age of 80, you should explore ways to reduce your risk of developing cancer. The following factors, which could make you vulnerable to cancer, can be controlled or at least recognized.

- *Know your family history.* You are the recipient of the genetic strengths and weaknesses of your biological parents and your more distant relatives. If you are able to determine that cancer is prevalent in your family medical history, you cannot afford to disregard this fact. It may be appropriate for you to be screened for certain types of cancer more often or at a young age. The importance of family history was clearly seen in our discussion of the *BRCA1/BRCA2* inheritance pattern and related decisions about prophylactic mastectomy and prophylactic oophorectomy.

- *Select and monitor your occupation carefully.* Because of recently discovered relationships between cancer and occupations that bring employees into contact with carcinogenic agents, you must be aware of the risks posed by certain job selections and assignments. Worksites where you will come into frequent contact with pesticides, strong solvents, volatile hydrocarbons, and airborne fibers could pay well but also shorten your life. The importance of this point is evident in reviewing the current list of environmental carcinogens studies funded by the National Cancer Institute. Included are studies that focus on indoor air pollution (tobacco smoke and cooking oils), dust (cotton, grain, plastic, and wood), organic solvents (benzene, carbon tetrachloride, toluene, xylene, and chlordane), organophosphates (diazinon, dichlorvos, malathion, triazines, and cyaniazine), polybrominated biphenyls, polychlorinated biphenyls, fumigants (ethylene), water pollution (chloride, phosphene, and fluoride), petroleum products (diesel fuel, gasoline, jet fuel), radiation (radon, neutron therapy, and reactor accidents), biological agents (chlamydia, HIV/HPV, helicobacter, hepatitis B and C) and radioisotopes (iodine and radium).

- *Do not use tobacco products.* You may want to review Chapter 9 on the overwhelming evidence linking all forms of tobacco use (including smokeless tobacco) to the development of cancer. Smoking, along with obesity, is so detrimental to health that it is considered a co-number-one preventable cause of death.

- *Monitor environmental exposure to carcinogens.* When one considers carcinogenic concerns related to types of employment, residential radon levels, ozone depletion leading to increased exposure to solar radiation, and environmental tobacco smoke, one realizes that the environment holds great potential as a source of carcinogenic exposure. To the extent to which it is possible to select the environment in which you will reside, work, and recreate, you should add selecting a low-risk environment to your list of cancer-prevention activities.

- *Follow a sound diet.* As mentioned in conjunction with folic acid and colorectal cancer and high-fat diets and prostate cancer, dietary patterns are known to play both a causative and a preventive role in cancer. (Review

Chapter 5 for information about dietary practices and the incidence of various diseases, including cancer. In that chapter, the role of fruits and vegetables known to be sources of cancer-preventing phytochemicals is introduced. Good sources include a wide variety of fruits and vegetables, particularly the cruciferous vegetables, including cauliflower, broccoli, and brussels sprouts, and fruits high in beta-carotene, vitamin C, and fiber.)

Should research demonstrate an even clearer role for nutrients, **chemoprevention** may become an even more widely practiced component of cancer prevention. Chemoprevention is not limited to food items and dietary supplements but can also involve pharmaceutical agents, such as aspirin, estrogen replacement therapy, and hormone replacement therapy.

- *Control your body weight.* For women, obesity is related to a higher incidence of cancer of the uterus, ovary, and breast because obesity correlates with high estrogen levels. Maintaining a desirable body weight could improve overall health and lead to more successful management of cancer should it develop. Additionally, consider carefully whether you want to follow the currently popular high-protein, high-fat diets (Chapter 6), given their recognized carcinogenic potential.

- *Exercise regularly.* Chapter 4 discusses in detail the importance of regular moderate exercise to all aspects of health, including reducing the risk of chronic illnesses. Moderate exercise increases the body's ability to deliver oxygen to its tissues and thus to reduce the formation of cancer-enhancing free radicals formed during incomplete oxidation of nutrients. Moderate exercise also stimulates the production of enzymes that remove free radicals.

- *Limit your exposure to the sun.* It is important to heed this message even if you enjoy many outdoor activities.

Particularly for people with light complexions, the radiation received through chronic exposure to the sun may foster the development of skin cancer.

- *Consume alcohol in moderation if at all.* People who consume a lot of alcohol have an increased prevalence of several types of cancer, including cancer of the oral cavity, larynx, and esophagus. Whether this results directly from the presence of carcinogens in alcohol or is more closely related to the alcohol user's tendency to smoke has not yet been established.

Cancer and Wellness

When you carefully consider the preceding suggestions, you will clearly see that you can do a great deal to prevent or at least minimize the development of cancer. A wellness-oriented lifestyle is the best weapon in your "personal war against cancer." However, all risk factor reduction is relative. Observation and experience tell us that life cannot be totally structured around the desire to achieve maximum longevity or reduce morbidity at all costs. Most people need to strike a balance between life that is emotionally, socially, and spiritually satisfying and life that is structured solely for the purpose of living a long time and minimizing exposure to illness. Regardless of our personal lifestyles, however, we can educate others, provide comfort and support to those

---

Key Terms

chemoprevention cancer prevention using food, food supplements, and medications thought to bolster the immune system and reduce the damage caused by carcinogens

---

who are living with cancer, and support the funding of continuing and innovative new cancer research.

Chronic Health Conditions

In addition to the two most widely recognized chronic health problems of adulthood—cardiovascular disease and cancer—adults can experience an array of other chronic health conditions. What all these chronic conditions have in common is the ability to cause significant change in the lives of people—both on the part of the affected person and his or her family members and friends (see Discovering Your Spirituality on page 293).

Some of these conditions are seen in early adulthood, such as lupus and Crohn's disease. Others, such as type 2 diabetes, generally do not appear until nearer middle age, although today it is appearing at much younger ages. However, some chronic diseases seen during adulthood have their origins in childhood, such as type 1 diabetes.

Systemic Lupus Erythematosus

Systemic lupus erythematosus (SLE), or simply *lupus*, is perhaps the most familiar of a class of chronic conditions known as **autoimmune** disorders, or connective tissue diseases. Collectively, these conditions reflect a concentrated and inappropriate attack by the body's immune system on its own tissues, which then serve as *self-antigens* (see Chapter 12 for a discussion of the immune response).

The name *systemic lupus erythematosus* reflects the widespread (systemic, or systemwide) destruction of fibrous connective tissue and other tissues and the appearance in some patients of a reddish rash (erythematosus) that imparts a characteristic "mask" to the face. Lupus is most often seen in women who developed the condition during young adulthood, although it is now known that autoantibodies may first appear in the blood as much as a decade before the first observable symptoms of SLE appear.[29] The course of the condition is gradual, with intermittent periods of inflammation, stiffness, fatigue, pleurisy (chest pain), and discomfort over wide areas of the body, including muscles, joints, and skin. Similar changes may also occur with tissue of the nervous system, kidneys, and heart.[30] Diagnosis is made on the basis of symptoms and several laboratory tests.

Why the immune system turns on the body in such an aggressive manner is not fully understood. It is likely, however, that a combination of genetic predisposition and an earlier viral infection or environmental exposure may be involved. Episodes (called *flares*) of lupus often follow exposure to the sun, periods of fatigue, or an infectious disease; all these should be avoided to the fullest extent possible. Management of the condition generally may involve long-term (and low-dose) use of prednisone (a corticosteroid) or newer medications, such as Plaquenil (hydroxychloroquine), may be employed.

Crohn's Disease

A wide array of chronic conditions that involve the gastrointestinal system are collectively referred to as *inflammatory bowel disease (IBD)*. One type of IBD is Crohn's disease, a deterioration of the inner surface and muscular layer of the intestinal wall that affects nearly 500,000 Americans, many of traditional college age. The disease commonly affects the terminal end of the small intestine and the beginning of the large intestine, or colon. When the disease is active (it frequently has long periods of remission), symptoms include abdominal pain, fever, diarrhea, weight loss, and rectal bleeding that leads to anemia.

Although the cause of Crohn's disease is not fully understood, a genetic predisposition and an autoimmune response are the principal factors. A variety of chromosomes are under investigation.[31] Multiple forms of Crohn's disease are thought to exist, with each reflecting different genetic components.

When a person reports the symptoms just described, the physician quickly suspects some form of IBD, such as Crohn's disease. Accordingly, blood tests and a complete series of gastrointestinal (GI) X-rays are undertaken. Additional diagnostic procedures could include a CT scan of the GI tract, endoscopic examination of the GI tract, and a biopsy of the intestinal wall. Positive results of these tests confirm the existence of Crohn's disease.

Today an array of medications is available or in development for use in management of Crohn's disease. Among these medications is infliximab (Remicade), an antibody to tumor necrosis factor (TNF) that has proven highly effective in managing some forms of the disease. Although still approved for use, Remicade now carries two new cautionary labels—one warning against an increased risk of fatal blood and central nervous system conditions and the second against an increased risk of lymphoma.

Although Crohn's disease can be well managed, intestinal obstructions can occur as a result of the progressive thickening of the intestinal wall in the areas of inflammation. Surgery may be necessary to remove the obstruction. People with Crohn's disease may encounter further complications, including gallstones, arthritis, and chronic irritation of the skin.

> **Key Terms**
>
> **autoimmune** an immune response against the tissues of a person's own body

Multiple Sclerosis

For proper nerve conduction to occur in the brain and the spinal cord, an insulating sheath of myelin must surround the neurons. In the progressive disease multiple sclerosis (MS), the cells that produce myelin are destroyed and myelin production ceases. Eventually, the vital functions of the body can no longer be carried out. The cause of MS is not fully understood. Research continues to focus on virus-induced autoimmune mechanisms in which T cells attack viral-infected myelin-producing cells. The virus most strongly suspected at this time is the Epstein-Barr virus, because antibodies for the Epstein-Barr Nuclear Antigen (EBNA) are found in higher than normal levels in people with diagnosed MS.[32] Some immune system evidence of this virus can be found in about 90 percent of all Americans, but not at the levels associated with MS.

Usually, MS first appears during the young adult years. It may take one of four forms, depending on the interplay of periods of stabilization (remitting), renewed deterioration (relapsing), continuous deterioration (progressive) or combinations of the above. The initial symptoms are often visual impairment, prickling and burning in the extremities, or an altered **gait.** Deterioration of nervous system function occurs in various forms during the course of MS. In the most advanced stages of MS, movement is greatly impaired, and mental deterioration may be present. It should be noted, however, that MS may be a "silent epidemic" among children, including those younger than 10 years of age. To facilitate a more timely diagnosis of MS, children showing mild tremors or reporting intermittent dimming of vision should be seen by a pediatric neurologist.[33] It is currently estimated that over 20,000 American children may have early-onset MS.

Treatment of MS involves reducing the severity of the symptoms and extending the periods of remission. Today a variety of therapies are used, including immune-targeted drugs, steroid drugs, drugs that relieve muscle spasms, injection of nerve blockers, and physical therapy.

The development of immune system–related medications is at the center of today's treatment of MS. Until very recently four immune system-related medications, Avonex, Betaserone, Coplaxone, and Tysabri (aka Antegren), were at the forefront of treating MS. Tydabri, however, was voluntarily withdrawn from the marketplace because of a small number of fatal reactions. The remaining three medications (sometimes called the A, B, C of MS treatment) remain highly effective, depending on the specific form of MS being addressed, in delaying the onset of the most debilitating symptoms.

Additional medications are available to address complications of MS, such as spasticity. Also, initial studies involving the implantation of stem cells into mice have proven promising in reducing the number of brain lesions, as has the use of statins (cholesterol-lowering drugs) in MS-developing laboratory mice.

In addition to drug therapy, psychotherapy is an important adjunct to the treatment of MS. Profound periods of depression often accompany the initial diagnosis of this condition. Emotional support is helpful in dealing with the progressive impairments associated with most forms of the condition.

Diabetes Mellitus

Before beginning a discussion of diabetes mellitus, we will review the names that have been used over the years to describe this serious and an increasingly widespread medical condition. There are two principal forms of diabetes mellitus: *type 2* (the most common form) and *type 1* (a less common form); this book uses these names. However, some older persons refer to diabetes mellitus in both of its principal forms simply as "sugar diabetes." Other people might be familiar with type 2, the form that usually begins during adulthood, as "adult-onset diabetes mellitus" and type 1 as "juvenile-onset diabetes mellitus," since this form most often begins during childhood. Persons with a fuller understanding of diabetes' physiology, might call type 2 "non-insulin-dependent diabetes mellitus," since extrinsic (outside) sources of insulin are not required; they might call type 1 "insulin-dependent diabetes mellitus," since it requires extrinsic sources of insulin in its management.

Type 2 Diabetes Mellitus

In people who do not have diabetes mellitus the body's need for energy is met through the "burning" of glucose (blood sugar) within the cells. Glucose is absorbed from the digestive tract and carried to the cells by the blood system. Passage of glucose into the cell is achieved through a transport system that moves the glucose molecule across the cell's membrane. Activation of this glucose transport mechanism requires the presence of the hormone insulin. Specific receptor sites for **insulin** can be found on the cell membrane. In addition to its role in the transport of glucose into sensitive cells, insulin is required for the conversion of glucose into glycogen in the liver and the formation of fatty acids in adipose cells. Insulin is produced in

---

Key Terms

gait pattern of walking

insulin a pancreatic hormone required by the body for the effective metabolism of glucose (blood sugar)

---

the cells of the islets of Langerhans in the pancreas. The release of insulin from the pancreas corresponds to the changing levels of glucose within the blood.[34]

In adults, and tragically in a rapidly increasing percentage of children and adolescents, with a **genetic predisposition** for developing type 2 diabetes, a trigger mechanism (most likely obesity) begins a process through which the body cells become increasingly less sensitive to the presence of insulin, although a normal (or slightly greater than normal) amount of insulin is produced by the pancreas. The growing ineffectiveness of insulin in getting glucose into cells results in the buildup of glucose in the blood. Elevated levels of glucose in the blood lead to *hyperglycemia*, a hallmark symptom of type 2 diabetes.

In response to this buildup, the kidneys begin the process of filtering glucose from the blood. Excess glucose then spills over into the urine. This removal of glucose in the urine demands large amounts of water, a second important symptom of adult-onset diabetes. Increased thirst, a third symptom of developing diabetes, results in response to the movement of fluid from extracellular spaces into the circulatory system to maintain homeostasis.

For many adults with diabetes or with a prediabetic status often referred to as having "glucose intolerance" or "insulin resistance," dietary modification (with an emphasis on monitoring total carbohydrate intake, not just sugar), weight loss, and regular exercise is the only treatment required to maintain an acceptable glucose level. Weight loss will improve the condition by "releasing" more insulin receptors, and exercise increases the actual number of receptor sites. With better insulin recognition, the affected person can better maintain glucose levels.

For people whose condition is more advanced, dietary modification, increased activity, and weight loss are not sufficient, and a hypoglycemia agent must be used. Increasingly, very aggressive management, including drugs and insulin, successfully reduces risks associated with the disease. Many people, however, have difficulty controlling blood sugar levels even with the help of insulin.

 TALKING POINTS You learn that two young women who are your coworkers have recently been diagnosed with lupus and Crohn's disease, respectively. How can you be supportive of them? What should you say to them about their conditions, particularly on days when it is obvious that they are not feeling well?

Key Terms

genetic predisposition an inherited tendency to develop a disease process if necessary environmental factors exist

---

Today, the role of obesity in the development of pre-diabetes and eventually type 2 diabetes mellitus is so well established, and the percentage of the population with these conditions is increasing so rapidly, that a new term, *diabesity*[35] (aka metabolic syndrome), is being used to call the public's attention even more closely to the need for better weight management.

In addition to genetic predisposition and obesity, unresolved stress appears to be involved in the development of hyperglycemic states. Although stress alone probably cannot produce a diabetic condition, it is likely that stress can create a series of endocrine changes that can lead to a state of hyperglycemia.

Diabetes, in both forms, can cause serious damage to several important structures within the body. The rate and extent to which people with diabetes develop these changes can be markedly influenced by the nature of their condition and their compliance with its management requirements. For those who already have diabetes, an understanding of the condition and a commitment to its management are important elements in living with diabetes mellitus.

In 2003, concern increased markedly regarding the alarming increase in the numbers of adults and even children who were diagnosed with either definitive type 2 diabetes mellitus or clear glucose intolerance, also called borderline diabetes mellitus. Today it is estimated that 18 million Americans are already diabetic (90 percent being type 2), and another 41 million are borderline. For the latter group, at least three of the five characteristics of the "metabolic syndrome" were found: abdominal obesity, elevated fasting blood triglycerides, low levels of HDL (the "good" cholesterol), high fasting blood glucose levels, and hypertension (high blood pressure). Underlying these factors and thus exposing millions to future diabetes mellitus and cardiovascular disease are excessive caloric intake and a sedentary lifestyle (see Chapters 4, 7, and 10 for information on reducing these risk factors).

Perhaps the most distressing aspect of this situation is the increasing number of young children, most often overweight or obese, accompanied by an equally overweight parent, presenting in pediatric offices across the country. Many of these children already have two or three of the five "metabolic syndrome" risk factors. As these children with diabesity progress into adulthood, the number of persons with type 2 diabetes mellitus could increase to 50 million by midcentury.

Type 1 Diabetes Mellitus

A second type of diabetes mellitus is insulin-dependent diabetes mellitus, or type 1 diabetes. The onset of this condition generally occurs before age 35, most often

Differences between Types of Diabetes Mellitus

Type 1 diabetes
(These symptoms usually develop rapidly.)

- Extreme hunger
- Extreme thirst
- Frequent urination
- Extreme weight loss
- Irritability
- Weakness and fatigue
- Nausea and vomiting

Type 2 diabetes
(These symptoms usually develop gradually.)

- Any of the symptoms for insulin-dependent diabetes
- Blurred vision or a change in sight
- Itchy skin
- Tingling or numbness in the limbs

If you notice these symptoms occurring, bring them to the attention of your physician.

during childhood. In contrast to type 2 diabetes, in which insulin is produced but is ineffective because of insensitivity, in type 1 diabetes the body does not produce insulin at all. Destruction of the insulin-producing cells of the pancreas by the person's immune system (possibly in combination with a genetic predisposition) accounts for this sudden and irreversible loss of insulin production.[36]

In most ways the two forms of diabetes are similar, with the important exception that type 1 diabetes mellitus requires the use of insulin from an outside source. Today this insulin is obtained either from animals or through genetically engineered bacteria. It is taken by injection (one to four times per day), through the use of an insulin pump that provides a constant supply of insulin to the body, by transdermal patch, or through nasal inhalation. An insulin pill, now under development, will hopefully be available within the next few years. The use of a glucometer, a highly accurate device for measuring the amount of glucose in the blood, allows for sound management of this condition and a life expectancy that is essentially normal. With both forms of diabetes mellitus, sound dietary practice, weight management, planned activity, and control of

Common Complications of Diabetes

- Cataract formation
- Glaucoma
- Blindness
- Dental caries
- Stillbirths/miscarriages
- Neonatal deaths
- Congenital defects
- Cardiovascular disease
- Kidney disease
- Gangrene
- Impotence

stress are important for keeping blood glucose levels within normal ranges. Without good management of diabetes mellitus, several serious problems can result, including blindness, gangrene, kidney disease, and heart attack. These and other common complications of diabetes are listed above. People who cannot establish good control are likely to live a shorter life than those who can.

Sickle-Cell Trait and Sickle-Cell Disease

Among the hundreds of human diseases, few are found almost exclusively in a particular racial or ethnic group. Such is the case, however, for the inherited condition *sickle-cell trait/sickle-cell disease*. In the United States, sickle-cell abnormalities are virtually unique to African Americans.

Of all the chemical compounds found in the body, few occur in as many forms as hemoglobin, which helps bind oxygen to red blood cells. Two forms of hemoglobin are associated with sickle-cell trait and sickle-cell disease. African Americans can be the recipients of either form of this abnormal hemoglobin. Those who inherit the trait form do not develop the disease but can transmit the gene for abnormal hemoglobin to their children. In the past, those who inherited the disease form faced a shortened life characterized by periods of pain and impairment. Today, however, with effective screening and new therapeutic approaches to treatment, life expectancy is being extended. Central to this progress has been the implantation of stem cells into young sickle cell victims that have been taken from the bone marrow of compatible donors, particularly siblings.[37] In the future, technological advances

will likely allow the use of embryonic stem cells, although probably not in the United States, and cells taken from unrelated donors.

About 8 percent of all African Americans have the gene for sickle-cell trait; they experience little impairment, but they can transmit the abnormal gene to their children. For about 1.5 percent of African Americans, sickle-cell disease is a painful, incapacitating, and life-shortening disease.

In the fully expressed disease form, red blood cells are elongated, crescent-shaped (sickled), and unable to pass through the body's minute capillaries. The body responds to the presence of these abnormal red blood cells by removing them very quickly. This sets the stage for anemia. Thus the condition is often called *sickle-cell anemia*. In addition to anemia, the disease form of the condition can cause many serious medical problems, including impaired lung function (including pulmonary hypertension), congestive heart failure, gall-bladder infections, bone changes, and abnormalities of the eye and skin.

If a key exists for preventing sickle-cell trait and disease, it lies in genetic counseling and testing in preparation for reproduction or in the use of **in vitro** fertilization followed by genetic testing of the embryo before implantation. At present, both of these preventive approaches are very expensive and limited in availability. However, further research and testing could make these methods more affordable and increase their availability to people who are at high risk.

Alzheimer's Disease

Although it affects less than 2 percent of the elderly, **Alzheimer's disease** is an incapacitating, emotionally painful, and costly affliction. It is the best known of the dementia disorders, affecting an estimated 4 to 5 million adults. Today, more than ever before, it is *the* disease associated with aging.

The first signs of Alzheimer's disease are often subtle and may be confused with mild depression. Initially, the person might have difficulty answering questions such as "What is today's date?" Over the next several months,

---

Key Terms

in vitro outside the living body

Alzheimer's disease gradual development of memory loss, confusion, and loss of reasoning; eventually leads to total intellectual incapacitation, brain degeneration, and death

greater memory loss, confusion, and *dementia* (or loss of normal thought processes) occur. In the advanced stages, people with Alzheimer's disease become incontinent, show infantile behavior, and finally become incapacitated as brain tissue is destroyed. With advanced Alzheimer's disease, institutionalization becomes necessary.

In the current classification system for AD, two principal categories are used, *early-onset AD* (before age 65) and *late-onset AD* (after age 65). Early-onset AD, encompassing types 1, 3, and 4, accounts for approximately 25 percent of all AD patients and is clearly an inherited form of the disease. Chromosomes 1, 14, and 21 have been identified as factors in this form of the disease. Late-onset AD, designated as type 2, the most prevalent form of the disease, is less clearly understood from a genetic point of view, although chromosome 19 is believed to be involved.[38]

Alzheimer's disease is difficult to diagnose because its symptoms are similar to those of other types of dementia. It is only after the person's death, if an autopsy is performed, that the characteristic changes in the brain can be used to make a definitive diagnosis. As a practical matter, a probable diagnosis of Alzheimer's disease is made by the process of elimination. Newer medical imaging technologies, such as MRI, have become so refined that it is now almost possible to confirm the diagnosis of Alzheimer's disease before death.

Medications to cure Alzheimer's disease do not exist at this time. However, four drugs (tacrine, donepezil, rivastigamine, and galantamine) provide temporary improvement in intellectual function during the early stages of the disease by inhibiting the breakdown of acetylcholine, whose diminished availability is the basis of the disease. A fifth medication, menantine, used in treating moderate to severe AD, functions by blocking glutamate, a substance capable of damaging neurons. Of these drugs, donepezil is most widely used; while galantamine influences receptors for three other neurotransmitters, as well as nicotine receptors, all of which play roles in the disease.

At this time, a wide array of studies attempting to link behavioral patterns to the prevention of cognitive decline with aging and the development of AD are underway. Among these are studies assessing the role of fatty acids (particularly n-3 omega fatty acid) in preventing cognitive decline, the role of exercise (particularly walking) in improving cognitive capabilities in aging adults, and the contributions of regular light alcohol consumption in protecting against Alzheimer's-like conditions. Additional studies in the same vein include those related to the effectiveness of NSAID (nonsteroidal anti-inflammatory drugs) in preventing cognitive decline, the ability of antioxidant vitamins (carotenes, vitamin C, and vitamin E) to prevent dementia, and the role of high-dose HRT in the cause or exacerbation of cognitive decline, including AD.

Taking Charge of Your Health

- Stay attuned to media reports about chronic conditions so that you can make informed choices.

- Support agencies devoted to the prevention of chronic health conditions.

- Monitor your work, home, and recreational environments to determine whether they are placing you at risk for cancer.

- Perform regular self-examinations for forms of cancer that can be detected through this technique.

- Undergo the recommended cancer screening procedures for your age and sex.

- If you have a chronic condition, participate actively in your own treatment.

SUMMARY

- More than one and a quarter million people in the United States develop cancer each year.
- Cancer is a condition in which the body is unable to control the specialization, replication, and repair of cells or the suppression of abnormal cell formation.
- Genes that control the replication, specialization, and repair of cells and the suppression of abnormal cellular activity have the potential to become oncogenes and thus can be considered proto-oncogenes.

- A variety of agents, including genetic mutations, viruses, and carcinogens, stimulate the conversion of regulatory genes (proto-oncogenes) into oncogenes.
- Cancer can be described on the basis of the type of tissue from which it originates, such as carcinoma, sarcoma, and melanoma.
- Cancer can be described on the basis of its location within the body, such as lung, breast, and prostate cancer.

- Cigarette smoking and genetic predisposition are both related to the development of lung cancer.
- Most cases of breast cancer do not demonstrate a clear familial pattern that suggests a genetic predisposition, although some do.
- Long-term exposure to high levels of estrogen is an important risk factor for breast cancer.
- Mammograms are an important component of breast cancer identification.
- Regular use of Pap tests is related to the early detection of cervical cancer. Sexually transmitted viral infections are strongly suspected of causing cervical cancer.
- The excessively long use of HRT is a strongly suspected cause of uterine cancer.
- Ovarian cancer is often "silent" in its presentation of symptoms.
- Prostate cancer is the second leading cause of cancer deaths in men.
- The PSA test improves the ability to diagnose prostate cancer.
- Regular self-examination of the testicles leads to early detection of testicular cancer. Environmental factors may be associated with an increasing rate of testicular cancer.
- Colorectal cancer has a strong familial link and is seen in populations that consume diets high in fat and low in fruits and vegetables. Polyp formation is associated with an increased risk of this form of cancer.
- Colonoscopy is the most effective method of detecting polyps and colorectal cancers.
- Pancreatic cancer is very difficult to survive, in part because of the absence of symptoms early in the disease's course.

- Lymphatic cancers display a wide array of initial symptoms that reflect failure of the immune system to function fully. Viral infections and environmental toxins are suspected causative agents.
- Basal cell and squamous cell carcinomas are highly curable forms of skin cancer when detected early. Malignant melanoma is life threatening if not detected early.
- Early detection based on self-examination and screening is the basis for the identification and successful treatment of many cancers.
- Risk reduction, through living a wellness lifestyle remains at the heart of cancer prevention.
- Chronic conditions may be lifelong or they may arise during later adulthood.
- In SLE the body's immune system attacks the body's connective tissues.
- Crohn's disease, a form of IBD, involves an autoimmune deterioration of the gastrointestinal wall.
- Multiple sclerosis is an autoimmune disorder in which the insulation on motor neurons and in the brain is destroyed, leading to a decreasing ability to control muscles.
- Type 1 and type 2 diabetes both involve the body's inability to utilize glucose but have different causes and usually require different forms of treatment.
- Sickle cell trait/disease is an inherited condition appearing in African Americans that results in abnormal hemoglobin.
- Alzheimer's disease reflects a progressive decline in cognitive function, leading eventually to death, and appears primarily in later life.

REVIEW QUESTIONS

1. What is the relationship between regulatory genes and tumor suppressor genes in the development of cancer? Why are regulatory genes called both proto-oncogenes and oncogenes?
2. What properties do cancer cells possess that are lacking in normal cells?
3. What are some types of cancer, based on the tissue from which they originate? What are some of the more familiar cancers based on organ of origin?
4. What are the principal factors that contribute to the development of lung cancer? Of breast cancer? What is prophylactic mastectomy and who might consider its use?
5. When should regular use of mammography begin, and which women should begin using it earliest?
6. What important information can be obtained with the use of Pap tests? What innovations are associated with the ThinPrep Pap Test?
7. How does the PSA test contribute to the early detection of prostate cancer?
8. What are the steps for effective self-examination of the breasts and testicles? What is the new status of Breast Self-Examination?
9. What signs indicate the possibility that a skin lesion has become cancerous?

10. Why is pancreatic cancer among the most lethal of all cancers?
11. What are the problems that arise with SLE and how is this autoimmune condition managed?
12. What larger family of conditions is Crohn's disease a part of, and what changes occur in the digestive tract when it is present?
13. What critically important material within the nervous system is eroded by the immune system in conjunction with multiple sclerosis? What are the consequences of losing the ability to continue production of this material?
14. How are type 1 and type 2 diabetes similar, and how are they clearly different conditions? What is the "metabolic syndrome," and how does it relate to type 2 diabetes mellitus?
15. What racial group is most susceptible to sickle cell trait/disease? What is sickle cell trait/disease? How could genetic counseling be used in the prevention of this condition?
16. In terms of Alzheimer's disease, what is the cause of its victims' cognitive decline? How effective are current medication used in the treatment of AD?

ENDNOTES

1. American Cancer Society. *Cancer Facts & Figures 2005.* American Cancer Society, 2005.

2. *Number of Americans without Insurance Reaches Highest Level on Record.* Center On Budget and Policy Priorities. www.cbpp.org/8-26-04health.htm. August 27, 2004.

3. *Estimated Cancer Cases and Deaths by Sex, for All Sites, US, 2005.* American Cancer Society, 2005. www.cancer.org/docroot/MED/content/downloads/MED_1_1xOFF2005_Estimated_New_Cases_Death_by_Sex_USasp.

4. Rieger PT. The biology of cancer genetics. 2004. *Semin Oncol Nursing.* Aug; 20(3):145–154.

5. Gilley D, Tanaka H, Herbert BS. Tolmere dysfunction in aging and cancer. 2005. *Int J Biochem Cell Biol.* May; 37(5): 1000–1013.

6. Bertino JR. (Ed.) *Encyclopedia of Cancer* (2nd ed.) (Vols 1–4.). New York: Academic Press, 2002.

7. Pope CA, et al. Lung cancer, cardiopulmonary mortality and long-term exposure to fine particulate air pollution. *JAMA,* 2002; 287(9):1132–1141.

8. Djousse L, et al. Alcohol consumption and risk of lung cancer: The Framingham Study. *J Natl Cancer Inst;* 2002, 94(24):1877–1882.

9. Nemunaitis J, et al. Granulocyte-marcophage colony-stimulating factor gene-modified autologous tumor vaccines in non-small-cell lung cancer. *J Natl Cancer Inst.* 2004; 96(4):326–331.

10. Collaborative Group on Hormonal Factors in Breast Cancer. Breast cancer and breast-feeding reanalysis of individual data from 47 epidemiological studies in 30 countries, including 50,302 women with the disease. *Lancet.* 2002. 360(9328):203–210.

11. Chlebowski RT. Influence of estrogen plus progestin on breast cancer and mammography in healthy postmenopausal women: The Women's Health Initiative Randomized Trial. *JAMA.* 2003. 289(24):3243–3253.

12. Folsom AR, et al. Association of general and abdominal obesity with multiple health outcomes in older women: The Iowa Women's Health Study. *Arch Intern Med.* 2000. 160(14):2117–2128.

13. Krainer M, et al. Differential contributions of BRCA1 and BRCA2 to early-onset breast cancer. *N Engl J Med.* 1997. 336(20):1416–1421.

14. McClain MR, et al. Adjusting the estimated proportion of breast cancer cases associated with BRCA1 and BRCA2 mutations: Public health implications. *Genet Med* 2005. Jan; 7(1):28–33.

15. Spear SL, Carter ME, Schwarz K. Prophylactic mastectomy: Indications, options, and reconstruction alternatives. *Plast Reconstr Surg.* 2005. 115(3):891–909.

16. McDonald S, Saslow D, Alciati MH. Performance and reporting of clinical breast examination: A review of the literature. 2004. *CA Cancer J Clin.* 54(6):345–361.

17. Henderson IC. Aromatase inhibitors in the management of early breast cancer: Optimizing the clinical benefit. *Semin Oncol.* 2004. 31(6 Suppl 12):31–34.

18. Harper DM, et al. Efficacy of a bivalent L1 viruslike particle vaccine in prevention of infection with human papillomavirus 16 and 18 in young women: A randomized controlled trial. *Lancet.* 2004. 364(9447):1757–1765.

19. American Cancer Society. Cancer *Facts & Figures 2003.* American Cancer Society, 2003.

20. Folsom AR, Anderson JP, Ross JA. Estrogen replacement therapy and ovarian cancer. *Epidemiology.* 2004. 15(1):100–104.

21. Yawn BP, Barrette BA, Wollan PC. Ovarian cancer: The neglected diagnosis. *Mayo Clin Proc.* 2004. 79(10):1277–1282.

22. Thompson IM, et al. The influence of finasteride on the development of prostate cancer. *N Engl J Med.* 2003. 349(3):215–224.

23. Ragde H, Cavanagh WA, Tjoa BA. Dendritic cell-based vaccines: Progress in immunotherapy studies for prostate cancer. *J. Urol.* 2004. 172(6 pt 2):2532–2538.

24. Brucker-Davis F, Pointis G, Fenichel P. Update on cryptorchidism: Endocrine, environmental, and therapeutic aspects. *Endocrinol Invest.* 2003. 26(6):575–587.

25. Collins JF, et al. Accuracy of screening for fecal occult blood on a single stool sample obtained by digital rectal examination: A comparison with recommended sampling practice. *Ann Intern Med.* 2005. 142(2):81–85.

26. Imperiale TF, et al. Fecal DNA versus fecal occult blood for coleroctal-cancer screening in an average-risk population. *N Engl J Med.* 2004. 351(26):2704–2714.

27. Feldman SR, et al. Ultraviolet exposure is a reinforcing stimulus in frequent indoor tanners. *Am Acad Dermatol.* 2004. 51(1):45–51.

28. *January 25, 2005 letter to The Honorable George W. Bush.* One Voice against Cancer. www.dragonflyde.com/ovac/link.html.

29. Arbuckle MR, et al. Development of autoantibodies before clinical onset of systemic lupus erythematosus. *N Engl J Med.* 2003. 349(16):1526–1533.

30. Kasper DL, et al. *Harrison's Principles of Internal Medicine* (16th ed.). New York: McGraw-Hill, 2004.

31. Pierik M, et al. The IBD international genetics consortium provides further evidence for linkage of IBD4 and shows gene-environment interaction. *Inflamm Bowel Dis.* 2004. 11(1):1–7.

32. Haahr S, et al. The role of late Epstein-Barr infection in multiple sclerosis. *Acta Neurol Scand.* 2004. 109(4):270–275.

33. Ruggieri M. Multiple sclerosis in children under 10 years of age. *Neurol Sci.* 2004. 25 Suppl 4:S326–335.

34. Saladin KS. *Anatomy and Physiology: The Unity of Form and Function* (4th ed.). New York: McGraw-Hill, 2007.

35. Kaufman F. *Diabesity.* New York: Bantam, 2005.

36. Rasilainen S, et al. Mechanisms of beta cell death during restricted and unrestricted enterovirus infection. *J Med Virol.* 2004. 72(3):451–461.

37. Gaziev J, Lucarelli G. Stem-cell transplantation and gene therapy for hemoglobinopathies. *Curr Hematol Rep.* 2005. 4(2):126–131.

38. U.S. National Library of Medicine. Alzheimer's disease—genetic home reference. www.ghr.nlm.gov/condition-alzheimerdisease. March 18, 2005.

Three respected health organizations (American Diabetes Association, European Association for the Study of Diabetes, and American Heart Association) are involved in a controversy regarding the role of "metabolic syndrome" in the prevention of heart disease. Metabolic syndrome (aka Syndrome X or diabesity) is a collection of conditions, including abdominal obesity, hypertension, elevated cholesterol, and glucose intolerance (insulin insensitivity), that is considered by cardiologists to be a "disease" that predisposes a person to cardiovascular disease. Cardiologists, and the American Heart Association, await the availability of a new medication, rimonabant (Acomplia), which will allow them to "treat" metabolic syndrome in a more comprehensive manner. Rimonabant has shown effectiveness in smoking abatement and weight management.

Aligned on the other side of the metabolic syndrome controversy are two diabetes groups that believe that the newly emerging emphasis on metabolic syndrome, as if it were a valid disease entity, is distracting the medical community's focus on more widely recognized cardiovascular disease, such as coronary artery disease, and perhaps is taking attention away from the focused attempt to deal with glucose insensitivity, a long-recognized indicator for diabetes mellitus.

personal assessment

Are you at risk for skin, breast, or cervical cancer?

Some people may have more than an average risk of developing particular types of cancer. These people can be identified by certain risk factors.

This simple self-testing method is designed by the American Cancer Society to help you assess your risk factors for three common types of cancer. These are the major risk factors but by no means represent the only ones that might be involved.

Check your response to each risk factor. Add the numbers in the parentheses to arrive at a total score for each cancer type. Find out what your score means by reading the information in the "Interpretation" section. You are advised to discuss the information with your physician if you are at a higher risk.

Skin Cancer

1. Frequent work or play in the sun
   A. Yes (10)
   B. No (1)
2. Work in mines, around coal tars, or around radioactivity
   A. Yes (10)
   B. No (1)
3. Complexion—fair skin or light skin
   A. Yes (10)
   B. No (1)

YOUR TOTAL POINTS _____

Explanation

1. Excessive ultraviolet light causes skin cancer. Protect yourself with a sunscreen.
2. These materials can cause skin cancer.
3. Light complexions need more protection than others.

Interpretation

Numerical risks for skin cancer are difficult to state. For instance, a person with a dark complexion can work longer in the sun and be less likely to develop cancer than can a light-complected person. Furthermore, a person wearing a long-sleeved shirt and a wide-brimmed hat may work in the sun and be less at risk than a person who wears a bathing suit and stays in the sun for only a short period. The risk increases greatly with age.

The key here is if you answered "yes" to any question, you need to realize that you have above-average risk.

Breast Cancer

1. Age group
   A. 20–34 (10)
   B. 35–49 (40)
   C. 50 and over (90)
2. Race/nationality
   A. Asian American (5)
   B. African American (20)
   C. White (25)
   D. Mexican American (10)
3. Family history of breast cancer
   A. Mother, sister, or grandmother (30)
   B. None or unknown (10)
4. Your history
   A. No breast disease (10)
   B. Previous noncancerous lumps or cysts (25)
   C. Previous breast cancer (100)
5. Maternity
   A. First pregnancy before age 25 (10)
   B. First pregnancy after age 25 (15)
   C. No pregnancies (20)

YOUR TOTAL POINTS _____

Interpretation

Under 100	Low-risk women should follow the 2005 ACS cancer screening guidelines. Note that the role of BSE has been redefined. Consult your physician for possible modifications to this protocol.
100–199	Moderate-risk women should consult their physicians to determine whether the ACS guideline should be followed as stated or, possibly, be modified in terms of scheduling or procedures employed. Note that the role of BSE has been redefined.
200 or more	High-risk women should consult their physicians to determine whether the ACS guidelines should be followed as stated or, very likely, be modified in terms of scheduling or procedures employed. Note that the role of BSE has been redefined.

Cervical Cancer*

1. Age group
   A. Less than 25 (10)
   B. 25–39 (20)
   C. 40–54 (30)
   D. 55 and over (30)
2. Race/nationality
   A. Asian American (10)
   B. Puerto Rican (20)
   C. African American (20)
   D. White (10)
   E. Mexican American (20)
3. Number of pregnancies
   A. 0 (10)
   B. 1 to 3 (20)
   C. 4 and over (30)
4. Viral infections
   A. Herpes and other viral infections or ulcer formations on the vagina (10)
   B. Never (1)
5. Age at first intercourse
   A. Before 15 (40)
   B. 15–19 (30)
   C. 20–24 (20)
   D. 25 and over (10)
6. Bleeding between periods or after intercourse
   A. Yes (40)
   B. No (1)

YOUR TOTAL POINTS _____

Explanations

1. The highest occurrence is in the 40-and-over age group. The numbers represent the relative rates of cancer for different age groups. A 45-year-old woman has a risk three times higher than that of a 20-year-old.
2. Puerto Ricans, African Americans, and Mexican Americans have higher rates of cervical cancer.
3. Women who have delivered more children have a higher occurrence.
4. Viral infections of the cervix and vagina are associated with cervical cancer.
5. Women with earlier intercourse and with more sexual partners are at a higher risk.
6. Irregular bleeding may be a sign of uterine cancer.

Interpretation/To Carry This Further . . .

40–69	This is a low-risk group. Ask your doctor for a Pap test. You will be advised how often you should be tested after your first test.
70–99	In this moderate-risk group, more frequent Pap tests may be required.
100 or higher	You are in a high-risk group and should have a Pap test (and pelvic examination) as advised by your doctor.

Regardless of score, you should discuss with your physician the desirability of the ThinPrep Pap test (or one similar to it), as it is designed to identify the presence of DNA from one or more of the HPV strains associated with cervical cancer.

_____

*Lower portion of uterus. These questions would not apply to a woman who has had a complete hysterectomy.

chapter twelve

Preventing Infectious Diseases

Chapter Objectives

On completing this chapter, you will be able to:

▌ describe the movement of a cold virus through each link in the chain of infectious disease.

▌ explain why persons with HIV/AIDS do not generally progress beyond the clinical stage of their disease.

▌ develop and then implement a plan to protect (or enhance) your immune system.

▌ assess your own immunizations status, and make arrangements for any additional immunizations such as flu shots.

▌ understand and describe the importance of frequent hand washing, particularly during the cold and flu season.

▌ recognize the importance of testing dead birds found on campus or in your neighborhood for the presence of the West Nile virus.

▌ identify those forms of hepatitis that are potentially sexually transmitted, in comparison to those that are not.

▌ take proper precautions to protect yourself from HIV/AIDS and other sexually transmitted diseases.

Eye on the Media

From Fear to Hope—AIDS in the News

In the early days of news coverage about AIDS, magazines like *Time* and *Newsweek* ran articles called: "The AIDS Epidemic," "Epidemic of Fear," "Plague Mentality," "Fear of Sex," "The Growing Threat," "A Spreading Scourge," "The New Untouchables," "AIDS Spreading Panic Worldwide," "A Grim Race Against the Clock," and "The Lost Generation." The titles reflected fear of the unknown, a new killer disease.

When the case of Kimberley Bergalis broke into the news in 1991, a routine visit to the dentist was suddenly fraught with risk. Bergalis was the first American to die of AIDS after being infected by her dentist, Dr. David Acer. Four of Acer's other patients became infected with AIDS—all traced back to Acer. The public's reaction was near-hysteria. *Time* ran an article called "Should You Worry About Getting AIDS from Your Dentist?" People started asking their dentists (and other doctors) about their use of sterile precautions and even whether they had been tested for HIV.

By 1996, when the "cocktail" approach to AIDS treatment started showing remarkably good results, Magic Johnson was on the cover of both *Time* and *Newsweek* the same week. After more than 4 years of retirement from pro basketball—and the announcement that he had tested positive for HIV—he was back in the game. The secret to his survival? New drug treatments, a healthy diet, regular exercise, support from family and friends, and a positive attitude.

By the late 1990s, many news articles reflected a more hopeful tone: "Living Longer with AIDS," "Hope with an Asterisk," "Are Some People Immune?" and "What—I'm Gonna Live?" Doctors, too, are feeling more positive about the disease. As one AIDS specialist said: "I go to work feeling like there's something I can do for my patients."

For people with HIV/AIDS in the most highly developed countries the future holds different things. For some, who can't afford or tolerate the new drugs, it's still a matter of waiting to die. Others feel that they've been given a second chance. They can think about having relationships again—something many put on hold when they learned they were HIV positive. They can make plans for what they want to do with the rest of their lives—however long that may be.

Most people with HIV/AIDS are buying time—hoping for the big breakthrough, the cure for AIDS. They're trying new drug treatments, hoping that one treatment won't disqualify them from the next one. They're watching TV news, reading the newspapers, and using the Internet with greater attention. Will protease-inhibiting drugs be the answer? Are the even newer antiviral medications the breakthrough hoped for? Is a vaccine on the horizon?

Today, the media are calling our attention to yet other aspects of the AIDS pandemic. For the more developed countries, the failure of younger gays and bisexuals to protect themselves from exposure to HIV has led to a reversal in the progress made over the last 20 years. In ways all too familiar to public health professionals, a younger generation can too

Eye on the Media *continued*
easily forget the progress against disease and premature death made by those who came before, and in doing so, unravel the threads of progress.

Increasingly, media attention has also been focused on the plight of the millions of HIV/AIDS victims in third world countries, particularly in Africa and areas of Asia. Television increasingly exposes the suffering in countries where diagnosis is inadequately undertaken and, once done, virtually no effective treatment exists for those infected. Beyond the suffering and limited hope for those infected, the media has also publicized the plights of the tens of thousands of orphaned children in these areas whose parents have died from AIDS. Our federal government and pharmaceutical industry has been exposed to this suffering as well, and initial responses are being mustered.

At the midpoint of the first decade of the new century, most major media outlets carry relatively little news regarding HIV/AIDS in the United States. Whether this situation reflects the transition of the disease from "infectious" to its present status of a "chronic condition," to date no vaccine has proven to be safe and effective against HIV in humans. Other than reporting on the global spread of HIV/AIDS and the recent discovery of a few cases of a drug-resistant form of the virus in persons either entering or reentering the country, the media has reduced its focus on HIV/AIDS.

In the 19th century, infectious diseases were the leading cause of death. These deaths came after exposure to the organisms that produced such diseases as smallpox, tuberculosis (TB), influenza, whooping cough (pertussis), typhoid, diphtheria, and tetanus. However, since the early 1900s, improvements in public sanitation, the widespread use of antibiotic drugs, and vaccinations have considerably reduced the number of people who die from infectious diseases. People now die more often from chronic disease processes.

Today, however, we have a new respect for infectious diseases. By the end of 2004, 39.4 million people worldwide were living with HIV/AIDS, with long-range projections pointing to 70 million in the absence of effective prevention programs. We are witnessing the resurgence of TB. We recognize the role of pelvic infections in infertility. We also know that failure to fully immunize children has laid the groundwork for a return of whooping cough, polio, and other serious childhood diseases. In fact, some experts suggest that because of HIV/AIDS and the emergence and reemergence of infectious diseases, today's young adults may have a lower life expectancy than did the generation immediately ahead of them.

Several new types of infectious disease have appeared, and new concerns have been raised about the spread of familiar infectious diseases.

Infectious Disease Transmission

Infectious diseases can generally be transmitted from person to person, although the transfer is not always direct. Infectious diseases can be especially dangerous because they can spread to large numbers of people, producing epidemics or **pandemics.** The following sections explain the process of disease transmission and the stages of infection.

Pathogens

For a disease to be transferred, a person must come into contact with the disease-producing agent, or **pathogen,** such as a virus, bacterium, or fungus. When pathogens enter our bodies, the pathogens can sometimes resist body defense systems, flourish, and produce an illness. We commonly call this an *infection*. Because of their small size, pathogens are sometimes called *microorganisms* or *microbes*. Table 12.1 describes infectious disease agents and some of the illnesses they produce.[1]

Chain of Infection

The movement of a pathogenic agent through the various links in the chain of infection (Figure 12-1) explains how diseases spread.[1] Not every pathogenic agent moves all the way through the chain of infection, because various links in the chain can be broken. Therefore, the presence of a pathogen creates only the potential for causing disease.

Agent

The first link in the chain of infection is the disease-causing **agent.** Whereas some agents are very **virulent**

Key Terms

pandemic an epidemic that has crossed national boundaries, thus achieving regional or international status (HIV/AIDS is a pandemic)

pathogen a disease-causing agent

agent the causal pathogen of a particular disease

virulent (**veer** yuh lent) capable of causing disease

Table 12.1 Pathogens and Common Infectious Diseases

Pathogen	Description	Representative Disease Processes
Viruses	Smallest common pathogens; nonliving particles of genetic material (DNA) surrounded by a protein coat	Rubeola, mumps, chicken pox, rubella, influenza, warts, colds, oral and genital herpes, shingles, AIDS, genital warts
Prion	Potentially self-replicating protein, lacking both DNA and RNA, viruslike in size, clinically called TSE (transmissible spongiform encephalopathies)	Creutzfeldt-Jakob disease, Gerstmann-Straussler-Scheinker syndrome, "mad cow" disease (bovine spongiform encephalopathy)
Bacteria	One-celled microorganisms with sturdy, well-defined cell walls; three distinctive forms: spherical (cocci), rod shaped (bacilli), and spiral shaped (spirilla)	Tetanus, strep throat, scarlet fever, gonorrhea, syphilis, chlamydia, toxic shock syndrome, Legionnaires' disease, bacterial pneumonia, meningitis, diphtheria, food poisoning, Lyme disease
Fungi	Plantlike microorganisms; molds and yeasts	Athlete's foot, ringworm, histoplasmosis, San Joaquin Valley fever, candidiasis
Protozoa	Simplest animal form, generally one-celled organisms	Malaria, amebic dysentery, trichomoniasis, vaginitis
Rickettsia	Viruslike organisms that require a host's living cells for growth and replication	Typhus, Rocky Mountain spotted fever, rickettsialpox
Parasitic worms	Many-celled organisms; represented by tapeworms, leeches, and roundworms	Dirofilariasis (dog heartworm), elephantiasis, onchocerciasis

and lead to serious infectious illnesses such as HIV, which causes AIDS, others produce far less serious infections, such as the common cold. Through mutation, some pathogenic agents, particularly viruses, can become more virulent.

Reservoir

Infectious agents require the support and protection of a favorable environment to survive. This environment forms the second link in the chain of infection and is called the *reservoir*. For many of the most common infectious

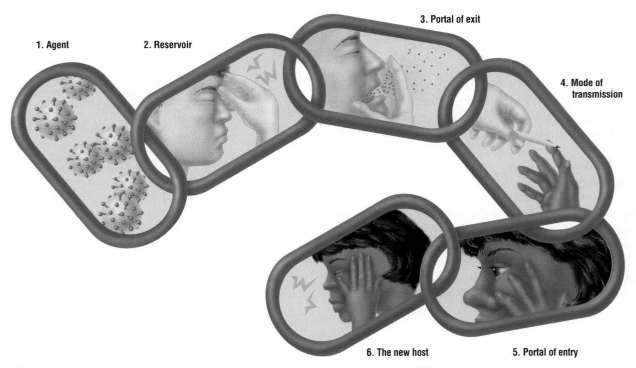

Figure 12-1   The six links in the chain of infection. The example above shows a rhinovirus, which causes the common cold, being passed from one person to another. 1. the *agent* (pathogen) is a rhinovirus; 2. the *reservoir* is the infected person; 3. the *portal of exit* is the respiratory system (coughing); 4. the *mode of transmission* is indirect hand contact; 5. the *portal of entry* is the mucous membranes of the uninfected person's eye; 6, the virus now has a *new host*.

diseases, the reservoirs are the bodies of people who are already infected. Here the agents thrive before being spread to others. These infected people are, accordingly, the hosts for particular disease agents. In some infectious illnesses a person's reservoir status may be restored after treatment and apparent recovery from the original infection. This is because some pathogens, particularly viruses, can remain sequestered (hidden), emerging later to give rise to another infection. The herpes viruses are often sequestered.

For other infectious diseases, however, the reservoirs are the bodies of animals. Rabies is a well-known animal-reservoir disease. The infected animals are not always sick and do not always show symptoms similar to those seen in infected people.

The third type of reservoir in which disease-causing agents can live is in a nonliving environment, such as the soil. The spores of the tetanus bacterium, for example, can survive in soil for up to 50 years, entering the human body in a puncture wound.

Portal of Exit

For pathogenic agents to cause diseases and illnesses in others, they must leave their reservoirs. Thus the third link in the chain of infection is the *portal of exit,* or the point at which agents leave their reservoirs.

The principal portals of exit are familiar—the digestive system, urinary system, respiratory system, reproductive system, and the blood, especially with infectious diseases that infect humans.

Mode of Transmission

The fourth link in the chain of infection is the *mode of transmission,* or the way in which pathogens move from reservoirs to susceptible hosts. Two principal methods are direct transmission and indirect transmission.

We see three types of direct transmission in human-to-human transmission. These include contact between body surfaces (such as kissing, touching, and sexual intercourse), droplet spread (inhalation of contaminated air droplets), and fecal-oral spread (feces on the host's hands are brought into contact with the new host's mouth), as could occur when changing the diaper of an infected infant.

Indirect transmission between infected and uninfected people occurs when infectious agents travel by means of nonhuman materials. Vehicles of transmission include inanimate objects (known as *fomites*), such as water, food, soil, towels, clothing, and eating utensils.

Infectious agents can also be indirectly transmitted through vectors. The term *vector* describes living things, such as insects, birds, and other animals, that carry diseases from human to human. An example of a vector is the deer tick, which transmits Lyme disease.

Airborne indirect transmission includes the inhalation of infected particles that have been suspended in an air source for an extended time. Unlike droplet transmission, in which both infected and uninfected people must be in close physical proximity, noninfected people can become infected through airborne transmission by sharing air with infected people who were in the same room hours earlier. Viral infections such as German measles can be spread this way.

Portal of Entry

The fifth link in the chain of infection is the *portal of entry.* As with the portals of exit, portals of entry have three primary methods that allow pathogenic agents to enter the bodies of uninfected people. These are through the digestive system, respiratory system, and reproductive system. In addition, a break in the skin provides another portal of entry. In most infectious conditions, the portals of entry are the same systems that served as the portals of exit from the infected people. In HIV, however, we see cross-system transmission. Oral and anal sex allow infectious agents to pass between the warm, moist tissues of the reproductive and digestive systems.

The New Host

All people are, in theory, at risk for contracting infectious diseases and thus could be called susceptible hosts. In practice, however, factors such as overall health, acquired immunity, health care services, and health-related behavior can affect susceptibility to infectious diseases.

Stages of Infection

When a pathogenic agent assaults a new host, a reasonably predictable sequence of events begins. That is, the disease moves through five distinctive stages.[1] You may be able to recognize these stages of infection each time you catch a cold.

1. *The incubation stage.* This stage lasts from the time a pathogen enters the body until it multiplies enough to produce signs and symptoms of the disease. The duration of this stage can vary from a few hours to many months, depending on the virulence of the organisms, the concentration of organisms, the host's level of immune responsiveness, and other health problems. This stage has been called a *silent stage.* The pathogen can be transmitted to a new host during this stage, but this is not likely. A host may be infected during this stage but not be infectious. HIV infection is an exception to this rule.

2. *The prodromal stage.* After the incubation stage, the host may experience a variety of general signs and symptoms, including watery eyes, runny nose, slight fever, and overall tiredness for a brief time. These symptoms are nonspecific and may not be severe enough to force the host to rest. During this

stage the pathogenic agent continues to multiply. Now the host is capable of transferring pathogens to a new host, but this is not yet the most infectious stage of an infectious disease. One should practice self-imposed isolation during this stage to protect others. Again, HIV infection is different in this stage.

3. *The clinical stage.* This stage, also called the *acme* or *acute stage,* is often the most unpleasant stage for the host. At this time the disease reaches its highest point of development. Laboratory tests can identify or analyze all of the clinical (observable) signs and symptoms of the particular disease. The likelihood of transmitting the disease to others is highest during this peak stage; all of our available defense mechanisms are in the process of resisting further damage from the pathogen.

4. *The decline stage.* The first signs of recovery appear during this stage. The infection is ending or, in some cases, falling to a subclinical level. People may suffer a relapse if they overextend themselves.

5. *The recovery stage.* Also called the *convalescence stage,* this stage is characterized by apparent recovery from the invading agent. The disease can be transmitted during this stage, but this is not probable. Until the host's overall health has been strengthened, he or she may be especially susceptible to another (perhaps different) disease pathogen. Fortunately, after the recovery stage, further susceptibility to the pathogenic agent is typically lower because the body has built up immunity. This buildup of immunity is not always permanent; for example, many sexually transmitted diseases can be contracted repeatedly.

We will discuss HIV/AIDS later in the chapter; for now, however, we need to note that this critically important pandemic infectious disease does not easily fit into the five-stage model of infectious diseases just presented. In individuals infected with HIV there is an initial asymptomatic *incubation stage,* followed by a *prodromal stage* characterized by generalized signs of immune system inadequacy. However, once the level of specific protective cells of the immune system declines to the point that the body cannot be protected from opportunistic diseases, and the label AIDS is assigned, the five-stage model becomes less easily applied.

Body Defenses: Mechanical and Cellular-Chemical Immune Systems

Much as a series of defensive alignments protect a military installation, so too is the body protected by sets of defenses. These defenses can be classified as either mechanical or cellular-chemical. Mechanical defenses are first-line defenses, because they physically separate the internal body from the external environment. Examples include the skin, the mucous membranes that line the respiratory and gastrointestinal tracts, earwax, the tiny hairs and cilia that filter incoming air, and even tears. These defenses serve primarily as a shield against foreign materials that may contain pathogenic agents. These defenses can, however, be disarmed, such as when tobacco smoke kills the cilia that protect the airway, resulting in chronic bronchitis, or when contact lenses reduce tearing, leading to irritation and eye infection.

The second component of the body's protective defenses is the cellular-chemical system or, more commonly, the **immune system.** The cellular-chemical component is far more specific than the mechanical defenses. Its primary mission is to eliminate microorganisms, foreign protein, and abnormal cells from the body. A wellness-oriented lifestyle, including sound nutrition, effective stress management, and regular exercise, supports this important division of the immune system. The microorganisms, foreign protein, or abnormal cells that activate this cellular component are collectively called *antigens.*[2]

Divisions of the Immune System

Closer examination of the immune system, or cellular-chemical defenses, reveals two separate but highly cooperative groups of cells. One group of cells originates in the fetal thymus gland and has become known as *T cell-mediated immunity,* or simply **cell-mediated immunity.** The second group of cells that makes up cellular immunity are the B cells (bursa of Fabricius), which are the working units of **humoral immunity.**[3] Cellular elements of both cell-mediated and humoral immunity can be found within the bloodstream, the lymphatic tissues of the body, and the fluid that surrounds body cells.

Although we are born with the structural elements of both cell-mediated and humoral immunity, developing

---

Key Terms

immune system the system of cellular and chemical elements that protects the body from invading pathogens, foreign protein, and abnormal cells

cell-mediated immunity also called *T cell-mediated immunity;* is principally provided by the immune system's T cells, both working alone and in combination with highly specialized B cells

humoral immunity also called *B cell-mediated immunity;* is responsible for the production of critically important immune system elements known as *antibodies*

an immune response requires that components of these cellular systems encounter and successfully defend against specific antigens. When the immune system has done this once, it is, in most cases, primed to respond quickly and effectively if the same antigens appear again. This initial confrontation produces a state of **acquired immunity (AI).**[1] Acquired immunity develops in different ways.

- **Naturally acquired immunity (NAI)** develops when the body is exposed to infectious agents. Thus when we catch an infectious disease, we fight the infection and in the process become immune (protected) from developing that illness if we encounter these agents again. For example, when a child catches chicken pox and then recovers, it is unlikely that the child will develop a subsequent case of chicken pox. Before the advent of immunizations, this was the only way of developing immunity.

- **Artificially acquired immunity (AAI)** occurs when the body is exposed to weakened or killed infectious agents introduced through vaccination or immunization. As in NAI, the body fights the infectious agents and records the method of fighting the agents. Young children, older adults, and adults in high-risk occupations should consult their physicians about immunizations.

- **Passively acquired immunity (PAI),** a third form of immunity, results when extrinsic antibodies are introduced into the body. These antibodies are for a variety of specific infections, and they are produced outside the body (either in animals or by the genetic manipulation of microorganisms). When introduced into the human body, they provide immediate protection until the body can develop a more natural form of immunity. This form of short-term but immediate protection is provided when the emergency room staff administers a tetanus-toxoid "booster." Note that in PAI no actual pathogenic agents are introduced into the body—only the antibodies against various forms of disease-causing agents.

Regardless of how infectious agents are acquired, either through naturally acquired immunity (NAI) or through artificially acquired immunity (AAI), the result is an "arming" of the body's own immune system. This process is frequently labeled as *active immunity*. This contrasts to passively acquired immunity (PIA) in which the body "borrows" another's immune elements, without actual involvement of the body's own immune system. This latter case is called *passive immunity*.[4]

In addition to the forms of immunity just described, unborn infants are also provided with a period of short-term immunity via the biological mothers' immune system elements crossing the placental barrier (see Chapter 14)

Are Americans Too Clean?

Infectious disease specialists are increasingly concerned about the widespread popularity and availability of antimicrobial cleaning products and the contribution they may be making to the development of antibiotic-resistant "super bugs." In fact, it is estimated that approximately 75% of all liquid hand soaps and nearly 30% of all bar soaps contain either triclocarban or triclosan, antibacterial chemicals to which pathogenic agents are already showing resistance.

As concern about our increasing reliance on antimicrobial products grows, we are reminded of the first personal hygiene rule that most Americans were taught as children at home and in school: Wash your hands thoroughly with soap and *hot water!* Even today, microbiologists remind us that nothing is more effective in cleaning our bodies, our homes, and our work places than "old-fashioned" soap and hot water.

and then following birth via breast milk. This *maternal immunity,* however, gradually deteriorates but is concurrently being replaced by the child's own increasingly functional immune system.

Collectively, these forms of immunity can provide important protection against infectious disease.

The Immune Response

Fully understanding the function of the immune system requires a substantial understanding of human biology and is beyond the scope of this text. Figure 12-2 presents a simplified view of the immune response.

Key Terms

acquired immunity (AI) the major component of the immune system; forms antibodies and specialized blood cells capable of destroying pathogens

naturally acquired immunity (NAI) a type of acquired immunity resulting from the body's response to naturally occurring pathogens

artificially acquired immunity (AAI) a type of acquired immunity resulting from the body's response to pathogens introduced into the body through immunizations

passively acquired immunity (PAI) a temporary immunity achieved by providing antibodies to a person exposed to a particular pathogen

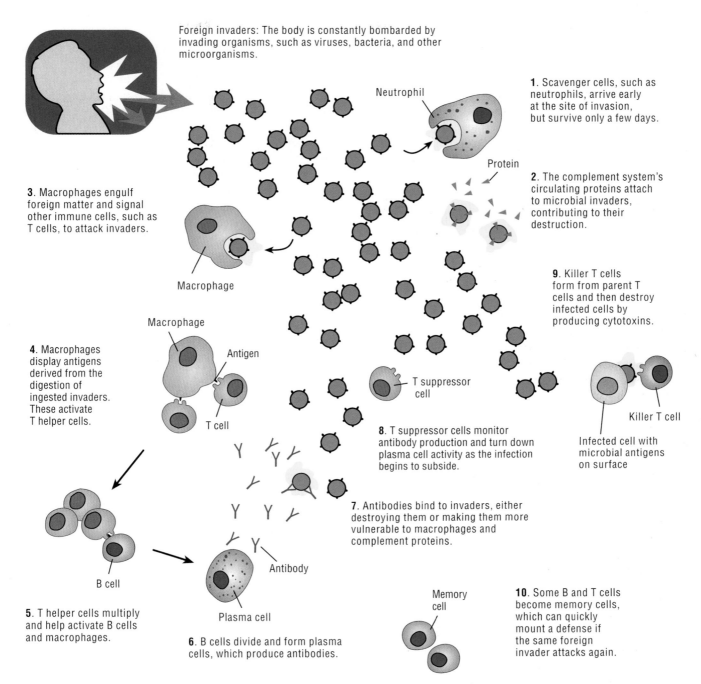

Foreign invaders: The body is constantly bombarded by invading organisms, such as viruses, bacteria, and other microorganisms.

Neutrophil

1. Scavenger cells, such as neutrophils, arrive early at the site of invasion, but survive only a few days.

Protein

2. The complement system's circulating proteins attach to microbial invaders, contributing to their destruction.

3. Macrophages engulf foreign matter and signal other immune cells, such as T cells, to attack invaders.

Macrophage

9. Killer T cells form from parent T cells and then destroy infected cells by producing cytotoxins.

Macrophage

Antigen

4. Macrophages display antigens derived from the digestion of ingested invaders. These activate T helper cells.

T cell

T suppressor cell

Killer T cell

Infected cell with microbial antigens on surface

8. T suppressor cells monitor antibody production and turn down plasma cell activity as the infection begins to subside.

7. Antibodies bind to invaders, either destroying them or making them more vulnerable to macrophages and complement proteins.

B cell

Antibody

5. T helper cells multiply and help activate B cells and macrophages.

Plasma cell

6. B cells divide and form plasma cells, which produce antibodies.

Memory cell

10. Some B and T cells become memory cells, which can quickly mount a defense if the same foreign invader attacks again.

Figure 12-2   Biological warfare The body commands an army of defenders to reduce the danger of infection and guard against repeat infections. Antigens are the ultimate targets of all immune responses

When antigens (whether microorganisms, foreign proteins, or abnormal cells) are discovered within the body, various types of white blood cells confront and destroy some of these antigens. Principal among these blood cells are the *macrophages* (very large white blood cells) that begin ingesting antigens as they are encountered. In conjunction with this "eating" of antigens, macrophages display segments of the antigen's unique protein coat on their outer surface. Now in the form of macrophage/antigen complexes, macrophages transport their captured antigen identifiers to awaiting T cells, whose recognition of the antigen will initiate the full cell-mediated immune response. This involves the specialization of "basic" T cells into four forms: helper T cells, killer T cells, suppressor T cells, and memory T cells.

Once helper T cells have been derived from the "parent" T cells by the presence of the macrophage/antigen complex, they notify a second component of cellular immunity, the killer T cells. Killer T cells produce powerful chemical messengers that activate specific white blood cells that destroy antigens through the production of caustic chemicals called cytotoxins, or "cell poisons." In addition to the helper T cells' activation of killer T cells, helper T cells also play a critical role in the activation of B cells, principal players in the expression of humoral immunity.

Activation of the humoral immunity component of the overall immune response involves the helper T cells' ability to construct a working relationship among themselves, the macrophage/antigen complexes (mentioned earlier), and the small B cells. Once these three elements have been constituted into working units, the B cells are transformed into *plasma cells*. Plasma cells then utilize the information about the antigen's identity to produce massive numbers of **antibodies.** On release from the plasma cells, these antibodies then circulate throughout the body and capture free antigens in the form of *antigen/antibody complexes*.[4] The "captured" antigens are now highly susceptible to a variety of white blood cells that ingest or chemically destroy these infectious agents.

To assure that the response to the presence of the antigen can be appropriately controlled, a third group of T cells, the suppressor T cells, have been formed by the activation of parent T cells. These suppressor T cells monitor the outcome of the humoral response (antibody formation) and, when comfortable with the number of antibodies produced, turn off further plasma cell activity. The fourth group of specialized T cells, the memory T cells, record this game plan for fighting the antigen invasion so that any subsequent similar invasion will be quickly fought.

An additional group of cells that operate independently from the T cell/B cell interplay just described are the *natural killer* (NK) cells. These immune cells continuously patrol the blood and intracellular fluids looking for abnormal cells, including cancer cells and viral-infected cells. When these are found, the NK cells attack them with destructive cytotoxins in a process called *lysing*.[4] (Can you think of a popular household sanitizing product that uses a version of *lysing* in its brand name?)

Clearly, without a normal immune system employing both cellular and humoral elements, we would quickly fall victim to serious and life-shortening infections and malignancies. As you will see later, this is exactly what occurs in many people infected with HIV (see Learning from Our Diversity on page 311).

Emerging medical technology holds promise for repairing damaged immune systems. In a current form of treatment, *adult stem cells* are harvested from non-diseased tissues of a person's body or from a biologically related family member and used to replace damaged or diseased cells within the immune system.[5] A second form of immune system repair involves harvesting *cord blood (stem) cells* taken from the umbilical cord blood collected and "banked" at birth. After careful matching, these cells can be transplanted into a recipient in anticipation that they will specialize into the cell type needed by the damaged or diseased immune system.[6] It is important to note that considerable controversy now surrounds the use of stem cells obtained from embryonic or fetal tissue sources. Even though these are considered to be the "best" stem cells, restrictions by the federal government (and several states) on their collection and use have forced clinicians to use stem cells from the sources mentioned earlier, as well as from cadavers. In spite of federal government restrictions on funding of embryonic stem cell research, however, some states have undertaken its funding to advance the application of this form of immune system–based therapy.

Immunizations

Although the incidence of several childhood communicable diseases is at or near the lowest level ever, we are risking a resurgence of diseases such as measles, polio, diphtheria, and rubella. The possible increase in childhood infectious illnesses is based on the disturbing finding that only 79 percent (range 67.5–93 percent, depending on state of residence) of American preschoolers are adequately immunized, which is principally due to the failure of many parents to complete their children's immunization programs. Today health professionals are attempting to raise the level of immunization to 90 percent of all children under the age of 2 years.

Vaccinations against several potentially serious infectious conditions are available and should be given. These include the following:

- *Diphtheria:* A potentially fatal illness that leads to inflammation of the membranes that line the throat, to swollen lymph nodes, and to heart and kidney failure

- *Whooping cough:* A bacterial infection of the airways and lungs that results in deep, noisy breathing and coughing

- *Hepatitis B:* A viral infection that can be transmitted sexually or through the exchange of blood or bodily fluids; seriously damages the liver

Key Terms

antibodies chemical compounds produced by the body's immune system to destroy antigens and their toxins

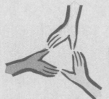
- *Haemophilus influenzae type B:* A bacterial infection that can damage the heart and brain, resulting in meningitis, and can produce profound hearing loss

- *Tetanus:* A fatal infection that damages the central nervous system; caused by bacteria found in the soil

- *Rubella (German measles):* A viral infection of the upper respiratory tract that can cause damage to a developing fetus when the mother contracts the infection during the first trimester of pregnancy

- *Measles (red measles):* A highly contagious viral infection leading to a rash, high fever, and upper respiratory tract symptoms

- *Polio:* A viral infection capable of causing paralysis of the large muscles of the extremities

- *Mumps:* A viral infection of the salivary glands

- *Chicken pox:* A varicella zoster virus spread by airborne droplets, leading to a sore throat, rash, and fluid-filled blisters

- *Pneumococcal infection:* A bacterium capable of causing infections, including pneumonia, heart, kidney, and middle ear infections

Parents of newborns should take their infants to their family-care physicians, pediatricians, or well-baby clinics operated by county health departments to begin the immunization schedule. The Children's' Immunization Schedule shown on the Online Learning Center is recommended by the American Academy of Pediatrics, the American Academy of Family Physicians, and the Centers for Disease Control and Prevention. As children quickly discover, and parents already know, most of today's immunizations are administered by injection. To improve compliance with the immunization schedule (some parents have a fear of "shots" resulting from early childhood experiences and thus avoid completing the schedule), researchers are attempting to develop a single immunization that would combine many individual vaccines. In addition, research is being conducted on new delivery systems, including a skin patch, nasal spray, and vaccine-enriched foods, such as potatoes.

 TALKING POINTS Through community service work, you meet a couple who say that they have not had their children immunized and don't see the reason for doing so. How would you explain the importance of having this done?

In recent years concern has arisen regarding the role of childhood immunizations in the development of other serious childhood physical and emotional health problems, such as type 1 diabetes mellitus, asthma, autism, and sudden infant death syndrome (SIDS). At this time studies investigating the possible relationship between recommended immunizations and conditions mentioned above have found no demonstrable cause-and-effect relationships. Persons interested in more in-depth information regarding adverse affects and contraindications associated with immunizations, the Vaccine Adverse Events Reporting System (VAERS), administered by the Food and Drug Administration (FDA) and the CDC, is in the public domain. Like other reporting systems, the VAERS has limitations; however, information from a wide array of research studies can be readily obtained through the system.[7]

Although immunization is universally viewed as important for infants and children, adults have immunization needs that can be unmet. Accordingly, the CDC's National Immunization Program has just released its first immunization schedule for adults. It recommends eight immunizations that should be updated or initially received by adults. (See Table 12.2.) Adults are particularly underprotected in regard to diphtheria and tetanus.[8,9]

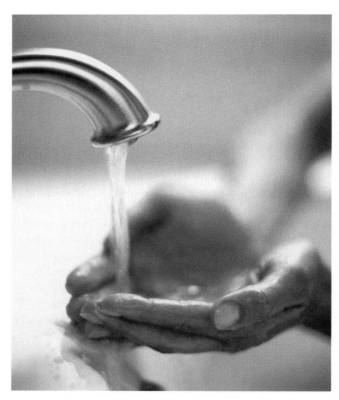

Washing your hands often is the best way to prevent the common cold.

Causes and Management of Selected Infectious Diseases

This section focuses on some of the common infectious diseases and some diseases that are less common but serious. You can use this information as a basis for judging your own disease susceptibility.

The Common Cold

The common cold, an acute upper-respiratory-tract infection, must reign as humankind's supreme infectious disease. Also known as **acute rhinitis,** this highly contagious viral infection can be caused by any of the nearly 200 known rhinoviruses. Colds are particularly common when people spend time in crowded indoor environments, such as classrooms.

The signs and symptoms of a cold are fairly predictable. Runny nose, watery eyes, general aches and pains, a listless feeling, and a slight fever all may accompany a cold in its early stages. Eventually the nasal passages swell, and the inflammation may spread to the throat. Stuffy nose, sore throat, and coughing may follow (Table 12.2 on page 313). The senses of taste and smell are blocked, and appetite declines.

When you notice the onset of symptoms, you should begin managing the cold promptly. After a few days, most of the cold's symptoms subside. In the meantime, you should isolate yourself from others, drink plenty of fluids, eat moderately, and rest.

At this time there is no effective way to prevent colds. In 1999 a medication, pleconaril, appeared to be effective in reducing the extent and duration of colds once initial symptoms had developed. However, in 2002 the FDA denied approval of pleconaril (brand name Picovir) owing, in part, to adverse reactions in some women using the drug and oral contraceptives; and the possibility of developing resistance to the drug within the family of viruses for which it is intended.

Some of the many OTC cold remedies can help you manage a cold. These remedies will not cure your cold but may lessen the discomfort associated with it. Nasal

---

Key Terms

acute rhinitis the common cold; the sudden onset of nasal inflammation

Table 12.2 Recommended Adult Immunization Schedule by Vaccine and Age Group. United States: October 2004—September 2005

Age group (yrs) ▶ Vaccine ▼	19–49	50–64	≥ 65
Tetanus, Diphtheria (Td)*	1 dose booster every 10 years[1]		
Influenza	1 dose annually	1 dose annually	
Pneumococcal (polysaccharide)	1 dose		1 dose
Hepatitis B*	3 doses (0, 1–2, 4–6 months)		
Hepatitis A*	2 doses (0, 6–12 months)		
Measles, Mumps, Rubella (MMR)*	1 or 2 doses[7]		
Varicella*	2 doses (0, 4–8 weeks)[8]		
Meningococcal (polysaccharide)	1 dose[9]		

*Covered by the Vaccine Injury Compensation Program.
www.cdc.gov/nip/recs/adult-schedule.pdf

For all persons in this group

For persons lacking documentation of vaccination or evidence of disease

For persons at risk (i.e., with medical/exposure indications)

The Recommended Adult Immunization Schedule is Approved by the Advisory Committee on Immunization Practices (ACIP), the American College of Obstetricians and Gynecologists (ACOG), and the American Academy of Family Physicians (AAFP)

This schedule indicates the recommended age groups for routine administration of currently licensed vaccines for persons aged ≥19 years. Licensed combination vaccines may be used whenever any components of the combination are indicated and when the vaccine's other components are not contraindicated. Providers should consult manufacturers' package inserts for detailed recommendations. Physicians should report all clinically significant postvaccination reactions to the Vaccine Adverse Event Reporting System (VAERS). Reporting forms and instructions on filing a VAERS report are available by telephone, 800-822-7967, or from the VAERS Web site at www.vaers.org.
Information on how to file a Vaccine Injury Compensation Program claim is available at www.hrsa.gov/osp/vicp or by telephone, 800-338-2382. To file a claim for vaccine injury, contact the U.S. Court of Federal Claims, 717 Madison Place, N.W., Washington, DC 20005, telephone 202-219-9657.
Additional information about the vaccines listed above and contraindications for immunization is available at www.cdc.gov/nip or from the National Immunization Hotline, 800-232-2522 (English) or 800-232-0233 (Spanish).

How to Wash Your Hands

The manner in which the hands are washed is as important as frequency is. Because of the preventive role of effective hand washing in the prevention of cold and influenza transmission, the CDC has formulated guidelines for hand washing.

1. Hands transmit infectious agents when they touch the eyes, nose, or mouth.
2. Hands should be washed:

   - before, during, and after you prepare food.
   - before you eat and after you use the bathroom.
   - after handling animals or animal waste.
   - when your hands are dirty.
   - more frequently when someone in your home is sick.
   - immediately following a period of frequent handshaking.
3. Effective handwashing involves the following steps:

   - First wet your hands and apply liquid soap or clean bar soap (place bar soap back on rack, thus allowing bar to dry).
   - Next, rub your hands vigorously together and scrub all hand surfaces.
   - Continue for 10–15 seconds.
   - Rinse well and dry with clean towel.

Source: "HandWashing: An Ounce of Prevention Keeps the Germs Away." National Center for Infectious Disease. CDC. 2000. www.cdc.gov/ncidod/op/handwashing.htm.

decongestants, expectorants, cough syrups, and aspirin or acetaminophen can give some temporary relief. Follow label directions carefully.

If a cold persists, as evidenced by prolonged chills, fever above 103 degrees Fahrenheit, chest heaviness or aches, shortness of breath, coughing up rust-colored mucus, or persistent sore throat or hoarseness, you should contact a physician. Because we now consider colds to be transmitted most readily by hand contact, you should wash your hands frequently.

Influenza

Influenza is also an acute contagious disease caused by viruses. Some influenza outbreaks have killed many people, such as the influenza pandemics of 1889 to 1890, 1918 to 1919, 1957 and 2003/2004. The viral strains that produce this infectious disease have the potential for more severe complications than the viral strains that produce the common cold. The viral strain for a particular form of influenza enters the body through the respiratory tract. After brief incubation and prodromal stages, the host develops signs and symptoms not just in the upper respiratory tract but throughout the entire body. These symptoms include fever, chills, cough, sore throat, headache, gastrointestinal disturbances, and muscular pain (Table 12.3).

Antibiotics are generally not prescribed for people with influenza, except when the patient has a possible secondary bacterial infection. Physicians may recommend only aspirin, fluids, and rest. Parents are reminded not to give aspirin to children because of the danger of Reye's syndrome. Reye's syndrome is an aspirin-enhanced complication of influenza in which central nervous system changes can occur, including brain swelling. For a person seeking a quicker resolution to the debilitating symptoms of flu, four antiviral medications are currently available; two are intended for influenza virus type A and two for both virus types A and B. Specific recommendations regarding use of these prescription medications, including age limitations, also exist.[10]

Most young adults can cope with the milder strains of influenza that appear each winter or spring. However, pregnant women and older people—especially older people with additional health complications, such as heart disease, kidney disease, emphysema, and chronic bronchitis—are not as capable of handling this viral attack. People who regularly come into contact with the general public, such as teachers, should also consider annual flu shots.

Today approximately 70 million Americans receive annual "flu shots." In past years, these annual immunizations, tailored to work against the flu viruses anticipated for the coming flu season, were principally received by adults over 50 years of age and others with special needs. During the flu epidemic of 2003/2004, younger adults moved into the recipient population, making the nation's supply of 89 million doses of vaccine inadequate.

The 2004/2005 flu season will go down as one of the most difficult in recent memory, because the anticipated supply of 100 million doses of vaccine that should have been in place for the beginning of the season did not materialize; the FDA curtailed production at a major facility in the United Kingdom. As a result, available vaccine was rationed, some vaccine was purchased from other countries, and, the amount of vaccine in each dose was reduced by one half and administered, with acceptable levels of protection, by under-the-skin injection rather than deep-muscle injection.[11]

Concern about coming flu seasons is beginning to shift focus from the more familiar viral strains to a possible pandemic involving mutating forms of the avian (bird) flu.[12]

Table 12.3 Is It a Cold or the Flu?

	Cold	Flu
Symptoms		
Fever	Rare	Characteristic, high (102°–104°+ F); lasts 3–4 days
Headache	Rare	Prominent
General aches, pains	Slight	Usual; often severe
Fatigue, weakness	Quite mild	Can last up to 2–3 weeks
Extreme exhaustion	Never	Early and prominent
Stuffy nose	Common	Sometimes
Sneezing	Usual	Sometimes
Sore throat	Common	Sometimes
Chest discomfort, cough	Mild to moderate; hacking cough	Common; can become severe
Complications	Sinus congestion, earache	Pneumonia, bronchitis; can be life threatening
Prevention	Avoidance of infected people	Annual vaccination; amantadine or rimantadine (antiviral drugs)
Treatment	OTC products for symptom relief	Amantadine or rimantadine within 24–48 hours after onset of symptoms

Note: The need to consult a physician as the result of complications that might arise during the course of a cold or flu is not unknown. During the course of a cold any of the following should be called to the attention of a physician: (1) when a cold fails to resolve within 5 to 7 days, (2) when an elevated temperature develops (above 103°F), or (3) when a "deep chest" cough develops that produces either a brownish-tinged sputum or does not respond to OTC cough medication. Similar complications can occur in conjunction with the flu and require consultation with a physician. In addition, prolonged vomiting and diarrhea also should be called to the attention of a physician. Upon contracting the flu, children, older adults, pregnant women, and all persons with chronic conditions such as diabetes mellitus, cardiovascular diseases, and malignancies should be carefully monitored and complications should be promptly reported to a physician.

This highly virulent form of flu is now primarily spread from birds (chickens and ducks) to humans (and other animals such as cats, pigs, and dogs) having contact with viral infested droppings (see page 322 for further information on bird influenza).

In June of 2003, the FDA approved the sale of Flumist, a nasal spray inhalation delivery system for influenza vaccine. Its use is approved for people ages 5 to 49. Its use is not, at this time, recommended for persons most in need of the highest level of protection.

Tuberculosis

Experts considered *tuberculosis* (*TB*), a bacterial infection of the lungs resulting in chronic coughing, weight loss, and sometimes death, to be under control in the United States until the mid-1980s. The number of cases surged then, however, with a peak of 26,283 cases in 1992. The number has declined since then, with 14,874 cases reported in 2003, a 9 percent decline from 2000.[13] However, public health officials must continually monitor this infectious disease, because people immigrate to the United States from areas of the world in which TB is considerably more common and because drug-resistant strains of the bacterium continue to develop. Drug-resistant TB takes two forms, monodrug resistant and multidrug resistant. The former involves a resistance to Isoniazidm (but not Rifampin), whereas the latter is resistant to both. The international medical community is calling for the development of additional drugs to treat TB in an attempt to control the growing drug-resistant populations. Worldwide TB infects 8.7 million people annually and kills 2 million.

Tuberculosis thrives in crowded places where infected people are in constant contact with others, since TB is spread by coughing. This includes prisons, hospitals, public housing units, and even college residence halls. In such settings, a single infected person can spread the TB agents to many others.

When healthy people are exposed to TB agents, their immune systems can usually suppress the bacteria well enough to prevent symptoms from developing and to reduce the likelihood of infecting others. When the immune system is damaged, however, such as in some older adults, malnourished people, and those who are infected with HIV, the disease can become established and eventually be transmitted to other people at risk.

A new serum-based TB screening test, ELISPOT, has been developed. Similar to the screening test used to detect HIV infection, this test identifies T cells that have been sensitized to an antigen component of the principal tuberculosis bacterium, mycobacterium. This test is more accurate in identifying infected persons than the older and more familiar skin tests.

Pneumonia

Pneumonia is a general term that describes a variety of infectious respiratory conditions. There are bacterial, viral, fungal, rickettsial, mycoplasmal, and parasitic forms of pneumonia. However, bacterial pneumonia is the most common form and is often seen with other illnesses that weaken the body's immune system. In fact, pneumonia is so common in the frail older adult that it is often the specific condition causing death. *Pneumocystis carinii* pneumonia, a parasitic form, is important today because it is a principal opportunistic infection associated with AIDS in HIV-infected people.

Older adults with a history of chronic obstructive lung disease, cardiovascular disease, diabetes, or alcoholism often encounter a potentially serious midwinter form of pneumonia known as *acute (severe) community-acquired pneumonia.* Characteristics of this condition are the sudden onset of chills, chest pain, and a cough producing sputum. In addition, a symptom-free form of pneumonia known as *walking pneumonia* is also commonly seen in adults and can become serious without warning.

As the number of older Americans grows, recommendations regarding immunization against pneumococcal pneumonia have been established and vaccination programs undertaken. Today, these recommendations encourage vaccination beginning at 50 years of age. The cost effectiveness of pneumonia immunizations for older adults, and particularly for minority older adults, is well established.

The first known drug-resistant strains of pneumonia have been identified in this country. As a result, some experts are calling for an even more comprehensive vaccination plan for older adults.

Mononucleosis

College students who contract **mononucleosis ("mono")** can be forced into a long period of bed rest during a semester when they can least afford it. Other common diseases can be managed with minimal disruption, but the overall weakness and fatigue seen in many people with mono sometimes require a month or two of rest and recuperation.

Mono is a viral infection in which the body produces an excess of mononuclear leukocytes (a type of white blood cell). After uncertain, perhaps long, incubation and prodromal stages, the acute symptoms of mono can appear, including weakness, headache, low-grade fever, swollen lymph glands (especially in the neck), and sore throat. Mental fatigue and depression are sometimes reported as side effects of mononucleosis. After the acute symptoms disappear, the weakness and fatigue usually persist—perhaps for a few months.

Mono is diagnosed by its characteristic symptoms. The Monospot blood smear can also be used to identify the prevalence of abnormal white blood cells. In addition, an antibody test can detect activity of the immune system that is characteristic of the illness.

This disease is most often caused by an Epstein-Barr virus (EBV), so antibiotic therapy is not recommended. Treatment usually includes bed rest and the use of OTC remedies for fever (aspirin or acetaminophen) and for sore throat lozenges. Corticosteroid drugs can be used in extreme cases. Rupture of the spleen is an occasional, but serious, consequence of the condition, particularly in persons who are too physically active during their recovery. Adequate fluid intake and a well-balanced diet are also important in the recovery stages of mono. Fortunately, the body tends to develop NAI (naturally acquired immunity) to the mono virus, so repeat infections of mono are unusual. However, persons on immunosuppressant drugs, such as Remicade for Crohn's disease, are more likely to experience a recurrence of mononucleosis or other EBV-related infections.

For years, mono has been labeled the "kissing disease"; however, mono is not highly contagious and is known to be spread by direct transmission in ways other than kissing. No vaccine has been developed for mononucleosis. The best preventive measures are the steps that you can take to increase your resistance to most infectious diseases: (1) eat a well-balanced diet, (2) exercise regularly, (3) sleep sufficiently, (4) use health care services appropriately, (5) live in a reasonably healthful environment, and (6) avoid direct contact with infected people.

Chronic Fatigue Syndrome

Chronic fatigue syndrome (CFS) may be the most perplexing "infectious" condition physicians see. First identified in 1985, this mononucleosislike condition is most often seen in women in their 30s and 40s. People with CFS, often busy professional people, report flulike symptoms, including severe exhaustion, fatigue, headaches, muscle aches, fever, inability to concentrate, allergies, intolerance to exercise, and depression. Examinations of the first people with CFS revealed antibodies to the Epstein-Barr

---

Key Terms

mononucleosis ("mono") a viral infection characterized by weakness, fatigue, swollen glands, sore throat, and low-grade fever

chronic fatigue syndrome (CFS) an illness that causes severe exhaustion, fatigue, aches, and depression; mostly affects women in their 30s and 40s

Living with an Infectious Disease—Life Is Not Over, Just Different

A chronic infectious disease can wear down your body and your spirit. First, you've got to deal with the pain, fatigue, and medicinal side effects associated with the condition. But you also need to learn to adapt everything—your routine, your relationships, and your work—to the illness. As the quality of your life changes dramatically, you may feel depressed, frustrated, and alone. What is the best way to handle the different aspects of your life as you learn to cope with a long-term illness such as chronic fatigue syndrome, hepatitis, or HIV? Will it ever be possible to enjoy a full life again?

Your workplace may present the first big challenge. Since your energy level will be decreased by your illness, you may have trouble completing tasks on time and handling your normal workload. Your allotted sick time and vacation days may be used up quickly for doctor's appointments, hospitalizations, and those days when you are simply too exhausted to go to work. Your coworkers and your supervisor may discriminate against you in subtle ways, making you feel that you're not doing your fair share. The best way to handle these challenges is to maintain a positive and friendly attitude, carefully manage your time off, promote open communication with your employer, and do your best to produce quality work even when you're not feeling well.

Your intimate relationships may also be strained. Your partner may not understand the new limits your illness places on your activities, especially if you were very active before. The best approach is open and honest communication. Try to dispel (or come to terms with) any fears your partner may have about your illness. Take all necessary precautions to avoid infecting your partner if the disease is transmissible. Also, reassure your partner that you're taking these precautions so that he or she won't become ill. Make a point of including your partner in your daily routines. Keep him or her informed of all doctor's appointments, procedures you must undergo, and any news of progress or setbacks. Share your feelings as a way of reducing anxiety for both of you. Create adaptations so that you can still enjoy a romantic relationship. Make the most of your time together, and find new ways to enjoy each other's company.

If you have children, they will also be affected by your illness. Young children may not understand why you can't take them for a sled ride when you feel sick or why you can't go to a school play because of a doctor's appointment. It's best to let children know that their fears and anxieties are valid and that you want them to share them with you. Tell them about your prognosis, taking care not to make any false promises of recovery if that is not expected. Spend time with each child—helping with homework, reading a story, or doing light chores around the house. Always allow the child to ask questions.

From your home to your workplace, your life will change along with your condition. As you adapt to your new situation, it is important to:

- *Be your own best friend.* Eat well, exercise as much as you can, rest when you need to, and follow the treatments prescribed by your physician.
- *Know and understand your limits.* Don't feel guilty about not doing things you used to do before you got sick. Instead, set goals and handle responsibilities as your condition allows.
- *Find new things to do for fun.* This is a good time to start a new hobby that's relaxing. You can also make adaptations so that you can continue activities you've always enjoyed. Maybe you can't run 3 miles a day, but an after-dinner walk might be a pleasant substitute.
- *Communicate openly with others.* Share your feelings respectfully, and allow others around you to share theirs. Together, you can calm your fears, instill hope in each other, and foster a sense of belonging.
- *Remain positive.* Remember, life is not over—just different. Look forward to the good days, when you feel well, and take advantage of them. Create new ways to fulfill your needs and desires. Remain positive about the future and your treatment. New discoveries do occur, and treatments are always evolving. However, be realistic about your situation. Joining a support group may be one of the best things you can do for yourself.

What you learn about yourself throughout your illness may surprise you. You may discover a strength of spirit you never knew you had. Some days may be very hard, but somehow you get through them. You may see life in a new way—slowing down and taking pleasure in a job well done, enjoying friendships more, listening to your inner voice, spending time with your children, taking a second look at nature, and being thankful for today and tomorrow.

---

virus. Thus observers assumed CFS to be an infectious viral disease (and initially called it *chronic Epstein-Barr syndrome*).

Since its first appearance, the condition has received a great deal of attention regarding its exact nature. Today, opinions vary widely as to whether the condition is a specific viral infection, a condition involving both viral infections and nonviral components, or some other disorder.[14]

In recent years it has been noted that another chronic condition, fibromyalgia, appears in a manner similar to CFS. As in CFS, the person with fibromyalgia demonstrates fatigue, inefficient sleep patterns, localized areas of tenderness and pain, morning stiffness, and headaches. The onset of this condition, like that of CFS, can follow periods of stress, infectious disease, physical trauma such as falls, thyroid dysfunction, or in conjunction with a connective tissue disorder.[15] Therefore, some clinicians believe that the two conditions might be very closely related; drawing on an explanation based on immune system involvement.

Regardless of its cause or causes, CFS is extremely unpleasant for its victims. Certainly, those experiencing the symptoms over an extended time need to be seen by a physician experienced in dealing with CFS.

Bacterial Meningitis

Since approximately 1995, a formerly infrequently seen but potentially fatal infectious disease, *meningococcal meningitis,* has appeared on college campuses, suggesting that college students are currently at greater risk of contracting the disease than are their noncollege peers. Particularly interesting is the fact that among college students, the risk of contracting this infection on campus is highest for those students living in residence halls, suggesting that close living quarters, as well as sharing cigarettes and beverages, kissing (exchanging infectious oral fluids), and contact with students from other areas of the world favor transmission of the bacteria. Since many colleges and universities require that first-year students reside in residence halls, it is in this group that the incidence of meningococcal meningitis is highest. Additionally, this group of students is most likely to be in large section lecture classes and take meals in large dining facilities. Some people, however, have questioned the cost-effectiveness of immunizing all entering students.[16] Annually, about 150 cases of meningococcal meningitis occur on American college campuses, resulting in 15 deaths per year. Understandably, more and more colleges and universities are requiring, as a condition of admission, documentation of immunization against bacterial meningitis.

Meningococcal meningitis is a bacterial infection of the thin membranous coverings of the brain. In its earliest stages, this disease can easily be confused with the flu. Symptoms usually include a high fever, severe headache, stiff neck, nausea with vomiting, extreme tiredness, and the formation of a progressive rash. For about 10 percent of people who develop this condition, the infection is fatal, often within 24 hours. Therefore the mere presence of the symptoms described above signals the need for immediate medical evaluation. If done promptly, treatment is highly effective.

Lyme Disease

Lyme disease is an infectious disease that has become a significant health problem in eastern, southeastern, upper Midwestern, and West Coast states, with 21,273 cases in 2003. The significant increase in the number of cases of Lyme disease since 1992 (when 9,909 cases were reported) most likely reflects widening geographical distribution of the disease, a greater awareness of its symptoms by the general public, and more consistent reporting by physicians. This bacterial disease results when infected black-legged ticks (also called deer ticks), usually in the nymph (immature) stage, attach to the skin and inject the infectious agent as they feed on a host's blood. The deer ticks become infected by feeding, as larvae, on infected white-footed mice.

The symptoms of Lyme disease vary but typically appear within 30 days as small red bumps surrounded by a circular red rash at the site of bites. The red rash has been described as being like a "bulls eye" in appearance—a pale center surrounded by a reddish margin. Flulike symptoms, including chills, headaches, muscle and joint aches, and low-grade fever, may accompany this acute phase. A chronic phase develops in about 20 percent of untreated infected persons. This phase may produce disorders of the nervous system, heart, or joints. Fortunately, Lyme disease can be treated with antibiotics. Unfortunately, however, no immunity develops, so infection can recur. Some physicians order tests and begin antibiotic therapy too quickly. The basis of treatment should be the appearance of clinical symptoms, not simply the reporting of a tick bite. Lyme disease may be more difficult to diagnose in children than in adults.

People who live in tick-prone areas, including near small urban/suburban wood lots, and participate in outdoor activities can encounter the nearly invisible tick nymphs. These people should check themselves frequently to be sure that they are tick-free. They should tuck shirts into pants, tuck pants into socks, and wear gloves and hat when possible. They should shower after coming inside from outdoors and check clothing for evidence of ticks. Pets can carry infected ticks into the house.

If you find ticks, carefully remove them from the skin with tweezers and wash the affected area. There is no vaccine available for humans, so prevention is very important. Repellants containing DEET or permethrin are effective in repelling ticks; they should be used according to directions on the label. A form of "natural" prevention seems to occur in conjunction with frequent noninfected tick exposure in the past, but this should not discourage persons from using preventive measures.[17]

Key Terms

Lyme disease a bacterial infection transmitted by deer ticks

Hantavirus Pulmonary Syndrome

Since 1993 a small but rapidly growing number of people have been dying of extreme pulmonary distress caused by the leakage of plasma into the lungs. In the initial cases, the people lived in the Southwest, had been well until they began developing flulike symptoms over one or two days, then quickly experienced difficulty breathing, and died only hours later. Epidemiologists quickly suspected a viral agent such as the *hantavirus,* known to exist in Asia and, to a lesser degree, in Europe. Exhaustive laboratory work led to the culturing of the virus and confirmed that all of these patients had been infected with an American version of the hantavirus.

Today hantavirus pulmonary syndrome has been reported in areas beyond the Southwest, including most of the western states and some of the eastern states. The common denominator in all these areas is the presence of deer mice. We now know that this common rodent serves as the reservoir for the virus. In fact, so common is the mouse that in 2000 the National Park Service began warning hikers, campers, and off-road bikers that hantavirus probably existed in every national park and that caution should be taken to avoid high-risk sites.

The virus moves from deer mice to humans when people inhale dust contaminated with dried virus-rich rodent urine or saliva-contaminated materials, such as nests. Health experts now warn people who live in areas with deer mouse populations (most of the United States) to be extremely careful when cleaning houses and barns in which deer mouse droppings are likely to be found. If you must remove rodent nests, wear rubber gloves, pour disinfectant or bleach on the nests and soak them thoroughly, and finally, pick up the nests with a shovel and burn them or bury them in holes that are several feet deep. These procedures should greatly reduce the airborne spread of the viral particles.

As humans and their domesticated animals encroach on the habitat of wild animals, which serve as reservoirs for infectious agents, transmission from wild animals to domesticated animals is also possible, if not probable.[18] In terms of hantavirus, curtailing the entry of domesticated animals into the nesting areas of deer mice, although difficult, may be prudent.

Because there is no vaccine for hantavirus pulmonary syndrome, people who likely have been exposed to the infected excrement of deer mice should seek early evaluation of flulike symptoms.

West Nile Virus

First detected in New York City in 1999, the *West Nile virus* was, by the summer of 2000, identified in six eastern states— New York, Connecticut, New Jersey, Maryland, Rhode Island, and Massachusetts. By the end of 2002 the West Nile virus had spread westward and to include 34 states. The West Nile virus was found in all but 2 of the 48 contiguous states by the end of 2003. During the summer and early fall months of 2002 and 2003, the number of newly reported cases and deaths doubled weekly. During the infectious season of 2004, the number of cases of West Nile decreased in comparison to the previous year (2003: 9,858 cases and 262 deaths / 2004: 2,282 cases reported and 77 deaths). A combination of temperature, rainfall, and aggressive community control of mosquitoes was a factor in the decline.

This vector-borne infectious virus is transmitted from a reservoir, most often birds, by mosquitoes that in turn infect humans.[1] Human to human transmission (via mosquitoes) apparently does not occur. West Nile virus infection involves flulike symptoms, including fever, headache, muscle ache, fatigue, and joint pain. In young children, persons with immune systems weakened by HIV, and older adults, West Nile virus infection may involve encephalitis, a potentially fatal inflammation of the brain. Physicians recommend that any unusual neurological symptoms be considered as a possible West Nile infection. The West Nile virus deaths that have occurred since the infection's initial appearance in 1999 have been the result of encephalitis.

In an attempt to determine the extent of the West Nile virus range, public health officials throughout the United States have tested mosquitoes, sentinel chickens, crows, other birds, cows, and other animals, including humans. Additionally, mosquito habitats are being treated in an attempt to reduce the vector population. Public service announcements focusing on protection against mosquito bites are routinely made in high-risk areas.

In the period 1999–2003, additional aspects of the disease were reported to the CDC, including the presence of the virus in blood transfusions. (Today, clinically recovered patients cannot give blood for 60 days following dismissal.) The West Nile virus has also been isolated from breast milk, and cases of prenatal transmission have been confirmed. Additionally, a new test to accurately screen for infected blood has been developed, as has a new diagnostic test, developed in Australia, that significantly reduces the time needed to obtain confirmation of the West Nile virus.

Tampon-Related Toxic Shock Syndrome

Toxic shock syndrome (TSS) made front-page headlines in 1980, when the CDC reported a connection between

---

Key Terms

toxic shock syndrome (TSS) a potentially fatal condition caused by the proliferation of certain bacteria in the vagina that enter the general blood circulation

Signs and Symptoms of Toxic Shock Syndrome

- Fever (102°F or above)
- Headache
- Vomiting
- Sore throat
- Diarrhea
- Muscle aches
- Sunburnlike rash
- Low blood pressure
- Bloodshot eyes
- Disorientation
- Reduced urination
- Peeling of skin on the palms of the hands and soles of the feet

TSS and the presence of a specific bacterial agent (*Staphylococcus aureus*) in the vagina associated with the use of tampons. (In addition to tampon misuse-induced TSS, the condition can be caused in conjunction with nasal packing following surgery, infected burns, and subcutaneous abscesses.)

TSS causes the signs and symptoms listed in the Star box. Superabsorbent tampons can irritate the vaginal lining three times more quickly than regular tampons do. This vaginal irritation is aggravated when the tampon remains in the vagina for a long time (more than five hours). When this irritation begins, the staphylococcal bacteria (which are usually present in the vagina) have relatively easy access to the bloodstream. When these bacteria proliferate in the circulatory system, their resultant toxins produce toxic shock syndrome. A woman with TSS can die, usually as a result of cardiovascular failure, if left untreated. Fortunately, less than 10 percent of women diagnosed as having TSS die.

In comparison to other infectious diseases, the incidence of TSS is limited. During the 1980s and through most of the 1990s, the rate of infection was 1/100,000 women. However, in recent years the rate of infections has increased to 5/100,000. This increase is believed to reflect the relaxed vigilance of women, in combination with earlier age of menstruation. Accordingly, premenopausal women should review (or learn anew) the recommendations for appropriate use of tampons. These recommendations include: (1) tampons should not be the sole form of sanitary protection used, and (2)

tampons should not remain in place for too long. Women should change tampons every few hours and intermittently use sanitary napkins. Tampons should not be used during sleep. Some physicians recommend that tampons not be used at all if a woman wants to be extraordinarily safe from TSS.

TALKING POINTS As a parent you are preparing yourself to discuss menstruation with your rapidly maturing daughter. What would you say regarding the safe use of tampons?

Hepatitis

Hepatitis is an inflammatory process in the liver that can be caused by several viruses. Types A, B, C (once called non-A and non-B), D, and E have been recognized. Hepatitis can also be caused indirectly from abuse of alcohol and other drugs. General symptoms of hepatitis include fever, nausea, loss of appetite, abdominal pain, fatigue, and jaundice (yellowing of the skin and eyes).[1]

Type A hepatitis is often associated with consuming fecal-contaminated food, such as raw shellfish raised in fecal-contaminated water, raw vegetables field-washed in contaminated water, or contaminated drinking water. As an example, in November of 2003, 520 patrons of a Chi-Chi's Mexican restaurant near Pittsburgh became ill, and 3 died as a result of eating contaminated green onions. Poor sanitation, particularly in the handling of food and diaper-changing activities, has produced outbreaks in child care centers. Experts estimate that up to 200,000 people per year experience this infection. This number far exceeds the reported 26,000 to 27,000 cases per year, suggesting that a very large reservoir exists among children, who are routinely asymptomatic before 6 years of age. Therefore, it is currently recommended that children living in states with high levels of reported hepatitis A be vaccinated, as well as children with weakened immune systems, and those who will travel outside the United States.

Type B hepatitis (HBV) is spread in various ways, including sexual contact, intravenous drug use, tattooing, body piercing, and even sharing electric razors. On the basis of these modes of transmission, college students should be aware of the potential risk that they too carry for HBV infection. Beyond the risk factors just identified, medical and dental procedures are also a potential means of transmitting the virus, including patient to practitioner, and practitioner to patient transmission. Chronic HBV infection has been associated with liver cirrhosis and is the principal cause of liver cancer. An effective immunization for hepatitis B is now available; thus, the incidence of HBV in children and adolescents has dropped by one-fifth since 1999. However, an increase has been noted in people over 19 years of age. Although it is given during childhood, it should be seriously considered for older unvaccinated people and college students. In 2002 the American Academy of Pediatrics recommended that all newborns be immunized before leaving the hospital. A new vaccine against both hepatitis A and B is now available. Earlier concerns regarding hepatitis B vaccine and multiple sclerosis have been largely dismissed.

Hepatitis C is contracted in ways similar to hepatitis B (sexual contact, tainted blood, and shared needles). In the absence of immunization, the pool of infected people is in excess of 4 million, and the death rate is expected to climb. Currently a dual-drug therapy for HCV involving multiple forms of interferon in combination with the drug ribavirin is the treatment of choice. Many infected persons remain asymptomatic for decades, and many persons infected with HCV recover from this liver-threatening infection. People in the latter group appear to have a genetically based ability to stimulate a high level of natural killer cells (NK cells) within the immune system (see Chapter 11).[19] In a recent study, a two-drug combination treatment resulted in a virus-free state for nearly 60 percent of a large group of infected persons treated for 1 year. In spite of encouraging news such as this, recovery from HCV infection seems less likely the case for infected African Americans, a phenomenon that cannot currently be explained.

The newly identified type D (delta) hepatitis is very difficult to treat and is found almost exclusively in people already suffering from type B hepatitis, since the hepatitis D virus requires the presence of the hepatitis B virus in order to gain full pathogenicity. This virus, like type B hepatitis and HIV, makes unprotected sexual contact, including anal and oral sex, very risky. Hepatitis E, associated with water contamination, is rarely seen in this country other than in people returning from hepatitis E virus-endemic areas of the world.

Sudden Acute Respiratory Syndrome (SARS)

In February 2003, the world became aware of a previously unknown respiratory disease, initially thought to be a form of pneumonia. This disease, characterized by high fever (100.4+°F), chills, headaches and, a few days later a dry cough, was, in fact, a new viral disease, *Sudden Acute Respiratory Syndrome* (*SARS*). First reported in Hanoi, then in Singapore, mainland China, and other Asian countries, the disease quickly presented in Europe and North America. In actuality, the disease had first appeared in a rural area of China, during the fall of 2002, but the Chinese government had apparently chosen not to disseminate this information.

With the rapid spread of SARS, the World Health Organization and CDC issued travel advisories against unnecessary travel to several areas and cities of Asia, as well as to Toronto, Canada. At the same time, scientists isolated the virus responsible for the respiratory disease and identified it as a member of the coronavirus family—a viral family with links to upper respiratory infection (colds). This particular virus, however, apparently entered the human germ pool in conjunction with the eating of civet cats—a delicacy in China—again demonstrating that many infectious conditions in humans have their origins in other animals— **zoonosis.** There still remains, however, some doubt as to whether the civet cat is the principal reservoir of the SARS virus or if rats or other rodents living in close proximity infect both the civet cat and humans.

With news of the SARS outbreak, the international scientific community began a cooperative effort to understand the disease's human-to-human transmission. It was quickly determined that the virus was transmitted by respiratory droplets. It was further determined that the frail, the elderly, and the young were at greatest risk, as well as persons in direct contact with symptomatic persons (family members and hospital staff). Soon thereafter, a diagnostic test was developed and treatment protocols became more focused and effective. These developments, in combination with concerted public health measures regarding the recognition of symptoms and curtailment of transmission opportunities, led to a rapid decline of reported new cases. On June 5, 2003, the World Health Organization declared that SARS had peaked and was subsiding in all infected areas. By the WHO-defined end of the pandemic, August 15, 2003, 33 people in the United States had been infected and none had died, while worldwide 8,422 had been infected and 916 had died.[20] Clearly, in terms of a potentially pandemic disease, the global village had been condensed in size by international travel and commerce.

> **Key Terms**
>
> **zoonosis** the transmission of diseases from animals to humans

However, between late summer of 2003 and early fall of 2004, evidence of a greater understanding of SARS virology, as well as its transmission, treatment and confinement became apparent. On October 6, 2004, the CDC announced that the outbreak of laboratory-acquired SARS cases in China had been controlled and that there were no known cases of SARS anywhere in the world.[21]

Bird (Avian) Influenza

As noted earlier in the chapter, countries are interconnected to such an extent that emerging infections can be spread globally in a matter of days, if not hours. Because of this, the probability of future pandemics—including one of *bird (avian) flu*—is nearing certainty. Based on extrapolations from the 1918 influenza pandemic and taking into account improvements in health care, the most conservative estimates of deaths if (some experts confidently say "when") avian flu reaches pandemic levels are a billion people ill, with 2 to 7 million deaths. Two highly respected experts in infectious disease epidemiology have separately predicted that one-quarter to one-third of the world's population would become ill and 180 million deaths would result. The financial costs would be in the tens of billions of dollars.[22]

Bird flu first reached the public in 2003 when health officials in Laos, Cambodia, Vietnam, and eventually nearly a dozen more Asian countries reported the wholesale death of millions of chickens, and by the end of 2004, the death of 45 humans—all infected with new orthomyxovirus, H5N1, a highly virulent mutated version of the avian virus associated with the Hong Kong bird flu epidemic of 1997. In this latest case, the 45 deaths represented about three-fourths of the infected people seen during that year.

Because the highly virulent H5N1 has now acquired genetic material from a widening array of animal hosts (chickens, ducks, turkeys, and other birds, and possibly cats) and could comingle with the less virulent but human-to-human transmissible avian virus (H7), the probability of a "super version" is high. To date killing or immunizing fowl has been the principal method of minimizing bird-to-human transmission,[23] but human-to-human transmission would be extremely difficult to curtail. Thus, as the world awaits coming flu seasons, vaccine experimentation is underway, and[24] several countries, including the United States and Canada, have begun stockpiling antiviral medications.

AIDS

AIDS (acquired immunodeficiency syndrome) has become the most devastating infectious disease in recent history and it is virtually certain to be among the most devastating diseases in history unless a cure is forthcoming. Setting aside for the present the international scope of the HIV/AIDS epidemic, statistics for the United States alone paint a distressing picture. On the basis of data reported through December 2003, a total of 934,485 Americans have been diagnosed with AIDS, and 524,060 have died from its effects (or 56.3 percent of all cases).[25]

Cause of AIDS

AIDS is the disease caused by HIV, a virus that attacks the helper T cells of the immune system (see pages 308–310). When HIV attacks helper T cells, people lose the ability to fight off a variety of infections that would normally be easily controlled. Because these infections develop while people are vulnerable, they are collectively called *opportunistic infections.* HIV-infected (HIV+) patients become increasingly vulnerable to infection by bacteria, protozoa, fungi, and several viruses. A variety of malignancies also develop during this period of immune-system vulnerability.

HIV+ with AIDS was originally diagnosed based on the presence of specific conditions. Among these were *Pneumocystis carinii* pneumonia and Kaposi's sarcoma, a rare but deadly form of skin cancer. Gradually, experts recognized that additional conditions were associated with advancing deterioration of the immune system and thus added them to the list of AIDS conditions. This list now includes almost 30 definitive conditions, with more conditions being added as they become apparent. Among the conditions found on the current version of the list are toxoplasmosis within the brain, cytomegalovirus retinitis with loss of vision, lymphoma involving the brain, recurrent salmonella blood infections, and a wasting syndrome that includes invasive cervical cancer in women, recurrent pneumonia, and recurrent tuberculosis. Today, however, experts tend to assign the label of HIV+ with AIDS to HIV-infected people when their level of helper T cells drops below 250 cells per cubic milliliter of blood, regardless of whether specific conditions are present.

Spread of HIV

HIV cannot be contracted easily in comparison to other infectious conditions such as colds, flu, and some childhood infections that can spread quickly within a classroom or office complex. The chances of contracting HIV through casual contact with HIV-infected people at work, school, or home are extremely low or nonexistent. HIV is known to be spread only by direct sexual contact involving the exchange of bodily fluids (including blood, semen, and vaginal secretions), the sharing of hypodermic needles, transfusion of infected blood or blood products, and perinatal transmission (from an infected mother to a fetus or newborn baby). For HIV to be transmitted, it must enter the bloodstream of the noninfected person, such as through needles or tears in body tissues lining the rectum, mouth, or reproductive system. Current research also indicates that HIV is not transmitted by sweat, saliva, tears, or urine, although the virus may be found in very low concentrations in these fluids. The virus cannot enter the body through the gastrointestinal system because digestive enzymes destroy the virus. An exception to this generalization, however, might exist, as studies conducted in Africa indicate that transmission can occur in conjunction with breast-feeding infants.[26] A second exception involves the transmission of HIV between infected persons and their uninfected sexual partners during episodes of unprotected oral sex when the uninfected persons have evident gingivitis and bleeding gums.[27]

Women are at much greater risk than men are of contracting HIV through heterosexual activity because of the higher concentration of lymphocytes in semen ($\pm$10 million lymphocytes/tsp) than in vaginal secretions ($\pm$1,200 thousand lymphocytes/tsp). This susceptibility is evidenced in part by the increasing percentage of women with AIDS who were infected through heterosexual contact—from 8 percent in 1981, to 19 percent in 1993, and 73 percent in 2003.[25] Women under age 25 contract the virus principally through heterosexual contact. Figure 12-3 shows the estimated number of new cases of HIV worldwide.

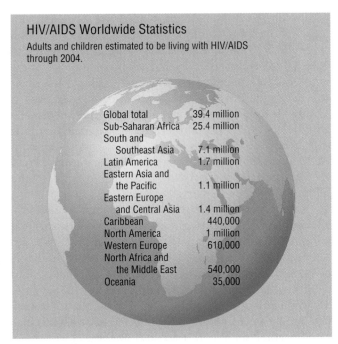

HIV/AIDS Worldwide Statistics

Adults and children estimated to be living with HIV/AIDS through 2004.

Global total	39.4 million
Sub-Saharan Africa	25.4 million
South and Southeast Asia	7.1 million
Latin America	1.7 million
Eastern Asia and the Pacific	1.1 million
Eastern Europe and Central Asia	1.4 million
Caribbean	440,000
North America	1 million
Western Europe	610,000
North Africa and the Middle East	540,000
Oceania	35,000

Figure 12-3 For every person counted in these statistics, there is a face and a story. What are you doing to protect yourself from HIV/AIDS?

Signs and Symptoms of HIV Infection

Most people infected with HIV initially feel well and have no symptoms (that is, they are asymptomatic). Experts generally consider the *incubation stage* for HIV infection to be 6 months to 10 or more years, with the average approximately 6 years. Despite the long period between infection and the first clinical observation of damage to the immune system, antibodies to HIV may appear within several weeks to three months of contracting the virus. Of course, relatively few people are tested for HIV infection at any time during the incubation period. Thus infected people could remain asymptomatic (currently described as HIV+ without symptoms) and be carriers of HIV for years before they experience signs of illness sufficient to warrant a physical examination. In light of the long incubation of HIV infection and the relatively small percentage of the general public yet tested, the cost-effectiveness of very widescale HIV screening has received renewed interest.[28] On the basis of new research, the CDC is reevaluating its current, and more restrictive, guidelines regarding screening populations.

Without symptoms of immune-system deterioration or AIDS-testing results, sexually active people need to redefine the meaning of monogamy. Couples must now account for the sexual partners they have both had over the past 10 years. Unfortunately, people do this so infrequently that some observers are labeling today's young adults "a generation in jeopardy."

Most people infected with HIV, in the absence of early screening and prophylactic drug treatment, eventually develop signs and symptoms of a more advanced stage of the disease. These signs and symptoms include tiredness, fever, loss of appetite and weight, diarrhea, night sweats, and swollen glands (usually in the neck, armpits, and groin). At this point, they are said to be HIV+ with symptoms. (See Table 12.4.)

Given sufficient time, perhaps as long as 15 years, most infected people without prophylactic drug treatment move beyond HIV with symptoms into the *acute stage*. At this point, the label HIV+ with AIDS is applied, either on the basis of clinically defined conditions or more likely on the basis of a helper T cell count below 250 per cubic milliliter of blood. A normal helper T cell range is 800 to 1,000. The efficacy of treatment is based in part on improvements in the T cell count over time.

A small percentage of infected people can suppress the infection and have survived for over two decades without developing AIDS, but experts do not fully understand this ability (possibly attributing it to a suppressor compound formed by specific immune system cells).

Diagnosis of HIV Infection

HIV infection is diagnosed through a clinical examination, laboratory tests for accompanying infections, and an initial

Table 12.4 The Spectrum of HIV Infection

	HIV+ without Symptoms (Asymptomatic)	HIV+ with Symptoms	HIV+ with AIDS
External signs	No symptoms Looks well	Fever Night sweats Swollen lymph glands Weight loss Diarrhea Minor infections Fatigue	Kaposi's sarcoma *Pneumocystis carinii* pneumonia and/or other predetermined illnesses Neurological disorders One or more of an additional 30+ diagnosable conditions or a helper T cell count falls below 250 per cubic milliliter of blood
Incubation	Invasion of virus to 10 years	Several months to 10 or more years	Several months to 10–12 or more years
Internal level of infection	Antibodies are produced Immune system remains intact Positive antibody test	Antibodies are produced Immune system weakened Positive antibody test	Immune system deficient Positive antibody test
Infectious?	Yes	Yes	Yes

screening test. Should the initial screening test produce a negative result, persons at risk for infection should be re-screened in 3 to 6 months. For persons reluctant to present themselves for screening in a clinical setting, home screening tests are also available. Regardless, once initial screening has been undertaken, to eliminate the small chance of a false positive having occurred, more sensitive tests can be administered, including the enzyme-linked immunosorbent assay (ELISA) and Western blot test. Although expensive and not completely reliable, even more recently developed tests are now available. One of these tests identifies the existence of viral mutations known to be drug resistant, while another helps determine whether a particular drug will function in suppressing the contracted viral strain. This information helps physicians structure treatment protocols.

Treatment of HIV and AIDS

There is no cure for HIV infection and the resultant AIDS. It is critically important, however, that treatment begin upon diagnosis or at least no later than the time at which the T cell count reaches 250/cubic milliliter of blood. Current treatment uses a combination of drugs drawn principally from two distinct groups: the *reverse-transcriptase inhibitors* (divided into two classes, nucleoside analogs and nonnucleoside analogs reverse-transcriptase inhibitors) and the *protease inhibitors.*

The reverse-transcriptase inhibitors block (or inhibit) the action of reverse transcriptase, an enzyme the virus requires to replicate itself within the host's infected T helper cells. Currently a combination of two of the many available reverse-transcriptase inhibitors is used to formulate a portion of the drug "cocktail" employed in treating HIV infection.

Introduction of the protease inhibitors, in combination with the reverse-transcriptase inhibitors, has revolu-

tionized the treatment of HIV infection. These drugs inhibit the ability of the virus to undertake the replication process. In most treatment protocols, one protease inhibitor is combined with two reverse-transcriptase inhibitors to complete the drug cocktail.

In addition to reverse-transcriptase inhibitors and protease inhibitors, three recently introduced types of medications have been developed to further enhance the battle against HIV/AIDS. Now, newer and even more potent "cocktails" are developed by combining both older and new medication. The treatment is deemed highly active antiretroviral therapy, or *HAART.* HAART has proven highly effective in extending the life of many persons with HIV/AIDS by significantly reducing the level of HIV (viral load) in the body. Decision as to what a given patients' HAART will consist of is determined by factors such as the viral load data and the presence of preexisting conditions.

In the final analysis, however, as effective as HAART is in improving the length and quality of life for persons with HIV/AIDS, mortality concerns remain, and life expectancy is compromised. The inability of persons with AIDS to move into and through the *decline stage* and on to the *recovery stage* reflects the relationship between the disease and the immune system itself.

In addition to the antiviral drugs, physicians also have a variety of medications to treat the symptoms associated with various infections and malignancies that make up AIDS. These drugs, of course, cannot reverse HIV status or cure AIDS. Researchers continue to search for vaccines to prevent HIV infection. Currently, several HIV vaccines are in the initial stage (Phase I) of human trial. One vaccine, under development by Merck Pharmaceuticals, has recently entered Phase II trials after showing considerable promise in initial trials. Of the two vaccines to reach Phase III trials (the most extensive trials before FDA approval for marketing), one was deemed unsuccessful, and trials using the second are ongoing.

The reality of HIV/AIDS in Africa and Asia is only now being recognized worldwide. With an estimated 25.4 million infected persons in sub-Saharan Africa and an additional 7.1 million infected persons in Southeast Asia, the need for a vaccine specific to the viral strains of these areas is growing rapidly.[29] In late 2000, a radically new and relatively inexpensive vaccine using segments of HIV DNA attached to salmonella bacteria underwent its initial human trials in Uganda. Should this innovative approach prove safe and effective, then progress can be made in quelling the potential catastrophe that is taking form on these two continents. Conversely, in the absence of a vaccine (and the inability to effectively treat those currently infected), it is projected that African life expectancy will drop to 29 years and that more than 29 million orphans will need care. Similar consequences would be expected in areas of Asia.

Prevention of HIV Infection

Can HIV infection be prevented? The answer is a definite yes. HIV infection rates on college campuses are considered low (approximately 0.2 percent), but students can be at risk. Every person can take several steps to reduce the risk of contracting and transmitting HIV. All these steps require understanding one's behavior and the methods by which HIV can be transmitted. Some appropriate steps for college-aged people are abstinence, safer sex, sobriety, and communication with potential sexual partners. To ensure the greatest protection from HIV, one should abstain from sexual activity. Other than this, Changing for the Better lists recommendations for safer sex, sobriety, and the exchange of honest, accurate information about sexual histories.

The role of prevention may become even more critical than it is now if an initial case of a drug-resistant form of HIV is proven to be more than an anomaly. This situation relates to an HIV infection in a New York City patient who failed to respond to three of the established drug protocols and progressed to AIDS within a few months.[30] The person involved was described as a male in his 40s, sexually promiscuous (anal intercourse), and a user of methamphetamine, but who apparently had a normal immune system before becoming infected. Clinicians in San Diego reported that they too may be dealing with a similar situation. Other HIV/AIDS experts believe that this situation does not represent the beginning of a drug-resistant form of the HIV-1 virus but is a true anomaly.

TALKING POINTS In a job interview with a representative from a large pharmaceutical company, you are asked about your feelings regarding the affordability of HIV/AIDS medications in third world countries. What would your response be?

Sexually Transmitted Diseases

Sexually transmitted diseases (STDs) were once called venereal diseases (for Venus, the Roman goddess of love). Today the term *venereal disease* has been superseded by the broader terms *sexually transmitted disease* or *sexually transmitted infection*. Experts currently emphasize the successful prevention and treatment of STDs rather than the ethics of sexuality. Thus one should consider the

Key Terms

sexually transmitted diseases (STDs) infectious diseases that are spread primarily through intimate sexual contact

following points: (1) By age 25 years approximately one-third of all adults will have contracted a sexually transmitted disease—most often chlamydia, herpes simplex, or human papillomavirus infection; (2) a person can have more than one STD at a time; (3) the symptoms of STDs can vary over time and from person to person; (4) the body develops little immunity for STDs; and (5) STDs can predispose people to additional health problems, including infertility, birth defects in their children, cancer, and long-term disability. In addition, the risk of HIV infection is higher when sexual partners are also infected with STDs.

This section focuses on the STDs most frequently diagnosed among college students (chlamydia, gonorrhea, human papillomavirus infection, herpes simplex, syphilis, and pubic lice). (Complete the Personal Assessment on page 335 to determine your risk of contracting an STD. See Changing for the Better on page 325 for safer sex practices.)

Chlamydia (Nonspecific Urethritis)

Chlamydia is thought to be the most prevalent STD in the United States today. Chlamydia infections occur an estimated 5 times more frequently than does gonorrhea and up to 10 times more frequently than syphilis. Because of its high prevalence in sexually active adolescents (310,505 cases in 2003),[31] they should be screened for chlamydia twice a year, even in the absence of symptoms. Because chlamydia frequently accompanies gonorrheal infections, a dual therapy is often appropriate when gonorrhea is found. Sexually active people in the 20- to 24-year age range (324,411 cases in 2003)[31] should also be considered for routine screening, particularly if they have a history of multiple sex partners and have not practiced a form of barrier contraception (also see Figure 12-4).[32]

Chlamydia trachomatis is the bacterial agent that causes the chlamydia infection. Chlamydia is the most common cause of nonspecific urethritis (NSU). NSU describes infections of the **urethra** and surrounding tissues that are not caused by the bacterium responsible for gonorrhea. About 80 percent of men with chlamydia display gonorrhea-like signs and symptoms, including painful urination and a whitish pus discharge from the penis. As in gonorrheal infections and many other STDs, most women report no overt signs or symptoms. A few women might exhibit a mild urethral discharge, painful urination, and swelling of vulval tissues. The recommended treatment for chlamydia is either a single dose of azithromycin (1 g) or doxycycline (100 mg) given orally twice a day for 7 days. The infected person should carefully comply with instructions to abstain from sexual intercourse.[32]

Both sexual partners should receive treatment to avoid the ping-pong effect—the back-and-forth reinfection that occurs among couples when only one partner receives treatment. Furthermore, as with other STDs, having chlamydia once does not effectively confer immunity.

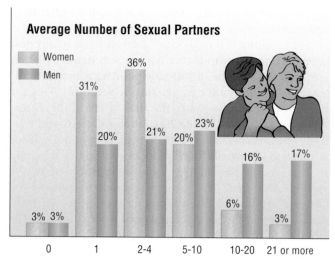

Average Number of Sexual Partners

Women
Men

0: 3% 3%
1: 31% 20%
2-4: 36% 21%
5-10: 20% 23%
10-20: 6% 16%
21 or more: 3% 17%

Figure 12-4 Average number of sexual partners men and women have had since age 18. The fewer the number of partners you've had, the lower your risk of contracting HIV or an STD.

Source: Michael RT, Gagnon JH, Laumann EO, Kolata G: *Sex in America: A definitive study.*

Unresolved chlamydia can lead to the same negative health consequences that result from untreated gonorrheal infections. In men the pathogens can invade and damage the deeper reproductive structures (the prostate gland, seminal vesicles, and Cowper's glands). Sterility can result. The pathogens can spread further and produce joint problems (arthritis) and heart complications (damaged heart valves, blood vessels, and heart muscle tissue).

In women the pathogens enter the body through the urethra or the cervical area. If the invasion is not properly treated, it can reach the deeper pelvic structures, producing a syndrome called **pelvic inflammatory disease (PID).** The infection may attack the inner uterine wall (endometrium), the fallopian tubes, and any surrounding structures to produce this painful syndrome. A variety of further complications can result, including

---

Key Terms

chlamydia the most prevalent sexually transmitted disease; caused by a nongonococcal bacterium

urethra (yoo **ree** thra) the passageway through which urine leaves the urinary bladder

pelvic inflammatory disease (PID) an acute or chronic infection of the peritoneum or lining of the abdominopelvic cavity and fallopian tubes; associated with a variety of symptoms or none at all and a potential cause of sterility

sterility, ectopic (tubal) pregnancies, and **peritonitis.** Infected women can transmit a chlamydia infection to the eyes and lungs of newborns during a vaginal birth. Detecting chlamydia and other NSUs early is of paramount concern for both men and women.

Human Papillomavirus

The appearance of another STD, **human papillomavirus (HPV),** is unwanted news. Because HPV infections are generally asymptomatic, the exact extent of the disease is unknown. A study of a group of sexually active college women found HPV infection in approximately 20 percent of the women. HPV-related changes to the cells of the cervix are found in nearly 5 percent of the Pap smears taken from women under age 30. Researchers currently believe that risk factors for HPV infection in women include: (1) sexual activity before age 20, (2) intercourse with three or more partners before age 35, and (3) intercourse with a partner who has three or more partners. The extent of HPV infection in men is even less clearly known, but it is probably widespread.

HPV infection is alarming because some of the more than 50 forms of the virus are strongly associated with precancerous changes to cells lining the cervix, illustrating the importance of new viral Pap smears (see Chapter 11). Additionally, visible genital warts (cauliflower-like, raised, pinkish-white lesions) are associated with viral forms 6 or 11, while viral forms 16, 18, 31, 33, and 35 foster changes in other areas[32] (Figure 12-5). Found most commonly on the penis, scrotum, labia, cervix, and around the anus, these lesions represent the most common symptomatic viral STD in this country. Although most genital wart colonies are small, they may become very large and block the anus or birth canal during pregnancy.

Treatment for HPV, including genital warts, may include patient-applied gels or creams or physician-administered cryotherapy, topical medication, or surgery. Regardless of treatment, however, the viral colonies will probably return. One should use condoms to attempt to prevent transmission of HPV.

As noted in Chapter 11, in conjunction with cervical cancer, a vaccine effective for HPV 16 and 18 has been approved for use. Several additional vaccines are under development, some intended for use in newly infected patients, some for long-established infections but before clear changes in the cervical lining cells occur, and others for more advanced cervical cancer.[33] Most of the last two classes of vaccines are for treatment rather than prevention of HPV infections.

Gonorrhea

Another extremely common (600,000 cases/year estimated and 335,104 cases/year reported) STD, *gonorrhea* is caused by a bacterium (*N. gonorrhoea*). The incidence of gonorrhea rose 18 percent between 1997 and 2003, perhaps, in part, because of decreasing fear of HIV/AIDS brought about by the effectiveness of the protease inhibitors being widely reported at that time. However, since 2001 the reported cases of gonorrhea have declined.[34] In men this bacterial agent can produce a milky-white discharge from the penis, accompanied by painful urination. About 80 percent of men who contract gonorrhea report varying degrees of these symptoms. This figure is approximately reversed for women: Only about 20 percent of women are symptomatic and thus report varying degrees of frequent, painful urination, with a slimy yellow-green discharge from the vagina or urethra. Oral sex with an infected partner can produce a gonorrheal infection of the throat (pharyngeal gonorrhea). Gonorrhea can also be transmitted to the rectal areas of both men and women.

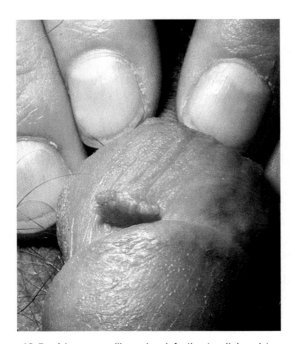

Figure 12-5 A human papillomavirus infection (genital warts).

> ## Key Terms
>
> **peritonitis** (pare it ton **eye** tis) inflammation of the peritoneum, or lining of the abdominopelvic cavity
>
> **human papillomavirus (HPV)** sexually transmitted viruses, some of which are capable of causing precancerous changes in the cervix; causative agent for genital warts

An interesting finding relative to gonorrhea in adolescents suggests that the incidence of gonorrhea within the adolescent population correlated closely with the consumption of beer, suggesting that alcohol consumption fosters a higher level of high-risk sexual behavior, including earlier onset of sexual activity, an increased number of partners, and less selectivity in choosing those partners. With heavy consumption of beer on many college campuses, this finding does not bode well for the highly asymptomatic female population.

Physicians diagnose gonorrhea by culturing the bacteria. Because of the paired occurrence of chlamydia and gonorrhea, dual therapy with doxycycline or azithromycin in combination with ofloxacin is used in susceptible populations, particularly adolescent women. Outside these groups, recommended treatment for uncomplicated cases involves the use of one of several antimicrobial drugs. Although prevalent in other areas of the world, drug-resistant strains are not extensive in the United States.[32] This said, however, it should be noted that a clear increase in drug-resistant strains has been reported along the west coast, in various Pacific areas, such as Hawaii, other Pacific Islands, and Asia. Infected persons who might have contracted the disease while in these areas should report this information to their physicians.

Testing for gonorrhea is included as a part of prenatal care so that infections in mothers can be treated before they give birth. If the birth canal is infected, newborns can easily contract the infection in the mucous membranes of the eye.

Herpes Simplex

Public health officials think that the sexually transmitted genital herpes virus infection rivals chlamydia as the most prevalent STD. To date about forty-five million Americans have been diagnosed, although the asymptomatic (thus undiagnosed) population could increase this figure substantially. *Herpes* is really a family of more than 50 viruses, some of which produce recognized diseases in humans (chicken pox, **shingles,** mononucleosis, and others). One subgroup, called herpes simplex 1 virus (HSV-1), produces an infection called *labial herpes* (oral or lip herpes). Labial herpes produces common fever blisters or cold sores around the lips and oral cavity. Herpes simplex 2 virus (HSV-2) is a different strain that produces similar clumps of blisterlike lesions in the genital region (Figure 12-6). Laypeople call this second type of herpes the STD type, but both types produce identical clinical pictures. About 5 to 30 percent of cases are caused by HSV-1. Oral-genital sexual practices most likely account for this crossover infection.

Herpes appears as a single sore or as a small cluster of blisterlike sores. These sores burn, itch, and (for some) become very painful. The infected person might also

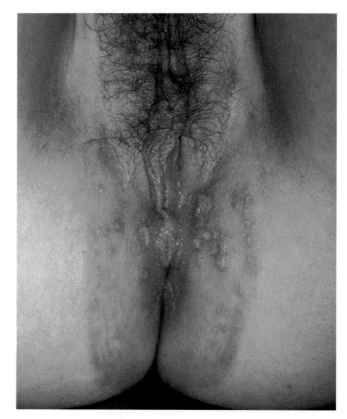

Figure 12-6 A severe herpes infection

report swollen lymph glands, muscular aches and pains, and fever. Some patients feel weak and sleepy when they have blisters. The lesions may last from a few days to a few weeks. Viral shedding lasts a week on average; then the blisters begin scabbing, and new skin is formed. Even when the patient has become asymptomatic, viral transmission is still possible.

Herpes is an interesting virus for several reasons. It can lie dormant for long periods. For reasons not well understood but perhaps related to stress, diet, or overall health, the viral particles can be stimulated to travel along the nerve pathways to the skin and then create an active infection. Thus herpes can be considered a recurrent infection. Fortunately for most people, recurrent infections are less severe than the initial episode and do not last as long. Recommended treatment for an initial outbreak of herpes calls for

> **Key Terms**
>
> **shingles**   painful fluid-filled skin eruptions along underlying sensory nerve pathways—due to reactivation of once-sequestered herpes zoster (chicken pox) viruses

the use of one of three medications: acyclovir, famciclovir, or valacyclovir. These medications are taken orally, multiple times each day, for 7 to 10 days. Because herpes may occur at intervals following initial treatment, two choices exist. One is to treat each recurrence as it arises (episodic recurrent treatment), and the second is to attempt to suppress recurrence through continuous use of medication (daily suppressive therapy). The treatment choices described above appear to be equally effective for HSV-1 and HSV-2.[32] Additionally, physicians may recommend other medications for relief of various symptoms. Genital herpes is almost always diagnosed through a clinical examination.

Currently, the best method of preventing herpes infection is to avoid all direct contact with a person who has an active infection. Do not kiss someone with a fever blister—or let them kiss you (or your children) if they have an active lesion. Do not share drinking glasses or eating utensils. Check your partner's genitals. Do not have intimate sexual contact with someone who displays the blisterlike clusters or rash. (Condoms are only marginally helpful and cannot protect against lesions on the female vulva or the lower abdominal area of men.) Be careful not to infect yourself by touching a blister and then touching any other part of your body. Changing for the Better gives helpful advice about talking with your partner if you have genital herpes.

Note that valacyclovir is now available and is more effective than earlier medications are. Intended as a prophylactic medication (to be taken daily), valacyclovir does reduce the incidence of viral shedding, but it does not completely suppress episodes of recurrent herpes.[35]

Syphilis

Like gonorrhea, *syphilis* is caused by a bacterium (*Treponema pallidum*) and is transmitted almost exclusively by sexual intercourse. The incidence of syphilis, a CDC-reportable disease, is far lower than that of gonorrhea. In 1950 a record 217,558 cases of syphilis were reported in this country. The number of cases then fell steadily to fewer than 80,000 cases in 1980. From 1980 through 1990 the incidence climbed, reaching nearly 140,000 cases in 1990. Another decline then began, and in 1993 the number of cases dropped to 101,259. In 2000 the CDC reported that syphilis had fallen to the lowest level (5,972) in 42 years. By 2003, however, reported syphilis cases had risen to 7,177, with increases across all racial and ethnic groups, with the exception of African Americans.[36]

Whether the upward trend in the number of reported syphilis cases continues remains to be seen. As has been true for most of the last decades a high percentage of cases have been associated with HIV infections, largely among gay men in several larger cities. (See the Star box on

page 330 for more information on this disease.) Observers have noted an alarming increase in infant syphilis in children born to mothers who use drugs and support their habit through sexual activity.

Pubic Lice

Three types of lice infect humans: The head louse, the body louse, and the pubic louse all feed on the blood of the host. Except for the relatively uncommon body louse, these tiny insects do not carry diseases. They are, however, very annoying.

Pubic lice, also called *crabs,* attach themselves to the base of the pubic hairs, where they live and lay their eggs (nits). These eggs move into a larval stage after one week; after two more weeks, they develop into mature adult crab lice.

Changing for the Better

Talking with Your Partner about Herpes

My girlfriend told me she has herpes and said she's "taking care of everything." What can I do to get things out in the open?

Although herpes rarely has serious consequences, the lesions are infectious and tend to reappear. It is important to talk openly with your partner about this sexually transmitted disease. Here are some tips to make things easier:

- *Educate yourself.*
  Be aware that herpes is rarely dangerous. Learn when the disease is most contagious (during the eruption and blister stage), and realize that herpes can be spread even during the noneruption, nonblister periods—traditionally defined as safe periods.
- *Choose the right time to talk.*
  Discuss herpes with your partner only after you have gotten to know each other.
- *Listen to your partner.*
  Be prepared to answer any questions that he or she may have.
- *Together, put things in perspective.*
  Keep a positive outlook.
  Remember that you are not alone.
  Be aware that using a condom and abstaining from coitus during the most infectious period can prevent transmission of the disease.
  Although there is no known cure, research continues on an antiviral drug.
  Join a local support group together.

www.herpeszone/MainMenu.htm

Syphilis

Syphilis is a serious disease that, left untreated, can cause death. The chance of contracting syphilis during a single sexual encounter with an infected partner is now about 30%. Syphilis takes a well-established course after it is contracted.

Infection

The syphilis bacterium, *Treponema pallidum,* is a spirochete. It is transmitted from an infected person to a new host through intimate contact. Moist, warm tissue, such as that lining the reproductive, urinary, and digestive tracts, offers an ideal environment for the agent.

Incubation

Syphilis incubates without symptoms for 10 to 90 days, followed by the characteristic primary stage of the disease.

Primary Stage

The primary stage of syphilis lasts 1 to 5 weeks. A small, raised, painless sore called a *chancre* forms at this time. This highly infectious lesion is not easily identified in 90% of women and 50% of men; thus these people generally do not seek treatment. The chancre heals in 4 to 8 weeks.

Secondary Stage

The extremely contagious secondary stage of the disease occurs 6 to 12 weeks after initial infection. The infectious agents are now systemic, so symptoms may include a generalized body rash, a sore throat, or a patchy loss of hair. A blood test (VDRL) will be positive, and treatment can be effectively administered. If untreated, the second stage subsides within 2 to 6 weeks. A pregnant woman can easily transmit syphilis to her fetus during this stage. Congenital syphilis often results in stillbirth or an infant born with a variety of life-threatening complications. Early treatment of infected pregnant women can prevent congenital syphilis.

Latent Stage

After the secondary stage subsides, an extended period of noninfectiousness occurs. The infectious agents remain dormant within the body cells, and the infected person displays few clinical signs during this state.

Late Stage

Syphilis can recur for a third time 15 to 25 years after initial contact. In late-stage syphilis, tissue damage is profound and irreversible. The person suffers damage to the cardiovascular system, central nervous system, eyes, and skin, and death from the effects of the disease is likely.

Treatment

Depending on the stage, syphilis is treated with varying doses of Benzathine penicillin G.

People usually notice they have a pubic lice infestation when they suffer intense itching in the genital region. Prescription and OTC creams, lotions, and shampoos are usually effective in killing both the lice and their eggs, although some reports suggest that lice are becoming resistant to OTC treatments.

Lice are not transmitted exclusively through sexual contact but also by contact with contaminated bedsheets and clothes. If you develop a pubic lice infestation, you must thoroughly treat yourself, your clothes, your sheets, and your furniture.

Vaginal Infections

Two common pathogens produce uncomfortable *vaginal infections.* The first is the yeast or fungus pathogen *Candida (Monilia) albicans,* which produces the yeast infection often called *thrush.* These organisms, commonly found in the vagina, seem to multiply rapidly when some unusual stressor (pregnancy, use of birth control pills or antibiotics, diabetes) affects a woman's body. This infection, now called *vulvovaginal candidiasis (VVC),*[32] is signaled by a white or cream-colored vaginal discharge that resembles cottage cheese. Vaginal itching and vulvar swelling are also commonly reported. Current treatment is based on the use of one of several prescription and OTC azole drugs. For women who have recurrent VVC, some degree of prophylactic suppression of candidiasis seems possible. Weekly use of a prescription antifungal medication (fluconazole) for periods of 6, 9, and 12 months managed to keep slightly over 40 percent of a group of women with recurrent[37] VVC free of infection for 12 months; higher percentages of infection-free patients were found at 6 and 9 months. Success after 12 months was not determined.

Nonprescription azole-based products offer effective home treatment. One should first consult with a physician before using these new products for the first time. (Men rarely report this monilial infection, although some may report mildly painful urination or a barely noticeable discharge at the urethral opening or beneath the foreskin of the penis.)

The protozoan *Trichomonas vaginalis* also produces a vaginal infection. This parasite can be transmitted through sexual intercourse or by contact with contaminated (often damp) objects, such as towels, clothing, or toilet seats, that may contain some vaginal discharge. In women, this infection, called *trichomoniasis,* or "trich," produces a foamy, yellow-green, foul-smelling discharge that may be accompanied by itching, swelling, and painful urination. Although topically applied treatments with limited effectiveness for trichomoniasis are available, only one highly effective oral medication is currently on the market.[32] Men infrequently contract trichomoniasis but may harbor the organisms without realizing it. They also should be treated to minimize reinfection of partners.

The vagina is warm, dark, and moist, an ideal breeding environment for a variety of organisms. Unfortunately, some highly promoted commercial products seem to increase the incidence of vaginal infections. Among these are tight panty hose (without cotton panels), which tend to increase the vaginal temperature, and commercial vaginal douches, which can alter the acidic level of the vagina. Both of these products might promote infections. Women are advised to wipe from front to back after every bowel movement to reduce the opportunity for direct transmission of pathogenic agents from the rectum to the vagina. Avoiding public bathrooms when possible is also a good practice. Of course, if you notice any unusual discharge from the vagina, you should report this to your physician.

Cystitis and Urethritis

Cystitis, an infection of the urinary bladder, and urethritis, an infection of the urethra, occasionally can be caused by a sexually transmitted organism. Such infections can also be caused by the organisms that cause vaginitis and organisms found in the intestinal tract. A culture is required to identify the specific pathogen associated with a particular case of cystitis or urethritis. The symptoms are pain when urinating, the need to urinate frequently, a dull aching pain above the pubic bone, and the passing of blood-streaked urine.

Physicians can easily treat cystitis and urethritis with antibiotics when the specific organism has been identified. The drug Monurol, which requires only a single dose,

has proved effective. Few complications result from infections that are treated promptly. If cystitis or urethritis is left untreated, the infectious agent could move upward in the urinary system and infect the ureters and kidneys. These upper-urinary-tract infections are more serious and require more extensive evaluation and aggressive treatment. Therefore one should obtain medical care immediately upon noticing symptoms.

A study involving urinary tract infections in mice, whose urinary tract infections are virtually identical to those in humans, demonstrated that the bacteria involved often avoid complete antibiotic elimination. This occurs when the bacteria clump into pods that are then covered by a "bio-film" produced by the organisms. The film retards further antibody effectiveness, allowing the infection to be re-established when antibiotics have been cleared from the body.

Preventing cystitis and urethritis depends to some degree on the source of the infectious agent. One can generally reduce the incidence of infection by urinating completely (to fully empty the urinary bladder) and by drinking ample fluids to flush the urinary tract. Drinking cranberry juice has been found to reduce urinary tract infections. Prevention of urinary tract infections cannot be disregarded, from both medical and cost perspectives. As noted, untreated cystitis and urethritis can be the basis of serious damage to the kidneys. These two infections combined are the second greatest cause of antibiotic use—which is both costly and increasingly losing effectiveness.

 TALKING POINTS Honesty regarding past sexual experiences is a critical issue in the decision to introduce sexual intimacy into a new relationship. What questions would you feel comfortable being asked by another person, and what questions would you be prepared to ask that person?

Taking Charge of Your Health

- Since microorganisms develop resistance to antibiotics, continue taking all such medications until gone, even when the symptoms of the infection have subsided.

- Check your current immunization status to make sure you are protected against preventable infectious diseases.

- If you are a parent, take your children to receive their recommended immunizations as necessary.

- Because of the possibility of contracting HIV/AIDS and sexually transmitted diseases, incorporate disease prevention into all your sexual activities.

- Use the Personal Assessment on page 335 to determine your risk of contracting a sexually transmitted disease.

- If you have ever engaged in high-risk sexual behavior, get tested for HIV.

SUMMARY

- We have made progress in reducing the incidence of some forms of infectious disease, but other infectious conditions are becoming more common.
- A variety of pathogenic agents are responsible for infectious conditions.
- A chain of infection with six potential links characterizes every infectious condition.
- One can acquire immunity for some diseases through both natural and artificial means. Children should be immunized according to a schedule.
- The immune system's response to infection relies on chemical-cellular and humoral elements.
- The common cold and influenza produce many similar symptoms but differ in their infectious agents, incubation period, prevention, and treatment.
- Tuberculosis and pneumonia are potentially fatal infections of the respiratory system.
- Mononucleosis and chronic fatigue syndrome are infections that produce chronic tiredness.
- Bacterial meningitis, a potentially fatal infection of the linings that cover the brain, is of increasing concern on college campuses.
- Lyme disease is a bacterial infection contracted through outdoor activities.
- Hantavirus pulmonary syndrome is caused by a virus carried by deer mice; human-to-human transmission has also been reported.

- West Nile virus is a vector-borne infection that is now widely distributed in the United States.
- Toxic shock syndrome is a bacterial infection generally arising from the improper use of tampons.
- Hepatitis B (serum hepatitis) is a bloodborne infectious condition that produces serious liver damage. Other varieties are hepatitis A, C, D, and E.
- SARS is a potentially fatal respiratory infection that reached North America from Asia.
- HIV/AIDS is a widespread, incurable viral disease transmitted through sexual activity, through intravenous drug use, in infected blood products, or across the placenta during pregnancy.
- The definitive diagnosis of AIDS can be based on the presence of specific conditions or a reduced number of helper T cells.
- HIV and AIDS are currently best treated with a drug cocktail, using protease inhibitors and reverse-transcriptase inhibitors; an effective vaccine for prevention has not been developed. Concerns are rising regarding the unchecked spread of HIV/AIDS in areas of Africa and Asia.
- There are a variety of sexually transmitted conditions, many of which do not produce symptoms in most infected women and many infected men.
- Safer sex practices can reduce the risk of contracting STDs.

REVIEW QUESTIONS

1. What are the agents responsible for the most familiar infectious conditions?
2. Describe the six links in the chain of infection.
3. What are the five stages that characterize the progression of infectious conditions?
4. What are the two principal chemical-cellular components of the immune system, and how do they cooperate to protect the body from infectious agents, foreign protein, and abnormal cells?
5. How are the common cold and influenza similar? How do they differ in their causative agents, incubation period, prevention, and treatment?
6. What symptoms make mononucleosis and chronic fatigue syndrome similar? What aspects of each are different?
7. Why is bacterial meningitis of greater concern on the college campus than elsewhere?
8. Why is outdoor activity a risk factor for contracting Lyme disease?
9. During what type of activities would persons most likely expose themselves to a hantavirus infection? What is the reservoir for the hantavirus?

10. What role do birds play in the transmission of the West Nile virus? What insect is the vector?
11. What group of persons seems most susceptible to the development of toxic shock syndrome? In what way is the infection most directly linked to the menstrual cycle?
12. How is hepatitis B transmitted, and which occupational group is at greatest risk of contracting this infection? How do forms A, C, D, and E compare with hepatitis B?
13. What is SARS? Where was the site of origin, and how did it most likely reach North America?
14. How is HIV transmitted? How are HIV/AIDS currently treated, and how effective is the treatment? In what areas of the world does the HIV/AIDS epidemic seem virtually unchecked? In terms of STD prevention, how can sexual practices be made safer?
15. Why are women more often asymptomatic for STDs than men?

ENDNOTES

1. Hamann B. *Disease Identification, Prevention, and Control* (2nd ed.). New York: McGraw-Hill, 2001.

2. Salidin KS. *Anatomy and Physiology: Unity of Form and Function* (4th ed.). New York: McGraw-Hill, 2007.

3. Parkham P. *The Immune System* (2nd ed.). New York: Garland Publishing, 2004.

4. Vander A, Sherman J, Luciano D. *Human Physiology: The Mechanisms of Body Function* (9th ed.). New York: McGraw-Hill, 2003.

5. Schonberger S, et al. Transplantation of haematopoietic stem cells derived from cord blood, bone marrow or peripheral blood: A single centre matched-pair analysis in a heterogeneous risk population. *Klin Padiatr.* 2004. 216(6):356–363.

6. Warwick R, Armitage S. Cord blood banking. *Best Pract Res Clin Obstet Gynaecol.* 2004. 18(6):995–1011.

7. Varricchio F, et al. Understanding vaccine safety information from the Vaccine Adverse Event Reporting System. *Pediatr Infect Dis* J. 2004. 23(4):287–294.

8. McQuillan GM, et al. Serologic immunity to diphtheria and tetanus in the United States. *Ann Intern Med.* 2002. 136(9);660–666.

9. Kruszon-Moran DM, McQuyillan GM, Chu SY. Tetanus and diphtheria immunity among females in the United States: Are recommendations being followed? *Am J Obstet Gynecol.* 2004. 190(4):1070–1076.

10. Guidelines & Recommendations. *Influenza antiviral medications: 2004–2005 interim chemoprophylaxis and treatment guidelines.* November 2004. www.cdc.gov/flu/professionals/treatment/0405/antiviralguide.htm.

11. Belshe RB, et al. Serum antibody responses after intradermal vaccination against influenza. *N Engl J Med.* 2004. 351(22):2286–2294.

12. Stohr K. Avian influenza and pandemics—research needs and opportunities. *N Engl J Med.* 2005. 352(4):405–407.

13. *Reported Tuberculosis in the United States, 2003.* U.S. Department of Health and Human Services, CDC. September 2004.

14. *Chronic Fatigue Syndrome, NIAID Fact Sheet.* 2004. National Institute of Allergy and Infectious Diseases. U.S. Department of Health and Human Services. www.niaid.nih.gov/factsheets/cfs.htm.

15. Fibromyalgia basics: Symptoms, treatments and research. 1999. www.fmnetnews.com/pages/basic.html.

16. Scott RD, et al. Vaccinating first-year college students living in dormitories for Meningococcal disease: An economic analysis. *Am J Prev Med.* 2002. 23(2):98–105.

17. Burke G, et al. Hypersensitivity to ticks and Lyme disease risk. *Emerg Infect Dis.* 2005. 11(1):36–41.

18. Zeier M, et al. New ecological aspects of hantavirus infection: A change of a paradigm and a challenge—a review. *Virus Genes.* 2005. 30(2):157–180.

19. Khakoo SI, et al. HLA and NK cell inhibitory receptor genes in resolving hepatitis C virus infection. *Science.* 2004. 305(5685):872–874.

20. World Health Organization. *Summary Table of SARS Cases by Country, 1 November 2002–7 August 2003.* www.who.int/entity/crs/sars/country/en/country200308_15.pdf. August 15, 2003.

21. Centers for Disease Control and Prevention. Department of Health and Human Services. *Current SARS Situation.* October 6, 2004. www/cdc.gov/ncidod/sars/situation.htm.

22. Specter M. Nature's bioterrorist: Is there any way to prevent a deadly avian-flu pandemic? *The New Yorker.* Feb. 28, 2005. pp 50–61.

23. Larkin M. Avian flu: Sites seek to respond and reassure. *Lancet Infect Dis.* 2005. 5(3):141–142.

24. Quirk M. USA to manufacture two million doses of pandemic flu vaccine. *Lancet Infect Dis.* 2005. 4(11):654.

25. Centers for Disease Control and Prevention, Department of Health and Human Services. *HIV/AIDS Surveillance Report. 2003* (Vol 15).

26. Coutsoudis A. Infant feeding dilemmas created by HIV: South African experiences. *J Nutr.* 2005. 135(4):956–959.

27. Edwards S, Crane C. Oral sex and the transmission of viral STIs. *JAMA.* 1998. 74(1):6–10.

28. Sanders GD, et al. Cost-effectiveness of screening for HIV in the era of highly active antiretroviral therapy. *N Engl J Med.* 2005. 352(6):570–585.

29. *Adults and Children Estimated to Be Living with HIV/AIDS, End 2004.* AIDS epidemic update: December 2004. www.unaids.org/wad2004/EPIupdate2004_html_enEPI04_13_en.htm.

30. Berkhout B, de Rhonde A, van der Hoek L. Aggressive HIV-1? *Retrovirology.* 2005. 2(1):13.

31. Centers for Disease Control and Prevention. *Chlamydia—Reported Cases and Rates per 100,000 Population by Age and Sex. United States 1999–2003.* www.cdc.gov/std/stats/tables/table10.htm.

32. Centers for Disease Control and Prevention. Sexually transmitted diseases treatment guidelines – 2002. *MMWR.* 2002. 51:(No.RR-6) 1–80.

33. American Cancer Society. What's new in cervical cancer research and treatment? *Cancer Reference Information.* www.cancer.org/docroot/CRI/content/CRI_2_4_6X_Whats_new_in_cervical_cancer.

34. Centers for Disease Control and Prevention. *Gonorrhea–Reported Cases and Rates per 100,000 Population by Age and Sex: United States 1999–2003.* www.cdc.gov/std/stats/tables/table20.htm.

35. Chakrabarty A, et al. Valacyclovir for the management of herpes viral infections. *Skin Therapy Lett.* 2005. 10(1):1–4.

36. Centers for Disease Control and Prevention. *Primary and Secondary Syphilis—Reported Cases by Race/Ethnicity, Age Group and Sex: United States 1999–2003.* www.cdc.gov/std/stats/tables/table34a.htm.

37. Sobel JD, et al. Maintenance fluconazole therapy for recurrent vulvovaginal candidiasis. *N Engl J Med.* 2004. 351(9):876–883.

Infectious diseases once common but now rare can, under certain circumstances, return with a vengeance. Cholera, a gastrointestinal bacterial infection that produces rapid and fatal diarrhea-induced dehydration is such a disease. When an outbreak of cholera develops it signals that human drinking water or food has been contaminated with human or animal waste. Cholera is currently occurring in several West African nations in conjunction with heavy rains that wash untreated sewage into wells and other drinking water sources. Compounding the problem are the mass migrations of displaced people fleeing politically induced hostilities and their settlement in overburdened refugee camps. Young children and the frail elderly are particularly vulnerable to the effects of cholera.

At the time of this writing, the United Nations describes the growing incidence of cholera as being an "upsurge" and is responding with antidiarrhea medications and, most important, uncontaminated drinking water supplies. Unfortunately, these supplies are not always effective, because of inadequately functioning health care delivery systems.

personal assessment

What is your risk of contracting a sexually transmitted disease?

A variety of factors interact to determine your risk of contracting a sexually transmitted disease (STD). This inventory is intended to provide you with an estimate of your level of risk.

Circle the number of each row that best characterizes you. Enter that number on the line at the end of the row (points). After assigning yourself a number in each row, total the number appearing in the points column. Your total points will allow you to interpret your risk for contracting an STD.

Age   **Points**

1	3	4	5	3	2	
0–9	10–14	15–19	20–29	30–34	35+	_____

Sexual Practices

0	1	2	4	6	8	
Never engage in sex	One sex partner	More than one sex partner but never more than one at a time	Two to five sex partners	Five to ten sex partners	Ten or more sex partners	_____

Sexual Attitudes

0	1	8	1	7	8	
Will not engage in nonmarital sex	Premarital sex is okay if it is with future spouse	Any kind of premarital sex is okay	Extramarital sex is not for me	Extramarital sex is okay	Believe in complete sexual freedom	_____

Attitudes toward Contraception

1	1	6	5	4	8	
Would use condom to prevent pregnancy	Would use condom to prevent STDs	Would never use a condom	Would use the birth control pill	Would use other contraceptive measure	Would not use anything	_____

Attitudes toward STD

3	3	4	6	6	6	
Am not sexually active so I do not worry	Would be able to talk about STD with my partner	Would check out an infection to be sure	Would be afraid to check out an infection	Can't even talk about an infection	STDs are no problem— easily cured	_____

YOUR TOTAL POINTS _____

Interpretation

5–8	Your risk is well below average
9–13	Your risk is below average
14–17	Your risk is at or near average
18–21	Your risk is moderately high
22+	Your risk is high

To Carry This Further . . .

Having taken this Personal Assessment, were you surprised at your level of risk? What is the primary reason for this level? How concerned are you and your classmates and friends about contracting an STD?

chapter thirteen

Understanding Sexuality

Chapter Objectives

On completing this chapter, you will be able to:

▌ explain the genetic basis and gonadal basis of sexuality.

▌ describe the psychosocial basis of sexuality, including gender identity, gender preference, gender adoption, and initial adult gender identification.

▌ define androgyny and discuss its role in our society.

▌ explain the components of the male and female reproductive systems.

▌ trace the menstrual cycle and identify the hormones that control the cycle.

▌ identify the four stages of the human sexual response pattern.

▌ discuss the refractory period and how it affects male sexual performance.

▌ discuss the effects of aging on both male and female sexual performance.

▌ define the three categories of sexual orientation.

▌ identify and discuss a few of the various lifestyles and relationships presented in this chapter.

Eye on the Media

Advertising to Gays and Lesbians

An evolving form of advertising is currently being seen in the United States and abroad. This approach depicts gays and lesbians in positive ways (that is, successful, attractive, happy); a far cry from historic, stereotypical views. What do these advertisements look like? You might be surprised, since the sexual orientation implications are frequently subtle and hidden.

To learn more about the blending of gay advertising into mainstream advertising, search the Web using "gay advertising" as the key words. One site you will likely find is the Web site for The Commercial Closet Association, a nonprofit educational and journalism organization that "works to improve public opinion of the lesbian, gay, bisexual, and transgender community through more informed GLBT portrayals in the powerful medium of advertising."[1] This Web site provides up-to-date reports, critiques, visitor reviews, live video lectures, and guidelines and resources for advertisers and the ad agencies they use. At this site, you can see The Commercial Closet's top 10 ads that feature advertising to gays and lesbians and see its list of "leaders and laggards" in gay advertising. You can also see video clips of many of these commercials. You might be surprised at how mainstream these commercials appear.

[1]The Commercial Closet. *Mission statement,* www.commercialcloset.com, May 1, 2005.

Early in the 21st century, we have reached an understanding of both the biological and psychosocial factors that contribute to the complex expression of our **sexuality.** As a society, we are now inclined to view human behavior in terms of a complex script written on the basis of both biology and conditioning. Reflecting this understanding is how we use the words "male" and "female" to refer to the biological roots of our sexuality and the words "man" and "woman" to refer to the psychosocial roots of our sexuality. This chapter explores human sexuality as it relates to the dynamic interplay of the biological and psychosocial bases that form your **masculinity** or **femininity.**

Biological Bases of Human Sexuality

Within a few seconds after the birth of a baby, someone—a doctor, nurse, or parent—emphatically labels the child: "It's a boy," or "It's a girl." For the parents and society as a whole, the child's **biological sexuality** is being displayed and identified. Another female or male enters the world.

Genetic Basis

At the moment of conception, a Y-bearing or an X-bearing sperm cell joins with the X-bearing ovum to establish the true basis of biological sexuality.[1] A fertilized ovum with sex chromosomes XX is biologically female, and a fertilized ovum bearing the XY sex chromosomes is biologically male. Genetics forms the most basic level of an individual's biological sexuality.

Gonadal Basis

The gonadal basis for biological sexuality refers to the growing embryo's development of **gonads.**[2] Male embryos develop testes about the 7th week after conception, and female embryos develop ovaries about the 12th week after conception.

Structural Development

The development of male or female reproductive structures is initially determined by the presence or absence of hormones produced by the developing testes—androgens and the müllerian inhibiting substance (MIS). With these hormones present, the male embryo starts to develop male reproductive structures (penis, scrotum, vas deferens, seminal vesicles, prostate gland, and Cowper's glands).

Because the female embryo is not exposed to these male hormones, it develops the characteristic female reproductive structures: uterus, fallopian tubes, vagina, labia, and clitoris.

Biological Sexuality and the Childhood Years

The growth and development of the child in terms of reproductive organs and physiological processes have traditionally been thought to be "latent" during the childhood years. However, a gradual degree of growth occurs in both girls and boys. The reproductive organs, however, will undergo more greatly accelerated growth at the onset of **puberty** and will achieve their adult size and capabilities shortly.

Puberty

The entry into puberty is a gradual maturing process for young girls and boys. For young girls, the onset of menstruation, called **menarche,** usually occurs at about age 12 or 13 but may come somewhat earlier or later.[3] Early menstrual cycles tend to be **anovulatory.** Menarche is usually preceded by a growth spurt that includes the budding of breasts and the growth of pubic and underarm hair.[4]

Young males follow a similar pattern of maturation, including a growth spurt followed by a gradual sexual maturity. However, this process takes place about 2 years later than it does in young females. Genital enlargement, underarm and pubic hair growth, and a lowering of the voice commonly occur. The male's first ejaculation is generally experienced by the age of 14, most commonly through **nocturnal emission** or masturbation. For many young boys, fully mature sperm do not develop until about age 15.

Key Terms

sexuality the quality of being sexual; can be viewed from many biological and psychosocial perspectives

masculinity behavioral expressions traditionally observed in males

femininity behavioral expressions traditionally observed in females

biological sexuality male and female aspects of sexuality

gonads male or female sex glands; testes produce sperm and ovaries produce eggs

puberty achievement of reproductive ability

menarche (muh **nar** key) time of a female's first menstrual cycle

anovulatory (an **oh** vyu luh tory) not ovulating

nocturnal emission ejaculation that occurs during sleep; "wet dream"

Reproductive capability declines only gradually over the course of the adult years. In the woman, however, the onset of **menopause** signals a more definite turning off of the reproductive system than is the case for the male adult. By the early to mid-50s, virtually all women have entered a postmenopausal period, but for men, relatively high-level **spermatogenesis** may continue for a decade or two.[4]

The story of sexual maturation and reproductive maturity cannot, however, be solely focused on the changes that take place in the body. The psychosocial processes that accompany the biological changes are also important.

Psychosocial Bases of Human Sexuality

If growth and development of our sexuality were to be visualized as a stepladder (Figure 13-1), one vertical rail of the ladder would represent our biological sexuality. The rungs would represent the sequential unfolding of the genetic, gonadal, and structural components.

Because humans, more than any other life form, can rise above a life centered on reproduction, a second dimension (or rail) to our sexuality exists—our **psychosocial sexuality.** The reason we possess the ability to be more than reproductive beings is a question for the theologian or the philosopher. We are considerably more complex than the functions determined by biology. The process that transforms a male into a man and a female into a woman begins at birth and continues to influence us through the course of our lives.

Gender Identity

Although expectant parents may prefer to have a child of a particular **gender,** they know that this matter is determined when the child is conceived. External genitals "cast the die," and femininity or masculinity is traditionally reinforced by the parents and society in general. By age 18 months, typical children have both the language and the insight to correctly identify their gender. They have established a **gender identity.** [5] The first rung rising from the psychosocial rail of the ladder has been climbed.

Gender Preference

During the preschool years, children receive the second component of the *scripting* required for the full development of psychosocial sexuality—**gender preference.** Gender preference refers to the emotional and intellectual acceptance of one's birth gender. Reaching this rung on the psychosocial rail of the ladder takes place during the preschool years, when nearly every boy prefers being a boy and nearly every girl prefers being a girl.

During the preschool years, parents typically begin to control the child's exposure to experiences traditionally reserved for children of the opposite gender. This is particularly true for boys; parents often stop a boy's play activities that they perceive to be feminine. (Note: The concept of gender preference is not to be confused with sexual preference. Sexual preference refers to a sexual and/or emotional attraction to sexual partners. Sexual preference is discussed later in this chapter in a section entitled "Sexual Orientation.")

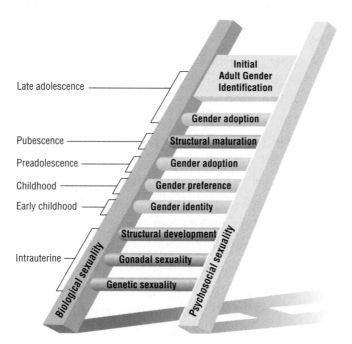

Figure 13-1 Our sexuality develops through biological and psychosocial stages.

Key Terms
menopause decline and eventual cessation of hormone production by the female reproductive system
spermatogenesis (sper mat oh **jen** uh sis) process of sperm production
psychosocial sexuality masculine and feminine aspects of sexuality
gender general term reflecting a biological basis of sexuality; the male gender or the female gender
gender identity recognition of one's gender
gender preference emotional and intellectual acceptance of one's own gender

Gender Adoption

The process of reaching an initial adult gender identification requires a considerable period of time. The specific knowledge, attitudes, and behavior characteristic of adults must be observed, analyzed, and practiced. The process of acquiring and personalizing these "insights" about how men and women think, feel, and act is reflected by the term **gender adoption,** the first and third rungs below the initial adult gender identification rail of the ladder in Figure 13-1.

In addition to developing a personalized version of an adult sexual identity, the child—and particularly the adolescent—must construct a *gender schema* for a member of the opposite gender. Clearly, the world of adulthood, involving intimacy, parenting, and employment, requires that men know women and women know men. Gender adoption provides an opportunity to begin constructing the equally valuable "pictures" of what the genders are like.

Initial Adult Gender Identification

By the time young people have climbed all of the rungs of the sexuality ladder, they have arrived at the chronological point in the life cycle when they need to construct an initial adult **gender identification.** You might notice that this label seems remarkably similar to the terminology used to describe one of the developmental tasks being used in this textbook. In fact, the task of forming an initial adult identity is closely related to developing an initial adult image of oneself as a man or a woman. Although most of us currently support the concept of "person" in many gender-neutral contexts (for some very valid reasons), we still must identify ourselves as either a man or a woman.

Transsexualism

Students are often intrigued by a gender identity variance that is first noticed during one or two of the psychosocial stages just discussed. Transsexualism is a variance of the most profound nature because it represents a complete rejection by an individual of his or her biological sexuality. The male transsexual believes that he is female and thus desires to be the woman who he knows he is. The female transsexual believes that she is male and wants to become the man who she knows she should be. Psychiatrists, sex therapists, and transexuals do not view transsexualism as a homosexual orientation.

For transsexuals, the periods of gender preference and gender adoption are perplexing as they attempt, with limited success, to resolve the conflict between what their mind tells them is true and what their body displays. Adolescent and young adult transsexuals often cross-dress, undertake homosexual relationships (which they view as being heterosexual relationships), experiment with hormone replacement therapy, and sometimes actively pursue a **sex reassignment surgery.** Thousands of these operations have been performed at some of the leading medical centers in the United States.

Androgyny: Sharing the Pluses

Over the last 25 years our society has increasingly accepted an image of a person who possesses both masculine and feminine qualities. This accepted image has taken years to develop because our society traditionally has reinforced rigid masculine roles for men and rigid feminine roles for women.

In the past, from the time a child was born, we assigned and reinforced only those roles and traits that were thought to be directly related to his or her biological gender. Boys were not allowed to cry, play with dolls, or help in the kitchen. Girls were not encouraged to become involved in sports; they were told to learn to sew, cook, and baby-sit. Men were encouraged to be strong, expressive, dominant, aggressive, and career oriented, and women were encouraged to be weak, shy, submissive, passive, and home oriented.

These traditional biases have resulted in some interesting phenomena related to career opportunities. Women were denied jobs requiring above-average physical strength, admittance into professional schools requiring high intellectual capacities, such as law, medicine, and business, and entry into most levels of military participation. Likewise, men were not encouraged to enter traditionally feminine careers, such as nursing, clerical work, and elementary school teaching.

For a variety of reasons, the traditional picture has changed. **Androgyny,** or the blending of both feminine

---

> ### Key Terms
>
> **gender adoption** lengthy process of learning the behavior that is traditional for one's gender
>
> **gender identification** achievement of a personally satisfying interpretation of one's masculinity or femininity
>
> **sex reassignment surgery** surgical procedures designed to remove the external genitalia and replace them with genitalia appropriate to the opposite gender
>
> **androgyny** (an **droj** en ee) the blending of both masculine and feminine qualities

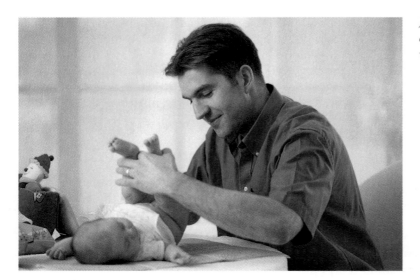

Just as women have broken into traditionally male careers, many men have taken on jobs and tasks that were once considered women's exclusive domain.

and masculine qualities, is more clearly evident in our society now than ever before. Today it is quite common to see men involved in raising children (including changing diapers) and doing routine housework. It is also quite common to see women entering the workplace in jobs traditionally managed by men and participating in sports traditionally played by men. Men are not scoffed at when they are seen crying after a touching movie. Women are not laughed at when they choose to assert themselves. The disposal of numerous sexual stereotypes has probably benefited our society immensely by relieving people of the pressure to be 100 percent "womanly" or 100 percent "macho."

Research data suggest that androgynous people are more flexible and independent, have greater self-esteem, have more positive attitudes toward sexuality, and show more social skills and motivation to achieve.[5] This finding should encourage you to be unafraid to break the gender role stereotype.

 TALKING POINTS How could you demonstrate to your grandmother that the blending of gender roles is a positive development?

Reproductive Systems

The most familiar aspects of biological sexuality are the structures that compose the reproductive systems. Each structure contributes to the reproductive process in unique ways. Thus, with these structures, males have the ability to impregnate. Females have the ability to become pregnant, give birth, and nourish infants through breast-feeding. Many of these structures are also associated with nonreproductive sexual behavior.

Male Reproductive System

The male reproductive system consists of external structures of genitals (the penis and scrotum) and internal structures (the testes, various passageways or ducts, seminal vesicles, the prostate gland, and the Cowper's glands) (Figure 13-2 A). The *testes* (also called *gonads* or *testicles*) are two egg-shaped bodies that lie within a saclike structure called the *scrotum.*[6] During most of fetal development, the testes lie within the abdominal cavity. They descend into the scrotum during the last 2 months of fetal life.

The testes are housed in the scrotum because a temperature lower than the body core temperature is required for adequate sperm development. The walls of the scrotum are composed of contractile tissue and can draw the testes closer to the body during cold temperatures (and sexual arousal) and relax during warm temperatures. Scrotal movements allow a constant, productive temperature to be maintained in the testes (Figure 13-2 B).

Each testis contains an intricate network of structures called *seminiferous tubules*. Within these 300 or so seminiferous tubules, the process of sperm production (*spermatogenesis*) takes place. Sperm cell development starts at about age 11 in boys and is influenced by the release of the hormone **ICSH (interstitial cell-stimulating hormone)** from the pituitary gland. ICSH does primarily what its

---

Key Terms

ICSH (interstitial cell-stimulating hormone) (in ter **stish** ul) a gonadotropic hormone of the male required for the production of testosterone

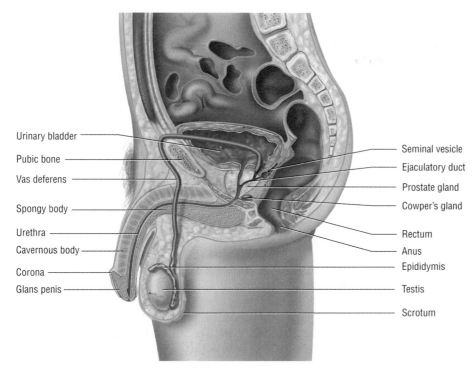

Figure 13-2 The male reproductive system.
A: Side view, B: Front view.

Urinary bladder

Pubic bone

Vas deferens

Spongy body

Urethra

Cavernous body

Corona

Glans penis

Seminal vesicle

Ejaculatory duct

Prostate gland

Cowper's gland

Rectum

Anus

Epididymis

Testis

Scrotum

A

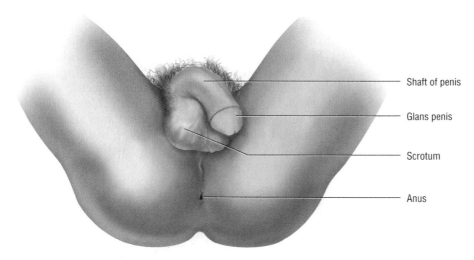

Shaft of penis

Glans penis

Scrotum

Anus

B

name suggests: it stimulates specific cells (called *interstitial cells*) within the testes to begin producing the male sex hormone *testosterone*. Testosterone in turn is primarily responsible for the gradual development of the male secondary sex characteristics at the onset of puberty. By the time a boy is approximately 15 years old, sufficient levels of testosterone exist so that the testes become capable of full spermatogenesis.

Before the age of about 15, most of the sperm cells produced in the testes are incapable of fertilization. The production of fully mature sperm *(spermatozoa)* is triggered by

another hormone secreted by the brain's pituitary gland— **FSH (follicle-stimulating hormone)**. FSH influences the

> **Key Terms**
>
> **FSH (follicle-stimulating hormone)** a gonadotropic hormone required for initial development of ova (in the female) and sperm (in the male)

seminiferous tubules to begin producing spermatozoa that are capable of fertilization.

Spermatogenesis takes place around the clock, with hundreds of millions of sperm cells produced daily. The sperm cells do not stay in the seminiferous tubules but rather are transferred through a system of *ducts* that lead into the *epididymis*. The epididymis is a tubular coil that attaches to the back side of each testicle. These collecting structures house the maturing sperm cells for 2 to 3 weeks. During this period the sperm finally become capable of motion, but they remain inactive until they mix with the secretions from the accessory glands (the seminal vesicles, prostate gland, and Cowper's glands).

Each epididymis leads into an 18-inch passageway known as the *vas deferens*. Sperm, moved along by the action of hairlike projections called *cilia*, can also remain in the vas deferens for an extended time without losing their ability to fertilize an egg.

The two vasa deferens extend into the abdominal cavity, where each meets with a *seminal vesicle*—the first of the three accessory structures or glands. Each seminal vesicle contributes a clear, alkaline fluid that nourishes the sperm cells with fructose and permits the sperm cells to be suspended in a movable medium. The fusion of a vas deferens with the seminal vesicle results in the formation of a passageway called the *ejaculatory duct*. Each ejaculatory duct is only about 1 inch long and empties into the final passageway for the sperm—the urethra.

The ejaculatory duct is located within the second accessory gland—the *prostate gland*. (See Figure 13–2.) The prostate gland secretes a milky fluid containing a variety of substances, including proteins, cholesterol, citric acid, calcium, buffering salts, and various enzymes. The prostate secretions further nourish the sperm cells and also raise the pH level, making the mixture quite alkaline. This alkalinity permits the sperm to have greater longevity as they are transported during ejaculation through the urethra, out of the penis, and into the highly acidic vagina.

The third accessory glands, the *Cowper's glands*, serve primarily to lubricate the urethra with a clear, viscous mucus. These paired glands empty their small amounts of preejaculatory fluid during the plateau stage of the sexual response cycle. Alkaline in nature, this fluid also neutralizes the acidic level of the urethra. Viable sperm cells can be suspended in this fluid and can enter the female reproductive tract before full ejaculation by the male.[7] This may account for many of the failures of the "withdrawal" method of contraception.

The sperm cells, when combined with secretions from the seminal vesicles and the prostate gland, form a sticky substance called **semen.**[8] Interestingly, the microscopic sperm actually makes up less than 5 percent of the seminal fluid discharged at ejaculation. Contrary to popular belief, the paired seminal vesicles contribute about 60 percent of the semen volume, and the prostate gland adds about 30 percent.[1] Thus the fear of some men that a **vasectomy** will destroy their ability to ejaculate is completely unfounded (see Chapter 14).

During *emission* (the gathering of semen in the upper part of the urethra), a sphincter muscle at the base of the bladder contracts and inhibits semen from being pushed into the bladder and urine from being deposited into the urethra.[9] Thus semen and urine rarely intermingle, even though they leave the body through the same passageway.

Ejaculation takes place when the semen is forced out of the *penis* through the urethral opening. The involuntary, rhythmic muscle contractions that control ejaculation result in a series of pleasurable sensations known as *orgasm*.

The urethra lies on the underside of the penis and extends through one of three cylindrical chambers of erectile tissue (two *cavernous bodies* and one *spongy body*). Each of these three chambers provides the vascular space required for sufficient erection of the penis. When a male becomes sexually aroused, these areas become congested with blood (*vasocongestion*). After ejaculation or when a male is no longer sexually stimulated, these chambers release the blood into the general circulation and the penis returns to a **flaccid** state.

The *shaft* of the penis is covered by a thin layer of skin that is an extension of the skin that covers the scrotum. This loose layer of skin is sensitive to sexual stimulation and extends over the head of the penis, except in males who have been circumcised. The *glans* (or head) of the penis is the most sexually sensitive (to tactile stimulation) part of the male body. Nerve receptor sites are especially prominent along the *corona* (the ridge of the glans) and the *frenulum* (the thin tissue at the base of the glans).

Female Reproductive System

The external structures (genitals) of the female reproductive system consist of the mons pubis, labia majora, labia minora, clitoris, and vestibule (Figure 13-3). Collectively

---

Key Terms

semen secretion containing sperm and nutrients discharged from the urethra at ejaculation

vasectomy surgical procedure in which the vasa deferens are cut to prevent the passage of sperm from the testicles; the most common form of male sterilization

flaccid (**fla** sid) nonerect; the state of erectile tissue when vasocongestion is not occurring

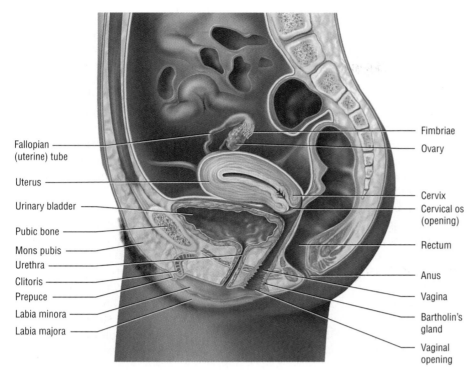

Figure 13-3 The female reproductive system.
A: Side view, **B:** Front view.

Fallopian (uterine) tube

Uterus

Urinary bladder

Pubic bone

Mons pubis

Urethra

Clitoris

Prepuce

Labia minora

Labia majora

Fimbriae

Ovary

Cervix

Cervical os (opening)

Rectum

Anus

Vagina

Bartholin's gland

Vaginal opening

A

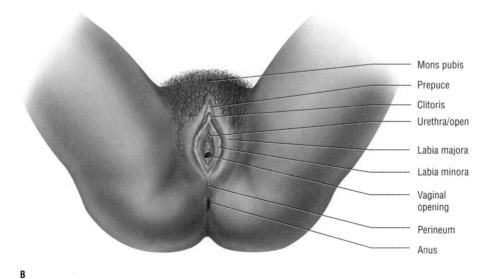

Mons pubis

Prepuce

Clitoris

Urethra/open

Labia majora

Labia minora

Vaginal opening

Perineum

Anus

B

these structures form the *vulva* or vulval area. The *mons pubis* is the fatty covering over the pubic bone. The mons pubis (or mons veneris, "mound of Venus") is covered by pubic hair and is quite sensitive to sexual stimulation. The *labia majora* are large longitudinal folds of skin that cover the entrance to the vagina, whereas the *labia minora* are the smaller longitudinal skin folds that lie within the labia majora. These hairless skin folds of the labia minora join at the top to form the *prepuce.* The prepuce

covers the glans of the *clitoris,* which is the most sexually sensitive part of the female body.

A rather direct analogy can be made between the penis and the clitoris. In terms of the tactile sensitivity, both structures are the most sensitive parts of the male and female genitals. Both contain a glans and a shaft (although the clitoral shaft is beneath the skin surface). Both organs are composed of erectile tissue that can become engorged with blood. Both are covered by skin folds (the clitoral prepuce of the female and the foreskin of the male), and both structures can collect **smegma** beneath these tissue folds.[5]

The *vestibule* is the region enclosed by the labia minora. Evident here are the urethral opening and the entrance to the vagina (or vaginal orifice). Also located at the vaginal opening are the *Bartholin's glands,* which secrete a minute amount of lubricating fluid during sexual excitement.

The *hymen* is a thin layer of tissue that stretches across the opening of the vagina. Once thought to be the only indication of virginity, the intact hymen rarely covers the vaginal opening entirely. Openings in the hymen are necessary for the discharge of menstrual fluid and vaginal secretions. Many hymens are stretched or torn to full opening by adolescent physical activity or by the insertion of tampons. In women whose hymens are not fully ruptured, the first act of sexual intercourse will generally accomplish this. Pain may accompany first intercourse in females with relatively intact hymens.

The internal reproductive structures of the female include the vagina, uterus, fallopian tubes, and ovaries. The *vagina* is the structure that accepts the penis during sexual intercourse. Normally the walls of the vagina are collapsed, except during sexual stimulation, when the vaginal walls widen and elongate to accommodate the erect penis. Only the outer third of the vagina is especially sensitive to sexual stimulation. In this location, vaginal tissues swell considerably to form the **orgasmic platform.** [10] This platform constricts the vaginal opening and in effect "grips" the penis (or other inserted object)—regardless of its size.[5] So the belief that a woman receives considerably more sexual pleasure from men with large penises is not supported from an anatomical standpoint.

The *uterus* (or *womb*) is approximately the size and shape of a small pear. This highly muscular organ is capable of undergoing a wide range of physical changes, as evidenced by its enlargement during pregnancy, its contraction during menstruation and labor, and its movement during the orgasmic phase of the female sexual response cycle. The primary function of the uterus is to provide a suitable environment for the possible implantation of a fertilized ovum, or egg. This implantation, should it occur, takes place in the innermost lining of the uterus—the *endometrium*. In the mature female, the endometrium undergoes cyclic changes as it prepares a new lining on a near-monthly basis.

The lower third of the uterus is called the *cervix*. The cervix extends slightly into the vagina. Sperm can enter the uterus through the cervical opening, or *cervical os.* Mucous glands in the cervix secrete a fluid that is thin and watery near the time of ovulation. Mucus of this consistency apparently facilitates sperm passage into the uterus and deeper structures. However, cervical mucus is much thicker during certain points in the menstrual cycle (when pregnancy is improbable) and during pregnancy (to protect against bacterial agents and other substances that are especially dangerous to the developing fetus).

The upper two thirds of the uterus is called the *corpus,* or *body*. This is where implantation of the fertilized ovum generally takes place. The upper portion of the uterus opens into two *fallopian tubes,* or *oviducts,* each about 4 inches long. The fallopian tubes are each directed toward an *ovary*. They serve as a passageway for the ovum in its week-long voyage toward the uterus. Usually, conception takes place in the upper third of the fallopian tubes.

The ovaries are analogous to the testes in the male. Their function is to produce the ovum, or egg. Usually, one ovary produces and releases just one egg each month. Approximately the size and shape of an unshelled almond, an ovary produces viable ova in the process known as *oogenesis*. The ovaries also produce the female sex hormones through the efforts of specific structures within the ovaries. These hormones play multiple roles in the development of female secondary sex characteristics, but their primary function is to prepare the endometrium of the uterus for possible implantation of a fertilized ovum. In the average healthy female, this preparation takes place about 13 times a year for a period of about 35 years. At menopause, the ovaries shrink considerably and stop nearly all hormonal production.

Menstrual Cycle

Each month or so, the inner wall of the uterus prepares for a possible pregnancy. When a pregnancy does not occur (as is the case throughout most months of a woman's fertile years), this lining must be released and a new one prepared. The breakdown of this endometrial wall and the resultant discharge of blood and endometrial tissue is known as *menstruation* (or *menses*) (Figure 13-4). The cyclic timing of menstruation is governed by hormones released from two sources: the pituitary gland and the ovaries.

Girls generally have their first menstrual cycle, the onset of which is called *menarche,* sometime around age

> ### Key Terms
>
> **smegma** cellular discharge that can accumulate beneath the clitoral hood and the foreskin of an uncircumcised penis
>
> **orgasmic platform** expanded outer third of the vagina that grips the penis during the plateau phase of the sexual response pattern

Menstrual cycle

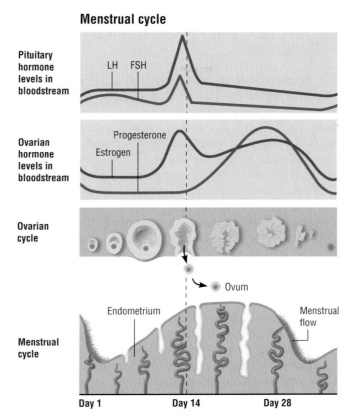

Figure 13-4 The menstrual cycle involves the development and release of an ovum, supported by hormones from the pituitary, and the buildup of the endometrium, supported by hormones from the ovary, for the purpose of establishing a pregnancy.

Endometriosis

Endometriosis is a condition in which endometrial tissue that normally lines the uterus is found growing within the pelvic cavity. Because the tissue remains sensitive to circulating hormones, it is the source of pain and discomfort during the latter half of the menstrual cycle. Endometriosis is most commonly found in younger women and is sometimes related to infertility in women with severe cases.

In addition to painful cramping before and during menstruation, the symptoms of endometriosis include low back pain, pain during intercourse, painful bowel movements, heavy menstrual flow, and difficulty becoming pregnant. Many women with endometriosis, however, experience no symptoms.*

Treatment of endometriosis largely depends on its extent. Drugs to suppress ovulation, including birth control pills, may be helpful in mild cases. For more severe cases, surgical removal of the tissue or a hysterectomy may be necessary. For some women, endometriosis is suppressed during pregnancy and does not return after pregnancy.

—————
*Health Guide A–Z: Endometriosis. Web MD Health. www.mywebmd.com/hw/endometriosis/hw/03000. September 5, 2005.

---

12 or 13. Over the past few decades, the age of menarche has been dropping gradually. This drop appears to be related to heredity, improved overall health, better childhood nutrition, and increased caloric intake. These factors in combination produce the increased body weight evident today in many young adolescent girls that seems to trigger an earlier menarche.

After a girl first menstruates, she may be anovulatory for a year or longer before a viable ovum is released during her cycle. This cyclic activity will continue until about age 45 to 55.

This text refers to a menstrual cycle that lasts 28 days. However, few women display perfect 28-day cycles. Most women fluctuate by a few days to a week around this 28-day pattern, and some women vary greatly from this cycle.

It is not uncommon for some women to experience irregular cycles (cycles that differ in length) and even occasional mid-cycle spotting (with small amounts of reddish discharge). These events are most likely to occur in young women who are just establishing their cycles, women who are approaching or moving through menopause, and women who are just starting to use hormone-based contraceptive methods. Major life changes, certain illnesses and medications, and unresolved stress can also affect the length of a woman's cycle. Any woman who experiences a significant, dramatic change from her usual pattern should contact her physician or health care practitioner.[5]

Your knowledge about the menstrual cycle is critical for your understanding of pregnancy, contraception, menopause, and issues related to the overall health and comfort of women (see the Star box for a discussion of endometriosis). Although at first this cycle may sound like a complicated process, each segment of the cycle can be studied separately for better understanding.

The menstrual cycle can be thought of as occurring in three segments or phases: the menstrual phase (lasting about 1 week), the preovulation phase (also lasting about 1 week), and the postovulation phase (lasting about 2 weeks). Day 1 of this cycle starts with the first day of bleeding, or menstrual flow.

The *menstrual phase* signals the woman that a pregnancy has not taken place and that her uterine lining is being sloughed off. During a 5- to 7-day period, a woman will discharge about ¼ to ½ cup of blood and tissue. (Only about 1 ounce of the menstrual flow is blood.) The menstrual flow is heaviest during the first days of this phase. Since the muscular uterus must contract to accomplish this tissue removal, some women have uncomfortable cramping during menstruation. Most women, however, report more pain and discomfort during the few days before the first day of menstrual flow. (See the following discussion of premenstrual syndrome [PMS].)

Today's methods of absorbing menstrual flow include the use of internal tampons and external pads. Caution must be exercised by the users of tampons to prevent the possibility of toxic shock syndrome (TSS) (see Chapter 12). Since menstrual flow is a positive sign of good health, women are encouraged to be normally active during menstruation.

The *preovulation phase* of the menstrual cycle starts about the time menstruation stops. Lasting about 1 week, this phase is first influenced by the release of FSH from the pituitary gland. FSH circulates in the bloodstream and directs the ovaries to start the process of maturing approximately 20 primary ovarian *follicles*. Thousands of primary egg follicles are present in each ovary at birth. These follicles resemble shells that house immature ova. As these follicles ripen under FSH influence, they release the hormone estrogen. Estrogen's primary function is to direct the endometrium to start the development of a thick, highly vascular wall. As the estrogen levels increase, the pituitary gland's secretion of FSH is reduced. Now the pituitary gland prepares for the surge of the **luteinizing hormone (LH)** required to accomplish ovulation.[11]

In the days immediately preceding ovulation, one of the primary follicles (called the *graafian follicle*) matures fully. The other primary follicles degenerate and are absorbed by the body. The graafian follicle moves toward the surface of the ovary. When LH is released in massive quantities on about day 14, the graafian follicle bursts to release the fully mature ovum. The release of the ovum is **ovulation.** Regardless of the overall length of a woman's cycle, ovulation occurs 14 days before her first day of menstrual flow.

The ovum is quickly captured by the fingerlike projections (*fimbriae*) of the fallopian tubes. In the upper third of the fallopian tubes, the ovum is capable of being fertilized in a 24- to 36-hour period. If the ovum is not fertilized by a sperm cell, it will begin to degenerate and eventually will be absorbed by the body.

After ovulation, the *postovulation phase* of the menstrual cycle starts when the remnants of the graafian follicle restructure themselves into a **corpus luteum.** The corpus luteum remains inside the ovary, secreting estrogen and a fourth hormone called *progesterone*. Progesterone, which literally means "for pregnancy," continues to direct the endometrial buildup. If pregnancy occurs, the corpus luteum monitors progesterone and estrogen levels throughout the pregnancy. If pregnancy does not occur, high levels of progesterone signal the pituitary gland to stop the release of LH and the corpus luteum starts to degenerate on about day 24. When estrogen and progesterone levels diminish significantly by day 28, the endometrium is discharged from the

uterus and out the vagina. The postovulation phase ends, and the menstrual phase begins. The cycle is then complete.

Premenstrual syndrome (PMS) PMS is characterized by psychological symptoms, such as depression, lethargy, irritability, and aggressiveness, or somatic symptoms, such as headache, backache, asthma, and acne, that recur in the same phase of each menstrual cycle, followed by a symptom-free phase in each cycle. Some of the more frequently reported symptoms of PMS include tension, tender breasts, fainting, fatigue, abdominal cramps, and weight gain.

The cause of PMS appears to be hormonal. Perhaps a woman's body is insensitive to a normal level of progesterone, or her ovaries fail to produce a normal amount of progesterone. These reasons seem plausible because PMS types of symptoms do not occur during pregnancy, during which natural progesterone levels are very high, and because women with PMS seem to feel much better after receiving high doses of natural progesterone in suppository form. When using oral contraceptives that supply synthetic progesterone at normal levels, many women report relief from some symptoms of PMS. However, the effectiveness of the most frequently used form of treatment, progesterone suppositories, is now being questioned.

Until the effectiveness of progesterone has been fully researched, it is unlikely that the medical community will deal with PMS through any approach other than a relatively conservative treatment of symptoms through the use of *analgesic drugs* (including *prostaglandin inhibitors*), diuretic drugs, dietary modifications (including restriction of caffeine and salt), vitamin B_6 therapy, exercise, and stress-reduction exercises.

Fibrocystic Breast Condition In some women, particularly those who have never been pregnant, stimulation of the breast tissues by estrogen and progesterone during the menstrual cycle results in an unusually high degree of secretory activity by the cells lining the ducts. The fluid released by the secretory lining finds its way into the fibrous connective tissue areas in the lower half of

---

Key Terms

luteinizing hormone (LH) (**loo** ten eye zing) a gonadotropic hormone of the female required for fullest development and release of ova; ovulating hormone

ovulation the release of a mature egg from the ovary

corpus luteum (**kore** pus **loo** tee um) cellular remnant of the graafian follicle after the release of an ovum

the breast, where in pocketlike cysts the fluid presses against neighboring tissues. This activity produces a benign fibrocystic breast condition characterized by swollen, firm or hardened, tender breast tissue before menstruation.

Researchers have begun to describe the importance of a healthy diet in preventing fibrocystic breast condition, in particular a low-fat, low-salt, low-red-meat diet that is rich in whole grains, fish, and poultry. The reduction or elimination of caffeine found in coffee, tea, soft drinks, and chocolate might also help reduce these benign breast changes. In some cases, vitamin E and vitamin B-complex supplementation have helped.[5]

Women who experience more extensive fibrocystic conditions can be treated with drugs that have a "calming" effect on progesterone production. In addition, occasional draining of the fluid-filled cysts can bring relief.

Menopause

For the vast majority of women in their late 40s through their mid-50s, a gradual decline in reproductive system function, called *menopause*, occurs. Menopause is a normal physiological process, not a disease process. It can, however, become a health concern for some middle-aged women who have unpleasant side effects resulting from this natural stoppage of ovum production and menstruation.

As ovarian function and hormone production diminish, a period of adjustment must be made by the hypothalamus, ovaries, uterus, and other estrogen-sensitive tissues. The extent of menopause as a health problem is determined by the degree to which **hot flashes,** night sweats, insomnia, vaginal wall dryness, depression and melancholy, breast changes, and the uncertainty of fertility are seen as problems.

In comparison with past generations, today's midlife women are much less likely to find menopause to be a negative experience. The end of fertility, combined with children leaving the home, makes the middle years a period of personal rediscovery for many women.

For women who are troubled by the changes brought about by menopause, physicians may prescribe **hormone replacement therapy (HRT).** This can relieve many symptoms and offer benefits to help reduce the incidence of osteoporosis (see Chapter 4). However, some forms of HRT have recently been found to increase the risk of breast cancer and cardiovascular problems.[12,13]

Human Sexual Response Pattern

Although history has many written and visual accounts of the human's ability to be sexually aroused, it was not until the pioneering work of Masters and Johnson[14] that the

events associated with arousal were clinically documented. Five questions posed by these researchers gave direction to a series of studies involving the scientific evaluation of human sexual response.

Do the Sexual Responses of Males and Females Have a Predictable Pattern?

The answer to the first question posed by the researchers was an emphatic yes. A predictable sexual response pattern was identified;[14] it consists of an initial **excitement stage,** a **plateau stage,** an **orgasmic stage,** and a **resolution stage.** Each stage involves predictable changes in the structural characteristics and physiological function of reproductive and nonreproductive organs in both the male and the female. These changes are shown in Figure 13-5.

Is the Sexual Response Pattern Stimuli-Specific?

The research of Masters and Johnson clearly established a no answer to the second question concerning stimuli specificity. Their findings demonstrated that numerous senses can supply the stimuli necessary for initiating the sexual response pattern. Although touching activities might initiate arousal in most people and maximize it for the vast majority of people, in both males and females, sight, smell, sound, and *vicariously formed stimuli* can also stimulate the same sexual arousal patterns.

Key Terms

hot flashes temporary feelings of warmth experienced by women during and after menopause, caused by blood vessel dilation

hormone replacement therapy (HRT) medically administered estrogen and progestin to replace hormones lost as the result of menopause

excitement stage initial arousal stage of the sexual response pattern

plateau stage second stage of the sexual response pattern; a leveling off of arousal immediately before orgasm

orgasmic stage third stage of the sexual response pattern; the stage during which neuromuscular tension is released

resolution stage fourth stage of the sexual response pattern; the return of the body to a preexcitement state

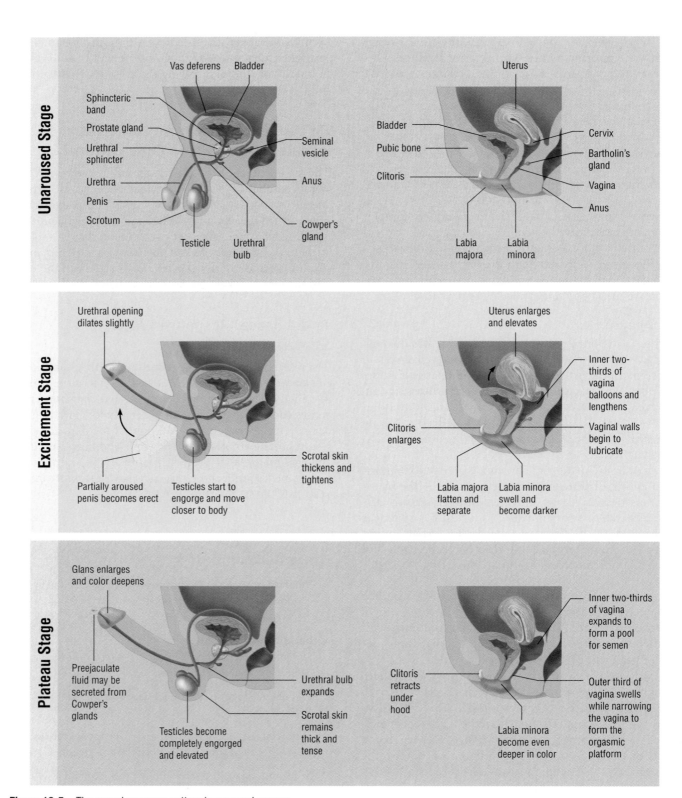

Figure 13-5   The sexual response pattern in men and women

Orgasmic Stage

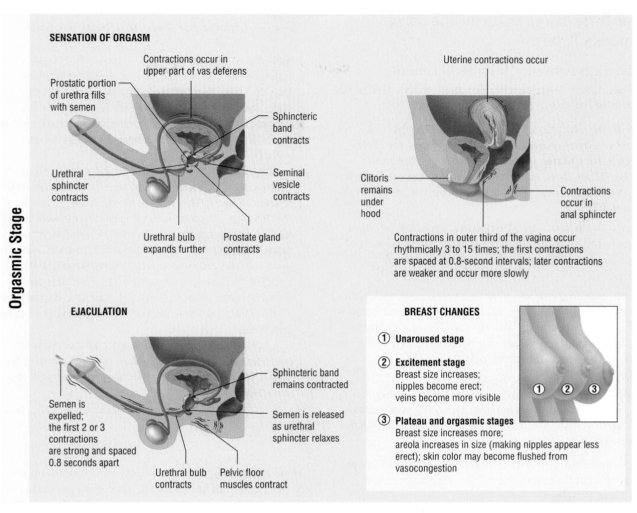

SENSATION OF ORGASM

Prostatic portion of urethra fills with semen

Contractions occur in upper part of vas deferens

Sphincteric band contracts

Urethral sphincter contracts

Seminal vesicle contracts

Urethral bulb expands further

Prostate gland contracts

Uterine contractions occur

Clitoris remains under hood

Contractions occur in anal sphincter

Contractions in outer third of the vagina occur rhythmically 3 to 15 times; the first contractions are spaced at 0.8-second intervals; later contractions are weaker and occur more slowly

EJACULATION

Semen is expelled; the first 2 or 3 contractions are strong and spaced 0.8 seconds apart

Sphincteric band remains contracted

Semen is released as urethral sphincter relaxes

Urethral bulb contracts

Pelvic floor muscles contract

BREAST CHANGES

① **Unaroused stage**

② **Excitement stage**
Breast size increases; nipples become erect; veins become more visible

③ **Plateau and orgasmic stages**
Breast size increases more; areola increases in size (making nipples appear less erect); skin color may become flushed from vasocongestion

① ② ③

Resolution Stage

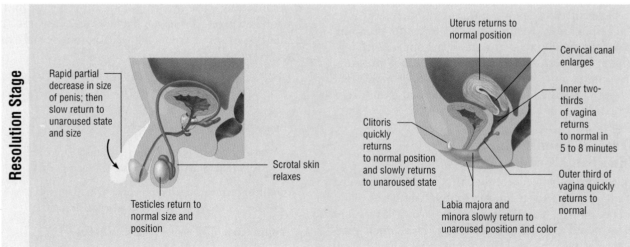

Rapid partial decrease in size of penis; then slow return to unaroused state and size

Scrotal skin relaxes

Testicles return to normal size and position

Uterus returns to normal position

Cervical canal enlarges

Clitoris quickly returns to normal position and slowly returns to unaroused state

Inner two-thirds of vagina returns to normal in 5 to 8 minutes

Outer third of vagina quickly returns to normal

Labia majora and minora slowly return to unaroused position and color

Figure 13-5   *Continued*

What Differences Occur in the Sexual Response Pattern?

Differences between Males and Females

Several differences are observable when the sexual response patterns of males and females are compared:

- With the exception of some later adolescent males, the vast majority of males are not multiorgasmic. The **refractory phase** of the resolution stage prevents most males from experiencing more than one orgasm in a short period, even when sufficient stimulation is available.

- Females possess a **multiorgasmic capacity.** Masters and Johnson found that as many as 10–30 percent of all female adults routinely experience multiple orgasms.

- Although they possess multiorgasmic potential, about 10 percent of all female adults are *anorgasmic*—that is, they never experience an orgasm.[14] For many anorgasmic females, orgasms can be experienced when masturbation, rather than **coitus,** provides the stimulation.

- When measured during coitus, males reach orgasm far more quickly than do females. However, when masturbation is the source of stimulation, females reach orgasm as quickly as do males.[14]

More important than any of the differences pointed out is the finding that the sexual response patterns of males and females are far more alike than they are different. Not only do males and females experience the four basic stages of the response pattern, but they also have similar responses in specific areas, including the **erection** and *tumescence* of sexual structures; the appearance of a **sex flush;** the increase in cardiac output, blood pressure, and respiratory rate; and the occurrence of *rhythmic pelvic thrusting.*[14] (See the Star Box for discussion about drugs that enhance penile erections.)

Differences among Subjects within a Same-Gender Group

When a group of subjects of the same gender was studied in an attempt to answer questions about similarities and differences in the sexual response pattern, Masters and Johnson noted considerable variation. Even when variables such as age, race, education, and general health were held constant, the extent and duration of virtually every stage of the response pattern varied.

Differences within the Same Individual

For a given person the nature of the sexual response pattern does not remain constant, even when observed over a

Drugs for Erectile Dysfunction

Within the last decade, three prescription drugs for erectile dysfunction (or ED) have been developed and marketed for men. The oldest drug, Viagra (Pfizer Pharmaceuticals), came on the market in 1998. A second drug, Levitra (GlaxoSmithKline), was approved by the Food and Drug Administration in 2003, and the newest drug, Cialis (Eli Lilly & Company), came on the market in 2004.

All three drugs act on an enzyme that helps relax small muscles in the penis and increase the flow of blood into the erectile chambers. Sexual stimulation is required for each of the drugs to work. The difference in the drugs is how long the drug can work and how quickly it produces an erection. Reportedly, Viagra can produce the desired effect within a 4-hour period, Levitra can work for about 5 hours, and Cialis can work for up to 36 hours. Viagra can work in as quickly as 30 minutes, Levitra in about 15 minutes, and Cialis around 30 minutes or more. Men are encouraged to discuss possible side effects and health risks with their physicians before using these drugs.

In the near future, be on the lookout for the development of prescription drugs that enhance sexual desire and performance in women. Pharmaceutical companies stand to reap tremendous sales with effective drugs in this area.

relatively short period. A variety of internal and external factors can alter this pattern. The aging process, changes in general health status, levels of stress, altered environmental settings, use of alcohol and other drugs, and behavioral changes in a sexual partner can cause one's own sexual response pattern to change from one sexual experience to another.

Key Terms

refractory phase that portion of the male's resolution stage during which sexual arousal cannot occur

multiorgasmic capacity potential to have several orgasms within a single period of sexual arousal

coitus (co ih tus) penile-vaginal intercourse

erection the engorgement of erectile tissue with blood; characteristic of the penis, clitoris, nipples, labia minora, and scrotum

sex flush the reddish skin response that results from increasing sexual arousal

What are the Basic Physiological Mechanisms Underlying the Sexual Response Pattern?

The basic mechanisms in the fourth question posed by Masters and Johnson are now well recognized. One factor, *vasocongestion*, or the retention of blood or fluid within a particular tissue, is critically important in the development of physiological changes that promote the sexual response pattern. The presence of erectile tissue underlies the changes that can be noted in the penis, breasts, and scrotum of the male and the clitoris, breasts, and labia minora of the female.

A second mechanism now recognized as necessary for the development of the sexual response pattern is that of *myotonia*, or the buildup of *neuromuscular tonus* within a variety of body structures.[9] At the end of the plateau stage of the response pattern, a sudden release of the accumulated neuromuscular tension gives rise to the rhythmic muscular contractions and pleasurable muscular spasms that constitute orgasm, as well as ejaculation in the male.[3]

What Role Is Played by Specific Organs and Organ Systems within the Sexual Response Pattern?

The fifth question posed by Masters and Johnson, which concerns the role played by specific organs and organ systems during each stage of the response pattern, can be readily answered by referring to the material presented in Figure 13-5. As you study this figure, remember that direct stimulation of the penis and either direct or indirect stimulation of the clitoris are the principal avenues toward orgasm. Also, intercourse represents only one activity that can lead to orgasmic pleasure.[15]

Patterns of Sexual Behavior

Although sex researchers may see sexual behavior in terms of the human sexual response pattern just described, most people are more interested in the observable dimensions of sexual behavior. (Complete the Personal Assessment on page 363 to determine whether your own attitudes toward sexuality are traditional or nontraditional.)

Celibacy

Celibacy can be defined as the self-imposed avoidance of sexual intimacy. It is synonymous with sexual abstinence. There are many reasons people could choose not to have a sexually intimate relationship. For some, celibacy is part of a religious doctrine. Others might be afraid of sexually transmitted diseases. For most, however, celibacy is preferred simply because it seems appropriate for them. Celibate people can certainly have deep, intimate relationships with other people—just not sexual relationships. Celibacy may be short-term or last a lifetime, and no identified physical or psychological complications appear to result from a celibate lifestyle.

 TALKING POINTS You have decided to remain celibate until you're ready to make a lifetime commitment to someone. How would you explain this to the person you are now dating?

Masturbation

Throughout recorded history, **masturbation** has been a primary method of achieving sexual pleasure. Through masturbation, people can explore their sexual response patterns. Traditionally, some societies and religious groups have condemned this behavior based on the belief that intercourse is the only "right" sexual behavior. With sufficient lubrication, masturbation cannot do physical harm. Today masturbation is considered by most sex therapists and researchers to be a normal source of self-pleasure.

Fantasy and Erotic Dreams

The brain is the most sensual organ in the body. In fact, many sexuality experts classify **sexual fantasies** and **erotic dreams** as forms of sexual behavior. Particularly for people whose verbal ability is highly developed, the ability to create imaginary scenes enriches other forms of sexual behavior.

When fantasies occur in conjunction with another form of sexual behavior, the second behavior may be greatly enhanced by the supportive fantasy. Both women and men fantasize during foreplay and intercourse. Masturbation and fantasizing are inseparable activities.

Key Terms

masturbation self-stimulation of the genitals

sexual fantasies fantasies with sexual themes; sexual daydreams or imaginary events

erotic dreams dreams whose content elicits a sexual response

Erotic dreams occur during sleep in both men and women. The association between these dreams and ejaculation resulting in a nocturnal emission (wet dream) is readily recognized in males. In females, erotic dreams can lead not only to vaginal lubrication but to orgasm as well.

Shared Touching

Virtually the entire body can be an erogenous (sexually sensitive) zone when shared touching is involved. A soft, light touch, a slight application of pressure, the brushing back of a partner's hair, and gentle massage are all forms of communication that heighten sexual arousal.

Genital Contact

Two important uses can be identified for the practice of stimulating a partner's genitals. The first is that of being the tactile component of **foreplay.** Genital contact, in the form of holding, rubbing, stroking, or caressing, heightens arousal to a level that allows for progression to intercourse.

The second role of genital contact is that of *mutual masturbation to orgasm.* Stimulation of the genitals so that both partners have orgasm is a form of sexual behavior practiced by many people, as well as couples during the late stage of a pregnancy. For couples not desiring pregnancy, the risk of conception is virtually eliminated when this becomes the form of sexual intimacy practiced.

As is the case of other aspects of intimacy, genital stimulation is best enhanced when partners can talk about their needs, expectations, and reservations. Practice and communication can shape this form of contact into a pleasure-giving approach to sexual intimacy.

Oral-Genital Stimulation

Oral-genital stimulation brings together two of the body's most erogenous areas: the genitalia and the mouth. Because oral-genital stimulation can involve an exchange of body fluids, the risk of disease transmission is real. Small tears of mouth or genital tissue may allow transmission of disease-causing pathogens. Only couples who are absolutely certain that they are free from all sexually transmitted diseases (including HIV infection) can practice unprotected oral sex. Couples in doubt should refrain from oral-genital sex or carefully use a condom (on the male) or a latex square to cover the female's vulval area. Increasingly, latex squares (dental dams) can be obtained from drug stores or pharmacies.

Three basic forms of oral-genital stimulation are practiced.[5] **Fellatio,** in which the penis is sucked, licked, or kissed by the partner, is the most common of the three. **Cunnilingus,** in which the vulva of the female is kissed,

licked, or penetrated by the partner's tongue, is only slightly less frequently practiced.

Mutual oral-genital stimulation, the third form of oral-genital stimulation, combines both fellatio and cunnilingus. When practiced by a heterosexual couple, the female partner performs fellatio on her partner while her male partner performs cunnilingus on her. Gay couples can practice mutual fellatio or cunnilingus.

Intercourse

Sexual intercourse (coitus) refers to the act of inserting the penis into the vagina. Intercourse is the sexual behavior that is most directly associated with **procreation.** For some, intercourse is the only natural and appropriate form of sexual intimacy.

The incidence and frequency of sexual intercourse is a much-studied topic. Information concerning the percentages of people who have engaged in intercourse is readily available in textbooks used in sexuality courses. Data concerning sexual intercourse among college students may be changing somewhat because of concerns about HIV infection and other STDs, but a reasonable estimate of the percentage of college students reporting sexual intercourse is 60–75 percent.

These percentages reflect two important concepts about the sexual activity of college students. The first is that a large majority of college students is having intercourse. The second concept is that a sizeable percentage (25–40 percent) of students is choosing to refrain from intercourse. Indeed, the belief that "everyone is doing it" may be a bit shortsighted. From a public health standpoint, we believe it is important to provide accurate health information to protect those who choose to have intercourse and to actively support a person's right to choose not to have intercourse.

Couples need to share their expectations concerning sexual techniques and frequency of intercourse.[6] Even the "performance" factors, such as depth of penetration, nature of body movements, tempo of activity, and timing of orgasm are of increasing importance to many couples.

Key Terms

foreplay activities, often involving touching and caressing, that prepare individuals for sexual intercourse

fellatio (feh **lay** she oh) oral stimulation of the penis

cunnilingus (cun uh **ling** gus) oral stimulation of the vulva or clitoris

procreation reproduction

Issues concerning sexually transmitted diseases (including HIV infection) are also critically important for couples who are contemplating intercourse. These factors also need to be explored through open communication.

There are a variety of books (including textbooks) that provide written and visually explicit information on intercourse positions. Four basic positions for intercourse—*male above, female above, side by side,* and *rear entry*—each offer relative advantages and disadvantages.

Anal Sexual Activity

Some couples practice **anal intercourse,** in which the penis is inserted into the rectum of a partner. Anal intercourse can be performed by both heterosexual couples and gay men. According to a year 2000 report in the journal *Archives of Sexual Behavior,* about 20–25 percent of college students have experienced anal intercourse.[16] The anal sphincter muscles contract tightly and tend to resist entry. Thus, couples who engage in anal intercourse must do so slowly, gently, and with adequate amounts of water-based lubricants. Because of the danger of tearing tissues in the rectal area, HIV transmission risk is increased if the inserting male is infected.[3] Unless it is absolutely certain that both partners are uninfected, the inserting male should always wear a condom. Even with a condom, disease transmission is possible, since during anal intercourse, condoms are more likely to tear than during penis-vaginal intercourse. Couples practicing anal sex must not follow anal insertion with insertion into the mouth or vagina because of the likelihood of transmitting infectious agents.

For many people, anal intercourse is not only unpleasant but simply unnatural. For others, the anal area is just another part of the human body that is especially sensitive to stimulation, and they enjoy the pleasurable sensations that come from intercourse or the insertion of a well-lubricated finger or sex toy. Some people enjoy kissing ("rimming") or touching in the anal area, but this should occur only when the anal area has been fully cleansed or covered with a sheet of protective plastic wrap. As with all sexual behavior, couples need to communicate clearly their feelings about any activity. If one partner is uncomfortable about an activity and wants to stop, his or her feelings must be supported by the other person. A desire for a particular sexual activity must not turn into sexual coercion or a sexual assault.

Until recently, 13 states had laws in effect that banned **sodomy** (another term for anal sex as well as certain other sexual practices). However, a U.S. Supreme Court ruling (*Lawrence and Garner v Texas*) in June 2003 invalidated a Texas law that banned private consensual sex (in this case, sodomy) between adults of the same sex. Legal experts expect this Texas ruling to eventually invalidate the laws of the 12 other states that banned sodomy in one form or another.[17]

Sexuality and Aging

Students are often curious about how aging affects sexuality. This is understandable because we live in a society that idolizes youth and demands performance. Many younger people become anxious about growing older because of what they think will happen to their ability to express their sexuality. Interestingly, young adults are willing to accept other physical changes of aging (such as the slowing down of basal metabolism, reduced lung capacity, and even wrinkles) but not those changes related to sexuality.

Most of the research in this area suggests that older people are quite capable of performing sexually. As with other aspects of aging, certain anatomical and physiological changes will be evident, but these changes do not necessarily reduce the ability to enjoy sexual activity.[5] Most experts in sexuality report that many older people remain interested in sexual activity. Furthermore, those who are exposed to regular sexual activity throughout a lifetime report being most satisfied with their sex lives as older adults.

As people age, the likelihood of alterations in the male and female sexual response cycles increases. In the postmenopausal women, vaginal lubrication commonly begins more slowly, and the amount of lubrication usually diminishes. However, clitoral sensitivity and nipple erection remain the same as in earlier years. The female capacity for multiple orgasms remains the same, although the number of contractions that occur at orgasm typically is reduced.

In the older man, physical changes are also evident. This is thought to be caused by the decrease in the production of testosterone between the ages of 20 and 60 years. After age 60 or so, testosterone levels remain relatively steady. Thus many men, despite a decrease in sperm production, remain fertile into their 80s.[5] Older men typically take longer to achieve an erection (however, they are able to maintain their erection longer before ejaculation), have fewer muscular contractions at orgasm, and ejaculate less forcefully than they once did. The volume of seminal

---

| Key Terms |

anal intercourse a sexual act in which the erect penis is inserted into the rectum of a partner

sodomy generally refers to anal or oral sex; a legal term whose definition varies according to state law

fluid ejaculated is typically less than in earlier years, and its consistency is somewhat thinner. The resolution phase is usually longer in older men. In spite of these gradual changes, some elderly men engage in sexual intercourse with the same frequency as do much younger men.

Sexual Orientation

Sexual orientation refers to the direction in which people focus their sexual interests. People can be attracted to opposite-gender partners (heterosexuality), same-gender partners (homosexuality), or partners of both genders (bisexuality).

The distinctions among the three categories of sexual orientation are much less clear than their definitions below will suggest. Most people probably fall somewhere along a continuum between exclusive heterosexuality and exclusive homosexuality. As far back as 1948, Kinsey presented just such a continuum.[18]

Heterosexuality

Heterosexuality (or heterosexual orientation) refers to an attraction to opposite-gender partners. (*Heteros* is a Greek word that means "the other.") A heterosexual person is sometimes called *straight*. Throughout the world, this is the most common sexual orientation. For reasons related to species survival, heterosexuality has its most basic roots in the biological dimension of human sexuality. Beyond its biological roots, heterosexuality has significant cultural and religious support in virtually every country in the world. Worldwide, laws related to marriage, living arrangements, health benefits, child rearing, financial matters, sexual behavior, and inheritance generally support relationships that are heterosexual in nature. However, this may be gradually changing. (See page 357 for an update on gay marriage.)

Homosexuality

Homosexuality (or homosexual orientation) refers to an attraction to same-gender partners. (*Homos* is a Greek word that means "the same.") The term *gay* refers either to males or females, whereas the word *lesbian* is used only in reference to females.

What percentage of the population is gay? This is difficult to determine accurately, since many people refuse to reveal their orientations and prefer to remain "in the closet." However, it is probably safe to say that the number of gay people in our society is probably much greater than most people realize. Kinsey estimated that about 2 percent of American females and 4 percent of American males were exclusively homosexual.[18,19] More recent estimates place the overall figure to be about 10 percent of the population. Clearly, the expression of same-gender attraction is widespread.

Bisexuality

People who have the ability to be attracted to either gender are referred to as *bisexual*. Bisexuals generally are in one of three groups: those who are (1) genuinely attracted emotionally and physically to both genders, (2) those who are gay but feel the need to behave heterosexually, and (3) those who are aroused physically by the same gender but attracted emotionally to the opposite gender. Some participate in a bisexual lifestyle for an extended period of time, while others move on more quickly to a more exclusive orientation. The size of the bisexual population is unknown. (See Learning from Our Diversity on page 355), which describes some of the challenges for bisexual men and women.)

Origins of Sexual Orientation

Students often wonder "what makes a person gay?" This question has no simple answer. (College sexuality textbooks devote entire chapters to this topic.) Some research has pointed to differences in the sizes of certain brain structures as a possible biological or anatomical basis for homosexuality.[20] Other research proposes possible genetic, environmental, hormonal, or other foundations.

However, for sexual orientation in general, no single theory has emerged that fully explains this complex developmental process. The consensus of scientific opinion is that people do not choose their sexual orientation. Thus, being straight or being gay is something that "just happens." Indeed, most gays and lesbians report that no specific event triggered them into becoming gay. Many gays also indicate that their orientations seemed different from those of other children as far back as their prepuberty years.

Given the many challenges of being gay in a mostly straight world, it would seem logical that gays and lesbians do not make conscious efforts to choose to become gay. (Who would want to be a magnet for taunts, discrimination, and physical violence?) In a similar manner, it is highly likely that heterosexual persons do not actually choose to become straight. Sexual orientation is something that just unfolds in a person's life. (See Discovering Your Spirituality on page 355 for insight into some of the issues that gays and lesbians face.)

Love

Love may be one of the most elusive yet widely recognized concepts that describe some level of emotional attachment to another. Various forms of love include

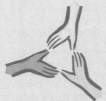

Learning from Our Diversity

The Challenges for Bisexuals

People whose sexual orientation is toward both men and women are termed bisexuals. This can be a confusing label, however. For example, if a man has had one sexual experience with a man, but all of his other sexual experiences are with women, does this mean he is bisexual? And what about the woman who has sequential relationships with men, followed by an occasional relationship with a woman? Is she bisexual? What about people who are sexually attracted to one gender, but are emotionally more attracted to the other gender? The labels can get confusing and can make one wonder about the value of any label describing sexual orientation. This is just one of the many challenges facing bisexual people.

Some experts suggest that bisexuals (those who have had at least one sexual experience with a man and one with a woman) probably outnumber exclusive homosexuals (those who have had sexual experience *only* with persons of their own gender).[1] One might think that this larger group would be better understood by society, but that seems not to be the case. Bisexuals may have a larger field of potential partners, but this benefit may be offset by the difficulty fitting into society.

Heterosexual people, gay males, and lesbians may not view bisexuality as acceptable, believing that the bisexual person is just incapable of making the decision to go one way or the other.[2] They may accuse the bisexual person of wanting the best of both worlds, as if "having it all" (in terms of sexual possibilities and experiences) is an inappropriate, bad

thing. Then there is the issue of telling a new dating partner that you are attracted to both men and women. Some new partners may find this reality a distinct "turnoff." The hostility that bisexual persons arouse can provide a real challenge.

For these reasons, numerous college and university counseling centers are expanding their outreach programs to include programs for bisexual students. If you are interested, you might check into the offerings of your campus counseling center to see if they provide educational information, support groups, or specialized counseling for bisexual students. Many campuses also have student groups that focus on gay, lesbian, bisexual, and transgendered students.

Interestingly, it appears that more and more bisexual students are "coming out" despite the challenges they may face. Perhaps this has been encouraged by the public pronouncements of bisexuality by well-known movie stars, such as Drew Barrymore.[3] In the near future, we may find more public acceptance for people who are bisexual. Would you consider increased public acceptance of bisexuality to be a good or bad thing?

[1]Hyde JS, DeLamater JD. *Understanding Human Sexuality,* 9th ed. New York: McGraw-Hill, 2006.
[2] Kelly GF. *Sexuality Today: The Human Perspective,* 8th ed. McGraw-Hill, 2006.
[3]Celebrity news. *Drew Barrymore: "I am bisexual,"* July 17, 2003, http://us.imdb.com/wn?20030717#6, July 23, 2003.

Discovering Your Spirituality

Coming Out—Then What?

If you are openly gay, when you finally told your family and friends about your sexual orientation, a lot of things changed. But one thing probably stayed the same—you still feel like an outsider. Most of the couples holding hands on campus are young men and women. TV sitcoms are centered on heterosexual couples. They may include a gay character, but usually in a minor role. Popular magazines—through their ads, their features, their entire focus—are telling you how to be attractive to the opposite sex.

Being openly gay has probably made you wonder about some of the mixed messages you receive. The person who says it's OK that you're gay also seems to feel sorry for you—because you can't have a "normal" life and enjoy some of the things she does. Your mother makes remarks that suggest she still has hopes that someday you'll marry her best friend's son.

Feeling good about being gay in a straight world doesn't come easily. You've got to work at it. Start by finding support among your gay friends. Knowing that you're not alone is important—especially right after coming out. Realizing that other good, whole people are gay helps to reinforce your self-esteem. Joining a campus gay organization is good for ongoing support, but don't limit yourself to that group. To grow

as an individual, you also need to interact with and be part of heterosexual society.

Focus on what you value about yourself. Are you creative? Someone who gets things accomplished? A dependable friend? Think about the contributions you make—to your family, school, friends, church, and community. Remind yourself that you're a worthy person.

What do your friends appreciate about you? Do they value your advice? Like your sense of humor? Admire your courage? Think you're a strong leader?

Reinforcing the fact that you're a whole, worthy person is up to you. Listen to the "tapes" that are constantly playing in your head—both positive and negative. Edit out the negative thoughts, and turn up the volume on the positive ones. Take charge of what you think about yourself, rather than accepting what others think you are or should be.

TALKING POINTS How would you react if a close family member told you that he or she was gay? How could you be supportive or at least communicate your feelings without anger or criticism?

friendship, erotic, devotional, parental, and altruistic love. Two types of love are most closely associated with dating and mate selection: *passionate love* and *companionate love.*

Passionate love, also described as romantic love or **infatuation,** is a state of extreme absorption in another person. It is characterized by intense feelings of tenderness, elation, anxiety, sexual desire, and ecstasy. Often appearing early in a relationship, passionate love typically does not last very long. Passionate love is driven by the excitement of being closely involved with a person whose character is not fully known.

If a relationship progresses, passionate love is gradually replaced by companionate love. This type of love is less emotionally intense than passionate love. It is characterized by friendly affection and a deep attachment that is based on extensive familiarity with the partner. This love is enduring and capable of sustaining long-term, mutual growth. Central to companionate love are feelings of empathy for, support of, and tolerance of the partner. (Complete the Personal Assessment on page 365 to determine whether you and your partner are truly compatible.)

Recognizing Unhealthy Relationships

Clearly, not all dating relationships will continue. Many couples recognize when a partnership is nearing an end, and they reach a mutual decision to break off the relationship. This is a traditional, natural way for people to learn about their interactions with others. They simply decide to split up and move on.

However, sometimes people do not recognize or heed the warning signs of an unstable relationship, so they stay involved long after the risks outweigh the benefits. These warning signs include abusive behavior, including both emotional and physical abuse (see Chapter 16). Another red flag is excessive jealousy about a partner's interactions with others. Sometimes excessive jealousy evolves into controlling behavior, and one partner attempts to manage the daily activities of the other partner. By definition, controlling behavior limits your creativity and freedom.

Other warning signs are dishonesty, irresponsibility, lack of patience, and any kind of drug abuse. We certainly do not want to see these qualities in those we have initially judged to be "nice people," even though these unappealing characteristics may be obvious to others. If you suspect that any of these problems may be undermining your relationship, talk about your concerns with one or two trusted friends, and seek the advice of a professional counselor at your college or university. Try to realize that

ending your relationship might be the best thing you could do for yourself.

 TALKING POINTS Your sister is in an unhealthy relationship but doesn't seem to see the warning signs. How could you alert her to the potential dangers?

Intimacy

When most people hear the word **intimacy,** they immediately think about physical intimacy. They think about shared touching, kissing, and even intercourse. However, sexuality experts and family therapists prefer to view intimacy more broadly, as any close, mutual, verbal or nonverbal behavior within a relationship. In this sense, intimate behavior can range from sharing deep feelings and experiences with a partner to sharing profound physical pleasures with a partner.

Intimacy is present in both love and friendship. You have likely shared intimate feelings with your closest friends, as well as with those you love. Intimacy helps us feel connected to others and allows us to feel the full measure of our own self-worth.

 TALKING POINTS Your teenage son equates intimacy with sex. How would you explain the emotional intimacy involved in marriage?

Lifestyles and Relationships

A variety of informal and formal lifestyles and relationships exist in our society. Here are a few of the most common ones.

Singlehood

One lifestyle option for adults is *singlehood.* For many people, being single is a lifestyle that affords the potential for pursuing intimacy, if desired, and provides an uncluttered path for independence and self-directedness. Other people, however, are single because of divorce, separation,

> **Key Terms**
>
> **infatuation** a relatively temporary, intensely romantic attraction to another person
>
> **intimacy** any close, mutual, verbal or nonverbal behavior within a relationship

death, or the absence of an opportunity to establish a partnership. The U.S. Census Bureau indicates that 43 percent of women and 39 percent of men over the age of 18 are currently single.[21]

Many different living arrangements are seen among singles. Some single people live alone and choose not to share a household. Other arrangements for singles include cohabitation, periodic cohabitation, singlehood during the week and cohabitation on the weekends or during vacations, or the *platonic* sharing of a household with others. For young adults, large percentages of single men and women live with their parents.

Like habitation arrangements, the sexual intimacy patterns of singles are individually tailored. Some singles practice celibacy, others pursue intimate relationships in a **monogamous** pattern, and still others may have multiple partners. As in all interpersonal relationships, including marriage, the levels of commitment are as variable as the people involved.

Cohabitation

Cohabitation, or the sharing of living quarters by unmarried people, represents another alternative to marriage. According to the U.S. Census Bureau, the number of unmarried, opposite-gender couples living together totals over 4.8 million couples. The number of reported same-gender couples totaled nearly 600,000 in the year 2000.[21]

Although cohabitation may seem to imply a vision of sexual intimacy between roommates, several forms of shared living arrangements can be viewed as cohabitation. For some couples, cohabitation is only a part-time arrangement for weekends, during summer vacation, or on a variable schedule. In addition, **platonic** cohabitation can exist when a couple shares living quarters but does so without establishing an intimate relationship. Close friends and people of retirement age might be included in a group called *cohabitants.*

How well do cohabitation arrangements fare against marriage partnerships in terms of long-term stability? A 2002 report prepared by the CDC's National Center for Health Statistics[22] indicated that unmarried cohabitations are generally less stable than marriages are. The probability of a first marriage ending in separation or divorce within 5 years was found to be 20 percent, but the probability of a premarital cohabitation breaking up within 5 years was 49 percent. After 10 years, the probability of a first marriage ending was 33 percent, compared to 62 percent for cohabitations.

Gay and Lesbian Partnerships

To believe that adult partnerships are reserved only for heterosexual couples is to avoid reality. In the United States and in many parts of the world, gays and lesbians are forming partnerships that, in many ways, mimic those of heterosexuals. It no longer is unusual to see same-sex men and women openly living together in one household. Gay and lesbian couples buy houses together and share property rights. As businesses restructure their employee benefits packages, gays and lesbians are covering their partners on health care plans and making them beneficiaries on their insurance policies and retirement plans.

A search of the literature indicates that gay and lesbian partnerships have many of the same characteristics and problems of heterosexual couples.[3] Like straight couples, they struggle with interpersonal issues related to their relationship and their lifestyle. They work to decide how best to juggle their financial resources, their leisure time, and their friends and extended families. If they live together in an apartment or house, they must decide how to divide the household tasks.

If children are present in the household, they must be cared for and nurtured. These children could have come from an adoption, a previous heterosexual relationship, or, in the case of a lesbian couple, from artificial insemination. Research indicates that children raised in lesbian or gay families overwhelmingly grow up with a heterosexual orientation, and are like other children from heterosexual families in terms of their adjustment, mental health, social skills, and peer acceptance.[3]

Same-Sex Marriage

One area in which gay and lesbian couples differ from heterosexual couples is in their ability to obtain a legal marriage. In the last few years, this inequity has been the focus of an intense national debate over same-sex marriage. The issues are complex, primarily because of the differences in state laws and the various courts' interpretations of those laws. At this point in the debate, here is where same-sex marriage stands.

If enacted, same-sex marriages would grant gay couples a legal marriage document that allows for an array of legal and economic benefits, including joint parental custody, insurance and health benefits, joint tax returns,

---

Key Terms

monogamous (mo **nog** a mus) paired relationship with one partner

cohabitation sharing of a residence by two unrelated, unmarried people; living together

platonic (pluh **ton** ick) close association between two people that does not include a sexual relationship

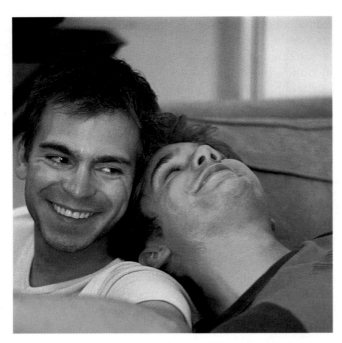

Legalization of same-sex marriage would grant gay couples a wide range of legal and economic rights.

alimony and child support, inheritance of property, hospital visitation rights, family leave, and a spouse's retirement benefits. (Social Security benefits come from a federal program and are not influenced by state laws.)

At the present time, only the state of Massachusetts has legalized gay marriage. The Massachusetts law came into effect in 2003, after a lengthy series of complex court battles. Ultimately, the Massachusetts Supreme Court determined that it was illegal (according to the state constitution) to deny gay couples the right to wed. In the year 2000, the Vermont legislature passed the nation's first "civil union" law, which granted legal status to gay and lesbian couples. Vermont's law confers on same-sex couples all the benefits that the state presently allows for heterosexual married couples. However, civil unions that take place in Vermont are not generally recognized in other states.

In early 2005, a San Francisco County Superior Court judge ruled that withholding marriage licenses from gay and lesbian couples constituted a violation of their civil rights under state law.[23] This ruling was expected to be appealed by those who felt it could undermine California's existing laws, which define marriage as between one man and one woman. Like Vermont, California already had a law that grants "domestic partner" benefits (but not marriage) to committed gay and lesbian couples who register with the state government. In April 2005, this law was upheld by the 3rd District Court of Appeal, thus keeping legal status for the 29,000 couples in California registered as domestic partners.[24]

In an attempt to counter the general push toward same-sex marriage, a number of states have passed so-called Defense of Marriage Acts (DOMAs). Voters in numerous states have passed laws that define marriage as the union between one man and one woman. It will be interesting to see how this debate evolves, since legal challenges to DOMAs are likely to occur in every state where these laws have been passed. The debate could encourage states to pass laws that support civil union or domestic partnerships, with the hopes of preserving bans on actual gay and lesbian marriages. Most observers believe that ultimately the U.S. Supreme Court will have to rule on the constitutionality of same-sex marriage.

Until that happens, some conservative members of the U.S. Congress are trying to rally support for a constitutional amendment that would ban gay marriage. This has been a challenging task indeed. While President George W. Bush has been somewhat reluctant to vigorously support such an amendment, he did "support the notion that marriage is between a man and a woman."[25]

Single Parenthood

Unmarried young women becoming pregnant and then becoming single parents is a continuing reality in the United States. A new and significantly different form of single parenthood is, however, also a reality in this country: the planned entry into a single parenthood by older, better educated people, the vast majority of whom are women.

In contrast to the teenaged girl who becomes a single parent through an unwed pregnancy, the more mature woman who desires single parenting has usually planned carefully for the experience. She has explored several important concerns, including questions about how she will become pregnant (with or without the knowledge of a male partner or through artificial insemination), the need for a father figure for the child, the effect of single parenting on her social life, and its effect on her career development. Once these questions have been resolved, no legal barriers stand in the way of her becoming a single parent.

A very large number of women and a growing number of men are becoming single parents through a divorce settlement or separation agreement. Additionally, increasing numbers of single persons are adopting children. In 2003, single women headed up 8.1 million households with children under age 18. In contrast, single men headed up 1.9 million households in 2003 with children under age 18.[21]

A few single parents have been awarded children through adoption. The likelihood of a single person's receiving a child this way is small, but more people have been successful recently in single-parent adoptions.

Marriage

Just as there is no single best way for two people to move through dating and mate selection, marriage is also a variable undertaking. In marriage, two people join their lives in a way that affirms each as an individual and both as a legal pair. Some are able to resolve conflicts constructively (see Changing for the Better). However, for a large percentage of couples, the demands of marriage are too rigorous, confining, and demanding. They will find resolution for their dissatisfaction through divorce or extramarital affairs. For most, though, marriage will be an experience that alternates periods of happiness, productivity, and admiration with periods of frustration, unhappiness, and disillusionment with the partner. Each of you who marries will find the experience unique in every regard. (Changing for the Better on this page presents some advice for improving marriage.)

Currently, certain trends regarding marriage are evident. The most obvious of these is the age at first marriage. Today men are waiting longer than ever to marry. The median age at first marriage for men is 27 years.[26] In addition, these new husbands are better educated than in the past and are more likely to be established in their careers. Women are also waiting longer to get married and tend to be more educated and career oriented than they were in the past. Recent statistics indicate that the median age at first marriage for women is 25 years.[26]

Marriage still appeals to most adults. Currently, 76 percent of adults age 18 and older are either married, widowed, or divorced.[21] Thus only about one-quarter of today's

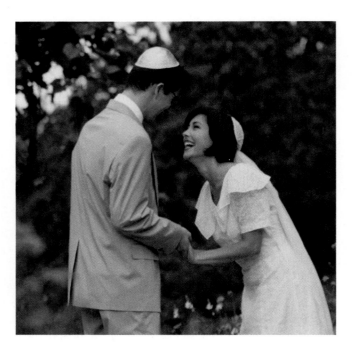

Marriage is a form of emotional and legal bonding.

adults have not married. Within the last decade, the percentage of adults who have decided not to marry has nearly doubled.

Divorce

Marriages, like many other kinds of interpersonal relationships, can end. Today, marriages—relationships begun with the intent of permanence "until death do us part"—end through divorce nearly as frequently as they continue.

Why should approximately half of marital relationships be so likely to end? Unfortunately, marriage experts cannot provide one clear answer. Rather, they suggest that divorce is a reflection of unfulfilled expectations for marriage on the part of one or both partners, including the following:

- The belief that marriage will ease your need to deal with your own faults and that your failures can be shared by your partner

- The belief that marriage will change faults that you know exist in your partner

- The belief that the high level of romance of your dating and courtship period will be continued through marriage

- The belief that marriage can provide you with an arena for the development of your personal power, and that once married, you will not need to compromise with your partner
- The belief that your marital partner will be successful in meeting all of your needs

If these expectations seem to be ones you anticipate through marriage, then you may find that disappointments will abound. To varying degrees, marriage is a partnership that requires much cooperation and compromise. Marriage can be complicated. Because of the high expectations that many people hold for marriage, the termination of marriage can be an emotionally difficult process to undertake.

Concern is frequently voiced over the well-being of children whose parents divorce. Different factors, however, influence the extent to which divorce affects children. Included among these factors are the gender and age of the children, custody arrangements, financial support, and the remarriage of one or both parents. For many children, adjustments must be made to accept their new status as a member of a blended family.

 TALKING POINTS A couple you know well is going through a divorce. How could you show support for each person without taking sides?

 Taking Charge of Your Health

- Take the Personal Assessment on page 363 to understand your sexual attitudes better.
- Use the Personal Assessment on page 365 to find out how compatible you and your partner are.
- If being around someone whose sexual orientation is different from yours makes you feel uncomfortable, focus on getting to know that person better as an individual.
- If you are in an unhealthy relationship, take the first step toward getting out of it through professional counseling or group support.

- If you are in a sexual relationship, communicate your sexual needs to your partner clearly. Encourage him or her to do the same so that you will both have a satisfying sex life.
- Consider whether your lifetime plan will involve marriage, singlehood, or cohabitation. Evaluate your current situation in relation to that plan.

SUMMARY

- Biological and psychosocial factors contribute to the complex expression of our sexuality.
- The structural basis of sexuality begins in the growing embryo and fetus. Structural sexuality changes as one moves through adolescence and later life.
- The psychosocial processes of gender identity, gender preference, and gender adoption form the basis for an initial adult gender identification.
- The complex functioning of the male and female reproductive structures is controlled by hormones.
- The menstrual cycle's primary functions are to produce mature ova and to develop a supportive environment for the fetus in the uterus.

- The sexual response pattern consists of four stages: excitement, plateau, orgasmic, and resolution.
- Three sexual orientations are heterosexuality, homosexuality, and bisexuality.
- Many older people remain interested and active in sexual activities. Physiological changes may alter the way in which some older people perform sexually.
- Abusive behavior, extreme jealousy, controlling behaviors, dishonesty, and drug abuse are warning signs of an unhealthy relationship.
- A variety of lifestyles and relationships exist in our society.
- A large majority of adults will marry at some time.
- Many marriages will end in divorce.

REVIEW QUESTIONS

1. Describe the following foundations of our biological sexuality: the genetic basis, the gonadal basis, and structural development.
2. Define and explain the following terms: gender identity, gender preference, gender adoption, initial adult gender identification, and transsexualism.
3. Identify the major components of the male and female reproductive systems. Trace the passageways for sperm and ova.
4. Explain the menstrual cycle. Identify and describe the four main hormones that control the menstrual cycle.

5. What similarities and differences exist between the sexual response patterns of males and females?
6. What is the refractory period?
7. How do myotonia and vasocongestion differ?
8. What are some of the dangers related to anal sex?
9. Approximately what percentage of today's college students report having had sexual intercourse?
10. Explain the differences between heterosexuality, homosexuality, and bisexuality. How common are each of these sexual orientations in our society?

ENDNOTES

1. Thibodeau GA, Patton KT. *Anatomy and Physiology* (5th ed.). St. Louis: Mosby, 2003.
2. Sherwood L. *Human Physiology: From Cells to Systems* (5th ed.). Belmont, CA: Brooks/Cole, 2004.
3. Hyde JS, DeLameter JD. *Understanding Human Sexuality* (9th ed.). New York: McGraw-Hill, 2006.
4. Allgeier ER, Allgeier AR. *Sexual Interactions* (5th ed.). Boston: Houghton Mifflin, 2000.
5. Crooks RL, Baur K. *Our Sexuality* (9th ed.). Belmont, CA: Wadsworth, 2005.
6. LeVay S, Valente SM. *Human Sexuality.* Sunderland, MA: Sinauer Associates, 2002.
7. Kelly GF. *Sexuality Today: The Human Perspective* (8th ed.). New York: McGraw-Hill, 2006.
8. Masters WH, Johnson VE, Kolodny RC. *Human Sexuality* (5th ed.). Upper Saddle River, NJ: Addison-Wesley, 1997.
9. Strong B, DeVault C, Sayad BW, Yarber WL. *Human Sexuality: Diversity in a Contemporary America* (5th ed.). New York: McGraw-Hill, 2005.
10. Greenberg JS, Bruess CE, Haffner DW. *Exploring the Dimensions of Human Sexuality* (2nd ed.). Boston: Jones and Bartlett, 2004.
11. Hatcher RA, et al. *Contraceptive Technology* (18th ed.). New York: Ardent Media, 2004.
12. Writing Group for the Women's Health Initiative Investigators. Risks and benefits of estrogen plus progestin in healthy postmenopausal women: Principal results from the Women's Health Initiative Randomized Controlled Trial. *Journal of the American Medical Association*, Vol. 288: No. 3 (July 17, 2002), 321–333.
13. Hormone therapy is no heart helper. *Harvard Heart Letter*, Vol. 13: No. 2 (October 2002), 2–4.
14. Masters WH, Johnson VE. *Human Sexual Response.* Philadelphia: Lippincott, Williams and Wilkins, 1966.
15. McAnulty RD, Burnette MM. *Exploring Human Sexuality: Making Healthy Decisions* (2nd ed.). Boston: Allyn and Bacon, 2004.
16. Baldwin JI, Baldwin JD. Heterosexual anal intercourse: An understudied, high-risk sexual behavior. *Archives of Sexual Behavior* 29(4):357–373, 2000.
17. *Supreme Court Strikes Down Texas Sodomy Law,* www.cnn.com, June 27, 2003.
18. Kinsey AC, Pomeroy WB, Martin CE. *Sexual Behavior in the Human Male*, reprint edition. Bloomington, IN: Indiana University Press, 1998.
19. Kinsey AC, et al. *Sexual Behavior in the Human Female*, reprint edition. Bloomington, IN: Indiana University Press, 1998.
20. Allen LS, Gorski RA. Sexual orientation and the size of the anterior commisure in the human brain. *Pract Nat Acad Sci USA* 89(15):7199–7202, 1992.
21. U.S. Census Bureau. *Statistical Abstract of the United States: 2004–2005*, ed.124, Washington, DC: 2004.

22. Bramlett MD, Mosher WD. *Cohabitation, Marriage, Divorce, and Remarriage in the United States.* U.S. Centers for Disease Control and Prevention, National Center for Health Statistics, Vital Health Statistics, 23(22), 2002.

23. *Same-Sex Marriage Ruling Foreshadows Legal War,* www.cnn.com, April 8, 2005.

24. *California Court Upholds Domestic Partner Law,* www.cnn.com, April 8, 2005.

25. *Bush Uncertain About Gay Marriage Ban,* www.cnn.com, July 22, 2003.

26. U.S. Census Bureau. *Current Population Survey, March and Annual Social and Economic Supplements:* 1970–2003, cited in Fields, J. America's families and living arrangements: 2003. *Current Population Reports* (U.S. Census Bureau), P20–553, p. 13, Washington DC: 2003.

personal assessment

Sexual attitudes: A matter of feelings

Respond to each of the following statements by selecting a numbered response (1–5) that most accurately reflects your feelings. Circle the number of your selection. At the end of the questionnaire, total these numbers for use in interpreting your responses.

1 Agree strongly
2 Agree moderately
3 Uncertain
4 Disagree moderately
5 Disagree strongly

Men and women have greater differences than they have similarities.   1   2   3   4   5

Homosexuality and bisexuality are immoral and unnatural.   1   2   3   4   5

Our society is too sexually oriented.   1   2   3   4   5

Pornography encourages sexual promiscuity.   1   2   3   4   5

Children know far too much about sex.   1   2   3   4   5

Education about sexuality is solely the responsibility of the family.   1   2   3   4   5

Dating begins far too early in our society.   1   2   3   4   5

Sexual intimacy before marriage leads to emotional stress and damage to one's reputation.   1   2   3   4   5

Sexual availability is far too frequently the reason that people marry.   1   2   3   4   5

Reproduction is the most important reason for sexual intimacy during marriage.   1   2   3   4   5

Modern families are too small.   1   2   3   4   5

Family planning clinics should not receive public funds.   1   2   3   4   5

Contraception is the woman's responsibility.   1   2   3   4   5

Abortion is the murder of an innocent child.   1   2   3   4   5

Marriage has been weakened by the changing role of women in society.   1   2   3   4   5

Divorce is an unacceptable means of resolving marital difficulties.   1   2   3   4   5

Extramarital sexual intimacy will destroy a marriage.   1   2   3   4   5

Sexual abuse of a child does not generally occur unless the child encourages the adult.   1   2   3   4   5

Provocative behavior by the woman is a factor in almost every case of rape.   1   2   3   4   5

Reproduction is not a right but a privilege.   1   2   3   4   5

YOUR TOTAL POINTS _____

Interpretation

20–34 points	A very traditional attitude toward sexuality
35–54 points	A moderately traditional attitude toward sexuality
55–65 points	A rather ambivalent attitude toward sexuality
66–85 points	A moderately nontraditional attitude toward sexuality
86–100 points	A very nontraditional attitude toward sexuality

To Carry This Further . . .

Were you surprised at your results? Compare your results with those of a roommate or close friend. How do you think your parents would score on this assessment?

personal assessment

How compatible are you?

This quiz will help test how compatible you and your partner's personalities are. You should each rate the truth of these 20 statements based on the following scale. Circle the number that reflects your feelings. Total your scores and check the interpretation following the quiz.

1 Never true
2 Sometimes true
3 Frequently true
4 Always true

We can communicate our innermost thoughts effectively.	1	2	3	4
We trust each other.	1	2	3	4
We agree on whose needs come first.	1	2	3	4
We have realistic expectations of each other and of ourselves.	1	2	3	4
Individual growth is important within our relationship.	1	2	3	4
We will go on as a couple even if our partner doesn't change.	1	2	3	4
Our personal problems are discussed with each other first.	1	2	3	4
We both do our best to compromise.	1	2	3	4
We usually fight fairly.	1	2	3	4
We try not to be rigid or unyielding.	1	2	3	4
We keep any needs to be "perfect" in proper perspective.	1	2	3	4
We can balance desires to be sociable and the need to be alone.	1	2	3	4
We both make friends and keep them.	1	2	3	4
Neither of us stays down or up for long periods.	1	2	3	4
We can tolerate the other's mood without being affected by it.	1	2	3	4
We can deal with disappointment and disillusionment.	1	2	3	4
Both of us can tolerate failure.	1	2	3	4
We can both express anger appropriately.	1	2	3	4
We are both assertive when necessary.	1	2	3	4
We agree on how our personal surroundings are kept.	1	2	3	4

YOUR TOTAL POINTS _____

Interpretation

20–35 points	You and your partner seem quite incompatible. Professional help may open your lines of communication.
36–55 points	You probably need more awareness and compromise.
56–70 points	You are highly compatible. However, be aware of the areas where you can improve.
71–80 points	Your relationship is very fulfilling.

To Carry This Further . . .

Ask your partner to take this test too. You may have a one-sided view of a "perfect" relationship. Even if you scored high on this assessment, be aware of areas where you can still improve.

chapter fourteen

Managing Your Fertility

Chapter Objectives

On completing this chapter, you will be able to:

▌ explain the difference between the terms *birth control* and *contraception.*

▌ define the *theoretical effectiveness* and the *use effectiveness* of contraceptive methods and why they differ.

▌ discuss the advantages and disadvantages of each form of birth control.

▌ identify the many ways in which contraceptive hormones can be delivered to females.

▌ identify the circumstances under which emergency contraception might be used.

▌ identify and explain the procedures for male and female sterilization.

▌ differentiate between the procedures involved in *human cloning* and *therapeutic cloning.*

▌ identify physiological obstacles and aids to fertilization.

▌ describe the events that take place during each of the three stages of labor.

▌ identify and explain the four procedures available through assisted reproductive technologies (ART).

Eye on the Media

Information Online: Birth Control and Sexuality

The Internet offers a number of resources for locating information about contraception, birth control and related topics. Planned Parenthood Federation of America provides one of the most comprehensive sites, at www.plannedparenthood.org. If you are looking for birth control information, click on this site's "Frequently Asked Questions," "Fact Sheets," "Sexual Health Glossary," and "Links." You will be able to learn about pregnancy determination, options concerning pregnancy, sexually transmitted diseases, laws in your state concerning teens' access to birth control and abortion services, and how to get access to contraception. Planned Parenthood believes that when people are empowered with knowledge, they are better able to make sound decisions about their health and sexuality.

Four other sites offer information about sexuality and reproductive choices. The Alan Guttmacher Institute site (www.agi-usa.org) is dedicated to protecting the reproductive choices of women and men throughout the world by disseminating the results of scientific research. The Guttmacher Institute's menu of options includes law and public policy, abortion, pregnancy and birth, prevention and contraception, sexual behavior, and STDs and youth.

The American Social Health Association (www.ashastd.org) is dedicated to stopping the spread of sexually transmitted diseases. ASHA's Web site provides comprehensive information about all aspects of STDs. Additionally, ASHA operates a network of national hotlines that answer over 2 million calls each year.

The Sex Information and Education Council of the United States (SIECUS) is a nonprofit organization dedicated to developing, collecting, and disseminating information about sexuality. This organization (www.siecus.org) promotes comprehensive sexuality education and distributes thousands of pamphlets, booklets, and bibliographies each year to professionals and the general public.

If you want to search for information about certain sexuality topics from a prolife perspective, you might wish to examine the Web site for The Ultimate Pro-life Resource List at www.prolifeinfo.org. This site is supported by the nonprofit Women and Children First organization and provides links to information related to abortion alternatives, *Roe v. Wade,* euthanasia and assisted suicide, pregnancy help, prolife news and prolife organizations.

How you decide to control your **fertility** will have an important effect on your future. Your understanding of information and issues related to fertility control will help you make responsible decisions in this complex area.

For traditional-age students, these decisions may be fast approaching. (See Discovering Your Spirituality for a discussion of decision making about sex and the spiritual dimension of sexuality.) Frequently, nontraditional students are parents who have had experiences that make them useful resources for other students in the class.

Birth Control versus Contraception

Any discussion about the control of your fertility should start with an explanation of the subtle differences between the terms **birth control** and **contraception.** Although many people use the words interchangeably, they reflect different perspectives about fertility control. *Birth control* is an umbrella term that refers to all the procedures you might use to prevent the birth of a child. Birth control includes all available contraceptive measures, as well as all sterilization and abortion procedures.

Contraception is a much more specific term for any procedure used to prevent the fertilization of an ovum.

Contraceptive measures vary widely in the mechanisms they use to accomplish this task. They also vary considerably in their method of use and their rate of success in preventing conception. A few examples of contraceptives are condoms, hormonal contraceptives, spermicides, and diaphragms.

Beyond the numerous methods mentioned, certain forms of sexual behavior not involving intercourse could be considered forms of contraception. For example, mutual masturbation by couples virtually eliminates the possibility of pregnancy. This practice, as well as additional forms of sexual expression other than intercourse (such as kissing, touching, and massage), has been given the

---

Key Terms

fertility the ability to reproduce

birth control all the methods and procedures that can prevent the birth of a child

contraception any method or procedure that prevents fertilization

---

Discovering Your Spirituality

There's More to Sex than You Thought . . .

Are you ready for sex? If you're not sure, take time to think it over. If you start having sex before you're ready, you might feel guilty. You might feel bad because you realize this step isn't right for you now. Or your religious upbringing may make you feel as though you're doing something wrong. You also may not be ready for the emotional aspects of a sexual relationship. Most important, you will probably have difficulty handling the complexities of an unplanned pregnancy or a sexually transmitted disease.

If you do feel ready for sex, you still have a choice. Sex may be OK for you now. It may be personally fulfilling, something that enhances your self-esteem. Alternatively, you can choose to abstain from sex until later—another way of enhancing your self-esteem. You'll feel empowered by making the decision for yourself, rather than doing what is expected. Being strong enough to say "no" can also make you feel good about yourself. For some, making this decision may reflect a renewed commitment to spiritual or religious concerns.

If you're married, sex is a good way of connecting as a couple. It's something that the two of you alone share. It's a time to give special attention to each other—taking a break from the kids, your jobs, and your other responsibilities. It's a way of saying: "This relationship is important—it's something I value."

Going through a pregnancy together is another opportunity for closeness. From the moment you know that you're going to be parents, you're connected in a new way. Your focus becomes the expected child. You'll watch the fetus grow on ultrasound, go to parenting and Lamaze classes together, visit the doctor together, mark the various milestones, and share new emotions. When your child is born, you'll be connected as never before.

Whether you're thinking about starting to have sex, making the decision to wait, or examining the sexual life you have now, you can't ignore the possibilities and the consequences. Is the time right for you? Are you doing this for yourself or for someone else? What do you think you will gain from waiting? Do you expect your future partner to also have made the decision to wait? What do you expect to get from a sexual relationship—pleasure, intimacy, love? What do you expect to give? Do you want an emotional commitment? Do you view sex and love as inseparable? Do you understand how sex can enhance your spirituality? Taking time to consider these questions can make you feel good about yourself—no matter what you decide.

generic term **outercourse.** Not only does outercourse protect against unplanned pregnancy, it may also significantly reduce the transmission of sexually transmitted diseases (STDs), including HIV infection.

Theoretical Effectiveness versus Use Effectiveness

People considering the use of a contraceptive method need to understand the difference between the two effectiveness rates given for each form of contraception. *Theoretical effectiveness* is a measure of a contraceptive method's ability to prevent a pregnancy when the method is used precisely as directed during every act of intercourse. *Use effectiveness,* however, refers to the effectiveness of a method in preventing conception when used by the general public. Use effectiveness rates take into account factors that lower effectiveness below that based on "perfect" use. Failure to follow proper instructions, illness of the user, forgetfulness, physician (or pharmacist) error, and a subconscious desire to experience risk or even pregnancy are a few of the factors that can lower the effectiveness of even the most theoretically effective contraceptive technique.

Effectiveness rates are often expressed in terms of the percentage of women users of childbearing age who do not become pregnant while using the method for 1 year. For some methods the theoretical-effectiveness and use-effectiveness rates are vastly different; the theoretical rate is always higher than the use rate. Table 14.1 presents data concerning effectiveness rates, advantages, and disadvantages of many birth control methods.

Selecting Your Contraceptive Method

In this section, we discuss some of the many factors that should be important to you as you consider selecting a contraceptive method. Remember that no method possesses equally high marks in all of the following areas. You and your partner should select a contraceptive method that is both acceptable and effective, as determined by your unique needs and expectations. Completing the Personal Assessment on page 395 will help you make this decision.

For a contraceptive method to be acceptable to those who wish to exercise a large measure of control over their fertility, the following should be given careful consideration:

- *It should be safe.* The contraceptive approach you select should not pose a significant health risk for you or your partner.

- *It should be effective.* Your approach must have a high success rate in preventing pregnancy.

- *It should be reliable.* The form you select must be able to be used over and over again with consistent success.

- *It should be reversible.* Couples who eventually want to have a family should select a method that can be reversed.

- *It should be affordable.* The cost of a particular method must fit comfortably into a couple's budget.

- *It should be easy to use.* Complicated instructions or procedures can make a method difficult to use effectively.

- *It should not interfere with sexual expression.* An ideal contraceptive fits in comfortably with a couple's intimate sexual behavior.

 TALKING POINTS The method of birth control your partner prefers doesn't allow for spontaneous sex. How would you explain that this decreases your enjoyment?

Current Birth Control Methods

Abstinence

Abstinence as a form of birth control has gained attention recently on college campuses. This method is as close to 100 percent effective as possible. There have been isolated reports in medical literature of pregnancy without sexual intercourse, usually involving ejaculation by the male near the woman's vagina. Avoiding this situation should raise the effectiveness of abstinence to 100 percent.

Abstinence as a form of birth control has additional advantages in that it gives nearly 100 percent protection from sexually transmitted diseases, it is free, and it does not require a visit to a physician or a health clinic.

However, some concerns exist about the effectiveness of educational programs that encourage abstinence. In a study of 12,000 adolescents published in 2005, Yale and Columbia University researchers found that teenagers who "pledged virginity until marriage" were more likely to participate in oral sex and anal sex than were nonpledging teens who had not had sexual intercourse. (Both oral and anal sex carry risks of STD transmission.) Additionally, the

---

Key Terms
outercourse sexual activity that does not involve intercourse

Table 14.1 Effectiveness Rates of Birth Control for 100 Women during 1 Year of Use

Method	Estimated Effectiveness		Advantages	Disadvantages
	Theoretical	Use		
No method (chance)	15%	15%	Inexpensive	Totally ineffective
Withdrawal	96%	73%	No supplies or advance preparation needed; no side effects; men share responsibility for family planning	Interferes with coitus; very difficult to use effectively; women must trust men to withdraw as orgasm approaches
Periodic abstinence Calendar Standard Days method Basal body temperature Cervical mucus method Symptothermal	91%–99%	75%	No supplies needed; no side effects; men share responsibility for family planning; women learn about their bodies	Difficult to use, especially if menstrual cycles are irregular, as is common in young women; abstinence may be necessary for long periods; lengthy instruction and ongoing counseling may be needed
Cervical cap (no previous births)	91%	85%	No health risks; helps protect against some STDs and cervical cancer	Limited availability in some areas
Spermicide (gel, foam, suppository, film)	92%	71%	No health risks; helps protect against some STDs; can be used with condoms to increase effectiveness considerably	Must be inserted 5 to 30 minutes before coitus; effective for only 30 to 60 minutes; some concern about nonoxynol-9
Diaphragm with spermicide	94%	84%	No health risks; helps protect against some STDs and cervical cancer	Must be inserted with jelly or foam and left in place for at least 6 hours after coitus; must be fitted by health care personnel; some women may find it awkward or embarrassing to use; some concern about nonoxynol-9
Sponge (no previous births) (previous births)	91% 80%	84% 77%	Easy to use; not messy; protection is good for 24 hours and multiple acts of intercourse; no prescription needed	Not reusable; contraceptive protection reduced for women with previous births; some concern about nonoxynol-9
Male condom	98%	85%	Easy to use; inexpensive and easy to obtain; no health risks; very effective protection against some STDs; men share responsibility for family planning	Must be put on just before coitus; some men and women complain of decreased sensation; some concern about nonoxynol-9
Male condom with spermicide	99%	95%		
Female condom	95%	79%	Relatively easy to use; no prescription required; polyurethane is stronger than latex; provides some STD protection; silicone-based lubrication provided; useful when male will not use a condom	Contraceptive effectiveness and STD protection not as high as with male condom; couples may be unfamiliar with a device that extends outside the vagina; more expensive than male condoms
IUD ParaGard (Copper T) Mirena (progestin)	99%+ 99%+	99%+ 99%+	Easy to use; highly effective in preventing pregnancy; does not interfere with coitus; repeated action not needed; depending on the device, can be effective for 5 or 10 years	May increase risk of pelvic inflammatory disease (PID) and infertility in women with more than one sexual partner; not usually recommended for women who have never had a child; must be inserted by health care personnel; may cause heavy bleeding and pain in some women
Contraceptive ring (estrogen-progestin)	99%+	92%	Easy to use after learning how to insert; remains in place for 3 weeks	Like other hormonal methods, does not protect against STDs; requires a physician's prescription; possibility of CV problems in a small percentage of users
Contraceptive patch (estrogen-progestin)	99%+	92%	Easy to apply; must be changed weekly for 3 weeks	(Same as above)
Combined pill	99%+	92%	Easy to use; highly effective in preventing pregnancy; does not interfere with coitus; regulates menstrual cycle; reduces heavy bleeding and menstrual pain; helps protect against ovarian and endometrial cancer	Must be taken every day; requires medical examination and prescription; minor side effects such as nausea or menstrual spotting; possibility of CV problems, in a small percentage of users
Minipill (progestin only)	99%+	92%		
Depo-Provera (3 month)	99%+	97%	Easy to use; highly effective for an extended period; continued use prevents menstruation	Requires supervision by a physician; administered by injection; some women experience irregular menstrual spotting and weight gain in early months of use
Tubal ligation	99%+	99%+	Permanent; removes fear of pregnancy	Surgery-related risks; generally considered irreversible
Vasectomy	99%+	99%+	Permanent; removes fear of pregnancy	Generally considered irreversible

Adapted from Hatcher RA et al: *Contraceptive Technology,* 18th ed, 2004. New York: Ardent Media, Inc.

Figure 14-1 Periodic abstinence (fertility awareness or natural family planning) can combine use of the calendar, basal body temperature measurements, and Billings mucus techniques to identify the fertile period. Remember that most women's cycles are not consistently perfect 28-day cycles, as shown in most illustrations. This figure is only an approximation of a woman's cycle.

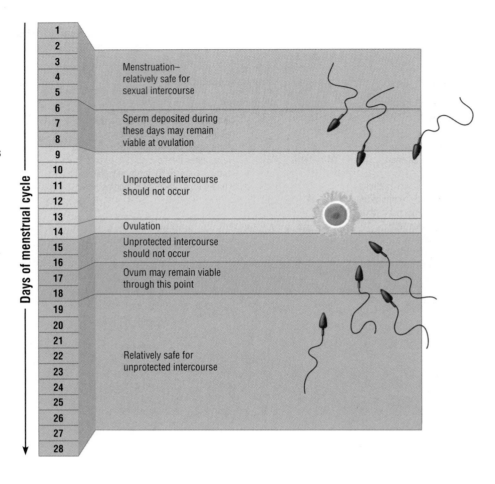

Days of menstrual cycle

Menstruation– relatively safe for sexual intercourse

Sperm deposited during these days may remain viable at ovulation

Unprotected intercourse should not occur

Ovulation

Unprotected intercourse should not occur

Ovum may remain viable through this point

Relatively safe for unprotected intercourse

researchers found that teens who pledged abstinence were less likely to use condoms during their first sexual intercourse and less likely to be tested for STDs than were nonpledging teens.[1] Abstinence works effectively only when it is broadly defined (to include many sexual behaviors) and used correctly and consistently. Abstinence is a challenging proposition for many adolescents and young adults.

Withdrawal

Withdrawal, or **coitus interruptus,** is the contraceptive practice in which the erect penis is removed from the vagina just before ejaculation of semen. Theoretically this procedure prevents sperm from entering the deeper structures of the female reproductive system. The use effectiveness of this method, however, reflects how unsuccessful this method is in practice (see Table 14.1).

There is strong evidence to suggest that the clear preejaculate fluid that helps neutralize and lubricate the male urethra can contain *viable* (capable of fertilization) sperm.[2] This sperm can be deposited near the cervical opening before withdrawal of the penis. This phenomenon may in part explain the relatively low effectiveness of

this method. Furthermore, withdrawal does not protect users from the transmission of STDs.

Periodic Abstinence

Five approaches are included in the birth control strategy called **periodic abstinence:** (1) the calendar method, (2) the Standard Days method, (3) the basal body temperature (BBT) method, (4) the Billings cervical mucus method, and (5) the symptothermal method.[3] All five methods attempt to determine the time a woman ovulates. Figure 14-1

Key Terms

withdrawal (coitus interruptus) a contraceptive practice in which the erect penis is removed from the vagina before ejaculation

periodic abstinence birth control methods that rely on a couple's avoidance of intercourse during the ovulatory phase of a woman's menstrual cycle; also called *fertility awareness, rhythm,* or *natural family planning*

★ Vaginal Contraceptive Film

A unique spermicide delivery system developed in England is vaginal contraceptive film (VCF). Vaginal contraceptive film is a sheet containing nonoxynol-9 that is inserted over the cervical opening. Shortly after insertion of the VCF, it dissolves into a gel-like material that clings to the cervical opening. The VCF can be inserted up to an hour before intercourse. Over the course of several hours, the material will be washed from the vagina in the normal vaginal secretions.

This spermicide is a nonprescription form of contraception that is as effective as other spermicidal foams and gels. Users should be aware that the nonoxynol-9 spermicide may not be as effective against STDs as was formerly thought. A box of 12 sheets costs about $12.

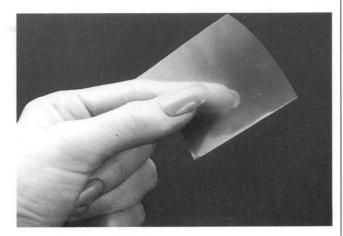

Vaginal contraceptive film

shows a day-to-day fertility calendar used to estimate fertile periods. Most research indicates that an ovum is viable for only about 24–36 hours after its release from the ovary. (Once inside the female reproductive tract, some sperm can survive up to a week.)

When a woman can accurately determine when she ovulates, she must refrain from intercourse long enough for the ovum to begin to disintegrate. *Fertility awareness, rhythm, natural birth control,* and *natural family planning* are terms interchangeable with periodic abstinence. Remember that periodic abstinence methods *do not* provide protection against the spread of STDs and HIV infection.

Periodic abstinence is the only acceptable method endorsed by the Roman Catholic Church. For some people who have deep concerns for the spiritual dimensions of their health, the selection of a contraceptive method other than periodic abstinence may indicate a serious compromise of beliefs.

The **calendar method** requires close examination of a woman's menstrual cycle for the last 6–12 cycles. Records are kept of the length (in days) of each cycle. A *cycle* is defined as the number of days from the first day of menstrual flow in one cycle to the first day of menstrual flow in the next cycle.

To determine the days she should abstain from intercourse, a woman should subtract 18 from her shortest cycle; this is the first day she should abstain from intercourse in an upcoming cycle. Then she should subtract 11 from her longest cycle; this is the last day she must abstain from intercourse in an upcoming cycle.[4]

The newest periodic abstinence approach is called the *Standard Days method.* This method is appropriate only for women who have menstrual cycles that are consistently between 26 and 32 days long. It is not to be used by women who have variable cycles that are shorter than

26 days or longer than 32 days. Having had just one cycle in the past year shorter than 26 days or longer than 32 days should encourage a woman NOT to use the Standard Days method. She should meet with her health care provider and discuss an alternative method.

To use this method, women must count the days of their menstrual cycle, with day 1 as the first day of menstrual bleeding. Women can have intercourse on days 1–7. On days 8–19, women should refrain from penis/vaginal intercourse or use a barrier method of contraception. Days 8–19 are the fertile days. From day 20 until the end of the cycle, unprotected intercourse can take place.[4] Keep in mind that the Standard Days method does not protect against the transmission of STDs.

The *basal body temperature method* requires a woman (for about 3 or 4 successive months) to take her body temperature every morning before she rises from bed. A finely calibrated thermometer, available in many drugstores, is used for this purpose. The theory behind this method is that a distinct correlation exists between body temperature and the process of ovulation. Around the time of ovulation, the body temperature rises at least 0.4° Fahrenheit and remains elevated until the start of menstruation. The woman is instructed to refrain from intercourse during the interval when the temperature change takes place.

Key Terms

calendar method a form of periodic abstinence in which the variable lengths of a woman's menstrual cycle are used to calculate her fertile period

Drawbacks of this procedure include the need for consistent, accurate readings and the realization that all women's bodies are different. Some women may not fit the temperature pattern projection because of biochemical differences in their bodies. Also, body temperatures can fluctuate because of a wide variety of illnesses and physical stressors. Temperature kits are available in drugstores and cost about $5–$8.

The *Billings cervical mucus method* (also called the *ovulation method*) is another periodic abstinence technique. Generally used with other periodic abstinence techniques, this method requires a woman to evaluate the daily mucous discharge from her cervix. Users of this method become familiar with the changes in both appearance (from clear to cloudy) and consistency (from watery to thick) of their cervical mucus throughout their cycles. Women are taught that the unsafe days are when the mucus becomes clear and is the consistency of raw egg whites. Such a technique of ovulation determination must be learned from a physician or family planning professional.

The *symptothermal method* of periodic abstinence combines the use of the BBT method and the cervical mucus method.[4] Couples using the symptothermal method are already using a calendar to chart the woman's body changes. Thus some family planning professionals consider the symptothermal method a combination of all of the periodic abstinence approaches.

Vaginal Spermicides

Spermicides are agents that are capable of killing sperm. When used alone, they offer a moderately effective form of contraception for the woman who is sexually active on an infrequent basis. Modern spermicides are generally safe (but see precaution below), reversible forms of contraception that can be obtained without a physician's prescription in most drugstores and supermarkets. Spermicides are relatively inexpensive. Applicator kits cost about $8, and refills cost around $4–$8 (Figure 14-2).

Spermicides, which are available in foam, cream, jelly, film, or suppository form, are made of water-soluble bases with a spermicidal agent in the base. Spermicides are commonly used with other contraceptives, such as diaphragms, cervical caps, and condoms.

Spermicides are not specific to sperm cells; they also attack other cells. Until recently, nonoxynol-9, the most commonly used spermicidal agent, was thought to protect women from developing **pelvic inflammatory disease (PID).** Health professionals believed that nonoxynol-9 provided this protection by attacking and killing pathogens which caused various STDs.

However, the latest research indicates that nonoxynol-9 is not very effective in killing other pathogens. Nonoxynol-9 may actually *increase* the likelihood of disease transmission,

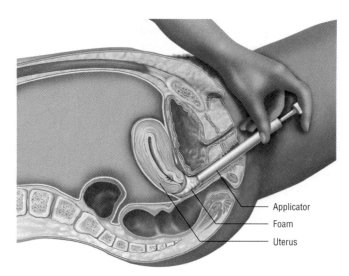

Figure 14-2 Spermicidal foams, gels, and suppositories are placed deep into the vagina in the region of the cervix no longer than 30 minutes before intercourse.

- Applicator
- Foam
- Uterus

including HIV transmission, because it can cause skin irritations and abrasions in a small percentage of users.[5] These irritated areas and abrasions can provide the avenue for passage into the bloodstream.

For this reason, couples should not depend on vaginal spermicides to stop the spread of infections from person to person. Condoms, when used consistently and correctly, provide much better disease protection and contraceptive effect than spermicides used alone. The latest research also indicates that condoms coated with nonoxynol-9 do not have enough of the spermicide to serve as a back-up contraceptive if the condom breaks.[6] Thus, some health centers and family planning agencies have stopped distributing condoms with nonoxynol-9 in the lubricant. If you and/or your partner have concerns about your use of spermicides, you should seek advice from your physician or health center.

Condoms

Colored or natural, smooth or textured, straight or shaped, plain or reservoir-tipped, dry or lubricated—the latex condom is approaching an art form. This is perhaps an

---

Key Terms

spermicides chemicals capable of killing sperm

pelvic inflammatory disease (PID) a generalized infection of the pelvic cavity that results from the spread of an infection through a woman's reproductive structures

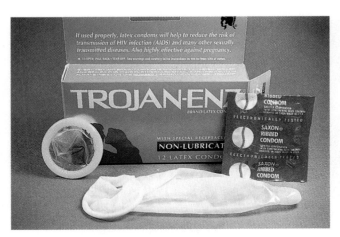

Male condoms

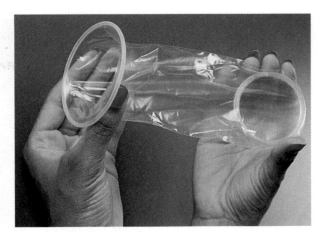

Female condom

exaggeration. Still, the familiar **condom** remains a safe, effective, reversible contraceptive device. All condoms manufactured in the United States must be approved by the FDA.[7]

For couples who are highly motivated in their desire to prevent a pregnancy, the effectiveness of a condom can approach that of an oral contraceptive—especially if condom use is combined with a spermicide. For couples who are less motivated, the condom can be considerably less effective. Condoms cost from 25¢ to $2.50 each.

The condom offers substantial protection against STDs. For both the man and the woman, chlamydial infections, gonorrhea, HIV infection, and other STDs are less likely to be acquired when the condom is used correctly (see Changing for the Better on page 375). Some lubricated condoms also contain a spermicide. However, recent research indicates that the use of the spermicide nonoxynol-9 may irritate tissues in some users and actually increase the likelihood of disease transmission.[6] Also, the small amount of spermicide present in the condom's lubricant is not enough to consistently prevent conception if the condom should break. Current recommendations are to use dry condoms or lubricated condoms without spermicide. Also, any additional lubricants used should be water-based lubricants.

The FDA has approved both male and female types of polyurethane condoms. At the time of this writing, at least three brands of polyurethane male condoms and one female condom (Reality) are available as one-time-use condoms.[3] These condoms are good alternatives for people who have an allergic sensitivity to latex estimated to be up to 7 percent of the population.[8] Also, they are thinner and stronger than latex condoms and can be used with oil-based lubricants. Currently, these condoms are believed to provide protection against STDs that is close to that of latex condoms. The contraceptive effectiveness of polyurethane condoms remains somewhat less than that of the male latex condom.[9,10]

The Reality female condom is a soft, loose-fitting polyurethane sheath containing two polyurethane rings

(see photo). Reality is inserted like a diaphragm to line the inner walls of the vagina. The larger ring remains outside the vagina, and the external portion of the condom provides some protection to the labia and the base of the penis. Reality is coated on the inside with a silicone-based lubricant. Additional lubricant is provided for the outside of the sheath. This lubricant does not contain a spermicide. Female and male condoms should not be used together since they might adhere to each other and cause slippage or displacement. Female condoms cost about $2.50.

Diaphragm

The **diaphragm** is a soft rubber cup with a springlike metal rim that, when properly fitted and correctly inserted by the user, rests in the top of the vagina. The diaphragm covers the cervical opening (Figure 14-3). During intercourse the diaphragm stays in place quite well and cannot usually be felt by either partner.

The diaphragm is always used with a spermicidal cream or jelly. The diaphragm should be covered with an adequate amount of spermicide inside the cup and around the rim. When used properly with a spermicide, the diaphragm is a relatively effective contraceptive, and when combined with the man's use of a condom, its effectiveness is even greater.

The diaphragm must be inserted before intercourse. It should provide effective protection for 6 hours. If this time interval extends beyond 6 hours, some clinicians

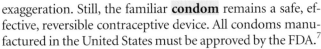

Key Terms
condom a latex shield designed to cover the erect penis and retain semen on ejaculation; "rubber"
diaphragm a soft rubber cup designed to cover the cervix

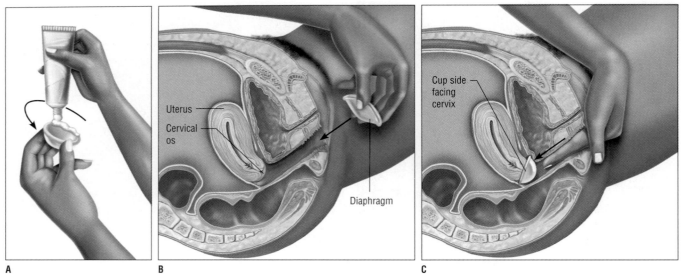

Figure 14-3 **A:** Spermicidal cream or jelly is placed into the diaphragm. **B:** The diaphragm is folded lengthwise and inserted into the vagina. **C:** The diaphragm is then placed against the cervix so that the cup portion with the spermicide is facing the cervix. The outline of the cervix should be felt through the central part of the diaphragm.

recommend that additional spermicide be placed in the vagina. Use of additional spermicide with multiple acts of intercourse is optional. After intercourse, the diaphragm must be left in place for at least 6 hours before it is removed. Because of the risk of toxic shock syndrome (TSS), the diaphragm must not remain in the vagina longer than 24 hours.[4] It is always best to ask a health care provider for specific instructions.

Diaphragms must always be fitted and prescribed by a physician. Typically, it costs $15–$75 for a diaphragm and $4–$8 for the spermicide. An examination may cost between $50 and $200, but it will be less at a family planning clinic.[11] Also, a high level of motivation to follow the instructions *exactly* is important.

Diaphragms and other vaginal barrier methods, such as the cervical cap, do not provide reliable protection against STDs and HIV infection. Recent concerns about the spermicide nonoxynol-9 should prompt users to ask their physicians to recommend a cream or jelly to use with a diaphragm. If you are concerned about possible infection, either avoid sexual activity or use a latex condom and spermicide in combination.

Cervical Cap

The **cervical cap** is a small, thimble-shaped device that fits over the entire cervix. The cap is held in place by suction rather than by pushing against anatomical structures (Figure 14-4). As with the diaphragm, a spermicide is used with the cervical cap. The use effective-

ness of the cervical cap appears to be approximately equal to that of the diaphragm. As with the diaphragm, the effectiveness of the cervical cap is much higher in women who have never had children. Cervical caps are

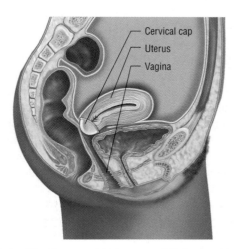

Figure 14-4 After the spermicidal cream or jelly is placed in the cervical cap, the cap is inserted into the vagina and placed against the cervix.

Key Terms

cervical cap a small, thimble-shaped contraceptive device designed to fit over the cervix

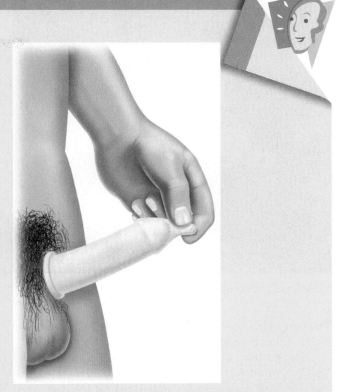
distributed in the United States through physician prescription.

The cervical cap comes in just four sizes and, thus, may be difficult to fit for some women.[4] A physician must prescribe the cervical cap and show the woman how to use it. The cervical cap is filled ⅓ full of spermicide before being placed snugly around the base of the cervix. The cap provides effective protection for 48 hours, no matter how many times intercourse occurs. Use of additional spermicide with repeated acts of intercourse is optional. Leave the cap in place for at least 6 hours after intercourse.[4] It is always best to ask a health care provider for specific instructions.

With new concerns about the use of the spermicide nonoxynol-9, women are advised to ask their physicians which contraceptive or cream or jelly they should use with their cervical cap. The cost of a contraceptive cap is similar to that for a diaphragm.

Lea's Shield and FemCap

The two newest barrier methods for women were approved by the FDA in 2002. Both methods are used with a spermicide. *Lea's Shield* is a reusable oval device made of silicone rubber that fits closely over the cervix. An attached loop helps in the removal from the vagina. The Lea's Shield works much like a diaphragm, but it has a central air valve that permits air to move out from beneath the shield and permit a closer fit. This device comes in only one size and must be prescribed by a physician.

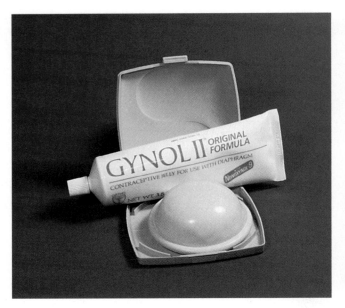

Diaphragm and contraceptive jelly

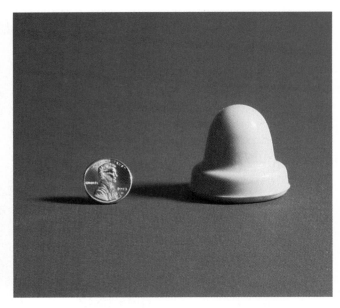

Cervical cap

The first year, use effectiveness of this device (85 percent) is about the same as that for diaphragms (84 percent).[11]

The *FemCap* is a reusable hat-shaped silicone rubber cap that completely covers the cervix. Coated with spermicide, the FemCap's brim fits snugly against the deep vaginal walls. An attached strap helps in the removal of this device. The FemCap must be prescribed by a physician and comes in three sizes. Among women who have never been pregnant or given birth vaginally, the first year use effectiveness of this device is 86 percent. Costs for these new devices are similar to those for diaphragms and caps.[11]

Contraceptive Sponge

The sponge is a small, pillow-shaped polyurethane device containing nonoxynol-9 spermicide. The sponge is dampened with tap water and inserted deep in the vagina to cover the cervical opening. This device provides contraceptive protection for up to 24 hours, regardless of the number of times intercourse occurs. After the last act of intercourse, the device must be left in place for at least 6 hours. Once removed, the sponge must be discarded. The sponge must not be left in place for longer than 24 to 30 hours because of the risk of toxic shock syndrome. Used alone, the sponge does not provide reliable protection against STDs and HIV infection.(Consult your physician if you are concerned about the use of nonoxynol-9.)

The sponge has an interesting history. Before its removal from the market in 1995, the sponge was the most popular female over-the-counter contraceptive in the United States. The sponge came off the market because the manufacturer decided it was too expensive to retool the manufacturing plant to meet governmental safety reg-

ulations. The removal of the sponge prompted the TV sitcom show *Seinfeld* to develop an episode in which the character Elaine Benes purchased as many sponges as she could before they disappeared from the New York City marketplace. She then used them sparingly and only with men she judged to be "spongeworthy."[12]

The company that originally manufactured the sponge sold the rights to Allendale Pharmaceuticals. In 2001, Allendale applied for FDA approval to start manufacturing and selling the sponge in the United States. In early 2005, the FDA granted its approval. It was anticipated that by August 2005, the sponge would again be on drugstore shelves in the United States. Interestingly, the sponge had been available in Canada for a couple of years. Sponges are expected to cost between $2.50 and $3.00 and come in packs of three.[12]

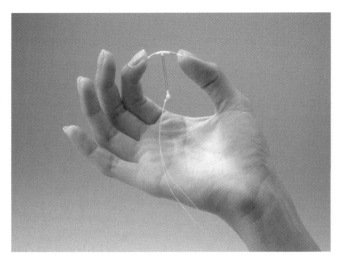

Mirena IUD

Intrauterine Device (IUD)

The **intrauterine device (IUD)** is the most popular reversible contraceptive method in the world, although the number of users in the United States is relatively small. The IUD is a safe, highly effective method of birth control. IUDs work by preventing sperm from fertilizing ova or by preventing a fertilized ovum from implanting in the uterus.

Two types of IUDs are available in the United States: a T-shaped one containing the hormone progestin (Mirena) and a T-shaped one wrapped with copper wire (ParaGard). The Mirena IUD works by thickening cervical mucus, inhibiting sperm survival, and producing a thin endometrial lining that will not support a fertilized ovum. The ParaGard works by releasing copper ions that impair sperm function and prevent fertilization.[4] The Mirena IUD substantially reduces menstrual flow, but the ParaGard may increase menstrual flow. About 20 percent of women who use the Mirena IUD stop having their periods altogether.[13]

The Mirena provides highly effective contraceptive protection for 5 years and the ParaGard for 10 years. Only a skilled physician can prescribe and insert an IUD. As with many other forms of contraception, IUDs do not offer protection against STDs, including the AIDS virus.[3]

As Table 14.1 indicates, IUDs are very effective birth control devices, surpassed in effectiveness only by abstinence, sterilization, and hormonal contraceptives. For many years, the public has been concerned about two potentially serious side effects: *uterine perforation* (in which the IUD embeds itself into the uterine wall) and pelvic inflammatory disease (PID, a widespread infection of the abdominal cavity). Recent research, however, indicates that these events rarely happen, especially when the IUD is inserted by a skilled clinician. Between 2 percent and 10 percent of IUD users experience *expulsion* (muscular contractions which force the IUD out of the uterus) within the first year of use.[4] The cost for an IUD ranges from $175 to $400, which includes an exam, insertion, and a follow-up visit.[11]

Oral Contraceptives

Introduced in the late 1950s, the **oral contraceptive pill** provides one of the highest effectiveness rates of any single reversible contraceptive method used today. Worldwide, more than 100 million women are currently using oral contraceptives.[4] A successful male version has not yet been developed. (See Learning from Our Diversity on page 378.)

Use of the pill requires a physical examination by a physician and a prescription. Since oral contraceptives are available in a wide range of formulas, follow-up examina-

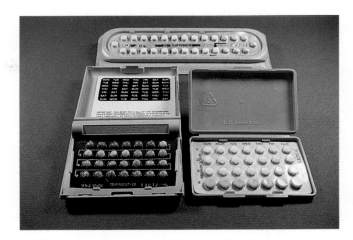

Oral contraceptives

tions are important to ensure that a woman is receiving an effective dosage with as few side effects as possible. Determining the right prescription for a particular woman may require a few consultations.

All oral contraceptives contain synthetic (laboratory-made) hormones. The typical *combined pill* uses both synthetic estrogen and synthetic progesterone in each of 21 pills. With *triphasic pills,* the level of estrogen remains constant, but the level of progestin varies every 7 days. In 2003 the FDA approved a new oral contraceptive (Seasonale) that contains active hormones for 84 days (12 weeks) followed by 1 week of pills containing inactive ingredients.[3] Women using this contraceptive pill would expect to have only four menstrual periods each year. This pill could become a highly popular choice for women. Estrogen levels remain constant during the cycle. As with many forms of contraception, *oral contraceptives do not provide protection from the transmission of STDs or HIV infection.* Furthermore, the use of antibiotics lowers the pill's contraceptive effectiveness.

Oral contraceptives function in several ways. The estrogen in the pill tends to reduce ova development. The progesterone in the pill helps reduce the likelihood of ovulation (by lowering the release of luteinizing hormone). The progesterone in the pill also causes the uterine wall to develop inadequately and helps thicken cervical mucus, thus making it difficult for sperm to enter the uterus.

Key Terms

intrauterine device (IUD) a small, plastic, medicated or unmedicated contraceptive device that prevents pregnancy when inserted in the uterus

oral contraceptive pill a pill taken orally, composed of synthetic female hormones that prevent ovulation or implantation; "the pill"

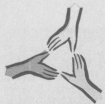
The physical changes produced by the oral contraceptive provide some beneficial side effects in women. Since the synthetic hormones are taken for 21 days and then are followed by **placebo pills** or no pills for 7 days, the menstrual cycle becomes regulated. Even women who have irregular cycles immediately become "regular." Since the uterine lining is not developed to the extent seen in a nonuser, the uterus is not forced to contract with the same amount of vigor. Thus menstrual cramping is reduced, and the resultant menstrual flow is diminished. Research indicates that oral contraceptive use can provide protection against anemia, PID, noncancerous breast tumors, acne, recurrent ovarian cysts, ectopic pregnancy, endometrial cancer, ovarian cancer, and endometriosis.[4]

The negative side effects of the oral contraceptive pill can be divided into two general categories: (1) unpleasant and (2) potentially dangerous. The unpleasant side effects generally subside within 2 or 3 months for most women. A number of women report some or many of the following symptoms:

- Tenderness in breast tissue
- Nausea
- Mild headaches
- Slight, irregular spotting
- Weight gain
- Fluctuations in sex drive
- Mild depression
- More frequent vaginal infections

 TALKING POINTS You've tried two different types of oral contraceptives and had unpleasant side effects with both. Your doctor says you should consider another birth control method, but you disagree. How could you talk to him about this in a matter-of-fact way?

The potentially dangerous side effects of the oral contraceptive pill are most often seen in the cardiovascular system. Blood clots, strokes, hypertension, and heart attack seem to be associated with the estrogen component of the combined pill. However, when compared with the risk to nonusers, the risk of dying from cardiovascular

---

Key Terms

placebo pills pills that contain no active ingredients

complications is only slightly increased among healthy young oral contraceptive users. Users of oral contraceptives are statistically more likely than nonusers are to develop cervical cancer. However, cervical cancer is also related to human papillomavirus (HPV) and unprotected intercourse with multiple partners. Additionally, over 50 scientific studies have determined that oral contraceptive use has little, if any, effect on the development of breast cancer, even among women with a family history of breast cancer.[4]

Most health professionals agree that the risks related to pregnancy and childbirth are much greater than those associated with oral contraceptive use. Certainly, a woman who is contemplating the use of the pill must discuss all of the risks and benefits with her physician.

There are some **contraindications** for the use of oral contraceptives. If you have a history of blood clots, migraine headaches, liver disease, a heart condition, high blood pressure, obesity, diabetes, breast cancer, hepatitis, or cirrhosis, or if you have not established regular menstrual cycles, the pill probably should not be your contraceptive choice. Providing a physician with a complete and accurate health history is important before a woman starts to take the pill.

Two additional contraindications are well understood by the medical community. Cigarette smoking and advancing age are highly associated with an increased risk of potentially serious side effects. Increasing numbers of physicians are not prescribing oral contraceptives for their patients who smoke. The risk of cardiovascular-related deaths is enhanced in women over age 35. The risk is even higher in female smokers over age 35.[4]

For the vast majority of women, however, the pill, when properly prescribed, is safe and effective. Careful scrutiny of a woman's health history and careful follow-up examinations when a problem is suspected are essential elements that can provide a good margin of safety. The ease of administration, the relatively low cost, and the effectiveness of the pill make it a sound choice for many women. Monthly pill packs cost $20–$35. An exam may cost $35–$125.[11]

Minipills

Some women prefer not to use the combined oral contraceptive pill. To avoid some of the potentially serious side effects of the combined pill, some physicians are prescribing **minipills.** These oral contraceptives contain no estrogen—only low-dose progesterone in all pills in a 28-day pill pack. The minipill seems to work by thickening cervical mucus, preventing ovulation, and producing a thin endometrial lining.[4] The effectiveness of the minipill is slightly lower than that of the combined pill. *Breakthrough bleeding* and **ectopic pregnancy** are more common in minipill users than in combined-pill users.

Injectable Contraceptives

Depo-Provera is a highly effective (99 percent+) injectable, progesterone contraceptive that provides protection for three months. This hormone shot works primarily by preventing ovulation and thickening the cervical mucus to keep sperm from joining the egg.

The most common side effects of Depo-Provera are irregular bleeding and spotting followed by *amenorrhea* (the absence of periods).[4] When the woman's body adjusts to the presence of this drug, breakthrough bleeding diminishes, and the most common side effect is amenorrhea. Many women see this as a desirable effect. Women who stop using Depo-Provera may experience infertility for a period of up to 1 year.[4] The cost of Depo-Provera ranges from $30 to $75 per injection.[11]

Contraceptive Ring

One of the newest contraceptives on the market is the vaginal **contraceptive ring** (NuvaRing). Available by prescription, NuvaRing is a thin polymer ring (2⅛ inches in diameter and ⅛ inch thick) that contains synthetic estrogen and progestin. Users insert this device deep into the vagina where it remains for 3 weeks. At the end of the third week, the device is removed for a week and the woman has her period. The NuvaRing provides effective contraception (99 percent+ effective when used perfectly) for the entire 4-week time frame.

The ring functions in a manner similar to the oral contraceptive pill: it reduces the chances of ovulation and thickens cervical mucus. Women who use the ring cannot at the same time use cervical caps or diaphragms as a backup method. The contraceptive ring does not protect against sexually transmitted diseases, including the virus that causes HIV/AIDS. The costs of the contraceptive ring are about $30–$35 per month for the device and $35–$125 for the exam.[11]

Key Terms

contraindications factors that make the use of a drug inappropriate or dangerous for a particular person

minipills low-dose progesterone oral contraceptives

ectopic pregnancy a pregnancy in which the fertilized ovum implants at a site other than the uterus, typically in the fallopian tubes

contraceptive ring thin, polymer contraceptive device containing estrogen and progestin; placed deep within the vagina for a 3-week period

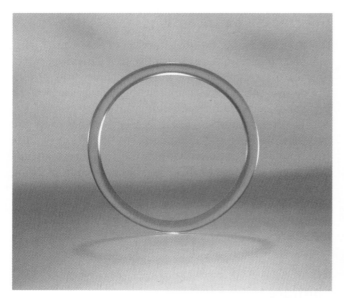
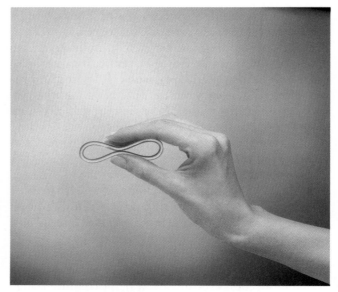

The NuvaRing contraceptive ring is a flexible ring about 2⅛ inches in diameter. When inserted into the vagina, it delivers a low dose of hormones similar to those found in oral contraceptives.

Contraceptive Patch

In 2002 the Ortho Evra **contraceptive patch** became available to women. This patch contains continuous levels of estrogen and progestin delivered from a 1¾-inch square patch that is applied weekly to one of four areas on the woman's body: the buttocks, abdomen, upper chest (front and back, excluding the breasts), or upper outer arm. The patch remains attached even while a woman bathes, swims, or exercises. After 3 weeks of patches, the woman uses no patch for the fourth week, during which time the woman has her period. The patch functions in a manner similar to the oral contraceptive pill. Like all hormonal measures of contraception, the patch does not protect against sexually transmitted diseases, including the virus that causes HIV/AIDS. The patch costs about $30–$35 per month and $35–$125 for the exam.[11]

Emergency Contraception

Emergency contraception is designed to prevent pregnancy after unprotected vaginal intercourse such as when a condom breaks, when a couple uses no method of contraception, or when someone forces another to have intercourse. This method is also called postcoital or "morning after" contraception. (Emergency contraception is not the "abortion pill" or RU-486.) Emergency contraception is available in two forms: emergency hormonal contraception and the insertion of an IUD. Both forms of contraception can be prescribed (or carried out) only by a physician.

As of May 2005, six states (Alaska, California, Hawaii, Maine, New Mexico, and Washington) had enacted laws that permit a pharmacist to provide emergency contraception to customers in the absence of a prescription by a physician. However, the pharmacist is required to act within a collaborative agreement with a physician or under state-approved protocols.[14]

Emergency hormonal contraception involves the use of one or two doses of certain oral contraceptives. Currently, only one FDA-approved oral contraceptive (Plan B) is available for emergency contraception, although physicians may prescribe other oral contraceptives for this purpose. (Previn, an FDA-approved combined estrogen-progestin pill was withdrawn from the market in 2004.) Plan B is a progestin-only pill whose first dose should be taken as soon as possible (but not later than 120 hours or 5 days) after unprotected intercourse. A second pill follows 12 hours after the first pill. This approach to emergency contraception reduces the risk of pregnancy after unprotected intercourse by 89 percent.[4]

Key Terms

contraceptive patch contraceptive skin patch containing estrogen and progestin; replaced each week for a 3-week period

emergency contraception contraceptive measures used to prevent pregnancy within 5 days of unprotected intercourse; also called *postcoital* or *"morning after"* contraception

The most commonly reported side effects of emergency hormonal contraception are nausea and vomiting. About 25 percent of users of progestin-only pills experience nausea, and 10 percent experience vomiting. Users of combined estrogen-progestin pills tend to experience more episodes of nausea and vomiting. The use of antinausea medication can help offset the nausea and vomiting. Some women also report fatigue, breast tenderness, abdominal pain, headaches, and dizziness. These side effects subside within a day or two after treatment.[4] Costs for Plan B are estimated to be $8–$35.[11]

The insertion of an IUD is a less commonly used, but highly effective, form of emergency contraception. To function as a contraceptive, however, the IUD must be inserted within 5 days after unprotected intercourse.

Sterilization

All the contraceptive mechanisms or methods already discussed have one quality in common: they are reversible. Although microsurgical techniques are providing medical breakthroughs, **sterilization** should generally be considered an irreversible procedure. When you decide to use sterilization, you are giving up control of your own fertility because you will no longer be able to produce offspring.

Therefore, couples considering sterilization procedures usually must undergo extensive discussions with a physician or family planning counselor to identify their true feelings about this finality. Sterilization does not protect one against sexually transmitted diseases, including HIV infection.

The male sterilization procedure is called a *vasectomy.* Accomplished with a local anesthetic in a physician's office, this 20- to 30-minute procedure consists of the surgical removal of a section of each vas deferens. After a small incision is made through the scrotum, the vas deferens is located and a small section is removed. The remaining ends are either tied or *cauterized* (Figure 14-5A).

Immediately after a vasectomy, sperm may still be present in the vas deferens. A backup contraceptive is recommended until a physician microscopically examines a semen specimen. This examination usually occurs about 6 weeks after the surgery. After a vasectomy, men can still produce male sex hormones, get erections, have orgasms, and ejaculate. (Recall that sperm account for only a small portion of the semen.) Some men even report increased interest in sexual activity, since their chances of impregnating a woman are virtually eliminated.

What happens to the process of spermatogenesis within each testicle? Sperm cells are still being produced, but they are destroyed by specialized white blood cells called *phagocytic leukocytes.* The cost of a vasectomy ranges from $350 to $1,000.[11]

The most common method of female sterilization is *tubal ligation.* During this procedure, the fallopian tubes

are cut and the ends are tied back. Some physicians cauterize the tube ends to ensure complete sealing (Figure 14-5B). The fallopian tubes are usually reached through the abdominal wall. In a *minilaparotomy,* a small incision is made through the abdominal wall just below the navel. The resultant scar is quite small and is the basis for the term *band-aid surgery.*

Female sterilization requires about 20 to 30 minutes, with the patient under local or general anesthesia. The use of a *laparoscope* has made female sterilization much simpler than in the past. The laparoscope is a small tube equipped with mirrors and lights. Inserted through a single incision, the laparoscope locates the fallopian tubes before they are cut, tied, or cauterized. When a laparoscope is used through an abdominal incision, the procedure is called a *laparoscopy.*

In 2002, a new method of female sterilization was approved by the FDA. This is a nonincision approach (the Essure coil), whereby a physician inserts a small, soft metallic coil into the vagina, through the cervix and directly into each fallopian tube. This procedure is done under local anesthetic and takes about a half-hour. Once inserted, the coils encourage scar tissue growth that eventually blocks the fallopian tubes. If the tubes are obstructed, sperm are blocked from meeting the ovum. After 3 months, a woman returns to her physician for an X-ray test that determines whether the tubes are fully obstructed. During these first 3 months, couples must use another form of birth control. Cramping is the most common side effect. In rare cases, Essure coils can be expelled or perforate the fallopian tube.[3] Reports indicate that Essure has a 99.8 percent effectiveness rate.[11]

Women who are sterilized still produce female hormones, ovulate, and menstruate. However, the ovum cannot move down the fallopian tube. Within a day of its release, the ovum will start to disintegrate and be absorbed by the body. Freed of the possibility of becoming pregnant, many sterilized women report an increase in sex drive and activity. Tubal ligation costs range from $1,500 to $6,000.[11]

Two other procedures produce sterilization in women. *Ovariectomy* (the surgical removal of the ovaries) and *hysterectomy* (the surgical removal of the uterus) accomplish sterilization. However, these procedures are used to remove diseased (cancerous, cystic, or hemorrhaging) organs and are not considered primary sterilization techniques.

Key Terms

sterilization generally permanent birth control techniques that surgically disrupt the normal passage of ova or sperm

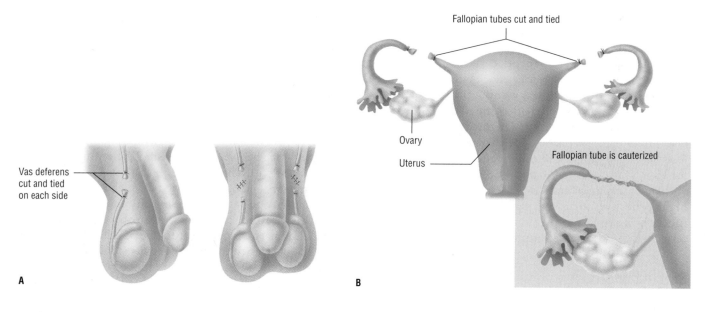

Fallopian tubes cut and tied

Ovary

Uterus

Fallopian tube is cauterized

Vas deferens cut and tied on each side

A

B

Figure 14-5 The most frequently used forms of male and female sterilization. **A:** Vasectomy. **B:** Tubal ligation.

 TALKING POINTS You and your husband have children, and you'd like to stop taking the pill for health reasons. Your husband says you're pressuring him to have a vasectomy. How can you keep the dialogue going in a cooperative way?

Abortion

Regardless of the circumstances under which pregnancy occurs, women may now choose to terminate their pregnancies. No longer must women who do not want to be pregnant seek potentially dangerous, illegal abortions. On the basis of current technology and legality, women need never experience childbirth. The decision is theirs to make.

Abortion should never be considered a first-line, preferred form of fertility control. Rather, abortion is a final, last-chance undertaking. It should be used only when responsible control of one's fertility could not be achieved. The decision to abort a fetus is a highly controversial, personal one—one that needs serious consideration by each woman.

On the basis of the landmark 1973 U.S. Supreme Court case *Roe v. Wade,* the United States joined many of the world's most populated countries in legalizing abortions.

In 2002, 1.29 million women in the United States made the decision to terminate a pregnancy.[15] Thousands of additional women probably considered abortion but elected to continue their pregnancies.

Clearly, abortion is a political issue. It will be interesting to see how future abortion-related decisions will unfold. Special interest groups on both sides of the issue, the Supreme Court, state legislatures, federal agencies (such as the FDA and the Department of Health and Human Services), the Congress, and the president all have a say in the abortion debate in this country. Regardless of the eventual outcomes of this debate, here are the present abortion procedures available in the United States.

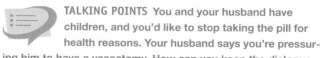 **TALKING POINTS** You're unexpectedly pregnant, but abortion doesn't seem like a good choice for you. Your boyfriend, your family, and your friends all have strong but conflicting opinions about the situation. How can you show that you value their advice but still make it clear that the final decision needs to be yours alone?

First-Trimester Abortion Procedures

The first trimester consists of the first 13 weeks (91 days) of pregnancy. During the first 49 days after a woman's last menstrual period, a woman has two options for terminating a pregnancy: *vacuum aspiration* or *medication abortion.* Once 63 days have passed, only vacuum aspiration is an abortion option.

Key Terms

abortion induced premature termination of a pregnancy

Vacuum Aspiration   There are two common methods of performing vacuum aspiration abortions. Both procedures can be performed in a physician's office or in a hospital. Both procedures require **dilation** of the cervix. The method used depends on how long the woman has been pregnant. Together, these methods represent the most widely used abortion procedures in the United States. In 1999, 96 percent of all abortions in the United States were performed through aspiration procedures.[4]

The **manual vacuum aspiration (MVA)** procedure can be performed in the earliest part of the first trimester, from the time a woman knows she is pregnant and up to 10 weeks after her last period. After a physician injects a local anesthetic into the cervix, dilators can be used to enlarge the cervical opening. The physician then inserts a small tube into the uterus and applies suction with a handheld instrument. By rotating and moving this small tube across the uterine wall, the physician can empty the uterus. A return visit to the physician is an important follow-up procedure.[4]

After the first month of pregnancy and throughout the first trimester, physicians typically select **dilation and suction curettage (D&C)** (frequently called *vacuum aspiration*) as the abortion procedure of choice. D&C is similar to the MVA, but the clinician uses a vacuum machine rather than a manually operated suction instrument. The clinician tends to use more sedation for the woman, in addition to the local cervical anesthetic. The cervix is stretched open with dilators that gradually enlarge the opening to permit the insertion of a tube into the cervix. This tube is attached to a vacuum machine that empties the uterus with gentle suction. If the physician believes that additional endometrial tissue remains in the uterus, he or she can use a **curette** to scrape the wall of the uterus. A subsequent visit to the clinician is an important follow-up procedure. Costs range from $225 to $575.[11]

Medication Abortion   Mifepristone and methotrexate are drugs that a woman can use under medical supervision to induce a **medication abortion** during the first trimester. Formerly known as RU-486, mifepristone blocks the action of progesterone and causes the uterine lining and any fertilized egg to shed.

Under FDA guidelines, women must use mifepristone within 49 days of their last menstrual period. Women take three pills at the first doctor visit and then return 48 hours later to take a second drug, misoprostol, which causes menstruation to occur, usually within about 5 hours. A third visit to a physician is necessary to ensure that the abortion was successful and the woman is recovering well from the procedure.

Methotrexate is a drug used since the 1950s for cancer treatment. However, physicians sometimes use this drug in an off-label manner to induce an abortion within the first 63 days.[3] Typically, a woman receives an injection of methotrexate and, during a second office visit 3 to 7 days later, receives misoprostol. The fetal contents are expelled, usually within a day, but some methotrexate abortions take up to a week to occur. A follow-up office visit is necessary. Medication abortions cost about the same as a first-term surgical abortion ($350–$650).[11]

Second-Trimester Abortion Procedures

When a woman's pregnancy continues beyond the 13th week of gestation, termination becomes a more difficult matter. The procedures at this stage are more complicated and take longer to complete.

Dilation and Evacuation   Between 13 and 16 weeks of pregnancy, the abortion method of choice is **dilation and evacuation (D&E).** Some physicians use this method up through 20 weeks or more of pregnancy.[4] The D&E is a more involved surgical procedure than is D&C and generally requires greater dilation of the cervix, larger medical instruments (including forceps), suction, and curettage. (See Figure 14-6.) Some women may be given a general anesthetic during D&E procedures. After D&E, a return visit to the clinician is an important follow-up procedure.

In the 1970s and the 1980s, it was not uncommon for women reaching the end of the second trimester of pregnancy to undergo an abortion using a **hypertonic saline procedure** or a *prostaglandin procedure*. In the saline procedure, a strong salt solution was injected directly into the amniotic sac. This caused the uterine contents to dehydrate

---

Key Terms

dilation   gradual expansion of an opening or passageway, such as the cervix

manual vacuum aspiration (MVA)   the abortion procedure performed in the earliest weeks after a pregnancy is established

dilation and suction curettage (D & C)   a surgical procedure in which the cervical canal is dilated to allow the uterine wall to be scraped

curette   a metal scraping instrument that resembles a spoon with a cup-shaped cutting surface on its end

medication abortion   an abortion caused by the use of prescribed drugs

dilation and evacuation (D&E)   a second-trimester abortion procedure that requires greater dilation, suction, and curettage than first-trimester vacuum aspiration procedures

hypertonic saline solution   a salt solution with a concentration higher than that found in human fluids

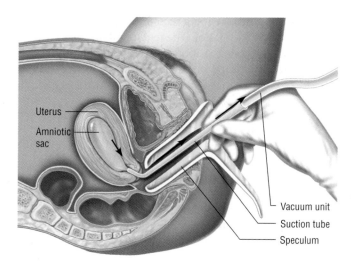

Figure 14-6 During dilation and evacuation, the cervix is dilated and the contents of the uterus are aspirated (removed by suction). This procedure is used to perform abortions up to 20 weeks' gestation.

Labels on figure: Uterus, Amniotic sac, Vacuum unit, Suction tube, Speculum

and be expelled from the uterus within 24–36 hours. In the prostaglandin procedure, an injection or a vaginal suppository of prostaglandin was administered. The prostaglandin produced strong uterine contractions that expelled the fetal contents. Both of these procedures are rarely used today.[4] The D&E remains the abortion method of choice for the second trimester.

Third-Trimester Abortion Procedures

If termination of a pregnancy is required in the latter weeks of the gestational period, a surgical procedure in which the fetus is removed (*hysterotomy*) or a procedure in which the entire uterus is removed (*hysterectomy*) can be undertaken. These procedures are more complicated and involve longer hospitalization, major abdominal surgery, and an extended period of recovery.

In the late 1990s, the U.S. House of Representatives and the U.S. Senate voted to ban a rarely used third-trimester abortion procedure referred to as dilation and extraction. Lawmakers felt that this procedure, also called *partial-birth abortion,* was too gruesome to be permitted. President Clinton vetoed this ban, and because the Senate failed to override his veto, the ban on partial birth abortion did not become law. Federal efforts to ban this procedure are continuing.

At the state level, however, many individual state governments had already passed laws banning partial-birth abortions. On June 30, 2000, the U.S. Supreme Court invalidated a Nebraska Law that prohibited this procedure. This ruling called into question the constitutionality of other existing states' laws concerning this third-trimester procedure.

Despite the tenuous nature of most state laws that banned partial-birth abortion procedures, President George W. Bush signed into law a federal ban passed in 2003 by the U.S. Congress. However, in 2004, this federal ban on partial-birth abortions was declared unconstitutional by three district courts because it shared the same constitutional flaws that the U.S. Supreme Court found in the 2000 Nebraska law that was struck down. These flaws included (a) not having an exception for the woman's health and (b) having language so broad as to potentially cover other abortion procedures.[16]

At the time of this writing (May 2005), 26 states have passed bans on partial-birth abortions that apply throughout pregnancy. Eighteen of these bans have been specifically blocked by a court, and 7 remain unchallenged but are likely to be unenforceable because they do not permit a health exception for the woman. Only Ohio's partial-birth abortion ban throughout pregnancy has been challenged and upheld by a court.[16] (For the current status of laws pertaining to partial-birth abortion, go to www.guttmacher.org.)

Post-Abortion Syndrome

Some women who have an abortion may be faced with the consequence of psychological difficulties in the years that follow the abortion. The term **post-abortion syndrome** refers to "the suggested long-term negative psychological effects of abortion."[17] These difficulties—if they occur—may arise soon after the abortion or may not surface until years later. The signs and symptoms of post-abortion syndrome are not unlike those of the more well-known post-traumatic stress disorder. (However, the American Psychiatric Association and other organizations do not recognize post-abortion syndrome as an identifiable illness.)

Women having post-abortion syndrome may experience some or all of the following effects: difficulties with personal relationships, substance abuse problems, nightmares, sexual difficulties, communication problems, damage to self-esteem, and, possibly, suicide.[17] These symptoms may range from mild to severe and may be lengthy in duration.

Fortunately, there are abortion follow-up services that can be helpful to women who believe they are suffering from the consequences of abortion. Individual and group counseling, as well as post-abortion support groups, can help women cope with difficult, complicated feelings. Look for these services through your medical care provider, or check your local phone book for helpful resources.

Key Terms

post-abortion syndrome the long-term negative psychological effects of abortion

---

A Final Word about Birth Control

In the heat of passion, people often fail to think rationally about the potential outcomes of unprotected sex. Therefore, the time to prepare for the romantic moment is *before* you are in a position where you don't want to think about the possibility of an unintended result. If you choose to be sexually active, find a form of protection that works well for you and use it consistently. If you choose not to be sexually active, realize that this is a viable choice that can be 100 percent effective.

Pregnancy

Pregnancy is a condition that requires a series of complex yet coordinated changes to occur in the female body. This discussion follows pregnancy from its beginning, at fertilization, to its conclusion, with labor and childbirth.

Physiological Obstacles and Aids to Fertilization

Many sexually active young people believe that they will become pregnant (or impregnate someone) only when they want to, despite their haphazard contraceptive practices. Because of this mistaken belief, many young people are not sold on the use of contraceptives. It is important for young adults to remember that from a species survival standpoint, our bodies were designed to promote pregnancy. It is estimated that about 85 percent of sexually active women of childbearing age will become pregnant within 1 year if they do not use some form of contraception.[4]

With regard to pregnancy, each act of intercourse can be considered a game of physiological odds. There are obstacles that may reduce a couple's chance of pregnancy, including the following:

Obstacles to Fertilization

1. *The acidic level of the vagina is destructive to sperm.* The low pH of the vagina kills sperm that fail to enter the uterus quickly.
2. *The cervical mucus is thick during most of the menstrual cycle.* Sperm movement into the uterus is more difficult, except during the few days surrounding ovulation.
3. *The sperm must locate the cervical opening.* The cervical opening is small compared with the rest of the surface area where sperm are deposited.
4. *Half of the sperm travel through the wrong fallopian tube.* Most commonly, only one ovum is released at ovulation. The two ovaries generally "take turns"

each month. The sperm have no way of "knowing" which tube they should enter. Thus it is probable that half will travel through the wrong tube.

5. *The distance sperm must travel is relatively long compared with the tiny size of the sperm cells.* Microscopic sperm must travel about 7 or 8 inches once they are inside the female.
6. *The sperm's travel is relatively "upstream."* The anatomical positioning of the female reproductive structures necessitates an "uphill" movement by the sperm.
7. *The contoured folds of the tubal walls trap many sperm.* These folds make it difficult for sperm to locate the egg. Many sperm are trapped in this maze.

There are also a variety of aids that tend to help sperm and egg cells join. Some of these are listed below.

Aids to Fertilization

1. *An astounding number of sperm are deposited during ejaculation.* Each ejaculation contains about a teaspoon of semen.[18] Within this quantity are between 200 and 500 million sperm cells. Even with large numbers of sperm killed in the vagina, millions are able to move to the deeper structures.
2. *Sperm are deposited near the cervical opening.* Penetration into the vagina by the penis allows for the sperm to be placed near the cervical opening.
3. *The male accessory glands help make the semen nonacidic.* The seminal vesicles, prostate gland, and Cowper's glands secrete fluids that provide an alkaline environment for the sperm. This environment helps sperm be better protected in the vagina until they can move into the deeper, more alkaline uterus and fallopian tubes.
4. *Uterine contractions aid sperm movement.* The rhythmic muscular contractions of the uterus tend to cause the sperm to move in the direction of the fallopian tubes.
5. *Sperm cells move rather quickly.* Despite their tiny size, sperm cells can move relatively quickly—just about 1 inch per hour. Powered by sugar solutions from the male accessory glands and the whiplike movements of their tails, sperm can reach the distant third of the fallopian tubes in less than 8 hours as they swim in the direction of the descending ovum.
6. *Once inside the fallopian tubes, sperm can live for days.* Some sperm may be viable for up to a week after reaching the comfortable, nonacidic environment of the fallopian tubes. Most sperm, however, will survive an average of 48 to 72 hours. Thus they

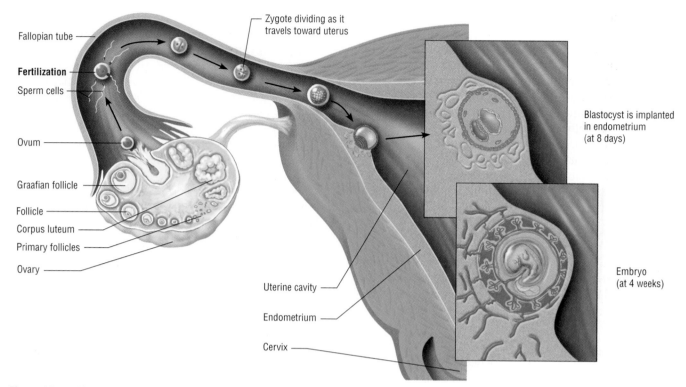

Figure 14-7 After its release from the follicle, the ovum begins its week-long journey down the fallopian tube. Fertilization generally occurs in the outermost third of the tube. Now fertilized, the ovum progresses toward the uterus, where it embeds itself in the endometrium. A pregnancy is established.

can "wait in the wings" for the moment an ovum is released from the ovary (Figure 14-7).

7. *The cervical mucus is thin and watery at the time of ovulation.* This mucus allows for better passage of sperm through the cervical opening when the ovum is most capable of being fertilized.

Human Cloning: An Ethical Dilemma?

Today's most controversial issue related to parenting is reproduction through **human cloning.** With the 1997 breakthrough cloning of the Scottish sheep Dolly, the possibility of human cloning emerged within the scientific community. To clone a human, the procedure would involve the following steps:[19]

- Doctors would surgically retrieve an egg from the female donor.
- The nucleus of this egg would be removed.
- A cell is taken from a cloning subject (a male or female).
- Through an electrical jolt, the cloning subject's cell is fused with the **enucleated egg.** This creates a clonal zygote. Shortly after, this clonal zygote divides over and over and develops into a clonal embryo.

- The clonal embryo is implanted in the womb of a surrogate mother.
- After 9 months, a genetically matched reproduction of the cloning subject is born.

Although this step-by-step process may seem simple, this has never been accomplished with human subjects.[19] In fact, to produce Dolly, the cloned sheep, it took scientists 277 attempts. The technical expertise to clone humans has not been fully developed, although some scientists believe it could be on the near horizon, if public policy would fully support this area of research.

However, public policy currently does not support human cloning. A few states have passed laws banning human cloning. The U.S. Food and Drug Administration (FDA) has warned researchers that any attempts at human cloning must first get FDA approval, which the FDA

Key Terms
human cloning the replication of a human being
enucleated egg an ovum with the nucleus removed

claims will not be forthcoming. Both the American Society for Reproductive Medicine and the National Academy of Sciences have voiced their opposition to human cloning.[20] Many public opinion polls have indicated that Americans are overwhelmingly against the use of cloning to produce babies.[21]

However, the potential use of a particular type of cloning has received much more popular public support in America. This is the use of cloning to reproduce body parts, tissues, and specific organs for use in medical transplant procedures. A baby is never reproduced in this cloning procedure.[20] In organ and tissue cloning, sometimes called **therapeutic cloning,** the clonal embryo is not implanted into a surrogate mother, but allowed to grow (divide) into a number of premature cells called **stem cells.** These stem cells have the potential to grow into any kind of body cell.

Theoretically, scientists could develop techniques that would cause these stem cells to grow into tissues or organs that would match the tissues or organs in the person who donated the genetic material. Because of this genetic match, these cloned organs would not be rejected after the transplant surgery. In essence, this technology permits a person's own body to be a human repair kit. Some predict that, in the not too distant future, scientists will be able to grow replacement organs like hearts, livers, and skin and replacement neurons for persons who suffer from diabetes, Parkinson's, or Alzheimer's disease.

And the future may be here sooner than we might think. In May 2005, South Korean scientists from Seoul National University reported that they had successfully taken the DNA from a sick patient's skin cells and injected this DNA into the stem cells taken from donated human embryos that had been cloned. These stem cells then evolved into new skin cells that were a genetic match with the original patient's skin cells. Dr. Hwang Woo-suk is the only scientist in the world acknowledged to have done this procedure. Not surprisingly, South Korea provides generous financial support for research into therapeutic cloning.[22]

On the other side of the fence are those who wonder if cloning represents "science gone mad." Some believe that any kind of cloning is unethical because it interferes with nature. Altering a woman's eggs, reprogramming cells, and tampering with embryos is something that is *simply wrong.* Regardless of the position you take on this issue, you can expect to see more scientific advances regarding cloning, especially therapeutic cloning.

Signs of Pregnancy

Aside from pregnancy tests done in a professional laboratory, a woman can sometimes recognize early signs and symptoms. The signs of pregnancy have been divided into three categories:

Presumptive Signs of Pregnancy

Missed period after unprotected intercourse the previous month

Nausea on awakening (morning sickness)

Increase in size and tenderness of breasts

Darkening of the areolar tissue surrounding the nipples

Probable Signs of Pregnancy

Increase in the frequency of urination (the growing uterus presses against the bladder)

Increase in the size of the abdomen

Cervix becomes softer by the sixth week (detected by a pelvic examination by clinician)

Positive pregnancy test

Positive Signs of Pregnancy

Determination of a fetal heartbeat

Feeling of the fetus moving (*quickening*)

Observation of fetus by ultrasound or optical viewers

Agents That Can Damage a Fetus

A large number of agents that come into contact with a pregnant woman can affect fetal development. Many of these (rubella and herpes viruses, tobacco smoke, alcohol, and virtually all other drugs) are discussed in other chapters of this text. The best advice for a pregnant woman is to maintain close contact with her obstetrician during pregnancy and to consider carefully the ingestion of any OTC drug (including aspirin, caffeine, and antacids) that could harm the fetus.

All pregnant women should also avoid exposure to radiation during pregnancy. Such exposure, most commonly through excessive X rays or radiation fallout from nuclear testing, can irreversibly damage fetal genetic structures. In addition, pregnant women should avoid taking Accutane, a drug prescribed for the treatment of cystic acne that can severely damage a fetus.

Key Terms

therapeutic cloning the use of certain human replication techniques to reproduce body tissues and organs

stem cells premature cells that have the potential to turn into any kind of body cell

Childbirth: The Labor of Delivery

Childbirth, or *parturition,* is one of the true peak experiences for both men and women. Most of the time, childbirth is a wonderfully exciting venture into the unknown. For the parents, this intriguing experience can provide a stage for personal growth, maturity, and insight into a dynamic, complex world.

During the last few weeks of the third **trimester,** most fetuses move deeper into the pelvic cavity in a process called *lightening.* During this movement, the fetus's body rotates and the head begins to engage more deeply into the mother's pelvic girdle. Many women will report that the baby has "dropped."

Another indication that parturition may be relatively near is the increased reporting of *Braxton Hicks contractions.*[3] These uterine contractions, which are of mild intensity and often occur at irregular intervals, may be felt throughout a pregnancy. During the last few weeks of pregnancy (*gestation*), these mild contractions can occur more frequently and may cause a woman to feel as if she is going into labor **(false labor).**

Labor begins when uterine contractions become more intense and occur at regular intervals. The birth of a child can be divided into three stages: (1) *effacement* and dilation of the cervix, (2) delivery of the fetus, and (3) delivery of the placenta (Figure 14-8). For a woman having her first child, the birth process lasts an average of 12 to 16 hours. The average length of labor for subsequent births is much shorter—from 4 to 10 hours on the average. Labor is very unpredictable: labors that last between 1 and 24 hours occur daily at most hospitals.

Stage One: Effacement and Dilation of the Cervix

In the first stage of labor the uterine contractions attempt to thin (efface) the normally thick cervical walls and to enlarge (dilate) the cervical opening. These contractions are directed by the release of prostaglandins and the hormone oxytocin into the circulating bloodstream.

The first stage of labor is often the longest. The cervical opening must thin and dilate to a diameter of 10 cm before the first stage of labor is considered complete.[23] Often this stage begins with the dislodging of the cervical mucous plug. The subsequent *bloody show* (mucous plug and a small amount of blood) at the vaginal opening may indicate that effacement and dilation have begun. Another indication of labor's onset may be the bursting or tearing of the fetal amniotic sac. "Breaking the bag of waters" refers to this phenomenon, which happens in various measures in expectant women.

The pain of the uterine contractions becomes more intense as the woman moves through this first stage of labor. As the cervical opening effaces and dilates 0–3 cm, many women report feeling happy, exhilarated, and confident. In the *early phase of the first stage* of labor, the contractions are relatively short (lasting 15–60 seconds), and the intervals between contractions range from 20 minutes to 5 minutes as labor progresses. However, these rest intervals will become shorter and the contractions more forceful when the woman's uterus contracts to dilate 4–7 cm.

In this *second phase of the first stage* of labor, the contractions usually last about 1 minute each, and the rest intervals drop from about 5 minutes to 1 minute over a period of 5–9 hours.

The *third phase of the first stage* of labor is called *transition.* During transition, the uterus contracts to dilate the cervical opening to the full 10 cm required for safe passage of the fetus out of the uterus and into the birth canal (vagina).[24] This period of labor is often the most painful part of the entire birth process. Fortunately, it is also the shortest phase of most labors. Lasting 15–30 minutes, transition contractions often last 60–90 seconds each. The rest intervals between contractions are short and vary from 30 to 60 seconds.

An examination of the cervix by a nurse or physician will reveal whether full dilation of 10 cm has occurred. Until the full 10-cm dilation, women are cautioned not to "push" the fetus during the contractions. Special breathing and concentration techniques help many women cope with the first stage of labor.

Stage Two: Delivery of the Fetus

Once the mother's cervix is fully dilated, she enters the second stage of labor, the delivery of the fetus through the birth canal. Now the mother is encouraged to help push the fetus out (with her abdominal muscles) during each contraction. In this second stage the uterine contractions are less forceful than during the transition phase of the first stage and may last 60 seconds each, with a 1- to 3-minute rest interval.

This second stage may last up to 2 hours in first births.[18] For subsequent births, this stage will usually be much shorter. When the baby's head is first seen at the vaginal opening, *crowning* is said to have taken place.

Key Terms

trimester a 3-month period; human pregnancies encompass three trimesters

false labor conditions that resemble the start of true labor; may include irregular uterine contractions, pressure, and discomfort in the lower abdomen

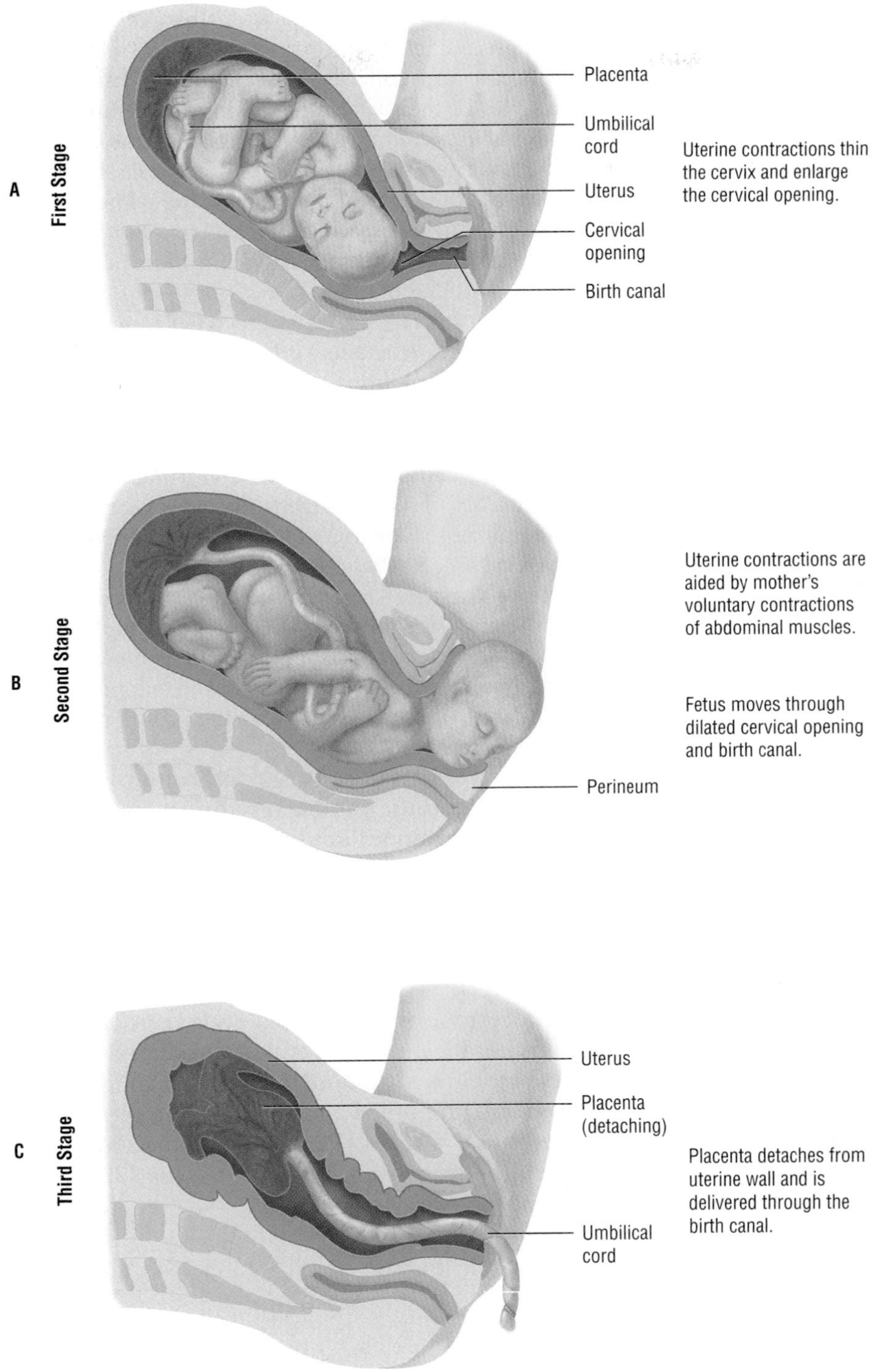

A First Stage

- Placenta
- Umbilical cord
- Uterus
- Cervical opening
- Birth canal

Uterine contractions thin the cervix and enlarge the cervical opening.

B Second Stage

Uterine contractions are aided by mother's voluntary contractions of abdominal muscles.

Fetus moves through dilated cervical opening and birth canal.

- Perineum

C Third Stage

- Uterus
- Placenta (detaching)
- Umbilical cord

Placenta detaches from uterine wall and is delivered through the birth canal.

Figure 14-8 Labor, or childbirth, is a three-stage process. During effacement and dilation, the first stage **A**: the cervical canal is gradually opened by contractions of the uterine wall. The second stage **B**: delivery of the fetus, encompasses the actual delivery of the fetus from the uterus and through the birth canal. The delivery of the placenta, the third stage **C**: empties the uterus, thus completing the process of childbirth.

Generally the back of the baby's head appears first. (Infants whose feet or buttocks are presented first are said to be delivered in a *breech position.*) Once the head is delivered, the baby's body rotates upward to let the shoulders come through. The rest of the body follows quite quickly. The second stage of labor ends when the fetus is fully expelled from the birth canal.

Stage Three: Delivery of the Placenta

Usually within 30 minutes after the fetus is delivered, the uterus again initiates a series of contractions to expel the placenta (or *afterbirth*). The placenta is examined by the attending physician to ensure that it was completely expelled. Torn remnants of the placenta could lead to dangerous *hemorrhaging* by the mother. Often the physician will perform a manual examination of the uterus after the placenta has been delivered.

Once the placenta has been delivered, the uterus will continue with mild contractions to help control bleeding and start the gradual reduction of the uterus to its normal, nonpregnant size. This final aspect of the birth process is called **postpartum.** External abdominal massage of the lower abdomen seems to help the uterus contract, as does an infant's nursing at the mother's breast.

Cesarean Deliveries

A **cesarean delivery** (cesarean birth, C-section) is a procedure in which the fetus is surgically removed from the mother's uterus through the abdominal wall. This type of delivery, which is completed in up to an hour, can be performed with the mother having a regional or a general anesthetic. A cesarean delivery is necessary when either the health of the baby or the mother is at risk.

Although a cesarean delivery is considered major surgery, most mothers cope well with the delivery and postsurgical and postpartum discomfort. The hospital stay is usually a few days longer than for a vaginal delivery. In 2003, the percentage of cesarean deliveries reached an all-time high of 27.1 percent of all births in the U.S.[25]

 TALKING POINTS Are there people in your life that you can comfortably ask, "What was it like to go through labor and delivery?" Will you feel open enough to express any personal concerns you might have about your own fears of this process?

Infertility

Most traditional-age college students are interested in preventing pregnancy. However, increasing numbers of other people are trying to do just the opposite: they are trying to become pregnant. It is estimated that about one in six couples has a problem with *infertility*. These couples wish to become pregnant but are unable to do so.

Why do couples experience infertility? The reasons are about evenly balanced between men and women. About 10 percent of infertility has no detectable cause.[2] The most common male complication is insufficient sperm production and delivery. A number of approaches can be used to increase sperm counts. Among the simple approaches are the application of periodic cold packs on the scrotum and the replacement of tight underwear with boxer shorts. When a structural problem reduces sperm production, surgery can be helpful. Frequent intercourse (more than once every 36 hours) tends to lower sperm counts.[26] Most experts (fertility endocrinologists) suggest

that couples have intercourse at least a couple of times in the week preceding ovulation.

Men can also collect (through masturbation) and save samples of their sperm to use in a procedure called *artificial insemination by partner.* Near the time of ovulation, the collected samples of sperm are then deposited near the woman's cervical opening. In the related procedure called *artificial insemination by donor,* the sperm of a donor are used. Donor semen is screened for the presence of pathogens, including the AIDS virus.

Causes of infertility in women center mostly on obstructions in the reproductive tract and the inability to ovulate. The obstructions sometimes result from tissue damage (scarring) caused by infections. Chlamydial and gonorrheal infections often produce fertility problems. Other possible causes of structural abnormalities include scar tissue from previous surgery, fibroid tumors, polyps, and endometriosis. A variety of microsurgical techniques may correct some of these complications.

One of the most recent innovative procedures involves the use of **transcervical balloon tuboplasty.** In this procedure, a series of balloon-tipped catheters are inserted through the uterus into the blocked fallopian tubes. Once inflated, these balloon catheters help open the scarred passageways.

When a woman has ovulation difficulties, pinpointing the specific cause can be very difficult. Increasing age produces hormone fluctuations associated with lack of ovulation. Being significantly overweight or underweight also has a serious effect on fertility. However, in women of normal weight who are not approaching menopause, it appears that ovulation difficulties are caused by lack of synchronization between the hormones governing the menstrual cycle. Fertility drugs can help alter the menstrual cycle to produce ovulation. Clomiphene citrate (Clomid), in oral pill form, or injections of a mixture of LH and FSH taken from the urine of menopausal women (Pergonal) are the most common fertility drugs available. Both are capable of producing multiple ova at ovulation.

Key Terms

postpartum the period after the birth of a baby, during which the uterus returns to its prepregnancy size

cesarean delivery surgical removal of a fetus through the abdominal wall

transcervical balloon tuboplasty the use of inflatable balloon catheters to open blocked fallopian tubes; a procedure used for some women with fertility problems

Assisted Reproductive Technologies (ART)

For couples who are unable to conceive after drug therapy, surgery, and artificial insemination, the use of one of four assisted reproductive technologies (ART) can be helpful. One option is *in vitro fertilization and embryo transfer (IVF-ET)*. This method is sometimes referred to as the "test tube" procedure. Costing around $10,000 per attempt, IVF-ET consists of surgically retrieving fertilizable ova from the woman and combining them in a glass dish with sperm. After several days, the fertilized ova are transferred into the uterus. IVF-ET accounts for 98 percent of all ART procedures.[27]

A second test tube procedure is called *gamete intrafallopian transfer (GIFT)*. Similar to IVF-ET, this procedure involves depositing a mixture of retrieved eggs and sperm directly into the fallopian tubes.

Fertilized ova (zygotes) can also be transferred from a laboratory dish into the fallopian tubes in a third procedure called *zygote intrafallopian transfer (ZIFT)*. One advantage of this procedure is that the clinicians are certain that ova have been fertilized before the transfer to the fallopian tubes. GIFT and ZIFT combined account for fewer than 2 percent of ART procedures.[27]

The fourth (and newest) procedure is *intracytoplasmic sperm injection* (ICSI). This is a laboratory procedure in which a single sperm cell is injected into a woman's retrieved egg. The fertilized egg is then transplanted into the woman's uterus. The cost and technical expertise involved in ICSI make it a seldom-used procedure for infertile couples.

Surrogate Parenting

Surrogate parenting is another option that has been explored, although the legal and ethical issues surrounding this method of conception have not been fully resolved. Surrogate parenting exists in a number of forms. Typically, an infertile couple will make a contract with a woman (the surrogate parent), who will then be artificially inseminated with semen from the expectant father. In some instances the surrogate will receive an embryo from the donor parents. In some cases, women have served as surrogates for their close relatives. The surrogate will carry the fetus to term and return the newborn to the parents. Because of the concerns about true "ownership" of the baby, surrogate parenting may not be a particularly viable or legal option for many couples.

TALKING POINTS You have tried for a couple of years to get pregnant, and now you are ready to consider some of the newest options to increase the chances of conception. Your partner seems unwilling to spend much money for these high-tech procedures. You are ready to spend some of your retirement savings in this effort. How can you and your partner best come to an agreement on this issue?

A Final Word about Infertility

The process of coping with infertility problems can be an emotionally stressful experience for a couple. Hours of waiting in physicians' offices, having numerous examinations, scheduling intercourse, producing sperm samples, and undergoing surgical or drug treatments place multiple burdens on a couple. Knowing that other couples are able to conceive so effortlessly adds to the mental strain. Fortunately, support groups exist to assist couples with infertility problems. Some of these groups are listed in the Star box above.

What can you do to reduce the chances of developing infertility problems? Certainly avoiding infections of the reproductive organs is one crucial factor. Barrier methods of contraception (condoms, diaphragm) with a spermicide reportedly cut the risk of developing infertility in half. The risk from multiple partners should encourage responsible sexual activity. Men and women should be aware of the dangers from working around hazardous chemicals or consuming psychoactive drugs. Maintaining overall good health and having regular medical (and, for women, gynecological) checkups are also good ideas. Finally, since infertility is linked with advancing age, couples may not want to indefinitely delay having children.

Taking Charge of Your Health

- Use the Personal Assessment on page 395 to help you determine which birth control method is best for you.
- Talk to your doctor about the health aspects of different types of birth control before making your decision.
- If the method of birth control you are currently using is unsatisfactory to you or your partner, explore other options.
- Reduce your risk of infertility by choosing a birth control method carefully, protecting yourself from infections of the reproductive organs, and maintaining good overall health.
- If you plan to have children, set a time frame that takes into account decreased fertility with advancing age.

SUMMARY

- *Birth control* refers to all the procedures that can prevent the birth of a child.
- *Contraception* refers to any procedure that prevents fertilization.
- Each birth control method has both a theoretical-effectiveness rate and a use-effectiveness rate. For some contraceptive approaches, these rates are similar (such as hormonal methods), and for others the rates are very different (such as condoms, diaphragms, and periodic abstinence).
- Many factors should be considered when deciding which contraceptive is best for you.
- Sterilization (vasectomy and tubal ligation) is generally considered an irreversible procedure.

- Currently, abortion remains a woman's choice under the guidelines of the 1973 *Roe v. Wade* decision.
- Abortion procedures vary according to the stage of the pregnancy.
- Several physiological factors can be either aids or obstacles to fertilization.
- Human cloning raises many ethical issues.
- Pregnant women should avoid agents that can harm the fetus.
- Childbirth takes place in three distinct stages.
- For couples with fertility problems, numerous strategies can be used to help conception take place.

REVIEW QUESTIONS

1. Explain the difference between the terms *birth control* and *contraception*. Give examples of each.
2. Explain the difference between theoretical and use-effectiveness rates. Which one is always higher?
3. Identify some of the factors that should be given careful consideration when selecting a contraceptive method. Explain each factor.
4. For each of the methods of birth control, explain how it works and its advantages and disadvantages.
5. How do minipills differ from the combined oral contraceptive?
6. How does the contraceptive patch differ from the contraceptive ring?

7. What is emergency contraception?
8. How are tubal ligation and vasectomy accomplished?
9. Identify and describe the different abortion procedures that are used during each trimester of pregnancy. What is a medication abortion?
10. What are some obstacles and aids to fertilization presented in this chapter? Can you think of others?
11. Identify and describe the events that occur during each of the three stages of childbirth. Approximately how long is each stage?
12. What can be done to reduce chances of infertility? Explain IVF-ET, GIFT, ZIFT, and ICSI procedures.

ENDNOTES

1. Bruckner H, Bearman P. After the promise: The STD consequences of adolescent virginity pledges. *Journal of Adolescent Health* (36) 271–278, 2005.

2. McAnulty RD, Burnette MM. *Exploring Human Sexuality: Making Healthy Decisions* (2nd ed.). Boston: Allyn and Bacon, 2004.

3. Crooks RL, Baur K. *Our Sexuality* (9th ed.). Belmont, CA: Wadsworth, 2005.

4. Hatcher RA, et al. *Contraceptive Technology* (18th ed.). New York: Ardent Media, Inc., 2004.

5. WebMD Medical News. *Warning for Spermicide Nonoxynol-9* (January 17, 2003), www.my.webmd.com, September 15, 2003.

6. Davis JL. WebMD Medical News. *Spermicide Promotes HIV* (September 26, 2002), www.webmd.com, September 15, 2003.

7. Allgeier ER, Allgeier AR. *Sexual Interactions* (5th ed.). New York: Houghton Mifflin, 2000.

8. DeNoon D. WebMD Health. *Best Condoms Still Latex,* (March 21, 2003), www.my.webmd.com, September 11, 2003.

9. Planned Parenthood Federation of America. *Your Contraceptive Choices,* www.plannedparenthood.org, September 10, 2003.

10. Steiner MJ, et al. Contraceptive effectiveness of a polyurethane condom and a latex condom: A randomized controlled trial. *Obstetrics and Gynecology* 101(3): 539–547, 2003.

11. Planned Parenthood Federation of America. *Health Info: Birth Control,* www.plannedparenthood.org, May 10, 2005.

12. Weise E. Contraceptive sponge is back, but why did it leave? *USA Today,* p. 7D, April 25, 2005.

13. Berlex Laboratories Web Site. *What Is Mirena?,* www.mirena-us.com, May 10, 2005.

14. The Alan Guttmacher Institute. *State Policies in Brief: Access to Emergency Contraception* (May 1, 2005), www.agi-usa.org, May 15, 2005.

15. The Alan Guttmacher Institute. *Facts in Brief: Induced Abortion in the United States* (May 2005), www.agi-usa.org, May 16, 2005.

16. The Alan Guttmacher Institute. *Facts in Brief: Bans on "Partial-Birth" Abortion* (May 1, 2005), www.agi.usa.org, May 17, 2005.

17. Blonna R, Levitan J. *Healthy Sexuality.* Belmont, CA: Wadsworth, 2005.

18. Hyde JS, DeLameter JD. *Understanding Human Sexuality* (9th ed.). New York: McGraw-Hill, 2006.

19. Bonsor K. *How Human Cloning Will Work,* www.science.howstuffworks.com/human-cloning.htm, September 24, 2003.

20. DeNoon D. *Cloning FAQs and Fiction,* www.my.webmd.com/content/article/57/66221.htm (January 6, 2003), September 24, 2003.

21. Warner J. *Most Americans against Human Cloning,* www.my.webmd.com/content/article/59/66746.htm (January 16, 2003), September 24, 2003.

22. Associated Press. Mandate lack, legal hurdles inhibit U.S. research on cloning, *The Muncie (IN) Star Press* (May 21, 2005), p. 8B.

23. Kelly GF. *Sexuality Today: The Human Perspective* (8th ed.). New York: McGraw-Hill, 2006.

24. Strong B, DeVault C, Sayad BW, Yarber WL. *Human Sexuality: Diversity in a Contemporary America* (5th ed.). New York: McGraw-Hill, 2005.

25. Hamilton BE, Martin JA, Sutton PD. Births: Preliminary data for 2003. (CDC: National Center for Health Statistics). *National Vital Statistics Reports* 53(9), November 23, 2004, p. 6.

26. WebMD. *Health Guide A–Z: Infertility—Home Treatment,* www.my.webmd.com/content/healthwise/130/32439, October 2, 2003.

27. WebMD. *A Couple's Guide: Trying to Conceive,* www.my.webmd.com/content/article/73/87996, October 3, 2003.

personal assessment

Which birth control method is best for you?

To assess which birth control method would be best for you, answer the following questions, and check the interpretation below.

Do I:	Yes	No
1. Need a contraceptive right away?		✓
2. Want a contraceptive that can be used completely independent of sexual relations?	✓	
3. Need a contraceptive only once in a great while?		✓
4. Want something with no harmful side effects?	✓	
5. Want to avoid going to the doctor?		✓
6. Want something that will help protect against sexually transmitted diseases?	✓	
7. Have to be concerned about affordability?		✓
8. Need to be virtually certain that pregnancy will not result?	✓	
9. Want to avoid pregnancy now but want to have a child sometime in the future?		✓
10. Have any medical condition or lifestyle that may rule out some form of contraception?		✓

Interpretation

If you have checked *Yes* to number:

1. Condoms and spermicides may be easily purchased without prescription in any pharmacy.
2. Sterilization, oral contraceptives, hormone injections, rings, or patches, cervical caps, and periodic abstinence techniques do not require that anything be done just before sexual relations.
3. Diaphragms, condoms, or spermicides can be used by people who have coitus only once in a while. Periodic abstinence techniques may also be appropriate but require a high degree of skill and motivation.

4. IUD use should be carefully discussed with your physician, although IUDs are quite safe for most users. Sometimes the use of oral contraceptives or hormone products results in some minor discomfort and, on rare occasions, may have harmful side effects.
5. Condoms and spermicides do not require a prescription from a physician.
6. Condoms help protect against some sexually transmitted diseases. Nonoxynol-9 may increase STD transmission in some users. No method (except abstinence) can guarantee complete protection.
7. Be a wise consumer: check prices, ask pharmacists and physicians. The cost of sterilization is high, but there is no additional expense for a lifetime.
8. Sterilization provides near certainty. Oral contraceptives, IUDs, hormone injections, rings or patches or a diaphragm-condom-spermicide combination also give a high measure of reliable protection. Periodic abstinence, withdrawal, and douche methods should be avoided. Outercourse may be a good alternative.
9. Although it is sometimes possible to reverse sterilization, it requires surgery and is more complex than simply stopping use of any of the other methods.
10. Smokers and people with a history of blood clots should probably not use oral contraceptives or other hormone approaches. Some people have allergic reactions to a specific spermicide or latex material. Some women cannot be fitted well with a diaphragm or cervical cap. The woman and her health care provider will then need to select another suitable means of contraception.

To Carry This Further . . .

There may be more than one method of birth control suitable for you. Always consider whether a method you select can also help you avoid an STD. Study the methods suggested above, and consult Table 14.1 to determine what techniques may be most appropriate.

chapter fifteen

Becoming an Informed Health Care Consumer

Chapter Objectives

On completing this chapter, you will be able to:

▮ identify several sources of reliable health information available to American consumers, and be able to discuss the health information you find through them with your health care provider.

▮ explain the role of the primary care physician as it relates to diagnosis, treatment, screening, consultation, and prevention.

▮ compare and contrast the medical training received by doctors of medicine with that received by doctors of osteopathy.

▮ explain the subtle but important differences between alternative medicine, integrative medicine, and complementary medicine.

▮ identify hospitals in your community and categorize them as public, voluntary, or private.

▮ describe the various health insurance plans available, and understand what deductibles, copayments, fixed indemnity, and exclusions are.

▮ talk to friends and family about their level of satisfaction with their own health care coverage.

▮ evaluate the health claims of various dietary supplements.

Eye on the Media

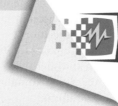

The Internet—Your Health Superstore

According to data collected by the Pew Internet & American Life Project (July 16, 2003), approximately 93 million Americans use the Internet as a source of health-related information. Most frequently, online users seek information regarding specific medical problems, followed by information regarding aspects of treatment and longer term management of these problems. The use of the Internet for health-related purposes is, however, not a daily occurrence for most Americans with Internet access. When the Internet is used for this purpose, women are more likely to be seeking information than are men, and they most often do so for other persons (spouses, children, and friends). If you are not already, it is highly probable that you too will be an online consumer of health-related information, products, or services.

The biggest challenge for you as a health consumer is determining the credibility of the information you find on the Internet. How can you know that this information (and accompanying products or services) is trustworthy and that the persons responsible for the information, products, or services are motivated by concern for your health and well-being rather than just by profit? Recognized authorities offer these guidelines to help you:

• Who does the Web site belong to? Is it sponsored by an institution of higher education, a professional society, a government or not-for-profit agency, or a recognized pharmaceutical company? If not, who is responsible for the information? Remember, virtually anyone can develop a web page and begin disseminating information.

• Is the information carefully referenced, showing sources such as government reports, professional journal articles, or respected reference publications? Are the references clearly documented and current? Is the Web page updated regularly? Does the information appear to agree with the titles of its own references?

• Does the content of the information seem to have a critical or negative bias toward a particular profession, institution, or treatment method? Does the information discredit others more than it supports its own position?

• Are "significant breakthroughs" promised in a way that suggests that only this source has the "ultimate answer" to certain problems? Does this answer involve throwing out your prescriptions, going against your physician's orders, or considering suicide as a way of escaping the pain and difficulties associated with your illness?

If you are skeptical about the credibility of any health care information you find online, submit the information to a respected health care professional or organization for assessment. If you and your physician find suspicious information or fraudulent health claims, report this to the Federal Trade Commission. Today, most health care practitioners feel comfortable with well-informed patients. Many will welcome the

Eye on the Media *continued*
chance to learn about your sources of information and share with you any concerns they
might have about them.

Once you feel secure about distinguishing
reliable and valid information from questionable or fraudulent information, you will be
able to make better judgments and choices.

Together, you and your health care provider
can use that information in the management
of your health care and in planning your
approach to a healthier lifestyle.

Health care providers often evaluate you by criteria from their areas of expertise. The nutritionist knows you by the food you eat. The physical fitness professional knows you by your body type and activity level. In the eyes of the expert in health consumerism, you are the product of the health information you believe, the health-influencing services you use, and the products you consume. When you make your decisions about health information, services, and products after careful study and consideration, your health will probably be improved. However, when your decisions lack insight, your health, as well as your pocketbook, may suffer.

Health Information

The Informed Consumer

As mentioned in *Eye on the Media* on page 396, the Pew Charitable Trust's on-going study of Internet use (Internet & American Life Project)[1] provides current information on health-related Internet use. The breadth of this interest is informative. Of the 93 million Americans who conducted health-related searches, 63 percent of the searchers sought information pertaining to specific conditions and problems, 47 percent to treatment and management of conditions, 44 percent to nutrition and diet, 36 percent to exercise and fitness, 34 percent to prescription medications and over-the-counter (OTC) products, and 28 percent to alternative treatments. Further, 25 percent sought information regarding health insurance, 17 percent investigated environmental health issues, and 10 percent pursued sexual health information. Among the 16 areas searched, only 8 percent sought information pertaining to drug and alcohol use, whereas 6 percent investigated information pertaining to smoking cessation, the area least visited.

In light of the breadth of these interest areas and the complexity associated with each, it is very likely that most people turn to a variety of sources for the information and access that they seek. In the section that follows you will be introduced to several sources of health-related information. (Complete the Personal Assessment on page 421 to rate your own skills as a consumer of health-related information, products, and services.)

Sources of Information

Your sources of information on health topics are as diverse as the number of people you know, the number of publications you read, and the number of experts you see or hear. No single agency or profession regulates the quantity or quality of the health-related information you receive. Readers will quickly recognize that all are familiar sources and that some provide more accurate and honest information than others.

Family and Friends

The accuracy of information you get from a friend or family member may be questionable. Too often the information your family and friends offer is based on "common knowledge" that is wrong. In addition, family members or friends may provide information they believe is in your best interest rather than facts that may have a more negative effect on you.

Advertisements and Commercials

Many people spend much of every day watching television, listening to the radio, and reading newspapers or magazines. Because many advertisements are health oriented, these are significant sources of information. The primary purpose of advertising, however, is to sell products or services. One newer example of this intertwining of health information with marketing is the "infomercial," in which a compensated studio audience watches a skillfully produced program that trumpets the benefits of a particular product or service. In spite of the convincing nature of these infomercials, however, the validity of their information is often questionable.

In contrast to advertisements and commercials, the mass media routinely offer public service messages, as mandated by the FCC, that give valuable health-related information. For example, the FCC ordered antismoking public-service announcements on television following the release of the first Surgeon General's Report on Smoking and Health (1964). These ads were powerful players in fostering a significant drop in smoking during the late 1960s and the 1970s.

Labels and Directions

Federal law requires that many consumer product labels, including all medications and many kinds of food (see Chapter 5), contain specific information. For example, when a pharmacist dispenses a prescription medication, he or she must give a detailed information sheet describing the medication.

Many health care providers and agencies give consumers informative information about their health problems or printed directions for preparing for screening procedures. Generally, information from these sources is accurate and current and is given with the health of the consumer foremost in mind.

Folklore

Because it is passed down from generation to generation, folklore about health is the primary source of health-related information for some people.

The accuracy of health-related information obtained from family members, neighbors, and coworkers is difficult to evaluate. As a general rule, however, one should exercise caution relying on its scientific soundness. A blanket dismissal is not warranted, however, because folk wisdom is occasionally supported by scientific evidence. In addition, the emotional support provided by the suppliers of this information could be the best medicine some people could receive. In fact, for some ethnic groups, indigenous health care is central to overall health care. Even though many Americans would consider this form of care "folk medicine," it is highly valued and trusted by those who find it familiar.

Testimonials

People eagerly want to share information that has benefited them. Others may base their decisions on such testimonials. However, the exaggerated testimonials that accompany the sales pitches of the medical quack or the "satisfied" customers appearing in advertisements and on commercials and infomercials should never be interpreted as valid endorsements.

Mass Media

Health programming on cable television stations, stories in lifestyle sections of newspapers, health care correspondents appearing on national network news shows, and the growing number of health-oriented magazines are sources of health information in the mass media.

In terms of the public's priority for specific media sources of health information, a gradual evolution is occurring. As recently as 1999, television, followed by magazines and newspapers, were the three principal sources of health-related news for American adults.[3] Now, with more than 110 million Americans having cable or phone access, these traditional sources of information are gradually losing popularity to the Internet. Most likely this trend will continue until a new information-sharing technology moves into the mainstream of American life.

Health-related information in the mass media is generally accurate, but it is sometimes presented so quickly or superficially that its usefulness is limited.

Practitioners

The health care consumer also receives much information from individual health practitioners and their professional associations. In fact, today's health care practitioner so clearly emphasizes patient education that finding one who does not offer some information to a patient would be difficult. Education improves patient **compliance** with health care directives, which is important to the practitioner and the consumer.

Online Computer Services

We have already discussed the rapidly growing utilization of the Internet as a primary source of health-related information. We have even, in a sense, concluded that you are or would be one of those users. This assumption may not, however, be as predictable as we believe. In fact, a study reported in 2003 concluded that the use of the Internet for accessing health-related information had been overstated in previous studies, perhaps by a factor of three.[3] In yet another study in which persons who were unable to afford Internet access were provided it at no cost, less than 25 percent accessed health information.[4] A similarly low level of Internet use was reported for persons who were afflicted with one of five major adult chronic conditions—although those who did access information about their illnesses reported that it was very helpful.[5]

How should health-related information gleaned from the Internet be used, particularly when communicating with health care providers? Consider the following suggestions:

- Inform your health care provider that you are accessing the Internet for information related to your particular area of concern. Know the name of the site you're using; your provider might already be familiar with the site, or wish to access it in preparation for your discussion.
- Do not bombard your provider with questions whenever you come across information that might

---

Key Terms

compliance willingness to follow the directions provided by another person

be related to your health concern. Keep notes and discuss all of your findings at one time.

- Be prepared to *discuss* your information with your provider; don't use Web information to second-guess his or her position. Bear in mind that health concerns are too complex to generalize from the kind of one-size-fits-all information provided by even the most reliable websites, and must be evaluated on a case-by-case basis by a physician who has actually examined you.

- Always recognize that health-related information involves knowledge from many disciplines and uses highly technical language; media-based sources may grossly oversimplify in an effort to be accessible to lay persons.

Health Reference Publications

A substantial portion of all households own or subscribe to a health reference publication, such as the *Encyclopedia of Complementary Health Practices,* the *Physicians' Desk Reference* (PDR), or a newsletter such as *The Harvard Medical School Health Letter* or *The Johns Hopkins Medical Letter: Health after 50.* Some consumers also use personal computer programs and videocassettes featuring health-related information.

Reference Libraries

Public and university libraries continue to be popular sources of health-related information. One can consult with reference librarians and check out audiovisual collections and printed materials.

 TALKING POINTS A family member considers herself good at diagnosing health problems. Since she hasn't been wrong in years, she no longer relies on physicians. What questions could you ask her to point out the dangers associated with her approach?

Consumer Advocacy Groups

A variety of nonprofit consumer advocacy groups patrol the health care marketplace—such as those listed in Table 15.1—These groups produce and distribute information designed to help the consumer recognize questionable services and products. Large, well-organized groups, such as The National Consumers' League and Consumers Union, and smaller groups at the state and local levels champion the right of the consumer to receive valid and reliable information about health care products and services.

Voluntary Health Agencies

Volunteerism and the traditional approach to health care and health promotion are virtually inseparable. Few

Communication between Patients and Their Health Care Providers

In the complex world of modern health care, it is of critical importance that patients communicate important information to their health care providers, and, in turn, that they understand as fully as possible the information that they receive from the providers. Below are ten valuable suggestions from the joint commission on Accreditation of Healthcare Organizations and the U.S. Government's Agency for Healthcare Research and Quality.

- Take part in every decision about your health care.

- If you are not prepared to ask questions on your own behalf, ask a family member or friend to fill this role for you.

- Tell your physician and pharmacist about every drug you are taking, including prescription drugs, OTC drugs, vitamins, supplements, and herbal products—bring them with you.

- Make certain that you get the results of every test and understand what they mean.

- If you do not hear about test results, never assume that everything is all right. Call your doctor's office and ask.

- Whenever possible, choose a hospital where many patients receive the same procedure that you are to receive. Ask your physician or the hospital for the actual numbers.

- Ask hospital personnel if they have washed their hands before they begin touching you.

- If you are having surgery, make sure that you, your physician, and your surgeon all agree on what will be done during the operation.

- Insist that your surgeon write his or her initials or words such as "yes" or "this side" on the part of the body to be operated on. Put "no" on the opposite body part.

- When you are discharged, ask your doctor to explain your treatment plan, including changes in medications, restrictions on activity, and additional therapies you will need.

In many situations involving medical care, carefully communicated comments and questions between providers and patients can be the basis of the successful resolution of a health problem, versus unnecessary delay, pain, discomfort, or even death.

Source: Ellis L. *How You Can Help Guard against Errors.* June 28, 2002. http://www.intelihealth.com.

countries besides the United States can boast so many national voluntary organizations, with state and local affiliates, dedicated to improving health through research, service, and public education. The American Cancer Society, the American Red Cross, and the American Heart Association are voluntary (not-for-profit)

Table 15.1 Consumer Protection Agencies and Organizations

These agencies and organizations can be found in a variety of forms. Many are located within the organizational makeup of various federal agencies, while others, taking the form of free-standing organizations, are sustained in part by the validity of products, services, and corporate "good citizenship" of companies engaged in retail sales. Yet a third arena of operation for consumer protective services is within the confines of a highly creditable professional organization, such as the American Medical Association. Several consumer protective agencies and organizations are listed below.

Federal Agencies

Office of Consumer Affairs, Food and Drug Administration

U.S. Department of Health and Human Services
5600 Fishers Lane
Rockville, MD 20857
(301) 827-5006

www.fda.gov/oca/aboutoca.htm

Federal Trade Commission
Consumer Inquiries
Public Reference Branch
6th Street and Pennsylvania Avenue
Washington, DC 20580
(202) 326-2222

www.ftc.gov

Fraud Division
Chief Postal Inspector
U.S. Postal Inspection Service
475 L'Enfant Plaza
Washington, DC 20260-2166
(202) 268-4299

www.usps.gov

Consumer Information Center
Pueblo, CO 81009
(719) 948-3334

www.pueblo.gsa.gov

U.S. Consumer Product Safety Commission Hotline
(800) 638-CPSC

Consumer Organizations

Consumers Union of the U.S., Inc.
101 Truman Avenue
Yonkers, NY 10703
(914) 378-2000

www.consumerreports.org

Professional Organizations

American Medical Association
515 N. State Street
Chicago, IL 60610
(312) 464-5000

www.ama-assn.org

American Hospital Association
1 N. Franklin Street
Chicago, IL 60606
(312) 422-3000

www.aha.org

American Pharmaceutical Association
2215 Constitution Avenue, NW
Washington, DC 20037
(202) 628-4410

www.aphanet.org

---

health agencies. Consumers can, in fact, expect to find a voluntary health agency for virtually every health problem. College students should also note that volunteerism on their part, perhaps with a health agency like the Red Cross or the AHA, is both a personally satisfying experience and an activity viewed favorably by potential employers.

Government Agencies

Government agencies are also effective sources of information to the public. Through meetings and the release of information to the media, agencies such as the Food and Drug Administration, Federal Trade Commission, United States Postal Service, and Environmental Protection Agency publicize health issues. Government agencies also control the quality of information sent out to the buying public, particularly through labeling, advertising, and the distribution of information through the mail. The various divisions of the National Institutes of Health regularly release

research findings and recommendations to clinical practices, which in turn reach the consumer through clinical practitioners.

State governments also distribute health-related information to the public. State agencies are primary sources of information, particularly in the areas of public health and environmental protection. (For an example of health care activism at work, see Learning from Our Diversity on page 401.)

Qualified Health Educators

Health educators work in a variety of settings and offer their services to diverse groups. Community health educators work with virtually all of the agencies mentioned in this section; patient educators function in primary care settings; and school health educators are found at all educational levels. Health educators are increasingly being employed in a wide range of wellness-based programs in community, hospital, corporate, and school settings.

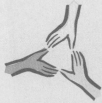

Learning from Our Diversity

Americans with Disabilities Act—New Places to Go

Although federal laws designed to end discrimination on the basis of gender and race were enacted in the United States decades ago, a law designed to address discrimination on the basis of physical and mental disabilities was not enacted until 1990. This law, the *Americans with Disabilities Act (1990),* has done a great deal to level the playing field for the disabled, both on the college campus and in the larger community. On campuses today, it's common to see students whose obvious disabilities would have prevented them from attending college before this law was enacted. Students with cerebral palsy, spina bifida, spinal cord injuries, sensory impairments, and orthopedic disabilities share living quarters, lecture hall seats, and recreational facilities with their nondisabled classmates.

Equally important are those students whose disabilities are largely unobservable. Students with learning disabilities, mental disabilities,

and subtle but disabling chronic health conditions such as Crohn's disease, lupus, and fibromyalgia may pass unnoticed. Yet their lives are equally challenged.

The Americans with Disabilities Act does not suggest that preferential treatment be given to students with disabilities, nor does it allow students to be unaccountable for their behavior. Instead, it seeks to create an environment—on the college campus and beyond—where people, regardless of disability, can learn new things, form meaningful relationships, and develop independence.

This law has the power to remove the physical and emotional barriers that can hinder a person with a disability from succeeding. For the first time, it allows students with disabilities to go where everyone else can—and beyond.

Health Care Providers

The sources of health information just discussed can greatly help us make decisions as informed consumers. The choices we make about physicians, health services, and medical payment plans will reflect our commitment to remaining healthy and our trust in specific people who are trained in keeping us healthy. (Refer to Changing for the Better on page 402 for tips on choosing a physician.)

Why We Consult Health Care Providers

Most of us seek care and advice from medical and health practitioners when we have a specific problem. A bad cold, a broken arm, or a newly discovered lump can motivate us to consult a health care professional. Yet *diagnosis* and *treatment* are only two reasons that we might require the services of health care providers.

We also might encounter health practitioners when we undergo *screening*. Screening most often involves a cursory (or noninvasive) collection of information that can quickly be compared to established standards often based on gender, age, race, or the presence of preexisting conditions. Your earliest experience with screening may have been in elementary school, where physicians, nurses, audiologists, and dentists sometimes examine all children for normal growth and development patterns. As an adult, your screening is more likely to be done on an individual

basis by a physician's staff as a routine portion of every office visit when they collect baseline information such as height, weight, and blood pressure measurements. You may also encounter community-based screening when you stop at your local shopping mall's health fair and have your blood pressure taken or cholesterol checked. Although

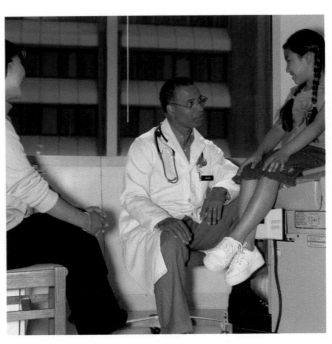

We often consult physicians for diagnosis and treatment of common ailments.

screening should be considered much less precise than actual diagnosis, screening serves to identify people who should seek further medical examination.

Consultation is a fourth reason that knowledgeable consumers seek health care providers. A consultation is the use of two or more professionals to deliberate a person's specific health problem or condition. Consultations are especially helpful when **primary care health providers,** such as family practice physicians, gynecologists, pediatricians, internists, and general practice dentists, require the opinion of specialists. Using additional practitioners as consultants can also help reassure patients who may have doubts about their own condition or about the abilities of their physician.

Prevention is a fifth reason we might seek a health care provider. With the current emphasis on trying to stop problems before they begin, using health care providers for prevention is becoming more common. People want information about how to prevent needless risks and promote their health, and they seek such advice from physicians, nurses, dentists, exercise physiologists, patient educators, and other health promotion specialists.

When prevention becomes a routine component of your personal health care, you will annually receive, in addition to the baseline measurements of height, weight, and blood pressure, more in-depth assessments such as a blood chemistry assessment, lipid profile, and cardiogram. Women will also likely receive a ViraPap test, breast examination, mammography, and pelvic examination, while men will likely receive a Prostate Specific Antibody

---

Key Terms

primary care health providers health care providers who generally see patients on a routine basis, particularly for preventive health care

(PSA) test, digital prostate examination, and testicular examination.

Physicians and Their Training

In every city and many smaller communities, the local telephone directory lists physicians in a variety of medical specialties. These health care providers hold the academic degree of Doctor of Medicine (MD) or Doctor of Osteopathy (DO).

At one time, **allopathy** and **osteopathy** were clearly different health care professions in terms of their healing philosophies and modes of practice. Today, however, MDs and DOs receive similar educations and engage in very similar forms of practice. Both can function as primary care physicians or as board-certified specialists. Their differences are in the osteopathic physician's greater tendency to use manipulation in treating health problems. In addition, DOs often perceive themselves as being more holistically oriented than MDs are.

Medical and osteopathic physicians undergo a long training process. After they are accepted into professional schools, students generally spend 4 or more years in intensive training that includes advanced study in the preclinical medical sciences and clinical practice. When they complete this phase of training, the students are awarded the MD or DO degree and then take the state medical license examination. Most newly licensed physicians complete a residency at a hospital. Residency programs vary in length from 3 to 4 years. When they conclude their residency programs, including board-related examinations, physicians are granted board-certified status. In addition to state and specialty board certification, comprehensive national certification of physicians is a frequently discussed possibility. At this time, no nationally required and all-encompassing certification of physician competency is required.

Complementary, Alternative, and Integrative Care Practitioners

In addition to medical and osteopathic physicians, several other forms of health care offer alternatives within the large health care market. Included within this group of complementary or alternative forms of practice are chiropractic, acupuncture, homeopathy, naturopathy, herbalism, reflexology, and ayurveda.[6] Although the traditional medical community has long scoffed at these fields of practice as ineffective and unscientific, many people use these forms of health care and believe strongly that they are as effective as (or more effective than) allopathic and osteopathic medicine. As a result of this belief, today many physicians are better informed about complementary care methods and more comfortable discussing them with patients. Following are brief descriptions of some of the more popular of these complementary care fields and the practitioners that function within them.

Chiropractic

Historically (and, to varying degrees, today) the underlying premise of chiropractic is that misalignment or subluxation of the spinal (vertebral) column is the primary cause of illness, and, thus, its realignment is the appropriate treatment for illness. Accordingly, chiropractic medical practice is primarily limited to vertebral adjustments, where manual manipulation of the spine its used to correct misalignments. Recent studies have shown that **chiropractic** treatment of some types of low-back pain can be more effective than conventional care.[7] With about 50,000 practitioners in the United States, chiropractic is the third-largest health profession, used by 15 to 20 million people. Some chiropractors use only spinal manipulation, whereas others use additional medical technologies, including dietary supplementation and various noninvasive technologies similar to those used by physical therapists and athletic trainers, including massage.

In spite of the fact that chiropractors undergo nearly the same number of years of training as do primary care physicians and take courses closely aligned with those taken by physicians, current laws restrict the scope of chiropractic practice to noninvasive techniques initially consistent with the original theoretical basis of their discipline, "one cause—one cure of all illnesses and diseases." In 1998 the National Center for Complementary and Alternative Medicine established a Comprehensive Center for Chiropractic Research (the 11th alternative medical field to receive such a center) to establish scientific standards for the study of chiropractic effectiveness.[8] Research is ongoing at five sites. Should careful study of chiropractic demonstrate limited effectiveness, beyond the area of low-back pain, then chiropractic medicine is

---

Key Terms

allopathy (ah **lop** ah thee) a system of medical practice in which specific remedies (often pharmaceutical agents) are used to produce effects different from those produced by a disease or injury

osteopathy (os tee **op** ah thee) a system of medical practice in which allopathic principles are combined with specific attention to postural mechanics of the body

chiropractic manipulation of the vertebral column to relieve misalignments and cure illness

likely to remain a user-friendly, highly popular but highly limited approach to health care.

Acupuncture

Acupuncture is, for Americans, the most familiar component of the 3,000-year-old Chinese medical system. This system is based on balancing the active and passive forces within the patient's body to strengthen the qi ("chee"), or life force. The system also employs herbs, food, massage, and exercise.

Acupuncturists place hair-thin needles at certain points in the body to stimulate the patient's qi. These points are said to correspond to different organs and bodily functions and, when stimulated, help the body's own defenses fight illness. More specifically, the scientific communities suggest that acupuncture speeds up the electrical conductivity within the central and peripheral nervous systems, enhances the production of biological opiates, and alters the production of specific neurotransmitters within various areas of the nervous system.[9]

Of all the Chinese therapies, acupuncture is the most widely accepted in the West. Researchers have produced persuasive evidence of acupuncture's effectiveness with treating low-back pain, adult postoperative pain, nausea and vomiting associated with chemotherapy, and pain following dental surgery. Acupuncture may also be effective in other areas such as addiction, headache, menstrual pain, fibromyalgia, osteoarthritis, and tennis elbow.[10]

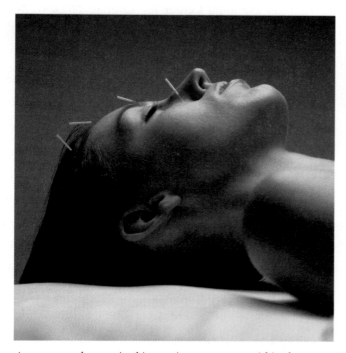

Acupuncture has received increasing acceptance within the Western medical community.

However, because of the difficulty of conducting double-blind research that involves the insertion of needles, acupuncture research is challenging to design, thus its use may remain largely complementary.

Reflexology

Reflexology uses principles similar to those of acupuncture but focuses on treating certain disorders through massage of the soles of the feet. To date, however, there is relatively little data regarding its effectiveness, when evaluated under carefully controlled conditions. The National Center for Complementary and Alternative Medicine is only now beginning to find research that holds some promise of being interpreted on the basis of acceptable research design. For example, in a recent Korean study, foot reflexology, in four sessions of 40 minutes each, was given to a group of women undergoing breast cancer chemotherapy.[11] In comparison to a control group, those receiving reflexology reported less nausea, vomiting, and fatigue. In a second study conducted in Israel, it was found that reflexology versus sham (calf area massage) was beneficial in alleviating motor, sensory, and urinary difficulties in persons with multiple sclerosis.[12] In contrast, a Danish study in which middle-ear infections in children were treated exclusively with reflexology (versus antibiotics) found reflexology to be ineffective.[13]

Homeopathy

Widely accepted in Europe, **homeopathy** is the leading alternative therapy in France. Homeopathy uses infinitesimal doses of herbs, minerals, or even poisons to stimulate the body's curative powers. The theory on which homeopathy is based, the *law of similars,* contends that if large doses of a substance can cause a problem, tiny doses can trigger healing. A few small studies showed homeopathy to be at least somewhat effective in treating hay fever, diarrhea, and flu symptoms, but members of the scientific community call the studies flawed or preliminary and suggest that the placebo effect was occurring. Much more informative, however, are reports

---

Key Terms

acupuncture insertion of fine needles into the body to alter electroenergy fields and cure disease

reflexology massage applied to specific areas of the feet to treat illness and disease in other areas of the body

homeopathy (hoe mee **op** ah thee) the use of minute doses of herbs, minerals, or other substances to stimulate healing

from three meta-analysis studies, funded by the National Center for Complementary and Alternative Medicine, involving the reassessment of 240 individual studies, in which it was concluded that major methodology weaknesses existed in most studies of homeopathy conducted to date. It was further concluded that on the basis of these studies there was no strong evidence in favor of homeopathy over conventional treatment methods. The Center recommended that larger, more carefully controlled studies be conducted.[14] Since the report on homeopathic medication was released by the National Center for Complementary and Alternative Medicine, recent studies continue to experience methodological difficulties, principally related to the small sample sizes used by researchers.[15]

Naturopathy

The core of naturopathic medicine is what Hippocrates called *medicatrix naturae,* or the healing power of nature. Proponents of naturopathy believe that when the mind and the body are in balance and receiving proper care, with a healthy diet, adequate rest, and minimal stress, the body's own vital forces are sufficient to fight off disease. Getting rid of an ailment is only the first step toward correcting the underlying imbalance that allowed the ailment to take hold, naturists believe. Correcting the imbalance might be as simple as rectifying a shortage of a particular nutrient, or as complex as reducing overlong work hours, strengthening a weakened immune system, and identifying an inability to digest certain foods.

Herbalism

Herbalism may be the world's oldest and most widely used healing form. Herbalists make herbal brews for treating a variety of ills, such as depression, anxiety, and hypertension. In some cases, scientific research supports the herbalists' beliefs. For example, studies have found St. John's wort to be more effective than a placebo and one of the older tricyclic antidepressants in alleviating mild depression, and that garlic reduces cholesterol and blood pressure, while black cohosh (a member of the buttercup family) and soy can relieve hot flashes and other menopause symptoms.

However, the potential side effects of many dietary supplements have raised questions about the dangers associated with particular herbs, especially of products containing ephedra, a stimulant used to enhance athletic performance or stimulate weight loss.[16] The Food and Drug Administration began to consider taking increased control over the testing and safety of all dietary supplements following the ephedra-related death of Baltimore Orioles pitcher Steve Belcher in February 2003; more than 150 deaths have been linked to the supplement. In December 2003, after extensive studies, the FDA officially banned the sale and use of ephedra and implemented the ban in April 2004.[17] However, most supplements are not studied in this manner, and virtually no regulation of the supplements industry currently exists.

Ayurveda

Even older than Chinese medicine, India's **ayurveda** takes a preventive approach and focuses on the whole person. This system employs diet, tailored to the patient's constitutional type, or dosha; herbs; yoga and breathing exercises; meditation; massages; and purges, enemas, and aromatherapy. Practitioners of ayurveda report success in treating rheumatoid arthritis, headaches, and chronic sinusitis.

If you would like to consult a practitioner in one of the alternative disciplines but you don't know where to start, see Changing for the Better on page 406 for some tips on choosing a provider in alternative medicine.

At the urging of many people in both the medical and complementary health care fields, the National Institutes of Health requested federal funding to establish a scientific center for the study of alternative medical care. Today the National Center for Complementary and Alternative Medicine assembles information about alternative approaches to medical care and provides a framework for well-controlled research into the effectiveness of each approach. The first substantial recommendation regarding an alternative form of care, acupuncture, was released in 1998.

It will be interesting to note whether all the branches of complementary medical care will want their theories of treatment and prevention tested under the rigorous criteria used by the National Center for Complementary and Alternative Medicine and to see how they respond if the results are not favorable.

Restricted-Practice Health Care Providers

We receive much of our health care from medical physicians. However, most of us also use the services of various health care specialists who also have advanced

---

Key Terms

naturopathy (na chur **op** ah thee) a system of treatment that avoids drugs and surgery and emphasizes the use of natural agents to correct underlying imbalances

herbalism an ancient form of healing in which herbal preparations are used to treat illness and disease

ayurveda (ai yur **vey** da) traditional Indian medicine based on herbal remedies

I'm interested in exploring complementary approaches to medicine, but I feel uncertain about how to proceed. What steps should I take?

Perhaps you are one of the millions of people who feel that their doctors don't encourage them to ask questions, don't seek their opinion about their medical condition, or don't take a thorough medical history. Perhaps you want advice on improving your health rather than just a quick diagnosis and prescription.

For whatever reasons, millions of Americans are turning to complementary medical practitioners, such as doctors of naturopathy, Chinese medicine, or ayurveda. Unfortunately, the patient looking for these alternatives faces other problems: practitioners' training may be weak, they might not be licensed or covered by insurance, they are hard to find, and they usually are not permitted to prescribe drugs unless they also happen to be medical doctors. This means that you must do some legwork to find a good provider who can meet your needs.

Consider the following tips for finding the practitioner who is right for you.

- *Don't forget the family physician.* Family-practice medicine is enjoying a surge in the United States, and many of these doctors tend to think holistically.
- *Find a physician who believes in complementary therapies.* Your doctor's attitude toward the treatment can be just as important as your own.
- *Give the treatment time.* Complementary therapies encourage the body to do its own healing. This often takes time. Seek a physician who is confident in your self-healing ability, so you won't become discouraged if it takes some time.

- *Request natural healing.* Natural healing tends to change the internal conditions so that pathogens are less likely to gain a foothold; conventional medicine seeks to destroy the pathogen. Natural healing searches for the causes of symptoms, while conventional medicine treats symptoms.
- *Know your disease.* Find books that describe your conditions and offer complementary as well as conventional treatments. This way you can discuss your treatment with your physician and create an effective treatment plan.
- *Treat yourself.* Don't overuse your health care provider, whether conventional or complementary. For many conditions, you can be your own best doctor; of course, persistent or severe symptoms should send you to the physician.
- *Learn whether the treatment is covered by insurance.* Coverage of complementary treatment differs sharply by state. Some insurance groups are beginning to pay for more complementary medicine, and HMOs are hiring some complementary specialists.
- *Talk to professional associations.* Most of the more established complementary fields have associations that can give you a list of providers. Use it as a start.
- *Interview the practitioner.* Before making an appointment, talk with the practitioner over the telephone. Then, in the practitioner's office, take notes; even use a tape recorder, to make certain you understand. Watch for a practitioner who is a good listener, a good communicator, and open-minded.

InfoLinks

http://nccam.nih.gov

---

graduate-level training. Among these professionals are dentists, psychologists, podiatrists, and optometrists.

Dentists (Doctor of Dental Surgery, DDS) deal with a wide range of diseases and impairments of the teeth and oral cavity. Dentists undergo undergraduate predental programs that emphasize the sciences, followed by 4 additional years of study in dental school and, with increasing frequency, an internship program. State licensure examinations are required. As with physicians, dentists can also specialize by completing a postdoctoral master's degree in fields such as oral surgery, **orthodontics,** and **prosthodontics.** Dentists are also permitted to prescribe therapy programs (such as the treatment of temporomandibular joint [TMJ] dysfunction) and drugs that pertain to their practices (primarily analgesics and antibiotics).

As discussed in Chapter 2, *psychologists* provide services to help patients understand behavior patterns or perceptions. More than 40 states have certification or licensing laws that prohibit unqualified people from using the term *psychologist*. The consumer should examine a psychologist's credentials. Legitimate psychologists have received advanced graduate training (often leading to a PhD or EdD degree) in clinical, counseling, industrial, or

Key Terms

orthodontics a dental specialty that focuses on the proper alignment of the teeth

prosthodontics a dental specialty that focuses on the construction and fitting of artificial appliances to replace missing teeth

educational psychology. Furthermore, these practitioners will have passed state certification examinations and, in many states, will have met further requirements that allow them to offer health services to the public. Psychologists may have special interests and credentials from professional societies in individual, group, family, or marriage counseling. Some are certified as sex therapists.

Unlike psychiatrists, who are medical physicians, psychologists cannot prescribe or dispense drugs. They may refer to or consult with medical physicians about clients who might benefit from drug therapy.

Podiatrists are highly trained clinicians who practice podiatric medicine, or care of the feet (and ankles). Although not MDs or DOs, doctors of podiatric medicine (DPM) treat a wide variety of conditions related to the feet, including corns, bunions, warts, bone spurs, hammertoes, fractures, diabetes-related conditions, athletic injuries, and structural abnormalities. Podiatrists perform surgery, prescribe medications, and apply orthotics (supports or braces), splints, and corrective shoes for structural abnormalities of the feet.

Doctors of podiatric medicine follow an educational path similar to that taken by MDs and DOs, consisting of a 4-year undergraduate preprofessional curriculum, 4 additional years of study in a podiatric medical school, and an optional residency of 1 or 2 years. Board-certified areas of specialization include surgery, orthopedics, and podiatric sports medicine. Hospital affiliation generally requires board certification in a specialized area.

Optometrists are eye specialists who primarily treat vision problems associated with **refractory errors.** They examine the eyes and prescribe glasses or contact lenses to correct visual disorders. Additionally, optometrists prescribe prescription medications, such as antibiotic drops for application in the eye. Optometrists sometimes attempt to correct certain ocular muscle imbalances with specific exercise regimens. Optometrists must complete undergraduate training and additional years of coursework at one of sixteen accredited colleges of optometry in the United States or two Canadian colleges before taking a state licensing examination.

Nurse Professionals

Nurses constitute a large group of health professionals who practice in a variety of settings. Their responsibilities usually depend on their academic preparation. Registered nurses (RNs) are academically prepared at two levels: (1) the technical nurse, and (2) the professional nurse. The technical nurse is educated in a 2-year associate degree program. The professional nurse receives 4 years of education and earns a bachelor's degree. Both technical and professional nurses must successfully complete state licensing examinations before they can practice as RNs.

In light of the important role that nurse professionals play in today's health care system, it is worrisome that a significant shortage of nurses exists. On the basis of enrollment data for nursing programs in this country, and the number of nurses who have apparently left the workforce for various reasons, the current shortage of registered nurses is estimated to be 110,000. Projecting through 2012, it is estimated that 1.1 million new and replacement openings for nurses will exist in the United States,[18] a need that will most likely not be met.

Compounding the shortage of nurses is an equally acute shortage of nursing faculty to staff the nursing education programs that currently exist. As can be imagined, the demand for nurses has increased salaries, generated competition between health care institutions to recruit nurses, and increased the nurse-to-patient ratio to dangerously high levels in many areas of the country. In this final regard, it is estimated that as many as 20,000 unnecessary deaths that occur annually in American hospitals and nursing facilities can be attributed to the shortage—about one-fifth of all deaths attributed to medical errors.[19]

Many professional nurses continue their education and earn master's and doctoral degrees in nursing or other health-related fields. Some professional nurses specialize in a clinical area (such as pediatrics, gerontology, public health, or school health) and become certified as *advanced practice nurses* (APNs). Currently four APN fields, including nurse midwives, nurse anesthetists, nurse practitioners, and nurse case managers, can be found in larger communities. Working in close association with physicians, APNs perform an array of diagnositic, treatment, and administrative activities once limited to physicians. The ability of these highly trained nurses to function at this level gives communities additional primary care providers and frees physicians to deal with more complex cases.

Licensed practical nurses (LPNs) are trained in hospital-based programs that last 12 to 18 months. Because of their brief training, LPNs' scope of practice is limited. Most LPN training programs are gradually being phased out.

Allied Health Care Professionals

Our primary health care providers are supported by a large group of allied health care professionals, who are often responsible for highly technical services and

> **Key Terms**
>
> **refractory errors** abnormal patterns of light wave transmission through the structures of the eye

procedures. These professionals include respiratory and inhalation therapists, radiographic technologists, nuclear medicine technologists, pathology technicians, general medical technologists, operating room technicians, emergency medical technicians, physical therapists, occupational therapists, cardiac rehabilitation therapists, dental technicians, physician assistants, and dental hygienists. Depending on the particular field, the training for these specialty support areas can take from 1 to 5 years of postsecondary school study. Programs include hospital-based training leading to a diploma through associate, bachelor's, and master's degrees. Most allied health care professionals must also pass state or national licensing examinations.

Self-Care/Home Care

The emergence of the **self-care movement** suggests that many people are becoming more responsible for maintaining their health. They are developing the expertise to prevent or manage many types of illness, injuries, and conditions. They are learning to assess their health status and treat, monitor, and rehabilitate themselves in a manner that was once thought possible only through a physician or some other health care specialist.

The benefits of this movement are that self-care can (1) reduce health care costs, (2) provide effective care for particular conditions, (3) free physicians and other health care specialists to spend time with other patients, and (4) increase interest in health-related activities.

Self-care is an appropriate alternative to professional care in three areas. First, self-care may be appropriate for certain acute conditions that have familiar symptoms and are limited in their duration and seriousness. Common colds and flu, many home injuries, sore throats, and nonallergic insect bites are often easily managed with self-care. That said, there are some symptoms that might seem somewhat familiar that should not be responded to through self-care, but rather by seeing a physician promptly. These include feeling of pressure or squeezing in the chest, a sudden severe headache, markedly blurred vision, difficulty talking or walking, dizziness and confusion, blood in urine or stool, unrelieved depression, and a cough with a yellow-green discharge. Self-care might be useful at some point, but not until the symptoms have been evaluated by a physician.

A second area in which self-care might be appropriate is therapy. For example, many people administer injections for diabetes mellitus, allergies, and migraine headaches and continue physical therapy programs in their homes. Asthma and hypertension are also conditions that can be managed or monitored with self-care.

A third area in which self-care has appropriate application is health promotion. Weight loss programs, physical conditioning activities, smoking cessation, and stress-reduction programs are particularly well suited to self-care (see Discovering Your Spirituality on page 409).

A potential fourth area in home care, self-diagnosis, is emerging, and not without some concern. Perhaps beginning with the thermometer, progressing to the home pregnancy test and the mail-in HIV diagnostic kit, today in-home genetic testing is available. These genetic screening tests are readily available and consist of a swab that is used to obtain a scraping of cells from the inner cheek and a mail-in envelope. Upon processing cells for their DNA, persons can obtain a genetic profile as it relates to specific disease predispositions. Principal concerns associated with the use of these tests are the shortcutting of primary care physicians (although some brands require physician consent) and the absence of genetic counselors to work with clients after they receive the results of their tests. Currently, in-home genetic screening tests cost $200–$400.

As the U.S. population ages, it is becoming increasingly common for family members to provide home care to older relatives. As the number of frail older people increases, home care can significantly reduce the need for institutional care. Home care also can be delivered by home health care specialists. In fact, this form of care is proving so cost-effective that some insurance programs, including *Medicare* and *Medicaid,* cover portions of the cost of home health care for older adults.

A decision to provide family-based home care, particularly for older adults, is often made for admirable and understandable reasons, including love for the relative who needs care and the high cost of professional home care and institutional care. For the millions of families who have made this decision, providing home health care can be highly rewarding. It also can be very demanding, however, because of the needs and limitations of the person who requires care and the compromises the caregivers must make.[20] Particularly when a spouse or family decides to provide care without the assistance of professional caregivers, they can jeopardize their own health long before the recovery or death of the person for whom they are caring.

Key Terms
self-care movement the trend toward individuals' taking increased responsibility for prevention or management of certain health conditions

Good Health—What's It Worth, Now and Later?

The average life expectancy for women in the United States today is 80 years. For men, it's 76 years. That's a dramatic change from just a century ago. Thanks to tremendous advances in medical science and technology, many people are enjoying healthy, happy, and spiritually fulfilling lives well into their final years.

But this longevity comes with a price tag. It means that making healthful choices every day—including eating a balanced diet, getting exercise and adequate rest, and making opportunities for emotional and spiritual expression—takes on new importance. If you're going to live 10 "extra" years, what do you want to do with that time? Probably many of the things you're doing now, plus some different ones. Are you going to be able to meet the challenge—healthwise?

Taking charge of your health right now, when you're young and healthy, can be one of the most empowering things you do. By consciously choosing a healthy lifestyle—limiting your intake of alcohol, avoiding drugs and cigarette smoking, and limiting your sexual partners—you are building the foundation for good health in your later years.

If you should ever have a serious health problem, you'll be better equipped to handle it if you're used to taking care of yourself. You'll feel comfortable being involved in your treatment decisions and doing whatever you can to control the quality of your life. You'll see your health crisis as a challenge you need to deal with, instead of viewing yourself as a helpless victim.

Taking charge of your own health—by being an informed health care consumer, by choosing a healthy lifestyle, and by fostering a positive attitude—brings a sense of peace. It's knowing that you're doing everything you can to take care of yourself. It's enhancing the quality of your life today and preparing for an active and rewarding tomorrow.

Health Care Facilities

Most of us have a general idea of what a hospital is. However, all hospitals are not alike. They usually fall into one of three categories—private, public, or voluntary. *Private hospitals* (or proprietary hospitals) function as profit-making hospitals. They are not supported by tax monies and usually accept only clients who can pay all their expenses. Although there are some exceptions, these hospitals are generally smaller than tax-supported public hospitals. Commonly owned by a group of business investors, a large hospital corporation, or a group of physicians, these hospitals sometimes limit their services to a few specific types of illnesses.

Public hospitals are supported primarily by tax dollars. They can be operated by government agencies at the state level (such as state mental hospitals) or at the federal level (such as the Veterans Administration Hospitals and various military service hospitals such as the National Naval Medical Center in Bethesda, Maryland). Large county or city hospitals are frequently public hospitals. These hospitals routinely serve indigent segments of the population.

The most commonly recognized type of hospital is the *voluntary hospital.* Voluntary hospitals are maintained as nonprofit public institutions. Often supported by religious orders, fraternal groups, or charitable organizations, these hospitals usually offer a wider range of comprehensive services than do private hospitals or clinics. Voluntary hospitals are supported by patient fees (covered by health insurance), Medicare reimbursement, and Medicaid and public assistance reimbursement.

In the last decade, hospitals, particularly private and voluntary hospitals, have expanded their scope of services. Today hospitals often operate *wellness centers,* stress centers, cardiac rehabilitation centers, chemical dependence programs, health education centers, and satellite centers for well-baby care and care for the homeless. During the 1990s two trends were observed in terms of hospital organization and ownership: the acquisition of small hospitals (such as county hospitals and smaller community hospitals) by larger regional hospitals and the reorganization of voluntary hospitals as for-profit hospitals. Both trends reflected the rapid movement of medical care in the direction of *managed care,* the term referring to the more profit-focused, cost-efficient, and third-party-controlled care reflective of the application of corporate strategies to the delivery of health care services.

Other health care facilities include clinics (both private and tax-supported), nursing homes (most of which are private enterprises), and rehabilitation centers. Rehabilitation centers are often supported by charitable organizations devoted to the care of chronically ill or handicapped people, orthopedically injured people, or burn victims.

In recent years, many private, 24-hour drop-in medical emergency and surgical centers have appeared. These clinics have their own professional staffs of physicians, nurses, and allied health professionals.

Another health care provider is the *hospice.* Hospices provide prescribed medical care (most often palliative or comfort care) for patients who have been deemed terminal by their health care provider. Although some

Table 15.2 Patients' Institutional Rights

Regardless of the type of institution in which you are a patient, you have a variety of rights. These are intended to protect you from unnecessary harm and financial loss. The hospital too can expect your cooperation as a patient.

As a patient, you can expect all of the following from the institution:

- To be treated with respect and dignity
- To be afforded privacy and confidentiality consistent with federal and state laws, institutional policies, and the requirements of your insurance carrier
- To be provided services on request, as long as they are reasonable and consistent with appropriate care
- To be fully informed of the identity of the physicians and staff providing care
- To be kept fully updated about your condition, including its management and your prognosis for recovery
- To be informed of any experimental or other research/educational projects that may be utilized in your treatment and to refuse such treatment
- To have the opportunity to specify advance directives (a living will, a life-prolonging statement, or the appointment of a health care representative) in order to facilitate health care decisions
- To receive an explanation of your bill for services regardless of the source of payment
- To present a complaint and receive a response about any aspect of your care or treatment and to have your complaint taken seriously
- To be involved in ethical considerations that arise during the course of your care

The institution can expect you, as a patient:

- To keep all appointments
- To provide all background information pertinent to your condition
- To treat hospital personnel with respect
- To ask questions and seek clarification about matters that affect you
- To follow the treatment prescribed by your physician
- To be considerate and respectful of other patients and to ensure that your visitors are considerate and respectful as well
- To satisfy your financial obligation to health care providers through the provision of insurance information and by arranging credit where applicable

As a patient, you may at any time:

- Refuse treatment
- Seek a second opinion
- Discharge yourself from the institution

hospices are housed within hospitals and provide in-hospital care, most provide home-based care, thus allowing the terminal patient the opportunity to die in familiar surroundings and in the presence of loving family members or friends. Many hospice models can be found within the United States, including those operated by hospitals (in-hospital care and/or home-based care), for-profit companies, charitable organizations, and those affiliated with religious bodies.

Although you might have no direct experience with the services of a hospice, you may recall that Terri Schaivo died in a hospice setting. The highly charged aspect of that particular person's life and death, however, should not distract from your appreciation of the compassionate care and dignity of death supported by virtually all hospices.

Regardless of the type of health care institutions in which you seek services, both you and the institutions have legally binding rights that structure your relationship. Table 15.2 details both your rights as a patient and their rights as licensed health care facilities.

Health Care Costs and Reimbursement

There are many avenues for receiving health care. However, being able to pay for quality care is one of the greatest concerns of the American public. In 2003 (the last year for which statistics are available) nearly 45 million American were without health insurance for the entire year.[21] Some believe that adding those people who lacked coverage for a portion of the year to the preceding figure would result in 75 million people with less than full health insurance coverage. No age group is more likely to be uncovered than are young adults between 18 and 24 years of age. American Indians and Alaskan Natives are the two racial groups least likely to have health insurance.[21] Employed persons, regardless of age or race, who work in the service sector and lack benefits, such as food workers, and the self-employed often find access to individual health insurance policies too expensive to own. Approximately 11.5 percent of all American children lack access to the fullest range of health services owing to a lack of health insurance.[21]

In addition to the availability of health insurance, the simple cost of health care is a major concern, even for those who have access to health insurance. It is estimated that in 2002 Americans spent $1.553 trillion on health care,[22] and by 2013 this expenditure will increase to $3.358 trillion.[23] Stated another way, in 2002 Americans incurred an average of $5,241 per person in health care-related costs.[24] This amount is expected to increase to $7,100 per person by the year 2007. No developed country spends a greater percent of its gross domestic product on health care than does the United States.

As a result of factors such as the high cost of modern medical technology, an emphasis on long life at any cost, the growing number of older people with chronic conditions that require expensive long-term care, and the AIDS epidemic, controlling the cost of medical care is one of the most complex problems facing the nation. Nevertheless, more than 40 different plans have been advanced since 1990 to respond to this problem. These range from only modest changes in the current system, to tax-credit strategies and mandatory employment-based insurance, to a federally controlled national health plan. Today government officials seem to be particularly interested in lowering the cost of prescription drugs for older Americans. Three models have received close attention. The first assigns some aspects of prescription drug coverage to Medicare, while the second relates to the development of prescription drug plans by the pharmaceutical industry, for those who qualify on the basis of need. The third model assigns an increased role for the health insurance industry in negotiating lower drug prices for its senior members. Both the first and second models, in various forms, are now in operation.

In December 2003, President Bush signed the Medicare Prescription Drug Improvement and Modernization Act. Hailed as an answer to rising drug costs for seniors, the act was widely criticized as still being too costly for many seniors.

Health Insurance

Health insurance is a financial agreement between an insurance company and an individual or group for the payment of health care costs. After paying a premium to an insurance company, the policyholder is covered for specific benefits. Each policy is different in its coverage of illnesses and injuries. Merely having an insurance policy does not mean that all health care expenses will be covered. Most health insurance policies require various forms of payments by the policyholder, which includes deductible amounts, fixed indemnity benefits, coinsurance, and exclusions. In 2000 Americans spent $372.8 billion on private health insurance, and they are expected to spend $643.4 billion by 2007.[25]

A *deductible* amount is an established amount that the insuree must pay before the insurer reimburses for services. For example, a person or family may have to pay the first $200 of the year's medical expenses before insurance begins providing any coverage.

A policy with *fixed indemnity* benefits will pay only a specified amount for a particular procedure or service. If the policy pays only $1,000 for an appendectomy and the actual cost of the appendectomy was $1,500, then the policy owner will owe the health care provider $500. A policy with full-service benefits, which pays the entire cost of a particular procedure or service, may be worth the extra cost.

Policies that have *coinsurance* features require that the policy owner and the insurance company share the costs of certain covered services, usually on a percentage basis. One standard coinsurance plan requires that the policyholder pay 20 percent of the costs above a deductible amount, and the company pays the remaining 80 percent.

An *exclusion* is a service or expense that is not covered by the policy. Elective or cosmetic surgery procedures, unusual treatment protocols, prescription drugs, and certain kinds of consultations are common exclusions. Illness and injuries that already exist at the time of purchase (preexisting conditions) are often excluded. In addition, injuries incurred during high-risk activities (ice hockey, hang gliding, mountain climbing, intramural sports) might not be covered by a policy.

Health insurance can be obtained through individual policies or group plans. Group health insurance plans usually offer the widest range of coverage at the lowest price and are often purchased cooperatively by companies and their employees. In 2004, companies with health insurance benefits spent on average $7,289 for each employee's family health insurance plan—an 11.8 percent increase over 2003 costs.[26] Fortunately, no employee is refused entry into a group insurance program. However, when employees leave the company, their previous group coverage can follow them for a prescribed period of time only, usually 18 to 24 months. Today, as many large American companies continue to lay off employees, the eventual loss of health insurance becomes a serious personal and family crisis.

Individual policies can be purchased by one person (or a family) from an insurance company. These policies are often much more expensive than group plans and may provide much less coverage. Still, people who do not have access to a group plan should attempt to secure individual policies, because the financial burdens resulting from a severe accident or illness that is not covered by some form of health insurance can be devastating. Many colleges and universities offer annually renewable health insurance policies that students can purchase. (Changing for the Better on page 412 gives the consumer some questions to consider before purchasing a health insurance policy.)

Medicare

Since it was established in 1965, *Medicare* has been a key provider of health care coverage for the nation's older adults. Medicare is a federally funded health insurance program for persons 65 years of age and older, as well as for persons of any age who have particular disabilities or permanent kidney failure. Funding for Medicare comes primarily from federal payroll taxes and is administered by the Health Care Financing Administration, within the Department of Health and Human Services.

In it current configuration Medicare is divided into two portions. Part A (the hospital insurance portion) helps pay for care while in hospitals, as well as for care in skilled nursing facilities and hospice care, and for some home health care. Persons become eligible for Part A coverage on turning 65 years of age, on the basis of having paid Medicare taxes while working.

Part B is an optional portion of Medicare that can be chosen at the time of becoming eligible for Part A. Unlike Part A, there is a monthly charge for Part B Coverage. Currently that charge is $78.20 per month but is subject to annual adjustment.[27] Part B helps pay for doctors' services, outpatient hospital care, and some home medical services not covered under Part A, including physical and occupational therapy, medical devices, and some home health. Routine dental and vision care are not covered.

Because of the universal nature of Medicare Part A and the affordable monthly charge for Part B, group health insurance plans to which many retirees belong require that Medicare be the "first player" for services, thus allowing the group plan to be responsible for only that portion of health-related charges not covered by Medicare.

The Medicare Prescription Drug Improvement and Modernization Act of 2003 (now referred to as Part D) provides new prescription coverage options for Medicare recipients. Beginning in 2006, it provides prescription coverage through third-party providers for a premium of about $35 per month. After meeting an annual deductible of $250, Medicare covers 75 percent of the costs of prescription drugs, up to $2,250 per year; there is then a gap in coverage until out-of-pocket expenses reach $3,500 in a single year, at which point Medicare kicks in again and covers 95 percent of further costs for the remainder of the year.[27] The Medicare prescription drug program is expected to cost the Medicare system $724 billion during the first decade of its existence.

Medicaid

Unlike Medicare, a program that is almost exclusively for persons 65 or older, *Medicaid* is a program designed to assist in meeting the health care needs of qualified persons regardless of age. Also unlike Medicare, which is a federal program entirely funded through Medicare tax withholdings (Part A) and user-paid elected enrollment fees (Part B), Medicaid is a federal- and state-funded program administered by each of the individual states.

Qualification for receiving Medicaid assistance can be perplexing. Federal Medicaid law sets mandatory eligibility standards, while optional eligibility standards allow each state to tailor many aspects of the program to fit its unique needs. Central to the majority of the federally mandated eligibility standards is the current Federal Poverty Level (FPL), as well as the standards related to the Aid to Families with Dependent Children (AFDC) program and the Temporary Assistance to Needy Families (TANF) program. Optional eligibility standards allow states to define some aspects of eligibility for pregnant women, disabled children, certain working disabled persons, and those designated as Medically Needy.

Federally mandated Medicaid services are wide ranging and include hospital services, physician services, laboratory/X-ray procedures, immunizations, family planning services, home health care services, transportation for medical care services, and nursing home services. This final service is of critical importance to older adults in that it pays for the majority of nursing home care required by this age group. Optional services, which are under state control, include prescription drugs, rehabilitation and physical therapy services, prosthetic devices, vision services, hearing services, and dental services, to include a few.

Health Maintenance Organizations

Health maintenance organizations (HMOs) are health care delivery plans under which health care providers agree to meet the covered medical needs of subscribers for a prepaid amount of money. For a fixed monthly fee, enrollees are given comprehensive health care with an emphasis on preventive health care. Enrollees receive their care from physicians, specialists, allied health professionals, and educators who are hired (group model) or contractually retained (network model) by the HMO.

Managed care, and HMOs in particular, was a reaction to the sharply climbing costs of health care that began in the 1980s. Businesses, which paid a large portion of health care costs through employee-benefit plans, complained that no one in the health care loop had an incentive to control costs. Employers complained that consumers paid only a deductible and a small copayment, giving them little cause to question prices; doctors faced little financial oversight; and insurance companies merely rubber-stamped the bills.

When HMOs presented an alternative, employers began offering their workers incentives to select HMOs over traditional fee-for-service coverage and thus attempted to rein in the runaway costs of health care. HMOs now cover nearly 70 million Americans. Increases in membership continued until 2000, when many HMOs that participated in Medicare supplement plans discontinued participation and, thus, discontinued service to their previously enrolled older adult members. The escalating cost of prescription medications was the principal factor in this decision. In all HMOs the annual cost of membership continues to rise, particularly for persons enrolled in the for-profit HMOs. This increase reflects the rising cost of services that must be provided to members.

HMOs are usually the least expensive but most restrictive type of managed care. The premiums are 8–10 percent lower than those for traditional plans, they charge no deductibles or coinsurance payments, and co-payments are $15–$20 per visit. However, you are limited to using the doctors and hospitals in the HMO's network, and you must get approval for treatments and referrals.

In theory, HMOs were to be the ideal blend of medical care and health promotion. Today, however, many observers are concerned that too many HMOs are being too tightly controlled by a profit motive in which physicians are being paid large bonuses to *not* refer patients to specialists or are prevented by "gag rules" from discussing certain treatment options with patients because of their costs to the HMOs.

Concerns, in addition to the "gag rules" mentioned above, have also arisen over the years. Among these have been concerns related to the right of members to sue their HMOs for medical negligence, the provision of better ob-gyn coverage, and the development of a more efficient mechanism to appeal denial of services. However, in the last regard, in 2004 the Supreme court ruled that HMO patients could not use more permissive state laws to sue HMOs for damages resulting from their refusal to approve particular medical services.

In spite of the problems just mentioned, HMOs remain, in theory, more cost-efficient than the tradiional fee-for-service healthcare model. Cost containment is achieved, in part, because most of the medical services within a group model HMO are centralized, there is little duplication of facilities, equipment, or support staff. Central filing of records gives all the HMO physicians access to a single file for each client. This saves time, administrative costs, and the overlapping of care. HMOs also routinely use health-promotion activities.[28]

Other new approaches to reducing health costs are independent practice associations (IPAs) and preferred provider organizations (PPOs). An IPA is a modified form of an HMO that uses a group of doctors who offer prepaid services out of their own offices and not in a central HMO facility. IPAs are viewed as "HMOs without walls." A PPO is a group of private practitioners who sell their services at reduced rates to insurance companies. When a policyholder chooses a physician who is in that company's PPO network, the insurance company pays the entire physician's fee, less the deductible and copay amounts. When a policyholder selects a non-PPO physician, the insurance company pays a smaller portion of that physician's fee. Today, more than 80 percent of Americans with health benefits are enrolled in a managed care plan (HMO, IPA, or PPO). In some areas of the country, such as California, Oregon, and Washington, over 90 percent of persons with benefits are in managed care plans.

Extended or Long-Term Care Insurance

With the aging of the population and the greater likelihood that nursing home care will be required (at nearly $61,665 per year in 2004 for a semi-private room), insurers have developed extended care policies.[29] When purchased at an early age (by mid-50s), these policies are much more affordable than if purchased when a spouse or family member will soon require institutional care. However, not all older adults will need extensive nursing home care, so an extended or long-term care policy could be an unnecessary expenditure.

Access to Health Care

With 45 million (or perhaps more) Americans lacking any health insurance and with nearly a quarter of those with insurance being underinsured, Americans are finding it increasingly difficult to access their country's highly sophisticated health care system. The unemployed poor, working poor, and minorities have the most difficulty accessing health care. African Americans, Hispanic Americans, and Native Americans have the worst health status of all Americans, yet they receive the fewest health care services. Even for older Americans with Medicare, gaping holes exist in the types of care covered (for example, glasses and hearing aids are not covered) and the prices of prescription medications far exceed the coverage provided. Thus, in America in the 21st century, its people are expressing growing concern about the extent to which their health care needs will be met. As political opposition remains strongly against a national health care system, the United States joins South Africa to make them the only two major industrialized nations lacking a comprehensive and unified approach to meeting the health care needs of their populations.

Health-Related Products

As you might imagine, prescription and over-the-counter (OTC) drugs constitute an important part of any discussion of health-related products.

Prescription Drugs

Caution: Federal law prohibits dispensing without prescription. This FDA warning appears on the labels of approximately three-fourths of all medications. Prescription drugs must be ordered for patients by a licensed practitioner. Because these compounds are legally controlled and may require special skills in their administration, the public's access to these drugs is limited.

Although the *Physicians' Desk Reference* lists more than 2,500 compounds that can be prescribed by a physician, only 200 drugs make up the bulk of the nearly 3,215 million new prescriptions and refills dispensed by online, mail-order, supermarket, mass-market, corporate, and independent pharmacies in 2003.[30] Total retail prescription sales of $203.1 billion for 2003 represents a 10 percent increase over the previous year's sales. This upward trend reflects in large part the greater variety of prescription medications being prescribed each year by physicians. It is projected that by the year 2012 approximately $446 billion will be spent on prescription medications.[31] The rapid expansion of online pharmacies now occurring is unlikely to influence the number of prescriptions filled, though their presence will likely affect the sales of "brick and mortar" drugstore chains.

Some consumers have fled the U.S. market altogether and chosen to purchase prescription medications in Canada, where prices are substantially lower. For example, a 90-day supply of the prescription drug Zocor, used to lower blood cholesterol, costs more than $350 at a typical American pharmacy; in Canada, a patient can purchase the same amount of the same medication for $140.

Research and Development of New Drugs

As consumers of prescription drugs, you may be curious about the process by which drugs gain FDA approval. The rigor of this process may be the reason that only about 100 new drugs are approved annually.

The nation's pharmaceutical companies constantly explore the molecular structure of various chemical compounds in an attempt to discover important new compounds with desired types and levels of biological activity. Once these new compounds are identified, companies begin extensive in-house research with computer simulations and animal testing to determine whether clinical trials with humans are warranted. Of the 125,000 or more compounds under study each year, only a few thousand receive such extensive preclinical evaluation. Even fewer of these are then taken to the FDA to begin the evaluation process necessary to gain approval for further research with humans. When the FDA approves a drug for clinical trials, a pharmaceutical company can obtain a patent, which prevents the drug from being manufactured by other companies for the next 17 years.

The $500 million price tag for bringing a new drug into the marketplace reflects this slow, careful process. If the 7 years of work needed to bring a new drug into the marketplace go well, a pharmaceutical company enjoys the remaining 10 years of legally protected retail sales. Today new "fast-track" approval procedures at the FDA are progressively reducing the development period, particularly for desperately needed breakthrough drugs like those used to treat AIDS. Concern was expressed in 2000 that this "rush to approval" forced the FDA to utilize the services of independent evaluators, many of whom had ties to the pharmaceutical industry that would have influenced their assessments of a drug's readiness for marketing.

A recent example of problems stemming from the FDA's approval process was seen in the later months of 2004 and the early months of 2005, when three extremely popular (and highly profitable) nonsteroidal anti-inflammatory drugs, used in the management of osteoarthritis, were called into question regarding their role in the development of heart disease. Of the three drugs in question (Vioxx, Celebrex, and Bextra), Vioxx was pulled from the market in September of 2004 when heart problems were reported among some longer-term users. Similar questions were quickly raised about Celebrex and Bextra, since all three drugs belong to the class of drugs called Cox-2 inhibitors. In response to rising levels of concern within the medical community and the general public, the FDA formed an advisory board to look at all safety-related information in the possession of the manufacturers. After three days of consideration, the 32-member advisory board issued its findings—all three drugs were deemed safe enough for continue sales. New concern immediately arose, however, when it was learned that 10 of the 32 board members had financial interests in one or both of the manufacturers of the medication under review.

Generic versus Brand Name Drugs

When a new drug comes into the marketplace, it carries three names: its **chemical name,** its **generic name,** and its **brand name.** While the 17-year patent is in effect, no other drug with the same chemical formulation can be sold. When the patent expires, other companies can manufacture a drug of equivalent chemical composition and market it under the brand name drug's original generic name. Because extensive research and development are unnecessary at this point, producing generic drugs is far less costly than is developing the original brand name drug. Nearly all states allow pharmacists to substitute generic drugs for brand name drugs, as long as the prescribing physician approves. For those interested in viewing all of the current approved generics, the FDA updates each month its Generic Drug Approvals list.[32]

 TALKING POINTS Your mother insists on using the brand-name drug that she has used for years to control her arthritis pain, even though her doctor has prescribed a generic version that has recently become available. What might you say to help her consider the less expensive option?

Today a variety of reference books are available to inform consumers about the availability of generic drugs and the prescription drugs that they can legally be substituted for. *Mosby's Drug Consult* series is highly recommended.[33]

Over-the-Counter Drugs

When people are asked when they last took some form of medication, for many the answer might be, "I took aspirin (or a cold pill, or a laxative) this morning." In making this decision, people engaged in self-diagnosis, determined a course for their own treatment, self-administered their treatment, and freed a physician to serve people whose illnesses are more serious than theirs. None of this would have been possible without readily available, inexpensive, and effective OTC drugs.

Although 2,500 prescription drugs are available, there are perhaps as many as 300,000 different OTC products, routinely classified into 26 different families. Like prescription drugs, nonprescription drugs are regulated by the FDA. However, for OTC drugs, the marketplace is a more powerful determinant of success.

The regulation of OTC drugs is based on a provision in a 1972 amendment to the 1938 Food, Drug, and Cosmetic Act. As a result of that action, OTC drugs were placed in three categories (I, II, and III) based on the safety and effectiveness of their active ingredient(s). Today, only category I OTC drugs that are safe, effective, and truthfully labeled are to be sold without a prescription. The FDA's drug-classification process also allows some OTC drugs to be made stronger and some prescription drugs to become nonprescription drugs by reducing their strength through reformulation.

Like the label shown in Figure 15-1, current labels for OTC products reflect FDA requirements. The labels must clearly state the type and quantity of active ingredients, alcohol content, side effects, instructions for appropriate use, warning against inappropriate use, and risks of using the product with other drugs (polydrug use). Unsubstantiated claims must be carefully avoided in advertisements of these products. In addition, under new labeling laws, following the controversy associated with Cox-2 medication, the use of Black Boxes will be required when it is known that OTC medications hold risks, particularly when used in combination with other medications. When used on a routine basis, OTC medications should be carefully discussed with a physician or a pharmacist.

> **Key Terms**
>
> **chemical name** name used to describe the molecular structure of a drug
>
> **generic name** common or nonproprietary name of a drug
>
> **brand name** specific patented name assigned to a drug by its manufacturer

Drug Facts

Active Ingredient (in each tablet)
Chlorpheniramine maleate 2 mg

Purpose
Antihistamine

Uses temporarily relieves these symptoms due to hay fever or other upper respiratory allergies:
■ sneezing ■ runny nose ■ itchy, watery eyes ■ itchy throat

Warnings

Ask a doctor before use if you have
■ glaucoma ■ a breathing problem such as emphysema or chronic bronchitis
■ trouble urinating due to an enlarged prostate gland

Ask a doctor or pharmacist before use if you are taking tranquilizers or sedatives

When using this product
■ you may get drowsy ■ avoid alcoholic drinks
■ alcohol, sedatives, and tranquilizers may increase drowsiness
■ be careful when driving a motor vehicle or operating machinery
■ excitability may occur, especially in children

If pregnant or breast-feeding, ask a health professional before use.
Keep out of reach of children. In case of overdose, get medical help or contact a Poison Control Center right away.

Directions

adults and children 12 years and over	take 2 tablets every 4 to 6 hours; not more than 12 tablets in 24 hours
children 6 years to under 12 years	take 1 tablet every 4 to 6 hours; not more than 6 tablets in 24 hours
children under 6 years	ask a doctor

Other information
■ store at 20-25° C (68-77° F) ■ protect from excessive moisture

Inactive ingredients D&C yellow no. 10, lactose, magnesium stearate, microcrystalline cellulose, pregelatinized starch

Figure 15-1 The FDA requires over-the-counter drugs to carry standardized labels, such as the one to the left.

Health Care Quackery and Consumer Fraud

A person who earns money by marketing inaccurate health information, unreliable health care, or ineffective health products is called a fraud, a **quack,** or a charlatan. **Consumer fraud** flourished with the old-fashioned medicine shows of the late 1880s. Unfortunately, consumer fraud still flourishes. You need look no further than large city newspapers to see questionable advertisements for disease cures and weight loss products. Quacks have found in health and illness the perfect avenues to indulge in **quackery**—to make maximum gain with minimum effort.

When people are in poor health, they may be afraid of becoming disabled or dying. So powerful are their desires to live and avoid suffering that people are vulnerable to promises of health improvement or a cure. Even though many people have great faith in their physicians, they also want access to experimental treatments or products touted as being superior to currently available therapies. When tempted by the promise of help, people sometimes abandon traditional medical care. Of course, quacks

Key Terms

quack a person who earns money by purposely marketing inaccurate health information, unreliable health care, or ineffective health products

consumer fraud marketing of unreliable and ineffective services, products, or information under the guise of curing disease or improving health; quackery

quackery the practice of disseminating or supplying inaccurate health information, unreliable health care, or ineffective health products for the purposes of defrauding another person

recognize this vulnerability and present a variety of "reasons" to seek their help (see Changing for the Better). Gullibility, blind faith, impatience, superstition, ignorance, or hostility toward professional expertise eventually carry the day. In spite of the best efforts of agencies at all levels, no branch of government can protect consumers from their own errors of judgment that so easily play into the hands of quacks and charlatans.

Regardless of the motivation that leads people into consumer fraud, the outcome is frequently the same. First, the consumer loses money. The services or products are grossly overpriced, and the consumers have little recourse to help them recover their money. Second, the consumers often feel disappointed, guilty, and angered by their own carelessness as consumers. Far too frequently, consumer fraud may lead to unnecessary suffering.

Taking Charge of Your Health

- Keep yourself well informed about current health issues and new developments in health care.
- Analyze the credibility of the health information you receive before putting it into practice.
- Select your health care providers by using a balanced set of criteria (see pages 402 and 406).

- Explore alternative forms of health care, and consider using them as a complement to traditional health care.
- In selecting a health care plan, compare various plans on the basis of several key factors, not simply cost (see page 412).
- Assemble a complete personal/family health history as soon as possible. Be sure

to include information from older family members.
- Comply with all directions regarding the appropriate use of prescription and OTC medications.

SUMMARY

- Sources of health information include family, friends, commercials, labels, the Internet, and information supplied by health professionals, as well as others.
- Physicians can be either Doctors of Medicine (MDs) or Doctors of Osteopathy (DOs). They receive similar training and engage in similar forms of practice.

- Although alternative health care providers, including chiropractors, naturopaths, herbalists, and acupuncturists, meet the health care needs of many people, systematic study of these forms of health care is only now under way.
- Restricted-practice health care providers play important roles in meeting the health and wellness needs of the public.

- Nursing at all levels is a critical health care profession. Advanced practice nurses represent the highest level of training within nursing.
- Self-care is often a viable approach to preventing illness and reducing the use of health care providers.
- Our growing inability to afford health care services has reached crisis proportions in the United States.
- More than 45 million Americans, not just the poor, have problems getting health care. Minorities have the most limited access to health care services of all Americans.
- Health insurance is critical to our ability to afford modern health care services.
- HMOs provide an alternative way of receiving health care services, although the influence of the profit motive in their operation is a concern.

- Medicare and Medicaid are governmental plans for paying for health care services.
- The development of prescription medication is a long and expensive process for pharmaceutical manufacturers. The cost of prescription medication is the most rapidly increasing aspect of health care affordability.
- OTC products have a role to play in the treatment of illness, but their safe use is based on following label directions.
- Critical health consumerism, including avoiding health quackery, requires careful selection of health-related information, products, and services.

REVIEW QUESTIONS

1. Determine how you would test the accuracy of the health-related information you have received in your lifetime.
2. Identify and describe some sources of health-related information presented in this chapter. What factors should you consider when using these sources?
3. Describe the similarities between allopathic and osteopathic physicians. What is an alternative health care practitioner? Give examples of the types of alternative practitioners.
4. What are the theories underlying acupuncture and ayurveda?
5. Describe the services that are provided by the following limited health care providers: dentists, psychologists, podiatrists, and optometrists. Identify several allied health care professionals. What levels of training and expertise exist within nursing?
6. In what ways is the trend toward self-care evident? What are some reasons for the popularity of this movement?
7. How do private, public, and voluntary (proprietary) hospitals differ.

8. What is health insurance? Explain the following terms relating to health insurance: deductible amount, fixed indemnity benefits, full-service benefits, coinsurance, exclusion, and preexisting condition.
9. What is a health maintenance organization? How do HMO plans reduce the costs of health care? What are IPAs and PPOs?
10. What do the chemical name, brand name, and generic name of a prescription drug represent? OTC drugs are approved for marketing on the basis of what three factors?
11. What role does Medicare and Medicaid play in meeting the health care needs of the American public? Which portion of Medicare is universal? What elective option does Medicare offer?
12. What are the three criteria that must be met by an OTC drug?
13. What is health quackery? What can a consumer do to avoid consumer fraud?

ENDNOTES

1. *Internet Health Resources.* Pew Internet & American Life Project. 2003. www.pewinternet.org/.
2. The National Council on the Aging. Media sources of health info. As reported in *USA Today.* 1999. 26 October, 9d.
3. Baker L, et al. Use of the Internet and e-mail for health care information: Results from a national survey. *JAMA.* 2003. 289(18):2400–2406.
4. Wagner TH, et al. Free internet access, the digital divide, and health information. *Med Care.* 2005. 43(4): 415–420.
5. Wagner TH, et al. Use of the Internet for health information by the chronically ill. *Prev Chronic Dis.* 2004. 1(4):A13. Epub 2004 September 15.
6. Sierpina VS. *Integrative Health Care: Complementary and Alternative Therapies for the Whole Person.* Philadelphia: F. A. Davis, 2001.
7. National Center for Complementary and Alternative Medicine. *About Chiropractic and Its Use in Treating Low-Back Pain.* Research Report. February 2004. www.nccam.nih. gov/health/chiropractic/chiropractic.pdf.
8. National Center for Complementary and Alternative Medicine. *Chiropractic Consortium Becomes OAM's Eleventh Research Center.* NIH News Release. March 1998. www. nccam.nih.gov/news/19972000/030398.htm.
9. National Center for Complementary and Alternative Medicine. *Acupuncture: Mechanism of Action.* September 2003. www.nccam.nih.gov/health/acupuncture/#nccam.
10. National Center for Alternative and Complementary Medicine. *Acupuncture.* December 2004. www.nccam.nih.gov/ health/acupuncture/.
11. Yang JH. The effects of foot reflexology on nausea, vomiting and fatigue of breast cancer patients undergoing chemotherapy. *Taehan Kanho Hakhoe Chi.* 2005. 35(1):177–185.
12. Siiev-Ner I, et al. Reflexology treatment relieves symptoms of multiple sclerosis: a randomized controlled study. *Mult Scler.* 2003. 9(4):356–361.

13. Kholler M. Children with ear disorders who are treated by reflexologists or general practitioners. *Ugeske Laeger.* 2003. 165(19):1994–1999.

14. National Center for Complementary and Alternative Medicine. *Questions and Answers about Homeopathy.* 2003. www.nih/gov/health/homeopathy/index.htm#al.

15. Jascobs J, et al. Homeopathy for menopausal symptoms in breast cancer survivors: A preliminary randomized controlled trial. *J Altern Complement Med.* 2005. 11(1):21–27

16. Shekelle PG, et al. Efficacy and safety of ephedra and ephedrine for weight loss and athletic performance: A meta-analysis. *JAMA.* 2003. 289(12):1537–1545.

17. FDA Statement. *FDA Announces Rule Prohibiting Sale of Dietary Supplements Containing Ephedrine Alkaloids Effective April 12.* April 12, 2004. www.fda.gov/bbs/topics/NEWS/2004/NEW01050.htm.

18. Department for Professional Employees. *Nurses: Vital Signs.* AFRL-CIO. 2004. www.dpeaflcio.org/policy/factsheets/fs_2004_nurses.htm.

19. Aiken LH, et al. Hospital nurse staffing and patient mortality, nurse burnout, and job satisfaction. *JAMA.* 2002. 288(16):1987–1993.

20. Sanders S. Is the glass half empty or full? Reflections on strain and gain in caregivers of individuals with Alzheimer's disease. *Soc Work Health Care.* 2005. 40(3):57–73.

21. National Coalition on Health Care. Health insurance coverage. 2004. www.nchc.org/facts/coverage.shtml.

22. U.S. Census Bureau. *National Health Expenditures by Type: 1900–2002 (No. 115).* Statistical Abstract of the United States: 2004–2005.

23. U.S. Census Bureau. *National Health Expenditures—Summary, 1960–2002, and Projections, 2003–2013 (No. 114).* Statistical Abstract of the United States: 2004–2005.

24. U.S. Census Bureau. *Health Services and Supplies—Per Capita Consumer Expenditures by Object: 1990 to 2002. (No. 117).* Statistical Abstract of the United States: 2004–2005.

25. Health Care Financing Administration. *Personal Health Care Expenditures Amounts, and Average Annual Percent Change, Percent Distribution, and Per Capita Amounts, by Source of Funds for Selected Calendar Years 1970–2007.* Table 2a. November 2000. www.chfa.gov/stats/NHE-proj/t02b.htm.

26. The Kaiser Family Foundation and Health Research and Education Trust. *Employer Health Benefits: 2004 Annual Survey.* 2004. www.kff.org.

27. Centers for Medicare & Medicaid Services. *Medicare and You—2005.* U.S. Department of Health and Human Services. 2005. Pub No. CMS-10050.

28. McKenzie JF, Pinger RR, Korwcki JE. *An Introduction to Community Health* (5th ed.). Boston: Jones and Bartlett.

29. The MetLife Mature Market Institute. *The MetLife Market Survey of Nursing Home & Home Care Costs—September 2005.* www.MatureMarketInstitute@metlife.com.

30. U.S. Census Bureau. *Retail Prescription Drug Sales: 1995–2003 (No. 122).* Statistical Abstract of the United States: 2004–2005.

31. Centers for Medicare & Medicaid Services. *National Health Care Expenditure Amounts, and Average Annual Percent of Change by Type of Expenditure (Table 2).* 2002. U.S. Department of Health and Human Services. www.hhs.gov/statistics/nhe/projections-2002/t2a.asp.

32. U.S. Food and Drug Administration. *Generic Drug Approvals.* 2005. Center for Drug Evaluation and Research. www.fda.gov/cder/ogd/approvals/default.htm.

33. *Drug Consult 2006: The Comprehensive Reference for Generic and Brand Name Drugs.* 2006. St. Louis: Mosby's Drug Consult, Mosby, 2006.

As We Go to Press

Does "wiring" a hospital make it a more effective institution for providers, patients, and families? A study was conducted that compared hospitals with highly developed computer accessibility to those with limited accessibility. Using data from a list of the 100 Most Wired Hospitals and similar data from hospitals not on the list, the study identified interesting differences in patient and physician practices. In the area of patient services, it found that patients able to access test results, renew prescriptions, schedule appointments, and request advice from physicians online were three to four times more likely to engage in these activities than patients who were required to use other means of communication. With respect to physicians, use of online access to clinical guidelines and the ability to order patient services (laboratory, radiography, and pharmacy) before patient admission, led these doctors to schedule such patient services two to three times more frequently than physicians who were required to use other modalities, such as the phone or fax.

Perhaps the most interesting observation involved patient surveillance by physicians using office or home computers in a secure manner. In those hospitals on the Most Wired Hospitals list, physicians used this technology to monitor patients in intensive care units, in postsurgical units, and on general medicine floors. Physicians who could monitor patients only via a telephone call or by direct observation were less inclined to engage in patient monitoring than were those in high-tech institutions.

personal assessment

Are you a skilled health consumer?

Circle the selection that best describes your practice. Then total your points for an interpretation of your health consumer skills.

1 Never
2 Occasionally
3 Most of the time
4 All of the time

1. I read all warranties and then file them for safekeeping.
   1   2   3   4
2. I read labels for information pertaining to the nutritional quality of food.
   1   2   3   4
3. I practice comparative shopping and use unit pricing, when available.
   1   2   3   4
4. I read health-related advertisements in a critical and careful manner.
   1   2   3   4
5. I challenge all claims pertaining to secret cures or revolutionary new health devices.
   1   2   3   4
6. I engage in appropriate medical self-care screening procedures.
   1   2   3   4
7. I maintain a patient-provider relationship with a variety of health care providers.
   1   2   3   4
8. I inquire about the fees charged before using a health care provider's services.
   1   2   3   4
9. I maintain adequate health insurance coverage.
   1   2   3   4
10. I consult reputable medical self-care books before seeing a physician.
    1   2   3   4
11. I ask pertinent questions of health care providers when I am uncertain about the information I have received.
    1   2   3   4
12. I seek second opinions when the diagnosis of a condition or the recommended treatment seems questionable.
    1   2   3   4
13. I follow directions pertaining to the use of prescription drugs, including continuing their use for the entire period prescribed.
    1   2   3   4
14. I buy generic drugs when they are available.
    1   2   3   4
15. I follow directions pertaining to the use of OTC drugs.
    1   2   3   4
16. I maintain a well-supplied medicine cabinet.
    1   2   3   4

YOUR TOTAL POINTS _____

Interpretation

16–24 points	A very poorly skilled health consumer
25–40 points	An inadequately skilled health consumer
41–56 points	An adequately skilled health consumer
57–64 points	A highly skilled health consumer

To Carry This Further . . .

Could you ever have been the victim of consumer fraud? What will you need to do to be a skilled consumer?

421

chapter sixteen

Protecting Your Safety

On completing this chapter, you will be able to:

▍ define the terms *intentional* and *unintentional injuries* and give three examples of each.

▍ discuss different types of domestic violence, including intimate partner violence, child maltreatment, and elder maltreatment.

▍ list some ways to reduce one's risk of becoming a victim of violent crime in your home, in your car, or on campus.

▍ explain the particular way guns contribute to violent crime statistics.

▍ name at least 5 groups who are targets of hate crimes.

▍ if you are male, list 5 things you can do to avoid perpetrating a date rape; if you are female, list 5 things you can do to reduce your risk of becoming a date rape victim.

▍ motor vehicle injuries are the leading cause of injury deaths in the United States. List 10 things you can do to reduce your risk of becoming seriously injured in a motor vehicle crash.

▍ compare the risk of a fatal injury occurring while riding a motorcycle to the risk of a fatal injury while riding in a car and explain the difference.

▍ list 10 things one can do to prevent injuries from occurring in the home.

▍ explain what identity theft is, and list several steps that you can take to protect yourself from it.

Eye on the Media

Terrorism on Television: The Tragedy of September 11/ The World Trade Center Disaster

Where were you on the morning of September 11, 2001? How did you hear the news about the terror attacks on New York and Washington? The entire nation stood stunned as TV cameras captured a passenger jet crashing into one of New York's twin towers, followed a few minutes later by a second plane that hit the second tower. Soon after, it was reported that a third plane had hit the Pentagon, and a fourth had crashed in a field in Pennsylvania.

Most of the day's horrors were captured by television cameras, as well as by a few film crews who happened to be filming in Manhattan that day. Americans watched in horror as networks played and replayed footage of each plane hitting the World Trade Center, and of the fires that ensued; they saw office workers running for their lives and witnessed firefighters and other rescue workers going back into buildings that were clearly unsound to guide people out of the burning towers. And finally, they saw the two towers crumble to the ground.

For three full days the major TV networks suspended their regular programming to cover the disaster in depth. No commercials, no sitcoms, no soap operas, and no David Letterman or Jay Leno for days. When Letterman returned to the air, it wasn't to tell jokes but to have Dan Rather talk about the tragic events, and viewers saw the normally staunch newsman's eyes fill with tears. When *Saturday Night Live* featured New York Mayor Rudolph Giuliani, it was as a respected guest, not as a target for a spoof. By Saturday morning the cartoons were back—for the children. In fact, many networks geared toward children— most notably PBS—tailored their programming to offer them more comforting fare, and provided special public service announcements advising parents on how to help their children feel safe despite their own uncertainty.

In the weeks and months that followed, the media helped provide a sense of unity to a vast, grieving nation. But the constant coverage of the tragedy and its aftermath— including footage of the attacks, and of rescue workers searching the rubble of Ground Zero for the bodies of their fallen comrades—took a toll on many people watching.

People lost sleep and felt depressed. Some worried about having to get on an airplane again. Young children had an especially difficult time—wondering why this happened and whether *they* would be victims of a terrorist attack. Some children touched buildings to make sure they were "safe" before going inside.

Today, Americans are acutely aware of the possibility of terror attacks on our soil. The international news media regularly report on anti-American sentiments in Middle Eastern countries. The Department of Homeland Security continually evaluates the national threat level, with a system ranging from Code Green (low) to Code Red (severe). When the national threat level was raised from Yellow (elevated) to Orange (heightened) in December

As recently as 25 years ago, the suspicious disappearance of a school-aged child or the death of a bystander during a drive-by shooting was virtually unheard of. However, violent crimes are committed so frequently in the United States that it is difficult to watch a television news report or read a newspaper without seeing headlines announcing some heinous murder or other senseless act of violence, including terrorist acts.

Although the overall crime rate has dropped in the last decade, domestic violence continues to be directed at women and children, and many people fear being a random victim of a homicide, robbery, or carjacking. Law enforcement officials contend that gang activities and hard-core drug involvement are significant factors related to continued violent behavior in our society.

Although violence may seem to be focused in urban areas, no community is completely safe. Even people who live in small towns and rural areas now must lock their doors and remain vigilant about protecting their safety. Crime on college campuses remains a threat for all students. (Complete the Personal Assessment on page 443 to see whether you are adequately protecting your own safety.)

Intentional Injuries

Intentional injuries are injuries that are committed on purpose. Except for suicide (which is self-directed), intentional injuries reflect violence committed by one person acting against another person. Examples include homicide, robbery, rape, assault, child abuse, spouse abuse, and elder abuse. Each year in the United States, intentional violence results in nearly 50,000 deaths and another 2 million nonfatal injuries.[1]

In 2003, more than 24 million crimes were committed against U.S. residents age 12 and older, according to data collected by the National Crime Victimization Survey. Of these, one in four (5.4 million) were violent crimes (rape, sexual assault, robbery, aggravated assault, and simple assault).[2] The good news is that these figures continue the downward trend in criminal victimization that began in 1994. The violent crime rate in 2003 was less than the rate in 1994.[3]

Homicide

Homicide, or murder, is the intentional killing of one person by another. The United States leads the industrialized world in homicide rates. The 2002 murder rate was 5.6 per 100,000 inhabitants. Fortunately, this rate reflected a decline since 1991, when the homicide rate was 9.8 per 100,000.[4]

Criminal justice experts are trying to pinpoint why U.S. homicide rates are dropping. No one answer has emerged, but speculation centers on better community policing efforts; the 1994 passage of the broad Federal Crime Bill; recent legislation, such as the Brady Law; and a variety of tough state laws, such as the "three strikes and you're out" provisions, that mandate life sentences without parole for repeat violent offenders. If recent incarceration rates do not change, an estimated 1 in 20 people (5.1 percent) will serve time in a state or federal prison. The chances of going to prison are higher for men (9 percent) than for women (1.1 percent).[5]

One continuing phenomenon is the extent to which illegal drug activity is related to homicide. A variety of research studies from large cities indicate that 25–50 percent of all homicides are drug related.[6] Most of these murders are associated with drug trafficking, including disputed drug transactions. Nationally, this figure is much lower; for 2003 only 4.6 percent of homicides were drug related.[7] Additionally, high percentages of both homicide assailants and victims have drugs in their systems at the time of the homicide.[6]

Key Terms

intentional injuries injuries that are purposely committed by a person

homicide the intentional killing of one person by another person

---

Handguns continue to be the weapon of choice for homicides. It was the proliferation of handguns and their use in violent crimes that led to the passage of the Brady Law.

Domestic Violence

Domestic violence refers to criminal acts of violence committed within a home or homelike setting by people that have some type of relationship with the victim. This text will discuss three forms of domestic violence: intimate partner violence, child maltreatment, and elder maltreatment.

Intimate Partner Violence

Intimate Partner Violence (IPV) refers to violence committed by a current or former spouse or boyfriend or girlfriend. IPV can include murder, rape, sexual assault, robbery, aggravated assault, and simple assault. Violent acts that constitute abuse range from a slap on the face to murder.

A 2001 report released by the Bureau of Justice Statistics revealed some slightly encouraging findings regarding IPV.[8] The report indicated that intimate nonlethal violence had declined 48 percent since 1993, from a rate of 5.8 nonfatal victimizations per 1,000 persons to just 3 per 1,000 persons. The rate of decline was greater for female victims (49 percent) than for male victims (42 percent). Two reasons have been proposed for the decline in intimate partner violence: better services for families at risk and an improved economy during the period covered by the report.[9] Actually, rates of IPV began to edge upward in 2001,[8] perhaps as a result of rising unemployment.

Murders by intimates in 2000 reached the lowest levels since 1976. In 2000 1,687 murders were reported among intimate partners, whereas nearly 3,000 such murders took place in 1976. As has been the case for many years, three of every four victims of intimate murder in 2000 were female.[8]

One serious issue related to domestic violence is the vast underreporting of this crime to law enforcement authorities. The U.S. Department of Justice estimates that about half of the survivors of domestic violence do not report the crime to police. Too many survivors view these violent situations as private or personal matters and not actual crimes. Despite painful injuries, many survivors view the offenses against them as minor.

It's easy to criticize the survivors of domestic violence for not reporting the crimes committed against them, but this may be unfair. Why do women stay in abusive relationships? Many women who are injured may fear being killed if they report the crime. They may also fear for the safety of their children. Women who receive economic support from an abuser may worry about being left with no financial resources.

Cell Phone Safety While Driving

Cell phones that fit easily into a pocket or purse are being used in every place imaginable, including restaurants, theaters, subways, parks, golf courses, and, of course, in cars. And it's in cars that the use of cellular phones is most controversial. A variety of studies and reports indicate a four- to nine-fold increase in the potential for car crashes associated with the driver's use of a cell phone. In July 2001, the state of New York passed the country's first *statewide ban* on the use of hand-held cellular phones while driving. Violators of this ban are subject to a $100 fine for the first offense. Since then, at least 24 other states have passed laws regulating cell phone use while operating a motor vehicle.

Research suggests the use of a cell phone decreases driver concentration and delays driver reaction time. The use of mounted, hands-free phones may improve safety, although the safety benefit has been controversial. Experts in traffic safety are careful to point out that there are too many other factors associated with driving to make it fair to blame behind-the-wheel phone use for all or most accidents. These complicating factors include adverse weather conditions, the structural integrity of the cars, the age and health of the drivers, radio, CD, or cigarette use, and interactions between drivers and passengers. The influence of other drivers on the road must also be considered.

If you must use your cell phone in a car, consider these common sense rules: Get off the main road to a safe parking area to make your call, especially if the call is an important one or one that might upset you. If you must talk while driving, opt for a hands-free phone. Dial when your car is stopped. Keep calls very brief. Don't try to dial or talk in heavy traffic. Keep your eyes on the road. (Or, let a passenger make the call!)

Source: Governors Highway Safety Association: Cell phone restrictions—state and local jurisdictions. 2003. www.statehighwaysafety.org/html/state_info/cellphone_laws.

However, help is available for victims of intimate abuse. Most communities have family support or domestic violence hot lines that abused people can call for help. Many have shelters where abused women and their children can seek safety while their cases are being handled by the police or court officials. If you are being abused or know of someone who is being injured by domestic violence, don't hesitate to use the services of these local hot

Key Terms

intimate partner violence (IPV) violence committed against a person by her or his current or former spouse, boyfriend, or girlfriend

lines or shelters. Also, check the resources listed in the Health Reference Guide at the back of this text.

 TALKING POINTS A close friend confides that her boyfriend sometimes "gets rough" with her. She's afraid to talk to him about it because she thinks that will make things worse. What immediate steps would you tell her to take?

Maltreatment of Children

Like intimate partner violence, **child maltreatment** tends to be a silent crime. It is estimated that nearly 1 million children are survivors of child abuse and neglect each year.[10] Some children are survivors of repeated crimes, and since many survivors do not report these crimes, the actual incidence of child abuse is difficult to determine.

Child maltreatment includes child abuse and child neglect. Children are abused in various ways. Physical abuse reflects physical injury, such as bruises, burns, abrasions, cuts, and fractures of the bones and skull. Sexual abuse includes acts that lead to sexual gratification of the abuser. Examples include fondling, touching, and various acts involved in rape, sodomy, and incest. Psychological abuse is another form of child abuse. Certainly, children are scarred by family members and others who routinely damage their psychological development. However, this form of abuse is especially difficult to identify and measure.

Child neglect is failure to provide a child with adequate clothing, food, shelter, and medical attention. The incidence of child neglect is approximately three times that of physical abuse and about seven times the incidence of child sexual abuse. Furthermore, child maltreatment deaths are more often associated with neglect than with any other type of abuse.[10] Educational neglect, such as failure to see that a child attends school regularly, is one of the most common types of child neglect. Each form of abuse can have devastating consequences for the child—both short term and long term.

Research studies in child abuse reveal some noteworthy trends. Abused children are much more likely than nonabused children to grow up to be child abusers. Abused children are also more likely to suffer from poor educational performance, increased health problems, and low levels of overall achievement. Recent research points out that abused children are significantly more likely than nonabused children to become involved in adult crime and violent criminal behavior. Finally, neglected children's rates of arrest for violence were almost as high as those for physically abused children.[11]

It is beyond the scope of this book to discuss the complex problem of reducing child maltreatment. However, the violence directed against children can likely be lessened through a combination of early identification measures and violence prevention programs. Teachers, friends,

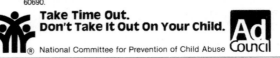

12 alternatives to lashing out at your child.

The next time everyday pressures build up to the point where you feel like lashing out—STOP! And try any of these simple alternatives.

You'll feel better . . . and so will your child.

1. Take a deep breath. And another. Then remember you are the adult . . .
2. Close your eyes and imagine you're hearing what your child is about to hear.
3. Press your lips together and count to 10. Or better yet, to 20.
4. Put your child in a time-out chair. (Remember the rule: one time-out minute for each year of age.)
5. Put yourself in a time-out chair. Think about why you are angry: Is it your child, or is your child simply a convenient target for your anger?
6. Phone a friend.
7. If someone can watch the children, go outside and take a walk.
8. Take a hot bath or splash cold water on your face.
9. Hug a pillow.
10. Turn on some music. Maybe even sing along.
11. Pick up a pencil and write down as many helpful words as you can think of. Save the list.
12. Write for parenting information: Parenting, Box 2866, Chicago, IL 60690.

Take Time Out. Don't Take It Out On Your Child.

National Committee for Prevention of Child Abuse

CHILD ABUSE PREVENTION CAMPAIGN
MAGAZINE AD NO. CA-2835-90—7" x 10"
Volunteer Agency: Lintas: Cambell-Ewald, Campaign Director: Beth M. Pritchard, S.C. Johnson & Son, Inc.

Figure 16-1 Alternatives to abusing your child

relatives, social workers, counselors, psychologists, police, and the court system must not hesitate to intervene as soon as child abuse is suspected. The later the intervention, the more likely that the abuse will have worsened. Once abuse has occurred, it is likely to happen again.

Violence prevention programs can help parents and caregivers learn how to resolve conflicts, improve communication, cope with anger, improve parenting skills, and challenge the view of violence presented in movies and television. Such programs may help stop violence before it begins to damage the lives of young children. Figure 16-1 provides simple alternatives parents can choose to avoid hitting a child.

Key Terms

child maltreatment the act or failure to act by a parent or caretaker that results in abuse or neglect of a child which places the child in imminent risk of serious harm

Maltreatment of Elders

Among the nation's 35 million elderly people, between 1 to 2 million, have been injured, exploited, or otherwise mistreated.[12,13] Particularly vulnerable are women over the age of 75 years. Nearly half of the abusers are the adult children of the victims, and 85 percent were family members.[14]

Many elderly people are hit, kicked, attacked with knives, denied food and medical care, and have their Social Security checks and automobiles stolen. This problem reflects a combination of factors, particularly the stress of caring for failing older people by middle-aged children who are also faced with the demands of dependent children and careers. In many cases, the middle-aged children were themselves abused, or there may be a chemical dependence problem. The alternative, institutionalization, is so expensive that it is often not an option for either the abused or the abusers.

Although protective services are available in most communities through welfare departments, elder abuse is frequently unseen and unreported. In many cases, the elderly people themselves are afraid to report their children's behavior because of the fear of embarrassment that they were not good parents to their children. Regardless of the cause, however, elder abuse must be reported to the appropriate protective service so that intervention can occur.

Violence at College

A recent report has summarized violent victimization of college students. Perhaps the most important finding was that college campuses are a relatively safe place to be. College students (ages 18–24 years) experience less violence than do nonstudents in the same age group. Violence rates have declined for both groups since 1995, when rates were 88 per 1,000 for college students and 102 per 1,000 for nonstudents. The 2002 rates are 41 and 56, respectively.[15]

During the period 1995–2002, simple assault (assault without a weapon) accounted for 63 percent of the violent victimizations, whereas rape/sexual assault accounted for 6 percent. Males were about twice as likely to be victims of violence as women were. About 93 percent of the crimes occurred off campus, 72 percent occurred at night, and 41 percent of victims perceived that the offenders were using alcohol or drugs at the time of the offense.[15]

Gangs and Youth Violence

In the last 30 years, gangs and gang activities have been increasingly responsible for escalating violence and criminal activity. Before that time, gangs used fists, tire irons, and, occasionally, cheap handguns ("Saturday night specials"). Now, gang members don't hesitate to use AK-47s (semiautomatic military assault weapons)

that have the potential to kill large groups of people in a few seconds.

The gang problem is most persistent in cities of greater than 25,000 population, where 66 percent of gang members live.[16] Here, socially alienated and economically disadvantaged youth come to believe that society has no significant role for them. So, they seek support from an association of peers that has well-defined lines of authority. Rituals and membership initiation rites are important in gang socialization. Gangs often control particular territories within a city. Frequently, gangs are involved in criminal activities, commonly illicit drug trafficking, and robberies.

Gangs and youth violence also occur in the suburbs. Sixty-one percent of large suburbs (greater than 100,000 population) reported gang activity. Only 13 percent of small cities and 7 percent of rural jurisdictions reported gang activity.[16]

Attempting to control gang and youth violence is expensive for communities. For every gang-related homicide, there are about 100 nonfatal gang-related intentional injuries, so gang violence becomes an expensive health-care proposition. Furthermore, gang and youth violence takes an enormous financial and human toll on law enforcement, judicial, and corrections departments. Reducing gang and youth violence is a daunting task for the nation.

Gun Violence

The tragic effect of gun violence has already been touched on throughout this chapter. Guns are being used more than ever in our society. Gun violence is a leading killer of American teenagers and young men, especially African American men, and the use of semiautomatic assault weapons by individuals and gang members continues. The fatality rate for gun injuries is 30 percent, much higher than the fatality rate for injuries of all causes (less than 1 percent).[17] Colleges and universities are not immune to gun violence. A recent study reported that 4.3 percent of college students had a working firearm at college; of these, nearly half stated that they had a gun for protection.[18] Accidental deaths of toddlers and young children from loaded handguns are another dimension of the violence attributable to guns in our society. In addition, guns are often used in **carjackings** (see Changing for the Better on page 428).

Key Terms

carjacking a crime that involves a thief's attempt to steal a car while the owner is behind the wheel; carjackings are usually random, unpredictable, and frequently involve handguns

---

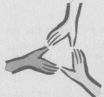

Learning from Our Diversity

Violence against the Disabled

No one is totally free from the risk of senseless violence—children, adults, or college students. No single group, however, is a more tragic target of violence than the disabled. Despite the protective efforts of laws such as the Fair Housing Amendments Act, the Americans with Disabilities Act, and the Rehabilitation Act, the disabled remain an easily victimized segment of the population.

Because of the high level of vulnerability that disabled persons face, national advocacy groups, such as All Walks Of Life, are working to assist the disabled, their caregivers, and the general population in reducing the risk of violence to this group. However, much can also be accomplished on an individual basis. If you are an able-bodied college student, you can probably implement the following suggestions on your campus:

- Encourage your disabled peers to remain vigilant by staying tuned in to their environment. Remind them that simply because they appear disabled does not guarantee that they will be protected from harm.
- Support your disabled friends in the challenges imposed by their limitations, particularly when they are in unfamiliar environments or experiencing unusual situations.
- Suggest that your peers with disabilities carry, or wear a personal alarm device. Such devices, also frequently carried by

able-bodied students, can be purchased in bookstores or sporting goods stores.

- Remind your disabled friends to inform others about their schedule plans, for example, when they will be away from school and when they are likely to return.
- Encourage people with disabilities to seek the assistance of an escort (security personnel) when leaving a campus building or a shopping mall to enter a large parking area.
- Be an advocate for your disabled friends. For example, if residence hall room doors do not have peepholes at wheelchair height, find out if the doors can be modified.

One additional approach remains controversial. That is the teaching of self-defense techniques to people with disabilities. Groups that advocate instruction to the disabled in the martial arts, such as judo, remind us that "doing nothing will produce nothing." Others contend that a limited ability to use a martial art leads to a false sense of confidence that encourages a disregard for other forms of protection. They further argue that if disabled persons try to counter aggression with ineffectively delivered martial arts techniques, they may anger their attacker and actually increase the aggression against themselves.

The growing use of firearms has prompted serious discussions about enactment of gun control laws. For years, gun control activists have been in opposition with the National Rifle Association (NRA) and its congressional supporters. Gun control activists want fewer guns manufactured and greater controls over the sale and possession of handguns. Gun supporters believe that such controls are not necessary and that people (criminals) are responsible for gun deaths, not simply the guns. This debate will certainly continue.

 TALKING POINTS At a campus talk on carjacking, one college student announced that he planned to carry a registered gun to protect himself. How would you respond to his position?

Bias and Hate Crimes

One sad aspect of any society is how some segments of the majority treat certain people in the minority. Nowhere is this more obvious than in **bias and hate crimes.** These crimes are directed at individuals or groups of people solely because of a racial, ethnic, religious, or other difference attributed to these minorities. The targeted individuals

are often verbally and physically attacked, their houses are spray painted with various slurs, and many are forced to move from one neighborhood or community to another.

According to Federal Bureau of Investigation (FBI) statistics, there are about 8,000 hate crime incidents in the United States each year. In 2003 more than half (52.3 percent) of all hate crimes were motivated by racial bias, followed by religious bias (16.4 percent), sexual orientation bias (16.4 percent), ethnic/national origin bias (14.2 percent), and disability bias (0.5 percent).[19]

Typically, the offenders in bias or hate crimes are fringe elements of the larger society who believe that the mere presence of someone with a racial, ethnic, sexual

Key Terms

bias and hate crimes criminal acts directed at a person or group solely because of a specific characteristic, such as race, religion, sexual orientation, ethnic background, disability, or other difference

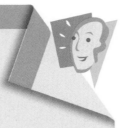
orientation, religious difference, or disability is inherently bad for the community, state, or country. Examples in the United States include skinheads, the Ku Klux Klan, and other white supremacist groups. (The case of Matthew Shepard—see the Star box on page 429—drew worldwide attention to hate crimes.) Increasingly, state and federal laws have been enacted to make bias and hate crimes serious offenses.

Road Rage

Within recent years, a phenomenon called "road rage" has been on the rise on the streets and highways of the United States. This violence occurs when a driver becomes enraged at the driving behavior of others—cutting off someone, driving too slowly, going through yellow lights and red lights, playing loud music, passing a long line of cars on the shoulder, playing "chicken" as two lanes merge into one. Toss in horn-honking, four-letter words, and hand gestures, and you have all the elements of the daily commuter.

Sometimes road rage has deadly results. It's not unusual for road ragers to force other cars into accidents. Since some drivers carry guns, they may injure or kill other drivers. These tragedies usually are not premeditated. They often happen when a driver loses control under the pressure of a triggering incident.

There is no typical profile of a person who expresses road rage. Although road ragers are frequently young adult, aggressive males, road rage can be displayed by anyone who drives and is stressed by time constraints, family problems, or job difficulties. One quick way to determine if you are prone to road rage is to tape record your voice while you're driving. If you hear yourself screaming and complaining, you could be considered an aggressive driver. You will need to find ways to calm yourself during your commute.

To avoid becoming a perpetrator or a victim of road rage, follow these recommendations:

- Avoid making hand gestures
- Use your horn sparingly
- Allow plenty of time to reach your destination
- Imagine yourself being videotaped while driving
- Avoid blocking the passing lane
- Avoid switching lanes without signaling
- Use only one parking place
- Avoid parking in a space for disabled people, unless you are disabled
- Refrain from tailgating
- Do not allow your door to hit the parked car next to you
- If you drive slowly, pull over and let others pass
- Avoid the unnecessary use of high-beam headlights
- Do not talk on a car phone while driving
- Avoid making eye contact with aggressive drivers
- Keep your music volume under control

Always drive defensively. Assume that a difficult situation may get out of hand, so conduct yourself in a calm, courteous manner. It's better to swallow your pride and preserve your health than to risk unnecessary danger to yourself or other people on the road.

 TALKING POINTS You're in a car with a friend when another driver starts tailgating you very closely. Your friend (the driver) slows down to annoy the tailgater. How would you convince your friend that his action is dangerous?

Violence Based on Sexual Orientation

Recent news reports indicate that violence based on sexual orientation continues to occur in the United States. Nowhere is this more clear than in the case of Matthew Shepard, an openly gay University of Wyoming freshman who was murdered in October 1998. Shepard was lured from a Laramie, Wyoming, bar by two young adult men posing as homosexuals. These men beat Shepard severely, stole $20 from him, and tied him to a fence post, where he was left to die. The men were later convicted of kidnapping and murder.

In July 1999, Barry Winchell, an Army private at Fort Campbell, Kentucky, was bludgeoned to death with a bat wielded by fellow private Calvin Glover. Glover, who said he was intoxicated when he committed the crime, was later convicted of premeditated murder in a military court and sentenced to life in prison, with the possibility of parole. Another soldier, charged as an accessory to the crime, apparently had spread rumors among members of the Army unit that Winchell was gay. This accomplice also tried to clean up the scene of the crime. He was sentenced to 12 years in prison.

The murder of Private Winchell prompted calls for a reevaluation of the military's 1993 "don't ask, don't tell" policy concerning homosexuals. Under this policy, gays can serve in the military as long as they do not disclose their sexual orientation. Superiors in the military cannot investigate or expel personnel who keep their sexual orientation to themselves. Some believe this "don't ask, don't tell" policy prevents military authorities from investigating complaints of harassment based on sexual orientation. This policy came up in the year 2000 presidential campaign and could be revised in the future.

Both of these deaths served as a reminder that the federal government has not yet passed the Hate Crimes Prevention Act. This proposed legislation would add acts of hatred motivated by sexual orientation, gender, and disability to the list of hate crimes already covered by federal law. Among these crimes already covered are ones motivated by prejudice based on race, religion, color, or national origin.

It will be interesting to see whether this proposed federal legislation will be enacted soon. The public outcry following the deaths of Matthew Shepard and Barry Winchell indicates that much support exists for some version of a Hate Crimes Prevention Act.

Stalking

In recent years the crime of stalking has received considerable attention. **Stalking** refers to an assailant's planned efforts to pursue an intended victim. Most stalkers are male. Many stalkers are excessively possessive or jealous and pursue people with whom they formerly had a relationship. Other stalkers pursue people with whom they have had only an imaginary relationship.

Stalkers often go to great lengths to locate their intended victims and frequently know their daily whereabouts. Although not all stalkers plan to batter or kill the person they are pursuing, their presence and potential for violence can create an extremely frightening environment for the intended victim and family. Some stalkers serve time in prison for their offense, waiting years to "get back at" their victims.

Virtually all states have enacted or tightened their laws related to stalking and have created stiff penalties for offenders. In many areas the criminal justice system is proactive in letting possible victims of stalking know, for example, when a particular prison inmate is going to be released. In other areas, citizens are banding together to provide support and protection for people who may be victims of stalkers. It should not come as a surprise that stalking occurs on college campuses. About 13 percent of college women are stalked in a given year.[20]

If you think you are or someone you know is being stalked, contact the police (or a local crisis intervention hot line number) to report your case and follow their guidance. Be on the alert if someone from a past relationship suddenly reappears in your life or if someone seems to be irrationally jealous of you or overly obsessed with you. Report anyone who continues to pester or intimidate you with phone calls, notes or letters, e-mails, or unwanted gifts. Report people who persist in efforts to be with you after you have told them you don't want to see them. Until the situation is resolved, be alert for potentially threatening situations and keep in close touch with friends. (Discovering Your Spirituality on page 430 deals with the question of dealing with fear in our lives.)

TALKING POINTS You suspect that someone is stalking you, but your friends think you're being dramatic. How would you get objective advice on what to do?

Key Terms

stalking a crime involving an assailant's planned efforts to pursue an intended victim

Your elderly neighbor stays locked in her house all day, afraid to open the door to anyone. Too many hours of watching local TV news, you think. But it's not just older people who are living in fear. Parents, women, gays, and minorities are all looking over their shoulders.

Some parents who walked to school when they were children wouldn't think of letting their kids do that. What about child molesters and kidnappers? A young woman at a party guards her drink all night—afraid that someone might put a drug in it. She's afraid of being raped. The gay person who goes to his old neighborhood to visit his grandmother feels uneasy. Is it his imagination, or are people looking at him in a threatening way? An African American man walking down the street hears a racial slur. Should he ignore it, or stop and say something?

All these situations call for caution. If you're a parent, you need to be careful about your child's safety. But your child can walk to school—accompanied by you, another parent, or an older child. If you're a woman, you can keep an eye on your drink at a party without making that the focus of your attention. If you're a gay man who feels uncomfortable in an unfamiliar part of town, stay focused on where you're going. Walk quickly and confidently, without being intimidated. If you're a minority who's being taunted, keep your dignity and remain calm.

Putting fear in perspective takes practice. First, stay reasonable. Recognize that acts of violence represent the extreme elements of society. There's a good reason you probably haven't met many (or any) murderers, robbers, or rapists. They make up a small segment of society. The people you usually encounter, who are basically good, represent the large majority. Second, be aware. Pay attention to what's going on around you. See things in a neutral way. If you do, you'll realize when an argument is about to turn into a fistfight or worse. Third, use common sense. Don't put yourself at risk, but don't stop living. You can't build your life around avoiding a potential act of violence. Fourth, trust your senses. If someone is walking too close to you and you feel uncomfortable, cross the street and go into a store. Last, practice what-if situations. For example, what would you do if you were in your car at a stoplight and someone held a gun up to your window? Considering your possible actions ahead of time, without dwelling on them, is one way of preparing yourself for real-life threats.

Living in fear is something that happens gradually—as fear takes control of a person's life. But that doesn't need to happen to you. You can take control of fear in a healthy, positive way—to build a life of rich experiences balanced by caution and good sense.

Sexual Victimization

Ideally, sexual intimacy is a mutual, enjoyable form of communication between two people. Far too often, however, relationships are approached in an aggressive, hostile manner. These sexual aggressors always have a victim—someone who is physically or psychologically traumatized. *Sexual victimization* occurs in many forms and in a variety of settings. This section takes a brief look at sexual victimization as it occurs in rape and sexual assault, sexual abuse of children, sexual harassment, and the commercialization of sex.

Rape and Sexual Assault

As violence in our society increases, the incidence of rape and sexual assault correspondingly rises. The victims of these crimes fall into no single category. Victims of *rape* and *sexual assault* include young and old, male and female. They can be the mentally retarded, prisoners, hospital patients, and college students. We all are potential victims, and self-protection is critical.

Table 16.1 covers some of the myths and facts relating to rape.

Sometimes a personal assault begins as a physical assault that turns into a rape situation. Rape is generally considered a crime of sexual aggression in which the victim is forced to have sexual intercourse. Current thought about rape characterizes this behavior as a violent act that happens to be carried out through sexual contact. (See the Changing for the Better boxes on pages 432 and 433 on rape awareness guidelines and help for the rape survivor.)

Acquaintance and Date Rape

In recent years, closer attention has been paid to the sexual victimization that occurs during relationships. *Acquaintance rape* refers to forced sexual intercourse between individuals who know each other. *Date rape* is a form of acquaintance rape that involves forced sexual intercourse by a dating partner. Studies on a number of campuses suggest that about 20 percent of college women reported having experienced date rape but a recent report issued by the Bureau of Justice Statistics puts the figure at about 3 percent per year. This figure includes completed and attempted rapes.[20] A higher percentage of women report being kissed and touched against their will. Alcohol is frequently a significant contributing factor in these rape situations. (See Chapter 8 concerning alcohol's role in campus crime.) Some men have reported being psychologically coerced into intercourse by their female dating partners. In many cases the aggressive partner will display

Table 16.1 Rape: Myth versus Fact

Only women are raped.	Nearly 10% of rape victims (19,670) in 2003 were males.
Most rapists are strangers.	Seventy-four percent of male victims and 70% of female victims describe the offender as a nonstranger (intimate, other relative, or friend/acquaintance).
Most rapes occur in streets, alleys, and deserted places.	Ninety percent of rapes occur in living quarters—60% in the victim's residence.
Rapists are easily identified by their demeanor or psychological profile	Most experts indicate that rapist do not differ significantly from nonrapists.
Rape is an overreported crime.	Only one in five rapes is reported.
Rape happens only to people in low socioeconomic classes.	Rape occurs in all socioeconomic classes. Each person, male or female, young or old, is a potential victim.
There is a standard way to avoid rape.	Each rape situation is different. No single method to avoid rape can work in every potential rape situation. Because of this we encourage personal health classes to invite speakers from a local rape prevention services bureau to discuss approaches to rape prevention.

certain behaviors that can be categorized (see Changing for the Better on page 433).

Psychologists believe that aside from the physical harm of date rape, a greater amount of emotional damage may occur. Such damage stems from the concept of broken trust. Date rape victims feel particularly violated because the perpetrator was not a stranger: it was someone they initially trusted, at least to some degree. Once that trust is broken, developing new relationships with other people becomes much more difficult for the date rape victim.

Nearly all victims of date rape seem to suffer from *posttraumatic stress syndrome.* They may have anxiety, sleeplessness, eating disorders, and nightmares. Guilt concerning their own behavior, loss of self-esteem, and judgment of other people can be overwhelming, and the individual may require professional counseling. Because of the seriousness of these consequences, all students should be aware of the existence of date rape.

Date Rape Drugs

As you may recall from Chapter 7, Rohypnol, GHB (liquid ecstasy, G), and ketamine (K, Special K, and Cat) have joined alcohol as forms of date rape intoxicants. For their own safety, students must be vigilant about being duped into consuming substances that increase the likelihood of sexual assault and violence.

Sexual Abuse of Children

One of the most tragic forms of sexual victimization is the sexual abuse of children. Children are especially vulnerable to sexual abuse because of their dependent relationships with parents, relatives, and caregivers (such as babysitters, teachers, and neighbors). Often, children are unable to readily understand the difference between appropriate and inappropriate physical contact. Abuse may range from blatant physical manipulation, including fondling, to oral sex, sodomy, and intercourse.

Because of the subordinate role of children in relationships involving adults, sexually abusive practices often go unreported. Sexual abuse can leave emotional scars that make it difficult to establish meaningful relationships later in life. For this reason, it is especially important for people to pay close attention to any information shared by children that could indicate a potentially abusive situation. Most states require that information concerning child abuse be reported to law enforcement officials.

Sexual Harassment

Sexual harassment consists of unwanted attention of a sexual nature that creates embarrassment or stress. Examples of sexual harassment include unwanted physical contact, excessive pressure for dates, sexually explicit humor, sexual innuendos or remarks, offers of job advancement based on sexual favors, and overt sexual assault. Unlike more overt forms of sexual victimization, sexual harassment may be applied in a subtle manner and can, in some cases, go unnoticed by coworkers and fellow students. Still, sexual harassment produces stress that cannot be resolved until the harasser is identified and forced to stop. Both men and women can be victims of sexual harassment.

Sexual harassment can occur in many settings, including employment and academic settings. On the college campus, harassment may be primarily in terms of the offer of sex for grades. If this occurs to you, think carefully about the situation and document the specific times, events, and places where the harassment took place. Consult your college's policy concerning harassment. Next, you could report these events to the appropriate administrative officer (perhaps the affirmative action officer, dean of academic affairs, or dean of students). You may also want to discuss the situation with a staff member of the university counseling center.

If harassment occurs in the work environment, the victim should document the occurrences and report them to the appropriate management or personnel official. Reporting procedures will vary from setting to setting. Sexual harassment is a form of illegal sex discrimination and violates Title VII of the Civil Rights Act of 1964.

In 1986 the U.S. Supreme Court ruled that the creation of a "hostile environment" in a work setting was sufficient evidence to support the claim of sexual harassment. This action served as an impetus for thousands of women to step forward with sexual harassment allegations. Additionally, some men are also filing sexual harassment lawsuits against female supervisors.

Not surprisingly, this rising number of complaints has served as a wake-up call for employers. From university settings to factory production lines to corporate board rooms, employers are scrambling to make certain that employees are fully aware of actions that could lead to a sexual harassment lawsuit. Sexual harassment workshops and educational seminars on harassment are now common and serve to educate both men and women about this complex problem.

Violence and the Commercialization of Sex

It is beyond the scope of this book to explore whether sexual violence can be related to society's exploitation or commercialization of sex. However, sexually related products and messages are intentionally placed before the public to try to sway consumer decisions. Do you believe that there could be a connection between commercial products, such as violent pornography in films and magazines, and violence against women? Does prostitution lead directly to violence? Do sexually explicit "900" phone numbers or Internet pornography cause an increase in violent acts? Can the sexual messages in beer commercials lead to acquaintance rape? What do you think?

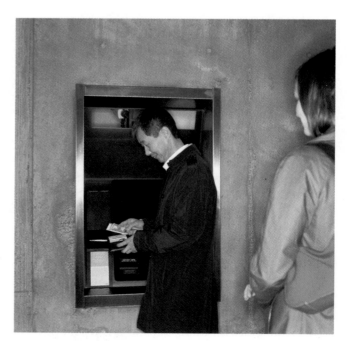

Being aware of your surroundings when using an ATM is important for personal safety.

Avoiding Date Rape

I've heard that there are warning signs for date rape. What signs should I be alert for?

First, consider your partner's behaviors. Many, but not all, date rapists show one or more of the following behaviors: a disrespectful attitude toward you and others, lack of concern for your feelings, violence and hostility, obsessive jealousy, extreme competitiveness, a desire to dominate, and unnecessary physical roughness. Consider these behaviors as warning signs for possible problems in the future. Reevaluate your participation in the relationship.

Following are some specific ways both men and women can avoid a date rape situation:

Men

- *Know your sexual desires and limits.* Communicate them clearly. Be aware of social pressures. It's OK not to score.
- *Being turned down when you ask for sex is not a rejection of you personally.* Women who say no to sex are not rejecting the person; they are expressing their desire not to participate in a single act. Your desires may be beyond control, but your actions are within your control.
- *Accept the woman's decision.* "No" means "No." Don't read other meanings into the answer. Don't continue after you are told "No!"
- *Don't assume that just because a woman dresses in a sexy manner and flirts that she wants to have sexual intercourse.*

Help for the Rape Survivor

If I should be in a position to help someone who has been raped, what information do we both need to know?

- *Call the police immediately to report the assault.* Police can take you to the hospital and start gathering information that may help them apprehend the rapist. Fortunately, many police departments now use specially trained officers (many of whom are female) to work closely with rape victims during all stages of the investigation.
- If you do not want to contact the police immediately, *call a local rape crisis center.* Operated generally on a 24-hour hot line basis, these centers have trained counselors to help the survivor evaluate her options, contact the police, escort her to the hospital, and provide aftercare counseling.

- *Don't assume that previous permission for sexual contact applies to the current situation.*
- *Avoid excessive use of alcohol and drugs.* Alcohol and other drugs interfere with clear thinking and effective communication.

Women

- *Know your sexual desires and limits.* Believe in your right to set those limits. If you are not sure, STOP and talk about it.
- *Communicate your limits clearly.* If someone starts to offend you, tell him so firmly and immediately. Polite approaches may be misunderstood or ignored. Say "No" when you mean "No."
- *Be assertive.* Often men interpret passivity as permission. Be direct and firm with someone who is sexually pressuring you.
- *Be aware that your nonverbal actions send a message.* If you dress in a sexy manner and flirt, some men may assume you want to have sex. This does not make your dress or behavior wrong, but it is important to be aware of a possible misunderstanding.
- *Pay attention to what is happening around you.* Watch the nonverbal clues. Do not put yourself into vulnerable situations.
- *Trust your intuitions.* If you feel you are being pressured into unwanted sex, you probably are.
- *Avoid excessive use of alcohol and drugs.* Alcohol and other drugs interfere with clear thinking and effective communication.

- *Do not alter any potential evidence related to the rape.* Do not change your clothes, douche, take a bath, or rearrange the scene of the crime. Wait until all the evidence has been gathered.
- *Report all bruises, cuts, and scratches, even if they seem insignificant.* Report any information about the attack as completely and accurately as possible.
- *You will probably be given a thorough pelvic examination.* You may have to ask for STD tests and pregnancy tests.
- Although it is unusual for a rape victim's name to appear in the media, you might *request that the police withhold your name* as long as is legally possible.

Identity Theft

Identity theft has been on the rise since the early 1990s. Thieves use falsely obtained names, addresses, and social security numbers to open credit card accounts and bank accounts, purchase cell phone services, and secure loans to buy automobiles and other big-ticket items. They

Key Terms

identity theft a crime involving the fraudulent use of a person's name, social security number, credit line, or other personal financial or identifying information

Reducing Your Risk for Identity Theft

The Federal Trade Commission outlines several steps to minimize your risk for identity theft:

- Order a copy of your credit report from each of the three major credit bureaus, and review it carefully to make sure it's accurate.

- Place passwords on your credit card, bank, and phone accounts. Avoid obvious passwords such as birthdays, mother's maiden name, or social security numbers.

- Keep personal information in your home secure. Be vigilant about guarding your mail and your trash; consider using a document shredder when discarding sensitive papers like credit card bills. Make sure your home computer has firewall protection.

- Ask about information security procedures in your workplace or at your school.

- Carefully read all your bills to make sure that you recognize all purchases and charges.

- Do not give out your personal information. Be especially wary of e-mail and phone solicitations requesting such information.

- Watch your wallet. Be wary of pickpockets, and carry only the identification and credit cards you need. Do not carry your social security card with you unless it is absolutely necessary.

- If you are a victim of identity theft, visit the FTC's Web site (www.consumer.gov/idtheft/) for valuable information on how to file a complaint and restore your credit.

Source: Federal Trade Commission. *ID Theft: When Bad Things Happen to Your Good Name.*

---

might even avoid paying taxes by working under false social security numbers, or use your identity for other purposes—if they are arrested, for example. Identity thefts can drain a person's bank account and ruin their credit rating before a person knows they've become a victim. Often the crime is not discovered until a person wants to make a major purchase—such as a house or a car—which requires a credit check.

There are several steps that you can take to avoid becoming a victim of identity theft. The most important step involves ordering copies of your credit reports each year to make sure that there are no fraudulent accounts in your name.[21] Other steps are outlined in the Star box.

Unintentional Injuries

Unintentional injuries are injuries that have occurred without anyone intending that any harm be done. Common examples include injuries resulting from car crashes, falls, fires, drownings, firearm accidents, recreational accidents, and residential accidents. Each year, unintentional injuries account for about 100,000 deaths and 27 million visits to hospital emergency departments.[22]

Unintentional injuries are very expensive for our society, both from a financial standpoint and from a personal and family standpoint. Fortunately, to a large extent it is possible to avoid becoming a victim of an unintentional injury. By carefully considering the tips presented in the safety categories that follow, you will be protecting yourself from many preventable injuries.

Since this section of the chapter focuses on a selected number of safety categories, we encourage readers to consider some additional, related activities. For further infor-

mation in the area of safety, consult a safety textbook. Finally, we encourage you to take a first aid course from the American Red Cross or the National Safety Council. These first aid courses incorporate a significant amount of safety prevention information along with the teaching of specific first aid skills.

Residential Safety

Many serious accidents and personal assaults occur in dorm rooms, apartments, and houses. As a responsible adult, you should make every reasonable effort to prevent these tragedies from happening. One good idea is to discuss some of the following points with your family or roommates and implement needed changes:

- Fireproof your residence. Are all electrical appliances and heating and cooling systems in safe working order? Are flammable materials safely stored?

- Prepare a fire escape plan. Install smoke or heat detectors.

- Do not give personal information over the phone.

- Use initials for first names on mailboxes and in phone books.

- Install a peephole and deadbolt locks on outside doors.

Key Terms

unintentional injuries injuries that have occurred without anyone's intending that harm be done

---

- If possible, avoid living in first floor apartments. Change locks when moving to a new apartment or home.
- Put locks on all windows.
- Require repair people or delivery people to show valid identification.
- Do not use an elevator if it is occupied by someone who makes you feel uneasy.
- Be cautious around garages, laundry rooms, and driveways (especially at night). Use lighting for prevention of assault.

Recreational Safety

The thrills we get from risk-taking are an essential part of our recreational endeavors. But a significant number of injuries occur in recreational settings. Bicycle riding accounted for 411,000 emergency department visits in 2002.[22] Some injuries occur because we fail to consider important recreational safety information. Do some of the following recommendations apply to you?

- Seek appropriate instruction for your intended activity. Few skill activities are as easy as they look.
- Always wear your automobile safety belt.
- Make certain that your equipment is in excellent working order. Use specific safety gear designed for cycling, in-line skating, and scooter use.
- Involve yourself gradually in an activity before attempting more complicated, dangerous skills.
- Enroll in an American Red Cross first aid course to enable you to cope with unexpected injuries.
- Remember that alcohol use greatly increases the likelihood that people will get hurt.

- Protect your eyes from serious injury.
- Learn to swim. Drowning occurs most frequently to people who never intended to be in the water.
- Obey the laws related to your recreational pursuits. Many laws are directly related to the safety of the participants.
- Be aware of weather conditions. Many outdoor activities turn to tragedy with sudden shifts in the weather. Always prepare yourself for the worst possible weather.

Firearm Safety

In 2003, 29,730 people died of firearm injuries in the United States. Of these, 16,859 were firearm-related suicides, 11,599 died as a result of homicides committed with a firearm, another 752 died from firearm-related accidents, 394 died from legal intervention, and 197 died from discharged firearms where intent was not determined.[23] Most murders are committed with handguns. (Shotguns and rifles tend to be more cumbersome than handguns and thus are not as frequently used in murders, accidents, or suicides.) Over half of all murders result from quarrels and arguments between acquaintances or relatives. With many homeowners arming themselves with handguns for protection against intruders, it is not surprising that over half of all gun accidents occur in the home. Children are frequently involved in gun accidents, often after they discover a gun they think is unloaded. Handgun owners are reminded to adhere to the following safety reminders:

- Consider every gun to be a loaded gun, even if someone tells you it is unloaded.
- Never point a gun at an unintended target.
- Keep your finger off the trigger until you are ready to shoot.

Wearing proper safety gear—including a helmet—is an essential safety measure when biking or skating. Obeying traffic laws and using proper hand signals are equally important.

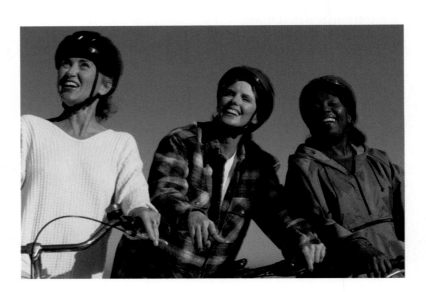

- When moving with a handgun, keep the barrel pointed down.
- Store your gun and ammunition safely in a locked container. Use a trigger lock on your gun when not in use.
- Never play with guns at parties. Never handle a gun when intoxicated.
- Make certain that your gun is in good mechanical order.
- Take target practice only at approved ranges.
- Load and unload your gun carefully.
- If you are a novice, enroll in a gun safety course. Gun safety courses are not the same as hunter safety courses. Your local police, sheriff, or fire department may offer such a course.
- Educate children about gun safety and the potential dangers of gun use. Children must never believe that a gun is a toy.
- Make certain that you follow the gun possession laws in your state. Special permits may be required to carry a handgun.

Motor Vehicle Safety

The greatest number of injury deaths in the United States take place on highways and streets. Young people (ages 16–24 years) are more likely to be involved in a fatal motor vehicle crash than persons of any other age. (Figure 16-2). The most dangerous time to drive is the period 12 A.M. to 3 A.M. Saturdays and Sundays.[24]

Motor vehicle accidents also cause disabling injuries. With nearly 2 million such injuries each year, concern for the prevention of motor vehicle accidents should be important for all college students, regardless of age. With this thought in mind, we offer some important safety tips for motor vehicle operators:

- Make certain that you are familiar with the traffic laws in your state.
- Do not operate an automobile or motorcycle unless it is in good mechanical order. Regularly inspect your brakes, lights, and exhaust system.
- Do not exceed the speed limit. Observe all traffic signs.
- Always wear safety belts, even on short trips. Require your passengers to buckle up. Always keep small children in child restraints.
- Never drink and drive. Avoid horseplay inside a car.
- Be certain that you can hear the traffic outside your car. Keep the car's radio/music system at a reasonable decibel level.
- Give pedestrians the right-of-way.
- Drive defensively at all times. Do not challenge other drivers. Refrain from drag racing.
- Look carefully before changing lanes.
- Be especially careful at intersections and railroad crossings.
- Carry a well-maintained first aid kit that includes flares or other signal devices.
- Alter your driving behavior during bad weather.
- Do not drive when you have not had enough sleep.
- Avoid distractions such as food, drink, cell phone use, and conversations with passengers. (See Star Boxes on pages 424 and 437.)

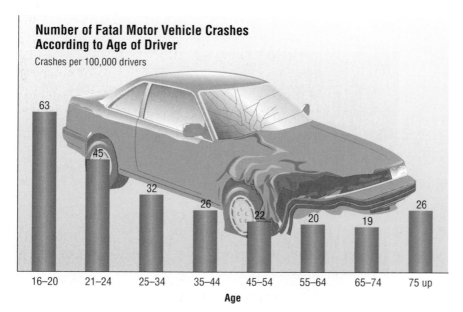

Number of Fatal Motor Vehicle Crashes According to Age of Driver

Crashes per 100,000 drivers

Age	
16–20	63
21–24	45
25–34	32
35–44	26
45–54	22
55–64	20
65–74	19
75 up	26

Figure 16-2 Driving is a dangerous activity for those under age 25. What could be done to reduce the number of driving fatalities among this age group?

Max Jones was a very popular youth soccer coach who was tragically killed when his car accidentally left the road while he was driving to an early morning practice. His family, his players, and their parents were all devastated when they heard the news. It was only later, after the funeral, when several of Max's close friends were chatting, that someone mentioned how Max would drive with a cup of coffee between his legs. Then another friend noted that Max had a habit of picking up fast food on his way to soccer practice. He would sometimes eat a breakfast sandwich and drink coffee while driving. His friends began to wonder whether if these distractions could have contributed to Max's crash.

A recent research study found that drivers are distracted an average of 16% of the time with activities that take their attention away from the road and their driving environment. Activities such as manipulating vehicle controls (air conditioning or windows), music/audio controls or talking to a child or baby in the car distracted drivers. Approximately three-fourths of those observed ate or drank something. Searching or reaching for an object while driving was also observed in a majority of the drivers who were observed. Forty percent were observed reading, writing, or grooming while the vehicle was moving.

To lower your risk of injuring yourself or others, avoid distractions while driving. Do not eat or drink while driving. If you are driving alone, make sure you have all of the vehicle's controls set appropriately before you embark on your trip. Use highway rest stops wisely to eat, read maps, arrange music, and reorganize the inside of your car so that you won't be distracted while at the wheel.

Source: Stutts J, Feaganes J, Rodgman E, Hamlett C, Meadows T, Reinfurt D, Gish K, Mercadante M, Staplin L. Distractions in Everyday Driving. Washington, DC: AAA Foundation for Traffic Safety, 2003.

Home Accident Prevention for Children and the Elderly

Approximately 1 person in 10 is injured each year at home. Children and the elderly spend significantly more hours each day at home than do young adults and adults. It is especially important that injury prevention be given primary consideration for these groups (see Changing for the Better on page 438). Here are some important tips to remember. Can you think of others?

For Everyone

- Be certain that you have adequate insurance protection.
- Install smoke detectors appropriately.
- Keep stairways clear of toys and debris. Install railings.
- Maintain electrical and heating equipment.
- Make certain that inhabitants know how to get emergency help.

For Children

- Know all the ways to prevent unintentional poisoning.
- Use toys that are appropriate for the age of the child.
- Never leave young children unattended, especially infants.
- Keep any hazardous items (guns, poisons, and so on) locked up.
- Keep small children away from kitchen stoves.

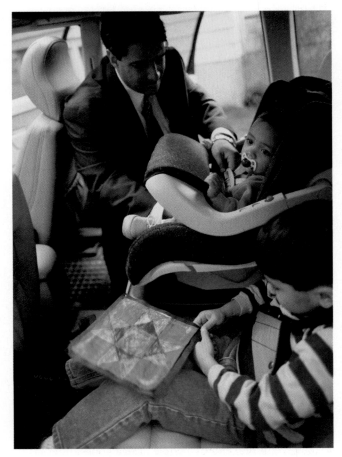

Consistent use of safety restraints during childhood can help make buckling up a lifelong habit.

Making Your Home Safe, Comfortable, and Secure

I take a common sense approach to safety, but I worry sometimes that I haven't thought about something important. What's the basic checklist for different areas?

Entry

- Install a deadbolt lock on the front door and locks or bars on the windows.
- Add a peephole or small window in the front door.
- Trim bushes so burglars have no place to hide.
- Add lighting to the walkway and next to the front door.
- Get a large dog.

Bedroom and Nursery

- Install a smoke alarm and a carbon monoxide detector.
- Remove high threshold at doorway to avoid tripping.
- Humidifiers can be breeding grounds for bacteria; use them sparingly and follow the manufacturer's cleaning instructions.
- In the nursery, install pull-down shades or curtains instead of blinds with strings that could strangle a child.

Living Room

- Secure loose throw rugs or use ones with nonskid backing.
- Remove trailing wires where people walk.
- Cover unused electrical outlets if there are small children in the home.
- Provide additional lighting for reading, and install adjustable blinds to regulate glare.

Kitchen

- To avoid burns, move objects stored above the stove to another location.
- Install ceiling lighting and additional task lighting where food is prepared.
- Keep heavy objects on bottom shelves or countertops; store lightweight or seldom-used objects on top shelves.
- Promptly clean and store knives.
- Keep hot liquids such as coffee out of children's reach, and provide close supervision when the stove or other appliances are in use.
- To avoid foodborne illness, thoroughly clean surfaces that have come into contact with raw meat.

Bathroom

- A child can drown in standing water; keep the toilet lid down and the tub empty.
- Clean the shower, tub, sink, and toilet regularly to remove mold, mildew, and bacteria that can contribute to illness.
- Store medications in their original containers in a cool, dry place out of the reach of children.
- Add a bath mat or nonskid strips to the bottom of the tub.
- Add grab bars near the tub or shower and toilet, especially if there are elderly adults in the home.
- Keep a first-aid kit stocked with bandages, first-aid ointment, gauze, pain relievers, syrup of Ipecac, and isotonic eyewash; include your physician's and a nearby emergency center's phone numbers.

Stairway

- Add a handrail for support.
- Remove all obstacles or stored items from stairs and landing.
- Repair or replace flooring material that is in poor condition.
- Add a light switch at the top of the stairs.
- If there is an elderly person in the home, add a contrasting color strip to the first and last steps to identify the change of level.

Fire Prevention Tips

- Install smoke detectors on every level of your home.
- Keep fire extinguishers handy in the kitchen, basement, and bedrooms.
- Have the chimney and fireplace cleaned by a professional when there is more than $1/4$ inch of soot accumulation.
- Place space heaters at least 3 feet from beds, curtains, and other flammable objects.
- Don't overload electrical outlets, and position drapes so that they don't touch cords or outlets.
- Recycle or toss combustibles, such as newspapers, rags, old furniture, and chemicals.
- If you smoke, use caution with cigarettes and matches; never light up in bed.
- Plan escape routes and practice using them with your family.

For the Elderly

- Protect from falls.
- Be certain that elderly people have a good understanding of the medications they may be taking. Know the side effects.
- Encourage elderly people to seek assistance when it comes to home repairs.
- Make certain that all door locks, lights, and safety equipment are in good working order.

Campus Safety and Violence Prevention

Although many of the topics in this chapter are unsettling, students and faculty must continue to lead normal lives in the campus environment despite potential threats to our health. The first step in being able to function adequately is knowing about these potential threats. You have read about these threats in this chapter; now you must think about how this information applies to your campus situation.

The campus environment is not immune to many of the social ills that plague our society. At one time the university campus was thought to be a safe haven from the real world. Now there is plenty of evidence to indicate that significant intentional and unintentional injuries can happen to anyone at any time on the college campus.

For this reason, you must make it a habit to think constructively about protecting your safety. In addition to the personal safety tips presented earlier in this chapter, remember to use the safety assistance resources available on your campus. One of these might be your use of university-approved escort services, especially in the evenings as you move from one campus location to another. Another resource is the campus security department (campus police). Typically, campus police have a 24-hour emergency phone number. If you think you need help, don't hesitate to call this number. Campus security departments frequently offer short seminars on safety topics to student organizations or residence hall groups. Your counseling center on campus might also offer programs on rape prevention and personal protection.

If you are motivated to make your campus environment safer, you might wish to contact an organization that focuses on campus crime. Safe Campuses Now is a nonprofit student group that tracks legislation, provides educational seminars, and monitors community incidents involving students. For information about Safe Campuses Now, including how to start a chapter on your campus, call (706) 354-1115, or see their Web page at www.uga.edu\~safe-campus. We encourage you to become active in making your campus a safer place to live.

Taking Charge of Your Health

- Use the Personal Assessment on page 443 to determine how well you manage your own safety.

- Assess your behaviors and those of your dating partners for signs of potential date rape by reviewing "Avoiding Date Rape" on page 433.

- Check your residence for the safety strategies listed on page 438. Make the necessary changes to correct any deficiencies.

- Review the motor vehicle safety tips on page 436. If you need to make changes to your car or your driving, begin working on them at once.

- Check the recommendations for recreational safety on page 435 and put them into practice. Be assertive about using these measures when you are participating in activities with others.

- Find out about the security services available on your campus, and take advantage of them. Post the 24-hour-help phone number in your room and carry it with you.

- Minimize your risk for identity theft by taking the steps outlined on page 434.

SUMMARY

- Everyone is a potential victim of violent crime.
- Each year in the United States, intentional injuries cause nearly 50,000 deaths and another 2 million nonfatal injuries.
- The homicide rate in the United States has declined significantly since the 1960s.
- Domestic violence includes intimate partner violence, child maltreatment, and elder maltreatment.
- Forms of child maltreatment include child abuse and child neglect. Child neglect is more common than child abuse.
- Youth violence and gang activity are serious social problems, especially in large cities.
- Gun violence continues to be a major contributor to the fatal injury statistics.
- Hate crimes are crimes motivated by bias against other races, religions, ethnicities, or sexual orientation.
- Rape, sexual assault, and sexual harassment are forms of sexual victimization in which victims are often both physically and psychologically traumatized.
- Unintentional injuries are injuries that occur without anyone intending that harm to be done.
- More people die from unintentional injuries than from intentional injuries.
- Motor vehicles are the leading cause of unintentional injury deaths.

REVIEW QUESTIONS

1. Identify some of the categories of intentional injuries. How many people are affected each year by intentional injuries?
2. What are some of the most important facts concerning homicide in the United States? How are most homicides committed?
3. Identify the three types of domestic violence discussed in the chapter.
4. What reasons might explain why so many people do not report domestic violence?
5. Aside from the immediate consequences of child maltreatment, what additional problems do many abused and neglected children face in the future?
6. Explain why gangs and gang activities continue to plague our large cities. How do gang activities lower the quality of life in communities?
7. List some examples of groups that are known to have committed bias or hate crimes.
8. Identify some general characteristics of a typical stalker.
9. Explain some of the myths associated with rape. How can date rape be prevented?
10. Identify some examples of behaviors that could be considered sexual harassment. Why are employers especially concerned about educating their employees about sexual harassment?
11. Identify some common examples of unintentional injuries.
12. List some places where unintentional injuries occur. Point out three safety tips from each of the safety areas listed at the end of this chapter.
13. Identify some precautions you can take to reduce your risk of becoming involved in a fatal motor vehicle crash.
14. In what ways can individuals minimize their risk for identity theft?

ENDNOTES

1. Center for Disease Control and Prevention, National Center for Injury Prevention and Control, WISQARS (Web-based Injury Surveillance Query and Reporting Systems), March 7, 2005, www.cdc.gov/ncipc/wisqars.
2. Bureau of Justice Statistics. *National Crime Victimization Survey: Criminal Victimization 2003*. U.S. Department of Justice, NCJ 205455, September 2004.
3. Bureau of Justice Statistics. U.S. Department of Justice, Office of Justice Programs, *National Crime Victimization Survey Violent Crime Trends, 1973–2003*, www.ojp.usdoj. gov/bjs/glance/tables/viortrdtab.htm.
4. Bureau of Justice Statistics. *Homicide Trends in the U.S., Long-Term Trends*, U.S. Department of Justice, Office of Justice Programs, November 2004, www.ojp.usdoj.gov/ bjs/homicide/tables/totalstab.htm.
5. Bureau of Justice Statistics. *Criminal Offenders Statistics: Lifetime Likelihood of Going to State or Federal Prison*, U.S. Department of Justice, November 2000.
6. Bureau of Justice Statistics. U.S. Department of Justice, Office of Justice Programs, *Homicide Trends in the United States*, November 21, 2002.
7. Bureau of Justice Statistics. U.S. Department of Justice, Office of Justice Programs, *Drug Use and Crime*, January 2005, www.ojp.usdoj.gov/bjs/dcf/duc.htm.
8. Bureau of Justice Statistics. U.S. Department of Justice, Office of Justice Programs, *Crime Data Brief, Intimate Partner Violence, 1993–2001*, NCJ 197838, February 2003.
9. McKenzie JF, Pinger RR, Kotecki JF. *An Introduction to Community Health* (5th ed.). Boston: Jones & Bartlett, 2005.
10. United States Department of Health and Human Services, Administration of Children, Youth and Families. *Child Maltreatment 2002*. Washington, DC: U.S. Government Printing Office, 2004, www.acf.hhs.gov/programs/cb/ publications/cm02/cm02.pdf.
11. National Institute of Justice. *The Cycle of Violence Revisited*. Washington, DC: U.S. Department of Justice, Office of Justice Programs, NIJ, Research in Progress Seminar Series, February 1996.
12. U.S. Census Bureau. *The 65 Years and Over Population: 2000, Census 2000 Brief*. U.S. Department of Commerce, Economics and Statistics Administration, 2001, www. census.gov/prod/2001pubs/c2kbr01-10.pdf.
13. National Research Council. *Elder Mistreatment: Abuse, Neglect, and Exploitation in an Aging America*. Washington, DC: The National Academies Press, 2003.
14. Office for Victims of Crime, Statistical Overviews. *Elder Abuse and Neglect*. Washington, DC: U.S. Department of Justice, Office of Justice Programs, 2001, www.ojp.usdoj. gov/ovc/ncvrw/2001/stat_over_7.htm.
15. Bureau of Justice Statistics. *Special Report: Violent Victimization of College Students, 1995–2002*. Washington, DC: U.S. Department of Justice, Office of Justice Programs, NCJ 206836, January 2005.
16. Office of Juvenile Justice and Delinquency Prevention. *OJJDP Fact Sheet: National Youth Gang Survey Trends from 1996 to 2000*. Washington, DC: U.S. Department of Justice, Office of Justice Programs, 2002.
17. Centers for Disease Control and Prevention. *Surveillance for Fatal and Nonfatal Firearm-Related Injuries—United States, 1993–1998. Morbidity and Mortality Surveillance Summaries* 50(ss02):1–32, 2001.
18. Miller M, Hemenway D, Wechsler H. Guns and Gun Threats at College. *J AM Coll Hlth* 51(2):57–65.
19. Federal Bureau of Investigation. *Hate Crime Statistics— 2003*. Washington, DC: November 2004, www.fbi.gov/ucr/ 03hc.pdf.
20. National Institute of Justice. *The Sexual Victimization of College Women*. U.S. Department of Justice, Bureau of Justice Statistics, Washington, DC, 2001.

21. Federal Trade Commission. ID THEFT: When bad things happen to your good name. www.consumer.gov/idtheft/index.html 2002.

22. National Safety Council. *Injury Facts, 2004 Edition.* Itasca, IL, 2004.

23. Hoyert DL, Kung HC, Smith BL. *Deaths: Preliminary Data for 2003.* National Vital Statistics Reports 53(15):1–48.

24. National Highway Traffic Safety Administration. *Traffic Safety Facts 2003.* Washington, DC, U.S. Department of Transportation. DOT HS 809 775, 2005.

As We Go to Press

Every person should be aware of the steps to take to guard against identity theft, but sometimes when it occurs it is beyond an individual's control. In October 2004, it was revealed that the database of 'ChoicePoint Inc., a national provider of identification and credential verification services,' had been breached. In February 2005, the company announced that personal information of as many as 145,000 people had been compromised. By March 2005, new information came forth that this was not the first time ChoicePoint Inc. had been victimized by criminals.

Consumers concerned about whether such a security breach may have harmed their credit rating can contact one of the major credit rating companies—Equifax, Experian, or Transunion. These companies usually offer a free trial period, or they may provide help in case you have had your identity stolen.

personal assessment

How well do you protect your safety?

This quiz will help you measure how well you manage your personal safety. For each item below, circle the number that reflects the frequency with which you do the safety activity. Then, add up your individual scores and check the interpretation at the end.

3   I regularly do this
2   I sometimes do this
1   I rarely do this

1. I am aware of my surroundings and do not get lost.
   3   2   1
2. I avoid locations in which my personal safety could be compromised.
   3   2   1
3. I intentionally vary my daily routine (such as walking patterns to and from class, parking places, and jogging or biking routes) so that my whereabouts are not always predictable.
   3   2   1
4. I walk across campus at night with other people.
   3   2   1
5. I am careful about disclosing personal information (address, phone number, social security number, my daily schedule, etc.) to people I do not know.
   3   2   1
6. I carefully monitor my alcohol intake at parties.
   3   2   1
7. I watch carefully for dangerous weather conditions and know how to respond if necessary.
   3   2   1
8. I do not keep a loaded gun in my home.
   3   2   1
9. I know how I would handle myself if I were to be assaulted.
   3   2   1
10. I maintain adequate insurance for my health and my property.
    3   2   1
11. I keep emergency information numbers near my phone.
    3   2   1
12. I keep my first aid skills up-to-date.
    3   2   1
13. I use deadbolt locks on the doors of my home.
    3   2   1
14. I use safety locks on the windows at home.
    3   2   1
15. I check batteries used in my home smoke detector.
    3   2   1
16. I have installed a carbon monoxide detector in my home.
    3   2   1

17. I use adequate lighting in areas around my home and garage.
    3   2   1
18. I have the electrical, heating, and cooling equipment in my home inspected regularly for safety and efficiency.
    3   2   1
19. I use my car seat belt.
    3   2   1
20. I drive my car safely and defensively.
    3   2   1
21. I keep my car in good mechanical order.
    3   2   1
22. I keep my car doors locked.
    3   2   1
23. I have a plan of action if my car should break down while I am driving it.
    3   2   1
24. I use appropriate safety equipment, such as flotation devices, helmets, and elbow pads, in my recreational activities.
    3   2   1
25. I can swim well enough to save myself in most situations.
    3   2   1
26. I use suggestions for personal safety each day.
    3   2   1

TOTAL POINTS _____

Interpretation
Your total may mean that:

72–78 points	You appear to carefully protect your personal safety.
65–71 points	You adequately protect many aspects of your personal safety.
58–64 points	You should consider improving some of your safety-related behaviors.
Below 58 points	You must consider improving some of your safety-related behaviors.

To Carry This Further . . .
Although no one can be completely safe from personal injury or possible random violence, there are ways to minimize the risks to your safety. Scoring high on this assessment will not guarantee your safety, but your likelihood for injury should remain relatively low. Scoring low on this assessment should encourage you to consider ways to make your life more safe. Refer to the text and this assessment to provide you with useful suggestions to enhance your personal safety. Which safety tips will you use today?

chapter seventeen

The Environment and Your Health

Eye on the Media

Hype versus Useful Information

An obscure scientist, an expert in an arcane subdiscipline of climatology, stands in front of his peers at a scientific conference and predicts a major shift in global climate. His warnings are brushed off by the powers-that-be. Within a month there are several massive polar hurricanes encircling the northern hemisphere of Earth. Within the following two weeks, the northern half of the United States is buried under ice and uninhabitable. Ten of millions of Americans are dead from storms and temperatures that dip to $-150°$ F. The survivors have moved to Mexico, probably permanently. Within two hours, *The Day After Tomorrow* has brought the complex, long-term process of global climate change to a tidy storyline conclusion. Television pundits predict the movie will raise public awareness of this looming environmental problem. A few weeks later the issue has fallen off the public radar.

"The Media" is one of the most powerful forces in American society, and its influence extends across most of the Earth's human population. As large multinational corporations have come to control many media producers, information and news are increasingly being filtered for their entertainment value. That which is deemed sufficiently interesting to be entertaining is often hyped, with the most titillating aspects repeated over and over. Information that is deemed uninteresting is simply ignored.

The "entertainment filter" of many media producers often does not interact well with issues of environmental health. Many environmental problems are complex and affect human health in subtle ways over long time periods. For example, likely effects of global climate change include expansion of tropical diseases into more northern latitudes, increased frequency of droughts and heat waves, gradual depletion of freshwater supplies, and extinctions of many species that cannot adapt to the changes. Compared to killer super polar storms and massive glaciers that appear in two weeks, these real-life issues have entertainment value similar to watching grass grow. The U.S. population is being exposed to hundreds, if not thousands of chemicals that have not been tested for human toxicity. They are found in our air, water, and food supply. They are found in our body fluids and hair. Some have been shown to cause cancer and birth defects in experimental animals. The U.S. Environmental Protection Agency estimates that air pollution in major U.S. cities contributes to thousands of deaths due to respiratory and cardiovascular disease each year. In the last 20 to 30 years, cancer rates in the U.S. population have increased substantially, while fertility of men as measured by sperm counts has been declining by 1–3 percent per year. When was the last time you heard anything about these issues on the evening news or read about them in a newspaper or magazine?

On the positive side, it has never been easier to obtain information about environmental health issues. The Internet provides a widely accessible means to obtain information on any topic. Just type a few words into the Google search line and you have more information at your finger tips than you can handle. Detailed reports from the U.S. Environmental Protection Agency and Centers for Disease Control can be copied from their Web sites to your computer in seconds.

When you "Google" an environmental health issue you need to exercise some judgment about what you read. Environmental advocacy groups, industrial groups, liberal and conservative think tanks all have their Web presence, where they promote their perspectives. The mainstream news media has self-correcting mechanisms; when someone makes inaccurate statements in public, someone else exposes the mistake. Similar mechanisms have not yet been fully developed for the Internet. When an industry group or environmental group criticizes some change in environmental regulations, you need to understand their motivations to assess the validity of their claims.

Another weakness of replacing professional news outlets with self-directed information searches on the Internet is that you need to know there is something you want to research before the process can even begin. If the mainstream news media is not talking about environmental health issues, how will you know what to type in the Google search line? We tend to seek information about topics that concern us. Without adequate news coverage we remain ignorant, blissfully or otherwise. As our lives become progressively more complex and busy, we rely more heavily on the news media to help us identify issues of importance. When news is screened for its entertainment value, environmental health issues are often ignored on the evening news. By the time an environmental health issue becomes "entertaining," the damage is often already done. No wonder that "The Environment" is not perceived as a high-priority issue when we elect our leaders.

Environmental issues are important concerns for many college-age students as they perceive disturbing trends that may affect their future health and well-being. News programs regularly present the latest bad news about over-population, pollution, global warming, damage to the ozone layer, loss of wilderness to economic exploitation, and endangered species. Movies such as *Water World, Blade Runner, Batman, The Matrix,* and *The Day After Tomorrow* depict fictional futures that are dismal environmental disasters. Some college students join environmental organizations that work to clean up litter, encourage recycling, regulate pollution, control human population growth, and protect endangered species and natural areas. Others feel there is nothing they can do about such monumental environmental issues. They lose hope for a future where the world will be a good place to live and raise a family, and may become depressed and apathetic. The impact of the environment on your health depends on the nature of your environment and your personal responses to that environment.

Your **environment** includes a range of conditions that can influence your health, such as the availability of resources (oxygen, water, food) and environmental characteristics, such as temperature, humidity, toxins, allergens, pathogens, noise, and radiation. Conditions in your environment operate across a wide range of spatial scales, from the air immediately surrounding your body to the global earth, air, and ocean system. Your physical health is influenced primarily by your *personal environment,* comprised of conditions in the home, neighborhood, and workplace, including indoor air, drinking water, toxic building materials and noise. This personal environment is influenced by conditions in the larger *community* and *regional environment,* including such conditions as air pollution and water pollution. These local and regional conditions are influenced by conditions of the *global environment,* such as climate and solar radiation.

The goal of this chapter is to help you identify aspects of your environment that can significantly affect your health, and to suggest ways that you can exert personal control over these environmental influences. Different environmental conditions and personal responses will be important at the various spatial scales (home/workplace, community/region, and global). Figure 17-1 displays some environmental problems at various spatial scales, and a range of personal responses that might be appropriate at each level.

The Personal Environment: Home, Neighborhood, Workplace

On average you spend about 90 percent of your time in your home, workplace, local stores, and entertainment venues.[1] The indoor air you breathe, the water you drink from the tap, and the radiation and noise in your immediate surroundings are environmental factors that have the most direct impact on your health. Some indoor environmental

---

Key Terms

environment the physical conditions (temperature, humidity, light, presence of substances) and other living organisms that exist around your body

Figure 17-1 Spatial scales of environmental health risks and appropriate personal responses to environmental problems

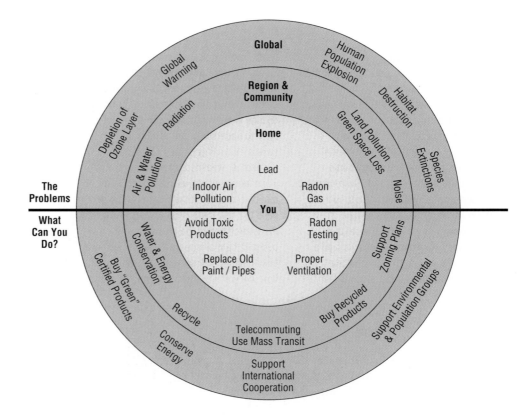

problems cause immediate health effects, such as headaches, dizziness, nausea, or allergic reactions. Other environmental problems act in subtle, cumulative ways, causing major health problems such as cancer or neurological damage that may not become apparent until permanent damage is done.

Of all the different environmental influences on your health, you have the greatest control over factors in your personal environment. You are responsible for maintaining your appliances so that they do not produce excessive air pollution. You control the ventilation in your home, allowing you to vent pollutants outside. You choose which products you will purchase, and can avoid products that contain toxic chemicals. You can eliminate tobacco smoke from your home and workspace. You can identify sources of health risk in the workplace and notify those responsible for environmental safety.

Indoor Air Quality

Indoor air quality within buildings can be influenced by a wide range of factors, including ventilation, humidity, gases given off by building construction materials, furniture and flooring materials, and combustion by-products from stoves and furnaces. When there is a problem with one or more of these factors, people in the affected building can experience a wide range of symptoms, from headaches and itchy eyes to unconsciousness

and death. This section covers some of the most important health risks associated with indoor air quality.

Carbon Monoxide

Carbon monoxide is a highly toxic gas that is colorless, odorless, and tasteless, and so is not detectable by the unaided senses. Health effects of carbon monoxide vary from mild discomfort (headaches, dizziness, mental confusion, and nausea) at concentrations below 70 parts per million (ppm) to death at concentrations above 150 ppm. Persons who suffer from heart disease may feel chest pain at low concentrations. Regular exposure to low levels in the home or workplace can cause flulike symptoms that rapidly disappear after you leave the location where you

---

Key Terms

indoor air quality characteristics of air within homes, workplaces, and public buildings, including the presence and amount of oxygen, water vapor, and a wide range of substances that can have adverse effects on your health

carbon monoxide a gaseous by-product of the incomplete combustion of natural gas, kerosene, heating oil, wood, coal, gasoline, and tobacco

Religious Perspectives on Human-Environment Relationships

In an article written by Lynn White (published in *Science,* 1967), he states that the root of all modern environmental problems can be found in Judeo-Christian (including Islamic) scripture. According to scripture of these religious traditions, the purpose of all of creation was to meet the needs and uses of humankind. This established a dualism (human versus not-human) that did not exist in earlier religions that perceived divinity in all of creation. Other passages in the Bible include statements that humankind should "go forth and multiply" and "subdue the Earth." These passages are often cited by those who seek a religious basis to justify unchecked human population growth and environmental destruction in pursuit of human goals. White proposed that the Judeo-Christian dualism encourages exploitation and dominion over nature by humans, resulting in the many environmental problems facing us today.

Earth-based religions of many indigenous cultures of the world (pre-Christian Europe, Native American, African religions) believed that many or all aspects of the natural world were manifestations of one or more gods. Humans were perceived as being at the mercy of these powerful, sometimes petty and vindictive natural forces, and often performed religious rituals to gain favors or atone for sins against Nature. Many of these cultures appear to have lived in ecological balance with their environment. Whether this balance was the consequence of their religious beliefs, their small populations, their limited technologies, or the combination of these factors is unknown.

Modern day Earth-based religions include Paganism, Wicca, Druidism (a resurrection of pre-Roman European Celtic religious traditions), and Goddess religions. These modern versions of ancient traditions also worship the natural world as a manifestation of the energy of God or Creation. People who follow these religious traditions are often dedicated to protecting the environment.[1]

Traditional Hinduism also lacks the distinction between humankind as separate from the rest of Creation. Hindus believe that humans, gods, and nature are all parts of a single organic whole. Many religious rituals serve to appease Mother Earth and seek forgiveness for any violations of Nature. Any abuse of Nature is considered a sacrilegious act.[2]

While traditional Earth-based and Hindu religious traditions encouraged followers to live in ecological balance with their environment, many of these cultures now face a modern dualism: economic development vs. environmental protection. In their efforts to develop a modern economic system in India, many Hindus have abandoned traditional beliefs. In recent decades India has suffered from the same environmental degradation as many other developed nations. Some Native American groups have made environmentally destructive management decisions in the interest of economic development on their reservations. In many cases these environmentally destructive decisions occur in the context of grinding poverty and a breakdown in traditional social systems. All too often, the economic benefits from such decisions are short-lived, while the environmental damage lasts for generations.

In the Islamic tradition, humankind is considered the most favored of God's creation, and all the rest of Creation is deemed subservient to human needs and uses. However, Islamic tradition also holds that all living things in Nature are partners of humankind, deserving of respect and their own existence. Passages in the Qur'an (Koran) state that it is the duty of humankind to deal with the environment and other species in a loving, caring, and respectful manner. Islamic tradition also stipulates that humankind should be good stewards of natural resources and should not pollute clean waters with their wastes. Muslims are encouraged to put the common good ahead of personal benefit and to be moderate in consumption, including the use of natural resources. Taken together, these passages from the Qur'an encourage Muslims to protect and manage their environment for the common good.[3]

While the Judeo-Christian and Islamic religious traditions have scriptural passages that could be seen as justifying environmentally destructive behavior, they also have distinctly environment-friendly teachings. All three of these religious traditions revere the biblical Old Testament, wherein God created the heavens and Earth, the land and waters, the plants and animals, and humankind. At the end of each day of creation, the Bible states that God saw each of his creations was "good." Some theologians interpret these statements to mean that the Creator valued all aspects of creation, not just humankind. In subsequent biblical passages, several references are made regarding human responsibility to be "good stewards" over the other parts of Creation.

The National Religious Partnership for the Environment is an umbrella organization for Christians and Jews who believe that protecting the environment is a mandate well-founded in their scriptural traditions.[4] This association of religious congregations works to increase awareness of the environmental message in the Bible and Torah. A main objective of this association is to enhance the activity of its members in the political process in support of environmental protection. For people who are committed to protecting the environment and dedicated to their Judeo-Christian religion, this organization offers a community of like-minded people working toward similar goals.

[1] *Pagan and Earth-Based Religions.* www.beliefnet.com/index/index_10015.html.

[2] Adhopia, A. 2001. *Hinduism Promotes Environmental Protection.* www.indianest.com/analysis/018.htm.

[3] Alhilaly, TH. 1993. *Islam and Ecology.* www.ummah.com/islam/taqwapalace/fitness/microcosmpage2.html.

[4] National Religious Partnership for the Environment. www.nrpe.org.

are exposed.[1] At high concentrations greater than 150 ppm, carbon monoxide poisoning can render you unconscious and then kill you.[2]

You can minimize your exposure to carbon monoxide and risk of poisoning by keeping all appliances that burn gas or other fuels in proper working order and ensuring proper ventilation. You should use the manufacturer-specified fuel in space heaters, and ensure proper ventilation of space heaters, woodstoves, charcoal and gas grills, and fireplaces. You should avoid letting your car idle inside a garage, especially if it is attached to your home.[1] Finally, you should install a carbon monoxide detector that will let you monitor levels of this gas in your home and will sound an alarm if levels exceed safety standards. Every year, 300 people in the United States die from carbon monoxide poisoning,[3] usually because of improperly maintained furnaces or incorrectly used space heaters. A carbon monoxide alarm can prevent this tragedy from happening to you.

Volatile Organic Compounds

Volatile organic compounds (VOCs) are emitted from products such as paint, paint stripper, cleaning solvents, wood preservatives, aerosol sprays, cleaners, disinfectants, insect repellents and pesticides, air fresheners, stored fuels and automotive products, hobby supplies such as wood glue, and recently dry-cleaned clothing. Formaldehyde is a specific VOC that commonly enters the indoor environment due to emissions from pressed wood products (hardwood plywood wall paneling, particleboard, fiberboard) and furniture made with these pressed wood products. Urea-formaldehyde foam used for home insulation can emit this gas into the indoor environment.[4]

The health effects of volatile organic compounds will vary, depending on which specific substance is involved. Immediate effects of many VOCs include irritation to the eyes, nose, and throat, headaches, loss of coordination, and/or nausea. Longer-term exposure to some VOCs can result in damage to the liver, kidneys, and central nervous system. Some VOCs are known or suspected carcinogens in animals and/or humans.

There are several ways you can limit your exposure to toxic volatile organic compounds. First, minimize your use of products that contain these substances by choosing cleaning supplies, paints, and glues that do not contain VOCs. If you must use a product that contains VOCs, follow directions and provide for plenty of ventilation. Also, you should buy only as much of the VOC-containing product as you will need for your current project and dispose of the unused portion in an appropriate manner as soon as possible.

Tobacco Smoke

Secondhand tobacco smoke is an indoor air pollutant widely recognized as a major health risk, especially for children. For example, this pollutant can increase the risk for acute asthma attacks that require hospital emergency care. There is some evidence that regular exposure to tobacco smoke increases the risk of developing asthma in the first place.[5] Exposure to tobacco smoke in the home is also associated with increased risk of Sudden Infant Death Syndrome (SIDS), childhood bronchitis, pneumonia and ear infections, cardiovascular disease, and cancer. The health effects of indoor tobacco smoke are covered in more detail in Chapter 9.

Asbestos

Asbestos is a building material that was widely used for insulation, floor tiles, and for its fire retardant and noise-dampening properties. Health effects of asbestos exposure include cancers of the lung and abdomen, and irreversible scarring of the lungs that can result in reduced respiratory function. These dire effects most commonly occur only after many years of exposure, usually in the workplace.[6] When the serious health risks associated with exposure to asbestos became known, governmental agencies banned several asbestos products, and manufacturers voluntarily limited other uses of asbestos. Today, asbestos is most commonly found in older buildings, including homes, schools, and factories. The greatest risk of exposure to asbestos occurs when insulation, floor tiles, and other asbestos-containing substances deteriorate, or are damaged during building renovation. These activities release the microscopic asbestos fibers into the air, from which they are inhaled into the lungs. However, intact and undisturbed, asbestos-containing products are relatively safe.[6]

You can minimize your risk of exposure to asbestos fibers by leaving undamaged asbestos-containing materials alone, and by hiring qualified contractors to remove damaged asbestos. Do not try to remove asbestos yourself. Never cut, rip, or use a sander on any material that contains asbestos. Follow manufacturer's recommendations for replacing and disposing of products that contain asbestos.[6]

Lead

Lead is a toxic metal that was widely used in house paint, as a gasoline additive, and in plumbing solder for metal pipes. As the health consequences of lead toxicity became

---

Key Terms

volatile organic compounds (VOCs) a wide variety of chemicals that contain carbon and readily evaporate into the air

asbestos a term used to refer to a class of minerals that have a fibrous crystal structure

better known, several of these uses of lead were banned, including lead-based house paint and leaded gasoline. However, lead is a very stable substance that remains in the environment today, long after its use was banned.

Lead exposure most commonly occurs in older homes, built before 1970. Many of these homes contain substantial amounts of lead-based paint, and older metal plumbing may contain lead solder. In late 1991, more than 10 years after lead-based paint was banned, the Secretary of the U.S. Department of Health and Human Services called lead, "the number one environmental threat to the health of children in the United States."[8] Exposure to lead from old paint occurs when the paint breaks down into paint flakes and dust, which are then inhaled or swallowed. This risk is especially high for young children who often put their hands into their mouth. Lead can also leach from solder in old plumbing and be ingested when people drink tap water.[7]

While lead additives in gasoline were banned by 1990, lead from automobile exhaust fumes was already deposited in soils and can still be found in high concentrations near major highways and city streets. Airborne dust from dirt tracked into the house on shoes can transfer this contaminant to the indoor environment.

Lead has serious health effects when ingested or inhaled, especially for children. Lead can affect virtually all organ systems of the body, but is particularly damaging to the nervous system, kidneys, and blood. *Acute lead toxicity* (blood lead level greater than 80 micrograms per deciliter) can lead to convulsions, coma, and death. However, blood lead levels as low as 10 micrograms per deciliter in children can delay physical and mental development, lower IQ, reduce attention span, and increase behavioral problems.[7]

You can minimize your exposure to lead by replacing deteriorated lead house paint and lead soldered plumbing, and by keeping your home clean of roadside dirt that may be contaminated with residual lead from automobile exhaust. If the lead-based paint in your old house is in good condition, leave it alone; it does not pose a hazard *if it is intact.* However, if the old paint is flaking or producing paint dust, you should have it removed by a contractor that is certified for lead abatement. Do not try to remove lead-based paint yourself, as you may inhale large amounts of paint dust or volatilized lead.

If you are exposed to lead contamination, eating a balanced diet that is rich in calcium and iron can reduce the effects of lead toxicity.[7] If you live in an older house with metal plumbing, you should have the tap water tested for lead. Lead is not readily excreted by the body, and will tend to accumulate over time. There are chelating drug treatments which help the body to excrete lead and reduce toxicity effects, but they have adverse side effects and are generally used only to treat acute lead toxicity.[8]

Biological Pollutants

There are many sources of **biological air pollutants** within your personal environment. Disease-causing viruses and bacteria (common cold, flu, measles) are put into the air when infected people or animals sneeze or cough. Contaminated central air handling systems can be breeding grounds for mold, mildew, and bacteria and can then distribute these contaminants throughout the home. Some people have allergic reactions (itchy eyes, runny nose, sneezing, coughing, stuffy chest, shortness of breath, headache, and/or dizziness) to spores from mold that grows on moist surfaces inside buildings. Some research indicates that exposure to indoor mold can more than double your risk of developing adult onset asthma.[5] Pollen from plants around the home or workplace can cause allergic reactions (hay fever) in many people. Household pets, rats, mice, and cockroaches are sources of saliva, urine, feces, and skin dander that can also stimulate strong allergic reactions.[9]

You can minimize your exposure to biological indoor air pollutants by maintaining the relative humidity in your home within the range of 30–50 percent. This will minimize the growth of many microorganisms that can cause health problems. Control indoor air humidity by installing exhaust fans in bathrooms and kitchens (major sources of water vapor), venting places where water vapor accumulates (attics, basements, and crawl spaces), and using air conditioning or a dehumidifier. You should also eliminate standing water, rugs that have been damaged by leaks or floodwater, and any other wet surfaces.[9]

To minimize allergic reactions to biological indoor air pollutants, you should regularly clean and vacuum your home. While this will not completely eliminate dust mites, pollen, and animal dander, cleaning can substantially reduce the amounts of these allergens and the severity of allergy symptoms. Allergic individuals should leave the house while it is being vacuumed because this may temporarily increase airborne levels of mite allergens and other biological contaminants. You

Key Terms

biological air pollutants living organisms or substances produced by living organisms that cause disease or allergic reactions, including bacteria, molds, mildew, viruses, dust mites, plant pollen, and animal dander, urine, or feces

should also try to keep your house free of rodents and cockroaches as these pests are sources of potent allergens.[9]

Radon

Radon is an environmental health risk that seeps into buildings from the soil surrounding their foundation. It is invisible, odorless, and tasteless, and can be detected only using radon detectors. Uranium, the source of radon, can be found in most parts of the world, and this element is present in rock and soil in parts of all fifty states of the United States. Once radon is produced by decay of uranium, this gas moves through the ground to the air above. Some radon gas may dissolve into groundwater.

It is estimated that indoor radon is at a level sufficient to increase risk of lung cancer in one of every fifteen homes in the United States.[10] The U.S. Surgeon General has warned that exposure to radon gas is the second leading cause of lung cancer in the United States. The National Academy of Sciences estimates that radon exposure causes about 15,000 lung cancer deaths in the United States every year.[11] This risk from radon is especially high for cigarette smokers. Lung damage is caused by radioactive particles formed as by-products from decay of radon that are inhaled and trapped deep within the lungs. As the particles continue the radioactive decay process, they emit bursts of energy that damage adjacent lung tissue. There are no obvious short-term effects from this damage, but long-term exposure can cause lung cancer.[11] There is some evidence that consuming water that is contaminated by radon gas can increase the risk of stomach cancer. The National Academy of Sciences estimates consumption of radon in drinking water causes 19 stomach cancer deaths per year in the United States.[12]

The key to minimizing the health risk of radon exposure is to have your home tested. You can purchase an inexpensive "do-it-yourself" test kit in some hardware stores and other retail outlets. If you can't find a radon test kit locally, you can purchase one from the National Safety Council's Radon Hotline (800-767-7236). After the kit is exposed to the air in your home for a specified time period, it must be returned to a laboratory for analysis.

If unsafe levels of radon are detected in your home, you should work with a contractor who is certified to install a radon reduction system. This will often involve installing a venting system just below the concrete slab of the house foundation. The venting system will intercept the radon gas before it enters your home and vent it outside, where it can be dissipated by wind. You should also have cracks in the slab, basement walls, or foundation of the home repaired to reduce seepage of radon gas through these spaces. However, just sealing the cracks, without installing the belowground venting system, will not adequately reduce indoor radon levels. If you live in a region where high radon levels are common and you plan to build a new home, you should work with your contractor to install radon-resistant features during construction. The average cost to install a radon venting system in an existing home is $800 to $2,500. The average cost to install radon-resistant features in a new home during construction is $350 to $500 (a 128–400 percent savings).[10] For a map of radon risk zones in the United States, see www.epa.gov/iaq/radon/zonemap.html.

Nonionizing Radiation

Radiation is a general term that refers to various forms of energy that are emitted by atoms and molecules when they undergo change, including radio waves, infrared, visible light, ultraviolet, X-rays, and gamma rays. Each kind of radiation has different effects on biological materials and health. **Nonionizing radiation** includes various forms of electromagnetic radiation that cannot break chemical bonds but may excite electrons (ultraviolet radiation) or heat biological materials (infrared, radio frequency, and microwave radiation). Common sources of nonionizing radiation are sunlight, electrical devices, electric power transmission lines, and cell phones. Most adverse health effects of nonionizing radiation are associated with heating tissues, resulting in burns.

Some experts have proposed that certain forms of nonionizing radiation may have more serious health effects. A small number of studies have documented DNA damage in brain cells of rats exposed to high levels of radiofrequency radiation (RFR) similar to that emitted by cell phones. Such DNA damage could initiate tumor development (cancer). However, other animal studies did not find similar effects. Some experiments have documented brain damage in rats exposed to cell phone RFR at levels analogous to those experienced by people who regularly use mobile phones.[13] Large-scale studies of brain cancer incidence among people who do and do not use cell phones have so far failed to document a link between RFR and increased incidence of brain cancer in humans.[14,15] However, cell phones are a relatively new technology, and there has not been sufficient time to study effects of long-term exposure to RFR. As people use

---

Key Terms

radon a naturally occurring radioactive gas that is emitted during the decay of uranium in soil, rock, and water

nonionizing radiation forms of electromagnetic radiation that cannot break chemical bonds but may excite electrons or heat biological materials

cell phones more, beginning at an increasingly younger age, some suggest that it may be prudent to reduce exposure to RFR from these devices.[16] This can be easily done by using a headset attachment to the cell phone so that there is greater distance between the cell phone transmitter and the brain. The intensity of RFR from cell phones decreases significantly over even small distances to levels so low that they are very unlikely to be a health risk.

Another common source of nonionizing radiation in the human environment is electricity flowing through wires and electronic devices, and electricity transmission lines. A few studies have suggested that exposure to nonionizing radiation around electric devices such as microwave ovens, televisions, tanning lamps, electric blankets, and electricity transmission lines may slightly increase risk for some cancers.[17,18,19] However, the vast majority of studies have failed to find any increased risk of adverse health effects associated with household electronics or living near power lines. (For a comprehensive review of the scientific literature, go to the Web site of J. E. Moulder, professor of radiation oncology at the Medical College of Wisconsin, www.mcw.edu/gcrc/cop/powerlines-cancer-FAQ/toc.html#C55.)

Drinking Water

The safety of drinking water in your home is affected by environmental factors both in the home or neighborhood and in the larger community. The water supply for rural homes is often a well that draws from groundwater, and can be much affected by environmental conditions around the home and neighborhood. In urban areas a municipal water supply system draws from rivers or lakes and then treats the water to make it safe to drink. The community/regional environment plays the dominant role in determining the safety of water from municipal suppliers. However, municipal water can be contaminated by the personal environment as it passes through pipes in the home. Environmental health issues relating to drinking water as influenced by conditions in your home and neighborhood will be covered here. Issues related to municipal water supply are presented later in this chapter.

Approximately 23 million people in the United States obtain their drinking water from groundwater (that is, from private wells), streams, or cisterns that collect rainwater.[20] These households are responsible for ensuring the safety of their own drinking water. Private drinking water supplies that rely on surface waters, or wells that tap shallow groundwater layers, are at risk of contamination by pathogens from home septic systems, contaminants from leaking underground fuel storage tanks, improper disposal of various household chemicals (cleaners, automotive fluids, and pesticides),

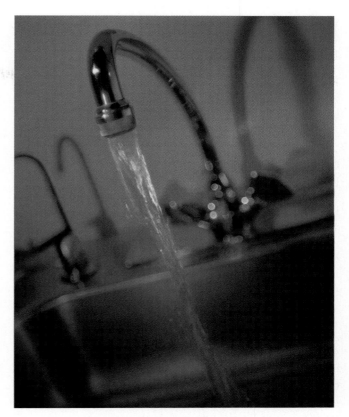

Tap water is a key source of pollutants in the home.

and agricultural chemicals applied to surrounding farm fields.

Nitrate from agricultural fertilizer that leaches into shallow groundwater supplies poses a widespread health risk in rural areas. The U.S. Geological Survey estimates that 10–20 percent of groundwater sources of drinking water may have levels of nitrate contamination that pose risks to human health.[21] Excessive consumption of nitrate in contaminated drinking water can cause serious illness and death. Nitrate interferes with the oxygen-transport function of the blood (methemoglobinemia). This effect is most pronounced in children, resulting in "blue-baby" syndrome.[21] Nitrate can also cause reproductive problems and is linked to development of several types of cancer.[22]

Rural wells contaminated by nitrate may also have high levels of other agricultural chemicals. Some researchers have suggested that agricultural pesticides and herbicides can contribute to the development of testicular cancer and reduced sperm production in men, breast cancer in women, and nervous system disorders in children.[22]

Leaching of substances from pipes in the plumbing of older homes is another potential source of contamination to drinking water in the home.[23] Metallic pipes can release toxic metals such as lead and copper into the water. Polyvinyl chloride (PVC) pipes manufactured before 1977 may release toxic vinyl chloride into the water. Vinyl chloride is a known human carcinogen.

Leaching of toxic substances from pipes into the drinking water supply is most problematic in small diameter pipes (less than a 2-inch diameter), with high water temperatures, and when the water is stagnant in the pipes for long periods (more than 24 hours).[23] A relatively easy way to reduce contaminants from household plumbing in your drinking water is to regularly flush fresh water through the plumbing. Let the water run from the tap for a couple of minutes before taking water to drink, especially first thing in the morning and if you have been away from home for long time periods. In some cases it may be advisable to replace the old plumbing, but this can be very expensive.

Private water supplies should be tested annually for nitrate and fecal coliform bacteria. If you suspect there may be a problem with radon or pesticide contamination, you may need to test your water even more frequently.[20] Testing generally requires that you send samples of your water to a laboratory that tests water quality. You can get a listing of local certified laboratories from your local or state public health department. Some local health departments test private water for free. A private laboratory will charge $10–$20 to perform a nitrate and bacteria test. Testing for pesticides or organic chemicals may cost from several hundred to several thousand dollars. Most laboratories mail back the sample results within a few days, or several weeks if the analyses are more complex. The results indicate the concentrations of contaminants and indicate whether each contaminant exceeds a drinking water quality standard.

If your drinking water contains contaminants that exceed safety standards, you should retest the water supply immediately and contact your public health department for assistance. High bacteria concentrations can sometimes be easily controlled by disinfecting a well. Water filters may also remove some contaminants. However, other problems may require a new source of water, such as a deeper well. Alternatively, you may need to rely on bottled water until a new water source can be obtained.[20] You can obtain technical assistance with residential drinking water supply problems from the organization Farm*A*Syst/Home*A*Syst (see the Web sites www.uwex.edu/farmasyst or www.uwex.edu/homeasyst).

Noise

Noise can be defined as any undesirable sound. What constitutes "undesirable sound" will vary from one person to the next, but it often involves loud sounds that occur at irregular intervals and are not controllable by the listener.[24] In the personal environment of the home, neighborhood, and workplace, noise may include overly loud music, barking dogs, motorcycles and cars with broken or missing muffler systems, loud machinery, appliances and power tools, airplanes flying overhead, and train whistles.

The health effects of environmental noise depend on the intensity, frequency, and nature of the noise. Excessively loud noise can cause physical damage to sensory tissues in your ears, resulting in partial or total hearing loss that can be temporary or permanent. This physical damage will depend on both the intensity (as measured in decibels) and the duration of exposure to the loud noise. For example, sitting in front of the speaker column at a large rock concert, with noise levels at 120 decibels for over 2 hours, can result in immediate pain and long-term or permanent hearing loss. Ironically, the tissues that are damaged by excessively loud sounds are those responsible for hearing high frequency sounds associated with normal conversation, not the tissues that actually hear the damaging sound. Loud noise sources rob you of one of your most important senses, the ability to hear the unamplified human voice.

Even noise at lower levels can cause adverse health effects. The American Speech-Language-Hearing Association reports that low level noise can elevate blood pressure, reduce sleep, cause fatigue, and disturb digestion. These physical effects of low level noise can impact emotional, intellectual, social, and occupational health. Effects reported by the World Health Organization include increased frustration and anxiety, impaired ability to concentrate, reduced productivity and ability to learn, and increased absenteeism and accidents.

These effects of noise can increase your feeling of stress and diminish your ability to tolerate minor irritations; you may exhibit anger and aggression that are out of proportion to the immediate source of your irritation.[24] This antisocial behavior may have negative consequences in your personal relationships and occupational health.

A common source of long-term exposure to loud sound that causes hearing loss in many young people is amplified music. Occasional loud rock music at 110–120 decibels may cause only temporary damage. However, daily exposure to such sound levels will cause permanent hearing loss. A number of aging rock stars have admitted to significant hearing loss that they attribute to standing in front of huge amplifiers night after night. Many rock musicians performing today stand behind the main speaker columns or wear ear protection. Jacking up the volume in your headphones, or the powerful amplifier in your car stereo, may be fun today, but is it worth a lifetime of incessant ringing in your ears and diminished hearing later in life? (See Changing for the Better for tips on reducing the health risks associated with noise pollution.)

 TALKING POINTS How can you encourage your children to develop sound habits regarding their environment and their personal health? What changes can you make in your own habits to serve as a better example for them?

The Community and Regional Environment

The community and regional environment is comprised of the outdoor air you breathe, local rivers and lakes that provide water and recreation opportunities, surrounding lands (urban, industrial, suburban, rural, agricultural, natural communities), and all the people and other species that live in these areas. A wide range of human activities can degrade this community environment in ways that affect personal health. Air, water, and land pollution include many substances that have significant negative effects on physical health. Loss of natural areas and other recreational and aesthetic "green space" to roads, cities, and industrial development can adversely affect your perceived quality of life, with negative effects on emotional and spiritual health. Degraded environmental conditions in many communities discourage new economic development and may limit occupational health.

While you can exert some influence on the environmental conditions in your community, the influence of any one individual is usually small. Your control over how the community environment affects your personal health is often limited to controlling your exposure to known health risks, such as contaminated water and land, or outdoor air pollution. You can also choose to reduce your own contributions to community/regional air, water, and land pollution through conservation of energy and water and recycling solid waste.

Because one person cannot have a significant impact on community environmental problems, many people join organizations that work to improve the environment and quality of life in their community. By working with others of like mind in the political process and in environmental organizations, you become "part of the solution" to major environmental problems that can affect your health and that of your family. For many people, getting involved in solving local environmental problems can provide significant benefits to emotional and spiritual health.

In this section you will learn about aspects of the community and regional environment that can affect your health, and what you can do to exert some level of personal control over these environmental influences.

Air Pollution

Air pollution includes substances that naturally occur in the air (pollen, microbes, dust, sea salt, volcanic ash) and substances produced by human activities (engine exhaust, ozone, various volatile organic compounds, and acid rain). In this section on community and regional environmental influences on health, we focus on those components of air pollution that are produced within a specific region and that have substantial health effects within that community or region.

The primary sources of human-caused air pollutants are various kinds of internal combustion engines associated with electric power plants, industry, and transportation (trucks, automobiles, and farm/construction equipment). Oil refineries and chemical production factories also contribute to air pollution in some communities. Electric power stations, industrial facilities, and chemical factories are classified as *point sources* that produce large amounts of pollution from a single location. Automobiles, trucks, heavy construction/farm equipment, gas stations, lawn mowers, and charcoal grills are *nonpoint sources* of air pollutants. Individually, nonpoint sources produce relatively small amounts of pollution, but when added together account for a large proportion of community air pollution.

Air pollutants that are directly produced by internal combustion engines include *carbon monoxide, nitrogen dioxide, sulfur dioxide, polycyclic aromatic hydrocarbons, and particulate matter.* Carbon monoxide is a toxic gas

that impairs respiration, as described under indoor air quality in the previous section. Nitrogen and sulfur oxides interact with water vapor in the air to form small particulates (diameter <2.5 μm) that are inhaled into the deepest parts of the lungs. These substances can damage lung tissues, reduce lung capacity, cause coughing and chronic bronchitis, and may worsen such ailments as hypersensitivity to allergens, asthma, emphysema, and heart disease. The U.S. Environmental Protection Agency estimates that over 70 million people in the United States live in counties where levels of small particulate air pollutants exceed human health standards for at least some part of the year.[25] It has been estimated that small-particulate air pollution causes as many as 50,000 to 100,000 premature deaths in the United States per year.[26]

Polycyclic aromatic hydrocarbons (PAHs) are widespread air pollutants from fossil fuel combustion in vehicles and residential furnaces, and from environmental tobacco smoke. These substances have been shown to be carcinogenic to both test animals and humans. Several new studies indicate that PAHs can cross the placenta and cause adverse health effects on a developing human fetus.[27,28] Increased maternal exposure to PAHs was associated with lower birth weight, smaller head circumference, and reduced birth length of newborn children.[27] A study of 867 mothers and 822 newborns living in large cities in the United States, Poland, and China documented a significant association between maternal exposure to PAHs and PAH-linked DNA damage in newborns that is associated with increased risk of cancer.[28] This type of DNA damage was detected in 42 percent and 61 percent of two groups of newborns in New York City (where PAH exposure was lowest), 71 percent of newborns in Krakow, Poland, and 80 percent of newborns in Tongliang, China (where PAH exposure was highest). Higher levels of DNA damage were also associated with higher PAH exposure. The prevalence and amount of DNA damage did not differ between mothers and their babies, despite the fact that fetal exposure was only 10 percent that of the mother. This indicates that the developing fetuses are 10 times more susceptible to DNA damage from PAHs than adult mothers are.[28]

Key Terms

air pollution refers to a wide variety of substances found in the atmosphere that can have adverse effects on human health, crop productivity, and natural communities

polycyclic aromatic hydrocarbons (PAHs) air pollutants from fossil fuel combustion

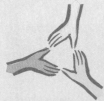

Learning from Our Diversity

Native Americans and the Environment

An essay by David Lewis, in *Native America in the Twentieth Century: An Encyclopedia,* published in 1994 by Garland Publishers of New York, describes the historical and modern environmental ethic of Native Americans. Many early environmentalists were inspired by their perceptions of the close relationship between Native Americans and their natural environment. Before contact with Euroamericans, Native American cultures perceived that their spiritual and physical universes were one. They felt connected with the animate and inanimate beings of their environment, and managed its bounty carefully so as not to upset the spirits who kept their world in balance and supplied all necessary resources. They acknowledged the power of the Earth and considered the hunter and hunted as equal partners in the larger scheme of things. They practiced rituals with the animals they killed, the agricultural fields they tended, and the resources they consumed to ensure a continued supply.

Romantic modern misconceptions that Native Americans "left no mark on the land" ignore much cultural and historical evidence that they used fire and water to transform their landscapes.[1] When necessary, Native Americans adjusted their environments to meet their cultural and material needs. However, Native Americans were careful students of their functional environments. They strived for maximum sustained yield, not maximum production. Their use of natural resources was based on reciprocity and balance.[1] This approach to stewardship of natural resources is certainly worthy of admiration, and a worthy goal for modern society.

Modern Native American communities are often far removed from their traditional land ethic, a fact that sometimes places them at odds with environmentalists. However, environmental problems on Native American lands must be placed in the perspective of the total destruction of their cultures and environment at the hands of Euroamericans. There are instances when control of natural resources on Indian reservations has been returned to Native Americans, with disastrous environmental consequences. However, these Native American communities have been forced to live on remote, marginal lands, with few apparent natural resources, and lacking virtually all the native plants and animal species upon which their traditional practices depended. These communities suffer in the depths of poverty, and sometimes seek any economic development regardless of the environmental cost. In desperation, some accept toxic waste dumps onto their lands, and others strip the land of its forests to meet the immediate needs of their communities. Often, these environmentally destructive decisions are made by Euroamerican government agents on behalf of their Native American clients.

Another point of disagreement between Native Americans and modern environmentalists involves traditional hunting of species that are now considered threatened or endangered, such as the bald eagle, bowhead whale, and Florida panther. The rights of Native Americans to these traditional hunting practices, intimately connected with their religion and culture, is protected by the American Indian Religious Freedom Act of 1978. Environmentalists who oppose these hunts seem to pick and choose which Native American traditions to admire and which to condemn. They fail to recognize that the religious practice of the hunts is part of a larger tradition that motivated Native Americans to seek balance with their environment.

As Native American communities struggle to meet their most basic needs and maintain their cultural traditions in a hostile modern world, we should be careful about harshly judging their departures from traditional land ethics. There is a diversity of opinion within Native American communities, just as in other communities. Some people seek to be modern, while others yearn for the traditional values of an earlier day. Traditional land ethics are much more recent history for Native Americans than are similar, pre-Christian, Earth-centered religions of Euroamericans. Nonetheless, both communities struggle with the question of how best to manage our environment for present and future generations.

[1] Lewis DR: Essay on Native American Environmental Issues. In: *Native Americans and the Environment.* 2000. http://www.cnie.org/nae/docs/intro.html

---

Tropospheric ozone is another important regional air pollutant that is linked to chemicals in exhaust fumes from internal combustion engines. This substance is produced when hydrocarbons, nitrogen oxides, and other small particle matter chemically interact in the presence of sunlight. The result is a brownish haze over affected cities, often called *smog.*

Ozone levels are particularly high in locations with warm, sunny climates (Southern California) and where natural vegetation produces volatile organic compounds that contribute to the photochemical process that produces ozone (eastern United States). The U.S. Environmental Protection Agency estimates that over 110 million people in the United States live in counties where ozone levels exceed human health standards for at least some part of the

Key Terms

tropospheric ozone ozone comprises three oxygen atoms that are bound into a single molecule; tropospheric ozone refers to this substance as it occurs in the lower layer of the atmosphere, close to the ground

Smog over Los Angeles, California

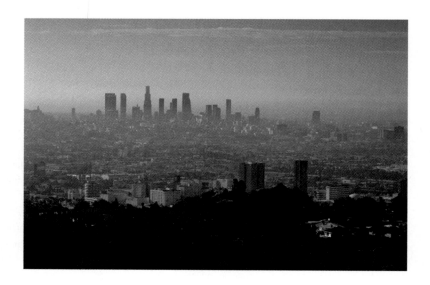

year.[25] Most of these people live in Southern California and near the East Coast between Virginia and southern Maine (see Figure 17-2).

Inhalation of ozone can cause lung damage that reduces lung capacity. This is a particular health risk to individuals who suffer from asthma, emphysema, or heart disease. On days when ozone concentrations are highest, local hospital emergency room visits associated with respiratory distress increase from 10–20 percent.[26] There is also some evidence that childhood exposure to ozone can actually cause children to become asthmatic.[29,30]

Air toxics are a diverse collection of hazardous air pollutants produced mainly by electric power plants and industrial sources that constitute a widespread environmental health risk in the United States. When lifetime cancer risks for all carcinogenic air toxics are combined, 20 million people live in areas where the risk exceeds 100 in one million.[31] However, these risk estimates are based on a lifetime of exposure to toxic air pollutant levels in 1996. With continued progress on reducing toxic air pollution, this risk is expected to decrease in the future. Since passage of the Clear Air Act in 1970, much progress has been made in reducing air pollution in the United States. However, further reduction of air pollution poses serious technological, economic, and political challenges. For more information about air toxics, go to the Web site www.epa.gov/ttn/atw.

Unfortunately, the degree to which you can control your own exposure to regional air pollution and the associated health risks is limited. In larger urban areas where air pollution levels are high, weather reports often include information about air pollution. If you live in a large city, you should pay attention to air pollution information, often conveyed in color-coded alerts. A "yellow" air pollution alert means people who suffer from respiratory or cardiac diseases, or hypersensitivity to allergens, should stay indoors. An "orange" alert indicates that everyone should limit their outdoor activities to the minimum possible.

You can also help to lower air pollution levels by limiting contributions from your own automobile, lawn mower exhaust, and charcoal grill. You can car pool, use mass transit, or telecommute (work at home via a computer network) to reduce air pollution associated with automobile exhaust. You can fill your car gas tank, mow your lawn, and use your grill during the cooler evening hours to reduce your contribution to tropospheric ozone. You can conserve electricity to reduce emissions from electric power plants. In areas of the United States where air pollution is especially problematic, local laws may require that you do some of these things on days when conditions result in a "pollution emergency."

Water Pollution

Humankind has had a very schizophrenic relationship with our rivers and lakes. Water is an essential resource for all living things on our planet, including humans and the plants and animals we use for food. We also value our rivers and lakes for their recreational opportunities and aesthetic benefits. Yet we used these water bodies as convenient dumps for sewage and industrial wastes.

> ### Key Terms
>
> **air toxics** a class of 188 toxic air pollutants identified by the U.S. Environmental Protection Agency as known or suspected causes of cancer or other serious health effects

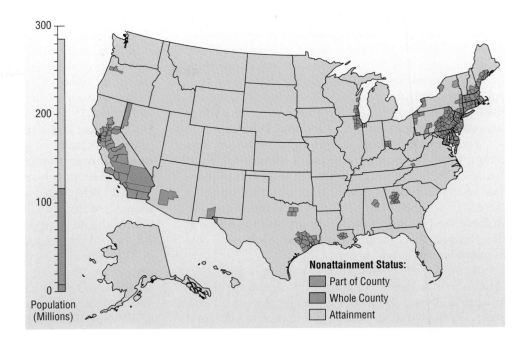

Figure 17-2 Counties classified by EPA as in "nonattainment" of ozone standards in the year 2003.

Population (Millions)

Nonattainment Status:
Part of County
Whole County
Attainment

The problem of water pollution came to national attention in 1968 when children playing with matches set on fire chemical pollutants that covered the Cuyahoga River in Ohio. The subsequent public outcry resulted in the Clean Water Act of 1972 and the Safe Drinking Water Act of 1974. Since then, substantial progress has been made in reducing water pollution and ensuring safe drinking water supplies.

The job of cleaning rivers and lakes in the U.S. is not complete, and people who come in close contact with contaminated waters or fish from these areas are still at risk for a variety of health problems. Water pollution comes from both point sources (sewer overflows, livestock feedlots, industrial areas, and mines) and from nonpoint sources such as runoff from urban streets and agricultural areas that carries chemicals and animal waste into rivers. Toxic air pollutants can be deposited into water bodies in rainfall. Some of the most troublesome water pollutants in the U.S. today are described below.

Biological water pollutants from untreated sewage and drainage from leaking home septic systems include various species of disease-causing viruses, bacteria, and protozoa. These organisms cause diseases that are at best uncomfortable (diarrhea) and at worst lethal (dysentery, hepatitis, typhoid fever, and cholera). In the late 1800s, diseases associated with contaminated drinking water were the third leading cause of death in the United States.[32]

The largest sources of biological water pollutants in surface waters of the U.S. today are overflows from old combined septic and storm sewers during heavy rainfall events, and animal wastes that are carried by runoff of rainfall from agricultural areas. While much has already been done to eliminate biological pollution, billions of dollars are still required to finish this task.

At present, your personal risk of exposure to biological water pollution in the United States is relatively small. Public health departments monitor local surface waters for the presence of **fecal coliform bacteria** in every county in the United States. These bacteria are an indicator that water has been contaminated by sewage. All municipal drinking water systems, and many private households, in the United States treat their water to kill pathogenic organisms. By the end of the 20th century, deaths due to water pathogens in the drinking water supply were very rare in the U.S.[32]

A wide variety of other **toxic pollutants** can be found in surface and groundwater sources of drinking water.

Key Terms

biological water pollutants disease-causing organisms that are found in water

fecal coliform bacteria a category of bacteria that live within the intestines of warm-blooded animals; the presence of these bacteria is used as an indicator that water has been contaminated by feces

toxic pollutants substances known to, or suspected of, causing cancer or other serious health problems

These substances include naturally occurring toxic elements (such as arsenic and mercury) produced by breakdown of minerals. Human activities produce a wide range of toxic chemicals, including metals, solvents, plastics, and PCBs (polychlorinated biphenols). Arsenic and mercury have both natural and human-caused sources. Runoff of *agricultural pesticides* carries toxic substances into rivers where large areas of land are used for crop production.

The dumping of toxic substances into surface waters is now illegal, but some of these toxins are very stable and can be found in large quantities in the sediments of rivers and lakes that were polluted before 1972. Cleaning up these toxic sediments can be very costly. A recent decision to dredge and dispose of PCB-contaminated sediments in the Hudson River near Albany, New York, will cost hundreds of millions of dollars.

Health effects of agricultural chemicals and other toxic substances depend on the specific chemical.[32] Taken as a group, these substances have been linked to adverse effects on the blood, liver, spleen, kidney, adrenal gland, thyroid gland, reproductive system (fertility), and cardiovascular system. Some are known or suspected human *carcinogens* (substances that cause cancer), *mutagens* (substances that cause cell mutations), or *teratogens* (substances that cause birth defects). The risks for these health effects are greatest for workers who come in direct contact with the concentrated chemicals. More insidious are health effects such as cancer and birth defects that develop imperceptibly, after long-term exposure to low concentrations of these chemicals in the environment.

The U.S. Environmental Protection Agency has set **maximum contaminant level (MCL)** standards for the amounts of the biological pollutants, pesticides, and toxic chemicals that are allowed in municipal drinking water supplies.[32] MCLs are set at levels that minimize human health risks, but also take into account the limits of available treatment technology and the costs of meeting the standards. Municipal water suppliers are required to report any violations of MCLs to state and federal environmental agencies.

The best way for you to minimize physical health risks posed by consuming biological or toxic contaminants is to be informed. Municipal water suppliers must report the amounts of biological contaminants, agricultural pesticides, and toxic substances that are detected in their water. You can access your supplier's annual report at www.epa.gov/safewater/dwinfo.htm. These reports list the mean and range (minimum and maximum) concentrations for all regulated contaminants for all samples analyzed in a year. Look at the maximum value to determine if your water system occasionally fails to meet health standards. If your water supplier fails to meet health standards, consider drinking bottled, boiled, or filtered water until the supplier fixes the problems.

You can also be exposed to toxic substances by eating contaminated fish or wild game. Some toxic substances, such as mercury and PCBs, accumulate to high levels in the bodies of shellfish, fish, and waterfowl. This problem can occur even in remote, apparently pristine areas. People who regularly consume wild food animals are at highest risk.

To reduce health risks associated with consuming wild game, you should be aware of health advisories for consuming contaminated fish or game, usually issued by the public health or fish and game state agencies. These advisories are often stated as limits on how much fish or meat should be consumed in a specified time period. Pregnant women should be especially careful of consuming shellfish, fish, or wild game; mercury and PCBs cause birth defects.

You can also be exposed to waterborne pollutants, with associated health risks, as a result of recreational activities. You should be aware of "Don't swim" warnings for your local rivers and lakes, usually issued by the public health department. When backpacking, always filter, boil, or chemically treat drinking water to kill pathogens, even in apparently pristine wilderness areas.

Land Pollution

We do not physically consume land or soil the way we do air and water, but pollution of land can still result in serious adverse health effects. Disposal of toxic wastes often involves burying them in the ground. When done with proper safeguards, this disposal method can be safe. If done improperly, toxic pollutants leach into groundwater or are carried by runoff into surface waters, resulting in significant human health risks.

Most land pollution today is associated with the disposal of **solid waste.** *Municipal solid waste* consists of everyday items such as product packaging, grass clippings, furniture, clothing, bottles, food scraps, newspapers, appliances, paint, and batteries. Other solid waste produced by business and industry includes waste tires, concrete, asphalt, bricks, lumber, and shingles from demolished

---

Key Terms

maximum contaminant level (MCL) the highest concentration of a contaminant that is allowed in drinking water, as established and regulated by the U.S. Environmental Protection Agency

solid waste pollutants that are in solid form, including nonhazardous household trash, industrial wastes, mining wastes, and sewage sludge from wastewater treatment plants

buildings, and *sewage sludge* (solids remaining after wastewater treatment). In 1999 the U.S. population produced 230 million tons of solid waste, or about 4.6 pounds of waste per person per day (or 1,680 pounds per person per year).[33]

Municipal sanitation departments and private disposal companies are very efficient at removing these wastes from our homes and businesses and putting them someplace where we don't see them. These waste disposal locations include sanitary landfills (wastes are compacted and buried under soil), ocean dumping in garbage barges (with trash sometimes escaping to wash up on beaches), and incinerators (where solid wastes are burned).

While out-of-sight often means out-of-mind, these solid wastes do not "go away," they accumulate. Many municipal and regional sanitary landfills are reaching their capacity and must be closed. As we run out of places to dump our solid waste, some have proposed that we burn it in large incinerators. However, incinerators release toxic substances into the air and their ash contains concentrated toxic chemicals.

Most of the potential health effects of land pollution have already been described in this chapter under the topics of air and water pollution. Most human exposure to pollutants that are deposited on land occurs when those toxic substances end up in the air or water. You can limit your risk of these health effects by being aware of where solid wastes are disposed, both at the present time and in the past. You should be particularly aware of proximity to a local landfill or waste disposal site if your water source is a private well that draws from groundwater that might be contaminated. In this situation, you should regularly monitor your water for pollutants.

You can reduce your personal contribution to the solid waste problem of your community by following the Three R's: Reduce, Reuse, Recycle. You can consume less and accept less packaging on the products you buy. You can compost yard waste or use a lawn mower with a mulching blade to eliminate grass clippings and leaves. Reusing bottles, zipper-closure storage bags, cloth shopping bags, and cloth diapers reduces solid waste. Newspapers, magazines, aluminum and steel cans, glass bottles, and many plastic containers can be recycled and the materials used to make new products. However, recycling will only work if you also buy products that are made from recycled materials, such as recycled paper and plastic "wood" products.

Loss of Green Space

Loss of **green space** represents another kind of land pollution that can affect your quality of life and health. In many parts of the United States, green space is being converted to housing developments, shopping malls,

industrial sites, and highways. Wildlife species disappear from your community and surroundings as their habitats are destroyed.

While development of green space for human uses may provide job opportunities and be beneficial for your occupational health, it can also detract from recreational and aesthetic aspects of your community. If you find that you must travel farther and longer from home or work to find a safe and enjoyable location to jog or bicycle, you may exercise less often. Your sense of "quality of life" is diminished when you no longer see wild animals in your backyard or you feel that your community is becoming ugly.

Some communities have created land-use (zoning) plans that allow for economic development while protecting recreational and aesthetic values in their communities. These zoning plans can be controversial, as they try to balance the rights of private property owners with the welfare of the entire community. You can contribute toward protecting environmental quality in your community by supporting land-use planning and enforceable zone laws that protect green space while allowing for responsible economic development.

Ionizing Radiation

Ionizing radiation, as opposed to nonionizing radiation, causes damage to biological structures such as DNA that can result in serious adverse health effects. Ionizing radiation is produced by nuclear reactions, and sources include medical X-rays, naturally occurring radioactive minerals such as uranium, various radioactive materials used by industry, nuclear reactors and their waste products, and nuclear bomb explosions.

The health effects of exposure to X-rays and gamma radiation depend on many factors, including the duration, type, and dose of radiation, and your individual sensitivity. Heavy exposure to these forms of radiation can occur if you are near a nuclear bomb blast or downwind of a major nuclear reactor accident. In such cases, exposure can cause *radiation sickness,* including intense fatigue, nausea, weight loss, hair loss, fever, bleeding from

---

Key Terms

green space areas of land that are dominated by domesticated or natural vegetation, including rural farmland, city lawns and parks, and nature preserves

ionizing radiation electromagnetic radiation that is capable of breaking chemical bonds, such as X-rays and gamma rays

The High-Tech Revolution and E-Waste

The high-tech revolution has a hidden dark side, mountains of accumulating obsolete electronic equipment that contain large amounts of toxic substances. During the period from 1997 to 2007, it is estimated that over 500 million computers must be disposed of. These computers will contain 6.2 billion pounds of plastic, 1.6 billion pounds of lead, 3 million pounds of cadmium, 1.9 million pounds of chromium, and 632,000 pounds of mercury. Lead, cadmium, chromium, and mercury are highly toxic metals, and can cause a wide range of severe health effects if they end up in the air, drinking water, or food supply.[1,2]

Computers contain over 1,000 different substances, many of which are toxic. This makes recycling a complex, labor-intensive process that can cost more than the value of the recycled materials. Only 6 percent of obsolete computers disposed of after 1998 were recycled. The remainder was deposited in landfills across the country. It is estimated that 70 percent of heavy metals such as lead and mercury going into U.S. landfills today comes from electronic waste. Several states, including California and Massachusetts, have banned disposal of computer monitors in landfills to protect groundwater.[1] While recycling of computers is seen as the ideal solution to the problem of waste disposal, it is estimated that

50 percent to 80 percent of computers "recycled" before the year 2002 were actually shipped to poor Asian countries. Workers in these countries disassemble computers to recover useful materials for very low wages and with minimal or no protection from the toxic materials to which they are exposed. These countries have weak or poorly enforced environmental regulations, so materials that cannot be recycled are dumped into rivers or burned in open air pits. These practices expose the recycling workers and surrounding local populations to toxic substances.[1]

The practice of shipping toxic computer waste to underdeveloped countries is now banned by an international treaty, but the United States is the only developed nation that has not ratified this treaty. The "free market" justification for the practice of shipping toxic computer waste to underdeveloped countries is that this provides jobs and helps poor people. The question is whether or not it is moral to give poor people the choice between poverty or poisons?[1]

Given that the use of computers and electronics will only increase in the future, many argue that we must develop environmentally responsible computer recycling systems. Recently proposed legislation would require the Environmental Protection Agency to

help set up computer recycling across the United States. The program would be funded by a fee of up to $10 on all retail sales of desktop and laptop PCs and computer monitors. Similar legislation is also appearing in many state legislatures. The electronics industry favors charging consumers the fee when they return their old computers to the manufacturer rather than on new computers. Some computer manufacturers are already initiating computer take-back programs. However, development of a comprehensive national strategy for responsibly addressing the computer waste problem continues as of this writing.

The other, and perhaps most important, approach to the computer waste problem is to develop electronic equipment that is less toxic and more easily recycled. This will require development of, and investment in, new technologies. In our free market system, this will happen only when the electronics manufacturers must share the cost of dealing with computer waste.

[1]Puckett J, et al: *Exporting Harm: The High-Tech Trashing of Asia.* The Basal Action Network and Silicon Valley Toxics Coalition, 2002.
[2]U.S. Environmental Protection Agency: *WasteWise Update: Electronics Reuse and Recycling.* 2003. www.epa.gov/wastewise/pubs/wwupda14.pdf.

---

the mouth, and compromised immune system, usually resulting in death. Exposure to ionizing radiation can also increase the occurrence of birth defects and cancer.

While your risk of exposure to ionizing radiation is very low, issues related to nuclear power plants and radioactive wastes are often very controversial. Nuclear reactors generate 20 percent of the electricity used in the United States. For decades, nuclear reactors in the United States have been accumulating highly radioactive wastes on site in shallow, water-filled temporary holding tanks. During this time, the U.S. government has been working to develop appropriate technologies and sites to store these wastes permanently. The most likely location is in underground salt caves below Yucca Mountain, Nevada. A major health concern raised about this nuclear waste disposal program is the need to transport large quantities of highly radioactive waste by truck or train across the United States. Many people do not want these wastes to be

transported through their community, but the current situation is not safe either. This problem will get only worse as older nuclear power plants are retired and hundreds of tons of radioactive concrete and steel must be disposed of.

 TALKING POINTS How can you approach your political representatives about environmental policy? What are some effective ways of keeping health-related environmental issues on the national agenda?

The Global Environment

The global environment is made up of the atmosphere, oceans, continental land masses, and all the living organisms that exist on Earth. Interactions among these components of the global environment influence the characteristics of solar radiation at the ground level, climate (temperature, precipitation, seasonal variation), production of food plants and animals, availability of freshwater, energy requirements for heating and cooling of human habitations, the geographic distribution of diseases, the composition of natural communities (deserts, tundra, rain forest), and the survival and extinction of species.

Some of the characteristics of the global environment have obvious and direct effects on human physical health, such as the presence of disease-causing organisms or solar UV radiation that can increase the risk of skin cancer. Other effects of the global environment on personal health are less well documented, such as the adverse effects on emotional or spiritual health associated with the extinction of species or destruction of beautiful natural communities. Many scientists warn that the global environment is being degraded by the combined forces of ever more powerful technology being used by a rapidly increasing global human population. In this section we briefly describe major concerns regarding the global environment and how these might affect personal health.

 TALKING POINTS Your sister is a sun worshipper who loves the look of a deep, dark tan. How might you persuade her to protect her skin from the rays of the sun?

Human Population Explosion

Many scientists warn that the human population is increasing at a rate that cannot be sustained by the resources of the Earth. (See Figure 17-3.) There are currently over 6 billion people in the global human population, and this is projected to increase to over 10 billion in the next 50 years. Every year the world's population grows by about 78 million people, with 97 percent born into the poorest countries.[34] Consider the vast problems we face with the current population, including depletion of natural resources (freshwater, food, and oil), air and water pollution, conflict and political upheaval, starvation, and destruction of natural communities. Now imagine trying to solve these problems in the 21st century with twice as many people trying to make a living and raise a family on the same Earth.

The effects of the human population explosion on personal health depend on who you are and where you live. Many of the poorer nations of Asia, Africa, and South America will not be able to feed their people; starvation and associated diseases will be major health problems for these populations. Growing populations in dry regions are exceeding their freshwater supply, and hundreds of millions of people must drink from contaminated water sources. Every year, 5 million children die from waterborne diarrhea diseases associated with unsanitary drinking water.[34] By 2025, 2.5 billion people may live in regions where available freshwater is insufficient to meet their needs.

In many extremely poor countries, hungry people will destroy most or all of the remaining natural communities (tropical rain forests, African savanna) in vain efforts to grow food on lands that are not suited for agriculture. Overcultivation of farmlands has already degraded the fertility of a land area equivalent to that of

Figure 17-3 Growth of the Earth's human population

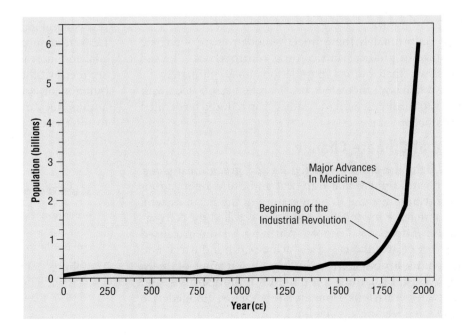

the United States and Canada combined.[34] Hungry people on oceanic islands destroy their coral reefs by using dynamite or cyanide to catch fish. In Africa hungry people hunt wild game for food, putting more species at risk of extinction.

Competition among nations for limited supplies of water and oil is often a root cause of political tensions, terrorism, and war. Political upheaval in the Middle East, recent terrorist attacks on U.S. targets, and the war in Iraq can be partially explained by competition for scarce resources (water, land, and oil). The genocide that killed hundreds of thousands in Rwanda in 1994–1995 has been traced to inequitable distribution of land and associated hunger in some parts of that country.[35]

The solutions to the human population growth problem are simple in theory, but often complex in their implementation. Basic population ecology theory states that the rate of population growth can be reduced if: (1) women have fewer children over their lifetime and (2) if they delay the start of their reproduction. A somewhat counterintuitive pattern is that population growth rate slows when infant survival rate is increased by better health care. Women choose to have fewer children if they are confident that the children they do have will survive.[34]

Simply providing education opportunities to girls can have major and long-lasting effects that act to reduce population growth. Girls who become educated delay having their first child; educated women have half the pregnancies of their uneducated sisters.[34] Educated women are more likely to be able to find employment outside the home. Working women usually have fewer children, and women with an independent income have a greater say about how many children they will have. Access to birth control information and affordable contraception is also needed to allow women to control their family size.

Unfortunately, these proactive initiatives are often held hostage to political and cultural controversies. The sad result is that human populations may ultimately be controlled by increased death rates associated with starvation, disease, and war, rather than reduced birth rates.

Global Climate Change

A wide range of human activities add **greenhouse gases** to the atmosphere that trap heat and cause a net gain of energy and increase in temperature in the Earth system. This increase in global temperature is called the "Greenhouse Effect" or "Global Warming." Human-caused sources of greenhouse gases include both industrial and agricultural activities, including the burning of fuels, conversion of natural communities to human uses, and methane emissions from livestock herds, flooded rice fields, and leaking gas pipelines.[36]

There is growing evidence that increases in atmospheric greenhouse gases are associated with changes in global climate. Chemical analyses of gas bubbles in glacial ice core samples from the polar ice caps indicate that over the past 420,000 years when carbon dioxide and methane concentrations increased, so did atmospheric temperature.[37] Coincident with the current increase in atmospheric concentrations of greenhouse gases, average global surface temperature was higher during the decade of the 1990s than at any other time in recorded history.[36] However, there is still controversy regarding the relative contributions of humans versus natural processes, and whether or not this warming trend is a short-term phenomenon or the beginning of a long-term trend.

Potential effects of climate change on human health include increased heat stress, loss of life in increasingly frequent severe storms and floods, expansion of the range of disease-carrying insects from subtropical regions into temperate regions (such as the United States), increased abundance of waterborne pathogens, decreased air and water quality, and decreased food availability associated with severe weather and water shortages.[36]

Ecological effects of global warming include increased frequency of wildfires and insect pest outbreaks that destroy forests, and widespread death of coral reefs associated with higher water temperature. Many scientists project large-scale decline and extinction of species that cannot adapt to changes in climate and cannot migrate to more suitable areas because of barriers associated with human roads, cities, and farms.[36] These ecological changes could adversely impact emotional and spiritual health as cherished natural wonders are degraded or disappear entirely under the onslaught of climate changes.

The primary means proposed for reducing and reversing global warming associated with human activities is to reduce the burning of fossil fuels such as oil and coal and increase the proportion of our energy needs that are met by other technologies. Many suggest that a combination of energy conservation, increased efficiency of automobiles and electrical appliances, and a gradual shift to alternate power sources for cars (fuel cells and/or

> ### Key Terms
>
> **greenhouse gases** a category of gases in the atmosphere that allow solar radiation to pass through the atmosphere to the Earth but then trap the heat that is radiated from the Earth back toward space; greenhouse gases include water vapor, carbon dioxide, methane, nitrous oxide, and tropospheric ozone

hydrogen) and electricity (photovoltaic cells, wind turbines, geothermal energy, nuclear power) can get this job done. These transitions will require major shifts in national and global economies, continuing innovation and technology development, and many small changes in everyday life of humans on planet Earth.

Your ability as an individual to take personal responsibility for addressing the global warming problem is limited, but all good things must start with individuals willing to do the right thing. You can reduce your personal contribution to global warming by conserving electricity at home, driving the most fuel-efficient automobile that meets your needs, using mass transit where available, recycling/reusing, and purchasing appliances that are rated as highly efficient. Government action will be required to support widespread conservation practices in industry and business. You could join and be active in environmental organizations that work to address global warming. When politicians see their constituents want to protect our common global environment, they may find the political will to do the right thing.

Stratospheric Ozone Depletion

The *stratospheric ozone layer* is a concentration of ozone molecules located about 10 to 25 miles above the Earth's surface. Stratospheric ozone is a naturally occurring gas formed by the interaction of atmospheric oxygen and components of solar radiation. The stratospheric ozone layer protects living organisms on the Earth's surface from harmful solar ultraviolet (UV) radiation. For people, overexposure to UV rays can lead to skin cancer, cataracts (clouding of the lens of the eye), and weakened immune systems. Increased UV can also lead to reduced crop yield and disruptions in the ocean's food chain.

It has been well-documented that chemical reactions between stratospheric ozone and certain human-made air pollutants can significantly reduce the ozone layer, causing increased UV radiation at the Earth's surface. The chemicals that cause ozone depletion include chlorofluorocarbons or CFCs (used as coolants in many air conditioning and refrigeration systems, in insulating foams, and as solvents), halons (used in fire suppression systems), and methyl bromide (used in pesticides).[38]

The vast majority of this depletion of the ozone layer occurs in the atmosphere above the north and south polar regions, with up to a 60 percent loss over Antarctica. These decreases in the stratospheric ozone layer have been associated with as much as a 50 percent increase in UV radiation at the ground level in Antarctica.[38] The ozone layer above the United States has decreased by 5–10 percent.[38]

In response to the well-documented links between certain air pollutants and depletion of the ozone layer, an international ban on the production of halons and CFCs

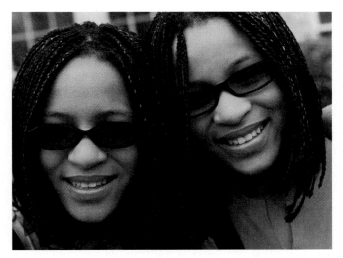

When you buy sunglasses, look for the UV-protection rating.

went into effect in the mid-1990s. As the amounts of ozone-depleting chemicals in the atmosphere decrease, the ozone layer is expected to recover to natural levels by the year 2050.[38]

To limit your risk of skin cancer and other UV-related health problems, limit your exposure to direct sunlight, and when you are outside wear sunscreen on exposed skin. You should also wear sunglasses that are rated as eliminating over 95 percent of UV radiation.

Loss of Natural Habitats and Species Extinctions

On every continent, an exploding human population armed with increasingly powerful technology is altering or completely taking over the habitats of other species that share our planet. Sixteen to 23 percent of the total land surface of Earth has been converted entirely for human uses, including row crop fields, grazing lands, and urban/industrial areas. As much as 40–50 percent of the land surface has been transformed or degraded by human activities.[39] Only 20 percent of the original forest cover on Earth remains ecologically intact and able to support its full complement of species, mostly in the northern parts of Canada and Siberia.[40] As much as 30 percent of the African continent is at risk for **desertification,** mainly

Key Terms

desertification a process that converts lands that historically supported grasslands, shrublands, or dry forest to nonproductive desert due to overgrazing by livestock, excessive brush and tree cutting for fuel, and inappropriate agricultural practices.[41]

The worldwide human population currently uses 50 percent of the Earth's freshwater runoff, 70 percent of which is used for agricultural irrigation. In some major river drainages—for example, the Colorado River in the southwest United States—water diversion is so great that no water reaches the ocean.

Human impact on the biosphere is not limited to the land. Sixty percent of the human population lives within 100 km of an ocean coast, and humans consume 25–35 percent of the energy flow in coastal ocean waters. As of 1995, 22 percent of all ocean fisheries for human consumption were overexploited (resulting in population crashes of the targeted fish species), and another 44 percent were being exploited at their maximum sustainable level.[39] In Indonesia, with the largest coral reef system in the world, 70 percent of the reefs have been severely degraded by dynamite fishing. Worldwide, 30 percent of all coral reefs have been destroyed by human activities, pollution, and coral bleaching that may be associated with global warming. Coastal water pollution has been linked to increased frequency of harmful algae blooms that cause extensive fish kills, massive "dead zones" where nothing else can live, and increased risk of shellfish poisoning for humans who eat seafood.[39]

The cumulative effects of all these human-caused changes to the Earth's land and oceans have increased the species extinction rate by 100 to 1,000 times over rates estimated for the period before human domination. The primary causes of these extinctions are habitat loss due to human transformations of land and water and overharvesting of species by humans.[40]

The effects on personal health associated with worldwide loss of natural communities and species extinctions are highly variable from person to person. Pharmaceutical companies have found many substances produced by species in various natural communities to be useful sources of drugs to treat human illnesses. As the richness of species on Earth is depleted by extinction, we lose a wealth of genetic material that could be of great importance to human health. The loss of natural ecosystems also undermines the systems that function to make Earth a livable planet, contributing to such problems as global climate change, freshwater shortages, and increased frequency of destructive flooding.

Some have proposed that human evolution predisposes us to desire green spaces and diverse biological systems; this is called the *Biophilia hypothesis*.[42] That is, we are most happy when we are surrounded by natural beauty. Many have written about the human psychological benefits from natural communities. John Muir, a famous early environmentalist in the United States, wrote:

Climb the mountains and get their good tidings. Nature's peace will flow into you as sunshine flows into trees. The winds will blow their own freshness into you, and the storms their energy, while cares drop off like autumn leaves.

Wallace Stegner wrote a passage that appears in the Wilderness Act passed by the U.S. Congress in 1964 to protect areas of intact ecosystems in the United States for the enjoyment of future generations:

It was a lovely and terrible wilderness, such a wilderness as Christ and the prophets went out into; harshly and beautifully colored, broken and worn until its bones are exposed, its great sky without a smudge or a taint from Technocracy, and in hidden corners and pockets under its cliffs, the sudden poetry of springs. Save a piece of country like that intact, and it does not matter in the slightest that only a few people every year will go into it. That is precisely its value . . . We simply need that wild country available to us, even if we never do more than drive to its edge and look in. For it can be a means of reassuring ourselves of our sanity as creatures, a part of the geography of hope.

Both Muir and Stegner refer to the psychological benefits that humans derive simply from the knowledge that natural communities and wildlife species still exist, as they always have, somewhere on our planet. For many, the loss of Earth's natural heritage would have profound adverse

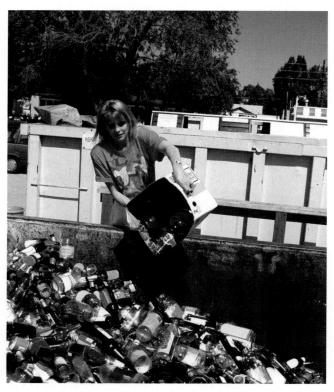

Recycling glass, paper, and metal can reduce land pollution and consumption of natural resources.

consequences for their emotional, psychological, and spiritual well-being. The thought of forever losing wilderness, coral reefs, rain forests, whales, pandas, tigers, and eagles can cause anger, frustration, depression, hopelessness, and despair.[43]

How can you or any one person exert any degree of personal control over such a great and complex threat to your physical, emotional, and spiritual health? Let's start with the little things: conserve energy, recycle and reuse what you can, limit your consumption of the world's resources to what you need, and join together with others of like mind to provide political and financial support to organizations that are working to solve these big problems (see the listing in the Star box below).

Another way you can reduce the negative environmental effects of your personal consumption of natural resources is to "buy green" when you can. In recent years, environmental organizations have begun certification programs so that the consumer can identify which products are produced by "Earth-friendly" means (for more information, go to www.newdream.org/buygreen/). Examples of such products include sustainably harvested timber, shade-grown coffee, and organic food and cotton. Many "buy green" organizations also work to improve the economic conditions of small rural villages where the producers of their products live. These efforts at economic development are often associated with improved education opportunities that lead to reduced birth rates,

Organizations Working to Address Environmental and Population Concerns

Population Issues
United Nations Family Planning Organization: www.unfpa.org
International Planned Parenthood Federation: www.ippf.org
The Population Institute: www.populationinstitute.org

Environmental Political Advocacy Groups
Sierra Club: www.sierraclub.org
Wilderness Society: www.wilderness.org

National Wildlife Federation: www.nwf.org
Natural Resources Defense Council: www.nrdc.org
Environmental Defense Fund: www.environmentaldefense.org
The League of Conservation Voters: www.lcv.org

Conservation of Natural Communities and Endangered Species
The Nature Conservancy: nature.org

World Wildlife Fund: www.panda.org

Source of Environmental Information
World Resources Institute: www.worldwatch.org
U.S. Environmental Protection Agency: www.epa.gov

slowing global human population growth that is the root cause for many environmental problems. For ideas on how to make environmentally sound choices in your life, see Changing for the Better on page 465.

The combined actions of 6 billion people making personal choices will determine the future of the Earth's environment and thus the future of humankind on Earth. The solutions to the great environmental problems looming in the future begin with you, today. Your positive actions and faith in fellow humans to do the right thing will not only benefit the future but also enhance your emotional well-being in the present.

Taking Charge of Your Health

- Protect yourself from ultraviolet light. Always wear sunscreen, and make sure your sunglasses filter out UV rays.

- Have your home tested for radon, and install a radon reduction system if necessary.

- Install a water filtration device to remove contaminants from your drinking water.

- Keep your car in proper running condition to reduce the amount of noise and air pollution it produces.

- Reduce your personal impact on the environment by reducing your consumption of energy and recycling and reusing what you can, and using Earth-friendly products in your home.

- Take personal action on environmental issues using the suggestions outlined in Changing for the Better on page 465.

SUMMARY

- Your environment contains a wide range of substances, living organisms, and forms of energy that may substantially impact one or more dimensions of your personal health.

- Environmental influences on personal health operate over a wide range of spatial scales, from the personal spaces of your home and workplace, to the common spaces of your community and region, to the global environment that supports all life on Earth.

- The most direct environmental health risks to your physical health are related to the presence of toxic substances or pathogenic organisms (pollutants) in the air and water of your personal and community environments.

- You can exert the greatest degree of control over your exposure to pollutants within the personal environment of your home and workplace. You can identify environmental health risks in your personal environment, and then eliminate or reduce these risks by changing your buying habits and eliminating pollutant sources.

- Air pollution in major urban areas can cause significant adverse health effects, especially for people who suffer from respiratory or cardiac disease.

- While you have no control over community air pollution, you can limit your exposure to these toxic substances by being aware of daily pollution levels and by restricting your outdoor activities when these levels are high.

- Much progress has been made in reducing community water pollution, but water in many rivers and lakes still contains chemicals and pathogens that can adversely affect your health.

- You should seek out information about any health advisories for wild foods you obtain from local rivers, and advisories regarding recreational use of those rivers.

- The U.S. Environmental Protection Agency monitors and regulates the quality of drinking water from municipal water suppliers, but it is up to you to ensure the safety of your drinking water if it comes from a private well.

- Improper disposal of toxic solid wastes in landfills designed for household waste is a major source of regional surface and groundwater pollution.

- You should never dispose of toxic household products (batteries, automotive fluids, pesticides, oil-based paint products) by simply putting them in the household trash or pouring them down a drain. Take them to specially designated toxic disposal locations.

- Loss of green space in your community and regional environment, associated with urban sprawl and unregulated land development, can diminish your perceived quality of life and reduce opportunities for exercise, which is important for maintaining good physical health.

- While you have limited personal control over the environment of your community and region, you can still work to enhance your environment by joining others of like mind in groups that advocate environmental protection through the democratic political process.

- At the current rate of human population growth, most scientists of the world warn of increased starvation and disease, decreased standards of living, and increased conflict over progressively decreasing supplies of natural resources.

- Human population growth can be substantially slowed by simply providing girls and women opportunities to become educated and gainfully employed, and access to contraception.
- Pollutants produced by humans are responsible for changes in the atmosphere that are altering climate patterns and allowing harmful solar radiation to reach the surface of the Earth.

- Changes in the global environment have potential to increase risks to human health, and to significantly harm many other species and natural communities.
- While individuals can do little to address global environmental problems, the solutions all start with individual choices about family size, resource consumption, and political candidates. The best path to a livable future for humankind is to do your part and have faith that others will do theirs.

REVIEW QUESTIONS

1. What is radon, and what are the health risks associated with it? What actions can you take to minimize the health risks of radon?
2. Identify the sources and the potential health effects of the following common indoor air pollutants: carbon monoxide, volatile organic compounds, and biological pollutants such as mold, mildew, pollen, and pet dander. Describe actions you could take to minimize health risks from these pollutants.
3. What health risks are associated with lead and asbestos? What actions can you take to minimize these risks?
4. Describe actions you should take to safeguard drinking from a well on your own property.
5. What are the physical and emotional health effects of noise? What actions could you take to minimize the health risks of noise?
6. Tropospheric ozone and small particulate matter are community and regional air pollutants that have been linked to serious health risks. For each of these substances, describe the main human source(s), the effect(s) on human physical health, and what actions you could take to minimize your own risk of adverse health effects from these air pollutants.
7. What are "air toxics" and where do you think you are most likely to be exposed to these substances? What do you think you could do to minimize your personal health risk from air toxics?
8. What is "biological water pollution" and what is the main source of this pollution in your community's rivers, streams, and/or lakes? What are the health risks associated with biological water pollution? What can you do to mini-

mize the risk to your personal health from this type of pollution?
9. Who is responsible for ensuring the safety of your drinking water if the source is a municipal water company? What can you do to minimize any health risks associated with your drinking water in this circumstance?
10. What is the main health risk associated with land pollution from solid waste landfills? What can you do to minimize your personal contribution to this type of pollution?
11. What is "green space," and why is it important to your personal health? What personal actions could you take to protect green space in your community or region?
12. What policies should the U.S. foreign aid agencies implement in poor underdeveloped countries to help them reduce their population growth rate? Explain how these policies would work toward this goal.
13. Global warming and stratospheric ozone depletion are large-scale changes in the global environment with uncertain, but potentially significant, health consequences. For each of these global changes, describe the cause(s) of environmental change, the potential health effects, and what might be done to minimize these effects.
14. Loss of natural habitats and species extinctions are major ecological problems, but do these phenomena represent any risk to *your* personal health? Your answer should reflect your own perceptions, and should provide some explanation for your assessment.
15. A well-known environmentalist slogan is, "Think globally, but act locally." Based on what you've learned in this chapter, describe how you think this slogan applies to your personal actions in response to environmental health risks.

ENDNOTES

1. U.S. Environmental Protection Agency. Healthy Buildings, Healthy People: A Vision for the 21st Century. 2003. www.epa.gov/iaq/hbhp/index.html.
2. Consumer Product Safety Commission. Carbon Monoxide Questions and Answers. CPSC Document #466. 2003. www.cpsc.gov/cpscpub/pubs/466.html.
3. U.S. Environmental Protection Agency. The Senseless Killer. 2003. www.epa.gov/iaq/pubs/senseles.html.
4. U.S. Environmental Protection Agency. The Inside Story: A Guide to Indoor Air Quality. 1995. www.epa.gov/iaq/pubs/insidest.html.
5. Thorn J, et al. Adult-onset asthma linked to mold and tobacco smoke exposure. *Allergy* 56: 287–292, 2001.

6. U.S. Environmental Protection Agency. Sources of Indoor Air Pollution: Asbestos. 2003. www.epa.gov/iaq/asbestos.html.
7. U.S. Environmental Protection Agency. Sources of Indoor Air Pollution: Lead (Pb). 2003. www.epa.gov/iaq/lead.html.
8. U.S. Department of Health and Human Services, Public Health Service, Agency for Toxic Substances and Disease Registry. Case Studies In Environmental Medicine: Lead Toxicity. 1995. www.atsdr.cdc.gov/HEC/HSPH/caselead.html.
9. U.S. Environmental Protection Agency. Sources of Indoor Air Pollution: Biological Pollutants. 2003. www.epa.gov/iaq/biologic.html.

10. National Safety Council. Radon. 2002. www.nsc.org/ehc/radon.htm.

11. National Academy of Sciences. Biological Effects of Ionizing Radiation (BEIR) VI Report: "The Health Effects of Exposure to Indoor Radon." 1998. National Academy Press. http://books.nap.edu/books/ 0309056454/html/.

12. National Academy of Science. Risk Assessment of Radon in Drinking Water. 1999. www.nap.edu/books/0309062926/html/index.html.

13. Salford LG, et al. Nerve cell damage in mammalian brain after exposure to microwaves from GSM mobile phones. *Environmental Health Perspectives* 111 (7): 881–883, 2003.

14. Foster KR. Are mobile phones safe? Institute of Electrical and Electronic Engineers (IEEE) *Spectrum Online,* 37 (8), 2000. www.spectrum.ieee.org/publicfeature/aug00/prad.html.

15. U.S. Food and Drug Administration. Cell Phone Facts: Consumer Information on Wireless Phones. 2002. www.fda.gov/cellphones/qa.html#25.

16. Health effects of radiofrequency exposure: A review. *Environmental Health Perspectives,* 112 (17), 2004.

17. UK Childhood Cancer Study Investigators. Childhood cancer and residential proximity to power lines. *Brit J Cancer* 83: 1573–1580, 2000.

18. Savitz DA, Loomis DP. Magnetic field exposure in relation to leukemia and brain cancer mortality among electric utility workers. *American Journal of Epidemiology* 141 (2):123–128, 1995

19. Greenland S, Sheppard AR, et al. A pooled analysis of magnetic fields, wirecodes, and childhood leukemia. *Epidemiology* 11: 624–634, 2000.

20. U.S. Environmental Protection Agency. Water on Tap: A Consumer's Guide to the Nation's Drinking Water. 2003. www.epa.gov/safewater/wot/howsafe.html.

21. U.S. Environmental Protection Agency. Technical Factsheet on: Nitrate / Nitrite. 2002. www.epa.gov/safewater/dwh/t-ioc/nitrates.html.

22. Gray LE, Ostby J. Effects of pesticides and toxic substances on behavioral and morphological reproductive development: Endocrine versus no-endocrine mechanisms. *Toxicology and Industrial Health* 14: 159–184, 1998.

23. U.S. Environmental Protection Agency. Permeation and Leaching. 2003. www.epa.gov/safewater/tcr/pdf/permleach.pdf.

24. Bell PA. Noise, pollution, and psychopathology. *In:* AMA Ghadirian and HE Lehmann (Eds.): *Environment and Psychopathology.* New York: Springer Publishing Co., 1993.

25. U.S. Environmental Protection Agency. Draft Report on the Environment: Outdoor Air Quality. 2003. www.epa.gov/indicators/roe/html/roeAirOut.htm.

26. Dockery DW, Pope CA, III. Acute respiratory effects of particulate air pollution. *Annual Review Public Health* 15, 107–132, 1994.

27. Perera F, et al. Effects of transplacental exposure to environmental pollutants on birth outcomes in a multiethnic population. *Environmental Health Perspectives* 111 (2): 201–205, 2003.

28. Perera F, et al. DNA damage from polycyclic aromatic hydrocarbons measured by Benzo[a] pyrene-DNA adducts in mothers and newborns from northern Manhattan, the World Trade Center area, Poland, and China. *Cancer, Epidemiology Biomarkers & Prevention* 14:709–714. 2005.

29. U.S. Environmental Protection Agency. Asthma Triggers—Related Topics—Ozone. 2003. www.epa.gov/iaq/asthma/triggers/ozone.html.

30. McConnell R, et al. Asthma in exercising children exposed to ozone. *The Lancet* 359: 386–391, 2002.

31. U.S. Environmental Protection Agency. The National Air Toxics Assessment. 2002. www.epa.gov/ttn/atw/nata.

32. U.S. Environmental Protection Agency. Drinking Water and Your Health, What You Need to Know, List of Drinking Water Contaminants & MCLs. 2003. www.epa.gov/safewater/mcl.html#1.

33. U.S. Environmental Protection Agency. Municipal Solid Waste: Basic Facts. 2003. www.epa.gov/epaoswer/non-hw/muncpl/facts.htm.

34. The Population Institute. www.populationinstitute.org/.

35. Gasana J. Remember Rwanda? *World Watch* 15(5): 24–33, 2002.

36. Intergovernmental Panel on Climate Change. Climate Change 2001: Summary Report: Synthesis for Policy Makers. 2001. www.ipcc.ch/pub/un/syreng/spm.pdf.

37. Petit JR, et al. Climate and atmospheric history of the past 420,000 years from the Vostok ice core, Antarctica. *Nature* 399: 429–436, 1999.

38. U.S. Environmental Protection Agency. The Science of Ozone Depletion. 2003. www.epa.gov/docs/ozone/science/index.html.

39. Vitousek P, et al. Human domination of Earth's ecosystems. *Science* 277: 494–499, 1997.

40. World Resources Institute. 2003. www.wri.org.

41. United Nations: Food and Agriculture Organization. www.fao.org/desertification/default.asp?lang=en.

42. Wilson E. *Biophilia: The Human Bond with Other Species.* Cambridge, MA: Harvard University Press, 1984.

43. Gardner GT, Stern PC. *Environmental Problems and Human Behavior.* Needham Heights, MA: Allyn & Bacon, 1996.

personal assessment

Are you an environmentalist?

When asked, many people will say that they are an "environmentalist," including political leaders who are widely criticized for decisions perceived by others to be environmentally destructive. So what is an "environmentalist"? One definition of environmentalism is that it is an ideology that values and reveres Nature, and works to protect and preserve natural systems for both ethical reasons and because humankind depends on these systems for life. However, beyond this general statement environmentalists encompass a wide diversity of beliefs and practices. For some, their environmental beliefs are a form of religion, others function mainly in the political process, and some operate like terrorist groups who use violence to fight human economic development on behalf of Earth.[1] The wide diversity of beliefs and practices encompassed under "environmentalism" creates a situation where almost anyone could claim to be an environmentalist. Perhaps more useful criteria for determining if you are an environmentalist would be (1) your awareness of how various human activities create environmental health hazards or degrade natural systems; (2) your willingness to consider your own role in creating environmental problems; and (3) your willingness to act in ways that reduce your personal risk from environmental hazards and your contribution to the causes of these hazards. These three criteria define a hierarchy of commitment to environmental protection. First you have to know a problem exists. Then you have to recognize your own part in creating that problem. The last, and most difficult, step is that you must be willing to reduce or eliminate your contribution to environmental problems. Your answers to the following questions will help you think about where you really stand on protecting the environment for yourself, your community, and all the rest of life on Earth.

Awareness of Environmental Problems

1. Have you ever read the water quality assessment provided by the supplier of your drinking water?
2. If your drinking water is from a well, do you know about potential sources of contamination (landfills or other waste disposal sites, large agricultural areas, confined feedlot livestock operations) in your watershed?
3. If your drinking water supply is from a well, do you know if your water contains potentially harmful contaminants?
4. Do you know whether or not your community wastewater treatment system occasionally dumps raw sewage into the local river during high rainfall events?

5. If you use a gas furnace or kerosene space heater, do you know whether or not these appliances are functioning properly so as to maximize energy efficiency and minimize risks from indoor air pollution?
6. Have you ever made a note of air pollution alerts or information about high ultraviolet radiation published in a local newspaper or presented on a local TV news program?
7. Have you ever searched for information on air, water, and land pollution in your community?
8. When you eat fish, are you aware of health advisories regarding contaminants in fish (for example, mercury, PCBs) and recommendations that you limit the amount of the fish you consume?
9. When you purchase products, do you look at packaging materials for warnings that the product contains toxic chemicals?
10. When you listen to loud music, do you think about potential long-term damage to your hearing and the nuisance noise you create for your neighbors?
11. Do you know if your community (city, county, state) has a land-use management (zoning) plan?
12. When you see new economic developments (malls, superstores, warehouses, suburban housing developments) being constructed, do you wonder if wildlife habitat is being destroyed?
13. Do you know the proposed human causes of global warming and the potential consequences of this change in climate?
14. Do you know the causes and potential health effects of depletion of the stratospheric ozone layer?
15. Do you know the link between the wood you buy at a store like Menard's, Lowe's, and Home Depot and species extinctions?

Willingness to Consider Your Personal Environmental Impact

16. When you think about having a family of your own, do you worry about contributing to a rapidly growing human population that is responsible for widespread environmental degradation?
17. When you think about purchasing a vehicle, do you consider fuel efficiency more important than "image" sold by advertisers?
18. When you consider purchasing any product, do you consider the resources used, and pollution created, to produce that product?

19. When you purchase an electric appliance or a gas-powered device, do you consider energy efficiency?

20. When planning to build a new home, do you consider how your choices regarding location and amount of land could contribute to loss of green space and natural habitat?

21. When you use or dispose of household, yard, and automotive chemicals and fluids, do you consider that you may be contributing to local water pollution?

22. When you hear about global warming, do you recognize that your own use of electricity and gas-powered vehicles contributes to this problem?

23. Did you know that if you vent your home or automotive air conditioning system coolant while performing do-it-yourself maintenance, you are contributing to the depletion of the stratospheric ozone layer?

24. When you purchase lumber, do you wonder if the wood you are buying was harvested using environmentally sound practices, or if critical wildlife habitats or wilderness was destroyed to produce the lumber?

25. Do you consider how your vote in public elections can affect government policies that impact the environment?

Willingness to Alter Your Lifestyle to Protect Yourself and the Environment

26. Would you limit the number of your own children to one or two so as to reduce your contribution to the problem of global human population explosion?

27. When you purchase a vehicle, is energy efficiency your main concern?

28. Would you use mass transit to travel from home to work, if it were available, to reduce your contribution to local air pollution and need for paving more land to expand highways?

29. When you buy a home, would you seek to minimize the distance from work and schools to reduce gas consumption, minimize air pollution, and reduce demand for construction of new roads?

30. When you buy a home, would you look for a smaller, energy-efficient home to minimize your contribution to natural resource exploitation and pollution associated with energy consumption?

31. When you buy lighting, do you buy energy-efficient lightbulbs (compact fluorescent and LED) that are initially more expensive, but more efficient and less expensive over the long term?

32. When furnishing your home, would you seek out water-efficient toilets, faucets, and shower heads that conserve freshwater and reduce demands on wastewater treatment systems?

33. Do you set the thermostat in your home to cooler temperatures in winter and warmer temperatures in summer to conserve energy?

34. Would you invest money and effort to better insulate your home so as to reduce energy needed for heating and cooling?

35. When buying food, would you be willing to pay more for organically grown foods that were produced without the use of pesticides and fertilizers that pollute the surrounding environment?

36. Would you buy locally grown foods to support farmers (and their green spaces) in your community and reduce energy spent on long-distance transport?

37. When purchasing wood products, would you buy more expensive wood that is certified to have been harvested using environmentally sound practices?

38. Would you be willing to have something less than the perfect lawn to avoid using fertilizers and pesticides that contaminate local waterways?

39. Would you limit your personal consumption of material goods to mainly those things you need, so as to reduce exploitation of natural resources?

40. When you dispose of household chemicals, automotive fluids, and spent batteries, do you make the extra effort to be sure they do not end up polluting the environment, like taking them to a Tox-Away Day location?

41. Do you make the effort to recycle paper, glass, plastic, and metals?

42. When you make purchases, do you look for products made from recycled materials (for example, post-consumer recycled paper, "plastic wood," fleece clothing made from recycled plastic)?

43. Do you limit the noise that you produce (loud music, loud car or motorcycle engines, barking dogs) to reduce noise pollution in your neighborhood?

44. Do you contribute financial support to environmental groups that promote conservation and protection of natural resources through the legal and political systems?

45. When you consider candidates for public office, do you vote for the candidates who have strong records or position statements for environmental protection?

If the majority of your answers to questions 1 to 15 are "Yes," you are likely "environmentally aware." That is, you pay attention to news stories about environmental issues or have taken an environmental science course.

If most of your answers to questions 16 to 25 are "Yes," you are "environmentally conscious." That is, you are not only aware of the problems, but beginning to think about how these problems are related to your own lifestyle.

If the majority of your answers to questions 26 to 45 are "Yes," you are likely "environmentally active." That is, you are personally involved in efforts to address environmental problems through your own lifestyle choices and through the political process.

[1]Wikipedia (The Free Encyclopedia). www.wikipedia.org/wiki/Environmentalism.

chapter eighteen

Accepting Dying and Death

Eye on the Media

The Controversy Surrounding the Death of Terri Schiavo

Terri Schiavo's death became a legal battle, a media event, religious debate, and was even brought into the political spotlight. She was 26 years old when she had heart failure because of a chemical imbalance that may have been caused by an eating disorder. This left her severely brain damaged for 15 years. While she was in hospice care in a vegetative state, her husband and her parents were in a legal battle over whether to remove the feeding tube that was keeping her alive. If she had had a living will, this would have helped to make her wishes more clear, but it may not have precluded the legal debate. Advance directives such as living wills and durable powers of attorney for health care are legal documents that communicate the person's wishes about being kept alive with life support should they become incapacitated.

Both Terri Schiavo's husband and her parents claimed to know her end-of-life wishes, but none of them was named as her health care agent or proxy, giving him or her a legal right to make this determination. Michael, her husband, stated that she had made casual comments about not wanting to be on life support if she were ever incapacitated. She had further stated to him that she didn't ever want to be a burden to him or her family. Her parents countered by saying that she was a devout Roman Catholic who believed in the sanctity of life. The publicity that this case received resulted in the America people becoming involved in this right-to-life battle, with a California businessman offering Michael Schiavo $1 million to walk away from Terri and allow her parents to have guardianship.

The tug of war that ensued between her family members, as well as the publicity surrounding her dying wishes, spurred thousands of people to consider completing living wills. In fact, the Aging with Dignity organization estimated that requests for advance directives increased 10-fold because of the Schiavo case. They further reported that they distributed over 1 million copies of living wills since this case, and orders for more living wills continued to flood in at a rate of 200 an hour.

Bitter legal battles continued for 12 years between these families. The case was brought to the U.S. Supreme court six times and refused each time. The Governor of Florida, Jeb Bush, sided with the parents and lobbied to have the tube reconnected after it had been removed. Even President Bush became involved in this volatile case, signing a law allowing transfer of jurisdiction of the case from Florida state court to a U.S. District Court so that federal judges could review the case. Again, the judges stated that any action on their part would be improper. There was a great deal of public outcry, with some referring to her death as "judicial homicide."

Terri Schiavo remained in hospice care for 5 years. There were further disputes over who was allowed to be at her bedside when she died, because her husband prohibited her parents and brother from being in the room saying he wanted her to have a peaceful environment for her death. Because she

The primary goal of this chapter is to help people realize that the reality of death can motivate us to live a more enjoyable, healthy, productive, and contributive life. Each day in our lives becomes even more meaningful when we have fully accepted the reality that someday we are going to die. We can then live each day to its fullest.

Our personal awareness of death can provide us with a framework from which to appreciate and conduct our lives. It helps us to prioritize our activities so that we can accomplish our goals (in our academic work, our relationships with others, and our recreation) before we die. Quite simply, death can help us to appreciate living.

Dying in Today's Society

Since shortly after the turn of the 20th century, the manner in which people experience death in this society has changed significantly. Formerly, most people died in their own homes, surrounded by family and friends. Young children frequently lived in the same home with their aging grandparents and saw them grow older and eventually die. Death was seen as a natural extension of life. Children grew up with a keen sense of what death meant, both to the dying person and to the grieving survivors.

Times have indeed changed. Today approximately 70 percent of people die in hospitals, nursing homes, and assisted living care facilities, not in their own homes. The extended family is seldom at the bedside of the dying person.[1] Frequently, frantic efforts are made to keep a dying person from death. Although medical technology has improved our lives, some people believe that it has reduced our ability to die with dignity. Some are convinced that our way of dying has become more artificial and less civilized than it used to be. The trend toward hospice care may be a positive response to this high-tech manner of dying.

As the baby boomers age over the next 30 years, the number of people age 85 and older will more than double to 9 million. This means that the topic of death and dying will become increasingly common and relevant for us all as we cope with the loss of our parents, grandparents, friends, and other family members.

Definitions of Death

Before many of the scientific advancements of the past 30 years, *death* was relatively easy to define. People were considered dead when a heartbeat could no longer be detected and when breathing ceased. Now, with the technological advancements made in medicine, especially emergency medicine, some patients who give every indication of being dead can be resuscitated. Critically ill people, even those in comas, can now be kept alive for years with many of their bodily functions maintained by medical devices, including feeding tubes and respirators.

Thus death can be a very difficult concept to define.[2] Numerous professional associations and ad hoc interdisciplinary committees have struggled with this problem and have developed criteria by which to establish death. Some of these criteria have been adopted by state legislatures, although there is certainly no consensus definition of death that all states embrace.

Clinical determinants of death refer to measures of bodily functions. Often judged by a physician, who can then sign a legal document called a *medical death certificate,* these clinical criteria include the following:

1. Lack of heartbeat and breathing.
2. Lack of central nervous system function, including all reflex activity and environmental responsiveness. Often this can be confirmed by an *electroencephalograph* reading. If there is no brain wave activity after

an initial measurement and a second measurement after 24 hours, the person is said to have undergone *brain death.*

3. The presence of *rigor mortis,* indicating that body tissues and organs are no longer functioning at the cellular level. This is sometimes referred to as *cellular death.*

The *legal determinants* used by government officials are established by state law and often adhere closely to the clinical determinants already listed. A person is not legally dead until a death certificate has been signed by a physician, *coroner,* or health department officer.

Psychological Stages of Dying

A process of self-adjustment has been observed in people who have a terminal illness. The stages in this process have helped form the basis for the modern movement of death education. An awareness of these stages may help you understand how people adjust to other important losses in their lives.

Perhaps the most widely recognized name in the area of death education is Dr. Elisabeth Kübler-Ross. As a psychiatrist working closely with terminally ill patients at the University of Chicago's Billings Hospital, Kübler-Ross was able to observe the emotional reactions of dying people. In her classic book *On Death and Dying,* Kübler-Ross summarized the psychological stages that dying people often experience.[6]

- *Denial.* This is the stage of disbelief. Patients refuse to believe that they actually will die. Denial can serve as a temporary defense mechanism and can allow patients the time to accept their prognosis on their own terms.

- *Anger.* A common emotional reaction after denial is anger. Patients can feel as if they have been cheated. By expressing anger, patients are able to vent some of their fears, jealousies, anxieties, and frustrations. Patients often direct their anger at relatives, physicians and nurses, religious figures, and normally healthy people.

- *Bargaining.* Terminally ill people follow the anger stage with a stage characterized by bargaining. Patients who desperately want to avoid their inevitable deaths attempt to strike bargains—often with God or a church leader. Some people undergo religious conversions. The goal is to buy time by promising to repent for past sins, to restructure and rededicate their lives, or to make a large financial contribution to a religious cause.

- *Depression.* When patients realize that, at best, bargaining can only postpone their fate, they may begin an unpredictable period of depression. In a sense, terminally ill people are grieving for their own anticipated death. They may become quite withdrawn and refuse to visit with close relatives and friends. Prolonged periods of silence or crying are normal components of this stage and should not be discouraged.

- *Acceptance.* During the acceptance stage, patients fully realize that they are going to die. Acceptance ensures a relative sense of peace for most dying people. Anger, resentment, and depression are usually gone. Kübler-Ross describes this stage as one without much feeling. Patients feel neither happy nor sad. Many are calm and introspective and prefer to be left either alone or with a few close relatives or friends.

One or two additional points should be made about the psychological stages of dying. Just as each person's life is totally unique, so is each person's death. Unfolding deaths vary as much as do unfolding lives. Some people move through Kübler-Ross's stages of dying very predictably, but others do not. It is not uncommon for some dying people to avoid one or more of these stages entirely or to revisit a stage more than once.

The second important point to be made about Kübler-Ross's stages of dying is that the family members or friends of dying people often pass through similar stages as they observe their loved ones dying. When informed that a close friend or relative is dying, many people also experience varying degrees of denial, anger, bargaining, depression, and acceptance. Because of this, as caring people we need to recognize that the emotional needs of the living must be fulfilled in ways that do not differ appreciably from those of the dying.

Advance Health Care Directives

Because some physicians and families find it difficult to support indirect euthanasia, many people are starting to use legal documents called *advance health care directives.*[4] One of these health care directives is the **living will** (see the Star Box on page 475). This is a document that confirms a dying person's desire to be allowed to die peacefully and with a measure of dignity if a time should arise when there is little hope for recovery from a terminal illness or severe injury. Living will statutes exist in all 50 states and the

---

Key Terms

living will legal document that requires physicians or family members to carry out a person's wish to die naturally, without receiving sustaining treatments

The Living Will

The living will is a legally binding document in all 50 states and the District of Columbia. This document allows individuals to express their wishes concerning dying with dignity. When such a document has been drawn, families and physicians are better able to deal with the wishes of people who are near death from conditions from which there is no reasonable expectation of recovery. Below is a sample living will for the state of Florida. However, people should use a living will that is specific for the state in which they live. For additional information and materials, contact the Partnership for Caring organization by using the toll-free number 1-800-989-9455 or by visiting Partnership for Caring Web site (www.partnershipforcaring.org). At this site, you can download state-specific packages for free.

Florida Living Will

Instructions	
Print the date	Declaration made this _____ day of _____, _____ .
	(day) _(month)_ _(year)_
Print your name	I, _____, willfully and voluntarily make known my desire that my dying not be artificially prolonged under the circumstances set forth below, and I do hereby declare that:
Please initial each that applies	If at any time I am incapacitated and
	_____ I have a terminal condition, or
	_____ I have an end-stage condition, or
	_____ I am in a persistent vegetative state
	and if my attending or treating physician and another consulting physician have determined that there is no reasonable medical probability of my recovery from such condition, I direct that life prolonging procedures be withheld or withdrawn when the application of such procedures would serve only to prolong artificially the process of dying, and that I be permitted to die naturally with only the administration or the performance of any medical procedure deemed necessary to provide me with comfort care or to alleviate pain.
	It is my intention that this declaration be honored by my family and physician as the final expression of my legal right to refuse medical or surgical treatment and to accept the consequences for such refusal.
	In the event that I have been determined to be unable to provide express and informed consent regarding the withholding, withdrawal, or continuation of life-prolonging procedures, I wish to designate, as my surrogate to carry out the provisions of the declarations:
Print the name, home address and telephone number of your surrogate	Name: _____
	Address: _____
	_____ Zip Code: _____
	Phone: _____

© 2000 Partnership for Caring, Inc.

Florida Living Will—Page 2 of 2

Print name, home address and telephone number of your alternate surrogate	I wish to designate the following person as my alternate surrogate to carry out the provisions of this declaration should my surrogate be unwilling or unable to act on my behalf:
	Name: _____
	Address: _____
	_____ Zip Code: _____
	Phone: _____
Add personal instructions (if any)	Additional instructions (optional):
	I understand the full import of this declaration, and I am emotionally and mentally competent to make this declaration.
Sign the document	Signed: _____
Witnessing Procedure	Witness 1:
Two witnesses must sign and print their addresses	Signed: _____
	Address: _____
	Witness 2:
	Signed: _____
	Address: _____

© 2000 Partnership for Caring, Inc.

Courtesy of **Partnership for Caring, Inc.** 6/00
1035 30th Street, NW Washington, DC 20007 800-989-9455

District of Columbia. The living will requires that physicians or family members carry out a person's wishes to die naturally, without receiving life-sustaining treatments. An estimated 25 percent of U.S. adults have signed living wills.[5] The Terri Schiavo case has drawn increased attention to health care advance directives, because she neither had a living will nor did she designate a health care agent. A bitter legal battle ensued between her husband and her parents regarding whether to keep her on life support while she lay in a vegetative state for 15 years.

A second important document that can assist terminally ill or incapacitated patients is the **durable power of attorney for health care** document. This legal document authorizes another person to make specific health care decisions about treatment and care under specified circumstances, most commonly when patients are in vegetative states and cannot communicate their medical wishes. This document helps inform hospitals

Key Terms

durable power of attorney for health care a legal document that designates who will make health care decisions for people unable to do so and physicians which person will help make the critical medical decisions. It is recommended that people complete both a living will and a durable power of attorney for health care document.

Coping with Specific Causes of Death

Coping with Terminal Illness

Watching a family member or friend slowly die can bring mixed emotions, from being glad to have that person with you as long as possible to wishing that the person would not have to suffer. It can be painful to see the person you know gradually slip away. In addition, he or she may become someone who seems more like a stranger to you and may not even recognize you or acknowledge your presence. Some people say that they are thankful for the time they have with this person and to be able to say good-bye. However, others may feel a false sense of hopefulness that the person is beating the illness only to feel shocked and devastated when the illness begins to progress at a faster rate. The research does suggest that we cope better with loss when we are expecting it, when we have time to prepare and take whatever action we feel necessary in response to it. In this way, a protracted illness can facilitate the ability to cope that people who experience loss through accidental death, natural disaster, suicide, or murder do not have.

Coping with Accidental Death, Natural Disasters, and Terrorism

Deaths that occur from natural disasters or accidental deaths bring some unique challenges. Accidental death is the number-one cause of death for 15- to 34-year-olds, and so college students may encounter this more often than terminal illnesses. Though any type of trauma or crisis is more difficult to deal with when it is unexpected, accidental death seems particularly devastating in that you are unprepared and shocked by the news. Often people have more trouble accepting this type of death because it is so unexpected that it seems unreal.

Death from natural disasters are typically uncommon and unlikely and so are even more difficult to comprehend and accept. We tend to cope better with events we can understand and explain. Yet this may be impossible to do with accidental deaths such as from a car accident or from incidents without a clear cause of death. Part of finding an explanation can also involve blaming someone: "I should have known he was too tired to

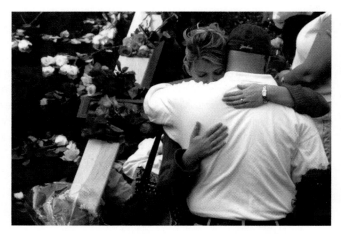

Grief is even harder to bear when loss happens suddenly, such as when a person commits suicide or dies in an accident. Family members of victims of the terrorist attacks on September 11, 2001, comfort each other.

drive." People can feel more vulnerable and fearful after accidents and disasters and become more hesitant in their day-to-day living. Things that you may not have questioned begin to seem potentially dangerous, such as going swimming after a friend has drowned or driving after a car accident.

Death associated with terrorism is something that Americans have not had to face, as other countries have, until 9/11. Since that time, Americans have felt less safe on their own soil and traveling abroad. People have changed their lifestyles in terms of the trips they take, having a survival kit at home, stockpiling food and water, and encountering stringent security. Organizations, hospitals, and government agencies are developing responses to bioterrorism and other types of terrorist attacks.

Coping with Death by Suicide

People react similarly to suicides as they do to accidental death, because both means of death are sudden and unexpected. Making sense of these types of death is difficult, and coping with a completed suicide brings the added burden of understanding the reason and motivation behind the death. If you hold religious beliefs that tell you committing suicide is a sin, this can lead to additional misunderstanding and anger. As with death by murder, this type of death is a crime, and so there are legal as well as religious and moral implications in accepting a person's decision to take his or her own life.

Family members frequently say they feel ashamed and embarrassed by the suicide because of these connotations.

They worry that others will see them and their family as crazy. These concerns usually mean that coping with death by suicide can be a longer process than coping with other types of death. It is helpful for people to understand the events that led up to and contributed to a person's choosing to take his or her life.

Chapter 2 discussed the warning signs and factors that contribute to suicide. Often people blame themselves for not seeing the warning signs or not acting on those they did see. There can also be a sense of feeling unimportant or unloved by this person because you tell yourself "if she really cared about me, she would have fought to stay with me and not left me." Survivors of suicide often feel abandoned and rejected. If your relationship with this person was distant, if you hadn't talked to him or her for awhile or you had recently had an argument, you may feel guilty and blame yourself, saying "if only I had been nicer or called her more often, this might not have happened."

Coping with Death by Murder

Shock, anger, guilt, confusion, and vulnerability are some of the emotions people commonly experience when they cope with a murder. Obviously, you don't expect murder to happen—certainly not to someone you know. It can be difficult to comprehend the taking of someone's life, which makes it even more difficult to accept such a loss. You may blame yourself for not protecting the victim in some way or not doing something to prevent it from happening. If the suspect hasn't been identified or apprehended, you may feel angry at the police for not doing more or feel frightened that you live in a world that seems suddenly very unsafe and frightening. If the murderer has been apprehended, it can take years before the trial is over, making it hard to have a sense of closure.

Euthanasia

There are two type of euthanasia: **indirect (passive) euthanasia** and **direct (active) euthanasia.** Indirect euthanasia is when people are allowed to die without being subjected to life-sustaining efforts such as being placed on life support. Examples of passive euthanasia include physicians' orders of "do not resuscitate (DNR)" and "comfort measures only (CMO)."

Indirect euthanasia is increasingly occurring in a number of hospitals, nursing homes, and medical centers. Physicians who withhold heroic lifesaving techniques or drug therapy treatments or who disconnect life support systems from terminally ill patients are practicing indirect euthanasia. Although some people still consider this form of euthanasia a type of murder, indirect euthanasia seems to be gaining legal and public acceptance for people with certain terminal illnesses—near-death cancer patients, brain-dead accident victims, and hopelessly ill newborn babies.

Direct euthanasia, or active euthanasia, is when people are intentionally put to death. It usually involves the administration of large amounts of depressant drugs, which eventually causes all central nervous system functioning to stop. Although direct euthanasia is commonly practiced on housepets and laboratory animals, it is illegal for humans in the United States, Canada, and other developed countries. However, in 1992, the Netherlands became the first developed country to enact legislation that permits euthanasia under strict guidelines.

TALKING POINTS You're having a class discussion on euthanasia. How would you argue different viewpoints—including euthansia as murder and euthansia as an act of mercy?

Physician-Assisted Suicide

In recent years, physician-assisted suicide has been the focus of some important news stories. In July 1997, the U.S. Supreme Court unanimously ruled that dying people have no fundamental constitutional right to physician-assisted suicide. In effect, this ruling left the decision to individual states to permit or prohibit physician-assisted suicide.

By April 1999, more than 30 states had enacted laws prohibiting assisted suicide, and many other states had essentially prohibited it through common law.[3] Only the state of Oregon had passed a law, in 1994, that legalized assisted suicide. This law is referred to as the Death with Dignity Act. It allows doctors to prescribe fatal doses of barbiturates and other drugs to adults of sound mind who have less than 6 months to live. It requires the patient to be at least 18 years of age and of sound mind, make two oral and one written request for the medication with 15 days between the first request and the final one, consult with two physicians, and notify pharmacists and state health authorities before proceeding with physician-assisted suicide. A fatal drug is prescribed, and the patient

---

Key Terms

indirect (passive) euthanasia allowing people to die without the use of life-sustaining procedures

direct (active) euthanasia intentionally causing death

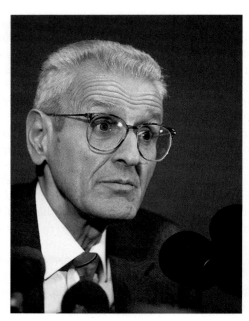

Dr. Jack Kevorkian was convicted of murder in 1999. How do you stand on the issue of physician-assisted suicide?

may ingest it orally at his or her discretion, with or without the doctor present. It remains illegal for physicians to administer lethal injections. To date, 70 people are known to have legally taken medication to hasten their death.

Even though physician-assisted suicide is legal in the state of Oregon, many physicians are unwilling to prescribe the lethal medication. Being confined to their bed or home, living a long way from a large urban area, experiencing difficulty finding a willing physician, dying before completing the requirements of the law, and encountering opposition from family and friends are some of the reasons why greater numbers of terminally ill patients are not obtaining medication to end their lives.

The third major news story concerned the April 1999 Michigan conviction of Dr. Jack Kevorkian, a retired pathologist who had aided in the suicides of over 100 people. Kevorkian was convicted of second-degree murder and delivery of a controlled substance in the assisted suicide of Thomas Youk, a 52-year-old patient with Lou Gehrig's disease. This suicide had been televised on the CBS show *60 Minutes*. Kevorkian is serving a 10- to 25-year sentence at a prison in Jackson, Michigan and could be eligible for parole in 2007 when he will be 79 years old.

Near-Death Experiences

As Bob lay on the gymnasium floor in apparent cardiac arrest, he watched from above as the team trainer and coaches performed CPR. After observing his own attempted resuscitation, he began walking in the direction of his uncle's voice. The last time he had heard his uncle's voice was a few days before his death 4 years earlier. Suddenly, his uncle instructed Bob to stop and turn back because Bob was not yet ready to join him. Over 24 hours later, Bob regained consciousness in the cardiac intensive care unit of The Ohio State University Hospital.

Death brings an end to our physical existence. Perhaps this is the ultimate connection between death and our physical dimension of health. Many people believe that, in a positive sense, death brings with it a sense of relief and comfort—two qualities that may be most needed when one is dying. The classic work of Raymond Moody,[7] who examined reports of people who had near-death experiences, suggests that we may have less to fear about dying than we have generally thought.

In a comprehensive study of more than 100 people who had near-death experiences, Kenneth Ring[8] reported that these people shared a core experience. This experience was composed of some or all of the following stages:

1. A sense of well-being and peace
2. An out-of-body experience in which the dying person floats above his or her body and is able to witness the activities that are occurring
3. A movement into extreme blackness or darkness
4. A shaft of intense light that generally leads upward or lies in the distance
5. A decision to enter into the light

Central to this experience is the need to make a decision to move toward death or to return to the body that has been temporarily vacated.

Experts are not in agreement as to whether near-death experiences are truly associated with death or more closely associated with the depersonalization that is experienced by some people during particularly frightening situations. In a scientific sense, near-death experiences are impossible to prove. Science can neither verify nor deny the existence of out-of-body experiences.[1]

Regardless, for those who have had near-death experiences, simply knowing that death might not be such an unpleasant experience appears to be comforting. Most seem to have formed a more positive orientation toward living.

Interacting with Dying People

Facing the impending death of a friend, relative, or loved one is a difficult experience. If you have yet to go through this situation, be assured that, as you grow older, your opportunities will increase. This is part of the reality of living.

Most counselors, physicians, nurses, and ministers who spend time with terminally ill people suggest that you display one quality when interacting with dying people: honesty. Just the thought of talking with a dying person may make you feel uncomfortable. (Most of us have had no training in this sort of thing.) Sometimes, to make ourselves feel less anxious or depressed, we may tend to deny that the person we are with is dying. Our words and nonverbal behavior indicate that we prefer not to face the truth. Our words become stilted as we gloss over the facts and merely attempt to cheer up both our dying friend and ourselves. This behavior is rarely beneficial or supportive—for either party.

As much as possible, we should attempt to be genuine and honest. We should not try to avoid crying if we feel the need to cry. At the same time, we can provide emotional support for dying people by allowing them to express their feelings openly. We should resist the temptation of trying to pull someone out of the denial, anger, or depression. We should not feel obliged to talk constantly and to fill long pauses with idle talk. Sometimes nonverbal communication, including touching, may be much more appreciated than mere talk. Since our interactions with dying people help fulfill our needs, we too should express our emotions and concerns as openly as possible.

Talking with Children about Death

Because most children are curious about everything, it is not surprising that they are also fascinated about death. From very young ages, children are exposed to death through mass media (cartoons, pictures in newspapers and magazines, and news reports), adult conversations ("Aunt Emily died today," "Uncle George is very ill"), and their discoveries (a dead bird, a crushed bug, the death of a pet). The manner in which children learn about death will have an important effect on their ability to recognize and accept their own mortality and to cope with the deaths of others.

Psychologists encourage parents and older friends to avoid shielding children from or misleading children about the reality of death. Young children need to realize that death is not temporary and it is not like sleeping. Parents should make certain they understand children's questions about death before they give an answer. Most children want simple, direct answers to their questions, not long, detailed dissertations, which often confuse the issues. For example, when a 4-year-old asks her father, "Why is Tommy's dog dead?" an appropriate answer might be, "Because he got very, very sick and his heart stopped beating." Getting involved in a lengthy discussion about "doggy heaven" or the causes of specific canine diseases may not be necessary or appropriate.

Parents should answer questions when they arise and always respond with openness and honesty. In this way, young children can learn that death is a real part of life and that sad feelings are a normal part of accepting the death of a loved one.

Death of a Child

Adults face not only the death of their parents and friends but perhaps also the death of a child. Whether because of sudden infant death syndrome (SIDS), chronic illness, accident, or suicide, children die and adults are forced to grieve the loss of someone who was "too young to die."

Coping with the death of a child is particularly difficult because it seems so unnatural and wrong for a child to precede his or her parents in death. Experts agree that grieving adults, particularly the parents, should express their grief fully and proceed cautiously on their return to normal routines. Many pitfalls can be avoided. Adults who are grieving for dead children should do the following:

- *Avoid trying to cope by using alcohol or drugs.*
- *Make no important life changes.* Moving to a different home, relocating, or changing jobs usually doesn't help parents deal any better with the grief they are experiencing.
- *Share feelings with others.* Grieving adults should share their feelings particularly with other adults who have experienced a similar loss. Group support is available in many communities.
- *Avoid trying to erase the death.* Giving away clothing and possessions that belonged to the child cannot erase the memories the adult has of the child.
- *Take the time and space to grieve.* On the anniversary of the child's death or on the child's birthday, grievers should give themselves special time just for grieving.
- *Don't attempt to replace the child.* Do not quickly have another child or use the deceased child's name for another child.

For most adults, grief over the death of a child will require an extended period. Eventually, however, life can return to normal.

Hospice Care for the Terminally Ill

The thought of dying in a hospital ward, with institutional furniture, medical equipment, and strict visiting hours, leaves many people with a cold feeling. Perhaps this thought alone has helped encourage the concept of

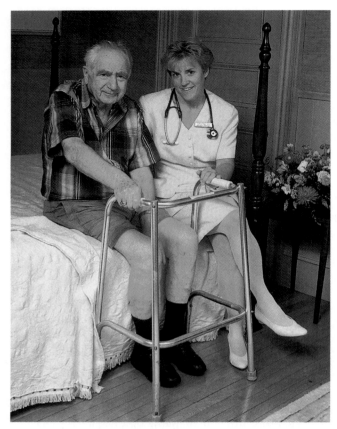

Hospice care allows terminally ill patients to spend their last days in a warm, homelike setting.

hospice care. Hospice care provides an alternative approach to dying for terminally ill patients and their families. The goal of hospice care is to maximize the quality of life for dying people and their family members. Popularized in England during the 1960s, yet derived from a concept developed during the Middle Ages (where *hospitable lodges* took care of weary travelers), the hospice helps people die comfortably and with dignity by using one or more of the following strategies:

- *Pain control.* Dying people are not usually treated for their terminal disease; they are provided with appropriate drugs to keep them free from pain, alert, and in control of their faculties. Drug dependence is of little concern, and patients can receive pain medication when they feel they need it.

- *Family involvement.* Family members and friends are trained and encouraged to interact with the dying person and with each other. Family members often care for the dying person at home. If the hospice arrangement includes a hospice ward in a hospital or a separate building (also called a hospice), the family members have no restrictions on visitation.

- *Multidisciplinary approach.* The hospice concept promotes a team approach.[9] Specially trained physicians, nurses, social workers, counselors, and volunteers work with the patient and family to fulfill important needs. The needs of the family receive nearly the same priority as those of the patient.

- *Patient decisions.* Contrary to most hospital approaches, hospice programs encourage patients to make their own decisions. The patient decides when to eat, sleep, go for a walk, and just be alone. By maintaining a personal schedule, the patient is more apt to feel in control of his or her life, even as that life is slipping away.

Another way in which the hospice differs from the hospital approach concerns the care given to the survivors. Even after the death of the patient, the family receives a significant amount of follow-up counseling. Helping families with their grief is an important role for the hospice team.

The number of hospices in the United States has climbed quickly to well over 3,300.[10] People seem to be convinced that the hospice system does work effectively. Part of this approval may be the cost factor. The cost of caring for a dying person in a hospice is usually less than the cost of full (inpatient) services provided by a hospital. Although insurance companies are delighted to see the lower cost for hospice care, many are still uncertain as to how to define hospice care. Thus not all insurance companies are fully reimbursing patients for their hospice care. Before discussing the possibility of hospice care for members of your family, you should consider the extent of hospice coverage in your health insurance policy.

Grief and the Resolution of Grief

The emotional feelings that people experience after the death of a friend or relative are collectively called *grief.* *Mourning* is the process of experiencing these emotional feelings in a culturally defined manner. (See the Star Box on page 481 for more information about the grieving process.) The expression of grief is seen as a valuable process that gradually permits people to accept the loss of the deceased. Expressing grief, then, is a sign of good health.

Key Terms

hospice care (**hos** pis) an approach to caring for terminally ill patients that maximizes the quality of life and allows death with dignity

The Grieving Process

The grieving process consists of four phases, each of which is variable in length and unique in form to the individual. These phases are composed of the following:

1. *Internalization of the deceased person's image.* By forming an idealized mental picture of the dead person, the grieving person is freed from dealing too quickly with the reality of the death.
2. *Intellectualization of the death.* Mental processing of the death and the events leading up to its occurrence move the grieving person to a clear understanding that death has occurred.

3. *Emotional reconciliation.* During this third and often delayed phase, the grieving person allows conflicting feelings and thoughts to be expressed and eventually reconciled with the reality of the death.
4. *Behavioral reconciliation.* Finally, the grieving person is able to comfortably return to a life in which the death has been fully reconciled. Old routines are reestablished and new patterns of living are adopted where necessary. The grieving person has largely recovered.

A mistake that might be made by the friends of a grieving person is encouraging a return to normal behavior too quickly. When friends urge the grieving person to return to work right away, make new friends, or become involved in time-consuming projects, they may be preventing necessary grieving from occurring. It is not easy or desirable to forget about the fact that a spouse, friend, or child has recently died.

Although people experience grief in remarkably different ways, most people have some of the following sensations and emotions:

- *Physical discomfort.* Shortly after the death of a loved one, grieving people display a rather similar pattern of physical discomfort. This discomfort is characterized by "sensations of somatic distress occurring in waves lasting from 20 minutes to an hour at a time, a feeling of tightness in the throat, choking with shortness of breath, need for sighing, and an empty feeling in the abdomen, lack of muscular power, and an intense subjective distress described as a tension or mental pain. The patient soon learns that these waves of discomfort can be precipitated by visits, by mentioning the deceased, and by receiving sympathy."[11]
- *Sense of numbness.* Grieving people may feel as if they are numb or in a state of shock. They may deny the death of their loved one.
- *Feelings of detachment from others.* Grieving people see other people as being distant from them, perhaps because the others cannot feel the loss. A person in grief can feel very lonely. This is a common response.
- *Preoccupation with the image of the deceased.* The grieving person may not be able to complete daily tasks without constantly thinking about the deceased.
- *Guilt.* The survivor may be overwhelmed with guilt. Thoughts may center on how the deceased was neglected or ignored. Sensitive survivors feel guilt merely because they are still alive. Indeed, guilt is a common emotion.
- *Hostility.* Survivors may express feelings of loss and remorse through hostility, which they direct at other family members, physicians, lawyers, and others.

- *Disruption in daily schedule.* Grieving people often find it difficult to complete daily routines. They can suffer from an anxious type of depression. Seemingly easy tasks take a great deal of effort. Initiation of new activities and relationships can be difficult. Social interaction skills can temporarily be lost.
- *Delayed grief.* In some people, the typical pattern of grief can be delayed for weeks, months, and even years.

The grief process continues until the bereaved person can establish new relationships, feel comfortable with others, and look back on the life of the deceased person with positive feelings (see Changing for the Better on page 482). Although the duration of the grief resolution process will vary with the emotional attachments one has to a deceased person, grief usually lasts for 18 months. Professional help should be sought when grieving is characterized by unresolved guilt, extreme hostility, physical illness, significant depression, and a lack of other meaningful relationships. Trained counselors, physicians, and hospice workers can all play significant roles in helping people through grief.

Rituals of Death

Our society has established a number of rituals associated with death that help the survivors accept the reality of death, ease the pain associated with the grief process, and provide a safe disposal of the body. Our rituals give us the chance to formalize our goodbyes to a person and to receive emotional support and strength from family members and friends. In recent years, more of our rituals seem to be celebrating the life of the deceased. In doing this, our rituals also reaffirm the value of our own lives.

I know someone whose brother just died. I want to help without getting in the way at this difficult time. What's the best approach?

Leming and Dickinson[1] point out that the peak time of grief begins in the week after a loved one's funeral. Realizing that there is no one guaranteed formula for helping the bereaved, you can help by performing some or all of the following:

- Make few demands on the bereaved; allow him or her to grieve.
- Help with the household tasks.
- Recognize that the bereaved person may vent anguish and anger and that some of it may be directed at you.
- Recognize that the bereaved person has painful and difficult tasks to complete; mourning cannot be rushed or avoided.

- Do not be afraid to talk about the deceased person; this lets the bereaved know that you care for the deceased.
- Express your own genuine feelings of sadness, but avoid pity. Speak from the heart.
- Reassure bereaved people that the intensity of their emotions is very natural.
- Advise the bereaved to get additional help if you suspect continuing severe emotional or physical distress.
- Keep in regular contact with the bereaved; let him or her know you continue to care about them.

Most of our funeral rituals take place in funeral homes, churches, and cemeteries. *Funeral homes* (or *mortuaries*) are business establishments that provide a variety of services to the families and friends of the deceased. The services are carried out by funeral directors, who are licensed by the state in which they operate. Most funeral directors are responsible for preparing the bodies for viewing, filing death certificates, preparing obituary notices, establishing calling hours, assisting in the preparation and details of the funeral, casket selection, transportation to and from the cemetery, and family counseling. Although licensing procedures vary from state to state, most new funeral directors must complete 1 year of college, 1 year of mortuary school, and 1 year of internship with a funeral home before taking a state licensing examination.

Full Funeral Services

An ethical funeral director will attempt to follow the wishes of the deceased's family and provide only the services requested by the family. Most families want traditional **full funeral services.** Three significant components of the full funeral services are as follows.

Key Terms

full funeral services all of the professional services provided by funeral directors

---

Several years ago, funeral homes wanted the public to feel they were not just focusing on the deceased but providing comprehensive service to the mourners. This sparked the concept of "after care," which refers to providing services to the family and friends of the deceased through the difficult times following the funeral. Funeral homes now offer counseling such as group meetings of widows or widowers where they can talk to one another about the difficulties they are having, especially during the holidays and special events of remembrance. They also coordinate special services in the cemetery or chapel during holidays such as Memorial Day or Mother's Day where everyone is invited and different ministers are invited to speak.

Some funeral homes offer seminars for the survivors on topics such as financial planning, cooking, auto and home repair, and parenting. Children are also provided supportive play therapy groups to give them a place to express their feelings of loss. Some advertise that they help with processing life insurance benefits, social security, and pension claims for deceased's family. They also act as a community referral and resource agency to assist other life transitions especially during the first year after the death. Thus the roles of funeral director and funeral home are expanding beyond helping to put the deceased to rest to also helping the survivors to live happy, fulfilling lives.

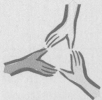
Death rituals vary considerably among ethnic and religious groups. Even within the broad categories of ethnic, racial, or religious distinction, differences exist in how groups of people dispose of their deceased. For example, funeral rituals may differ between Orthodox Jews and Conservative Jews. Furthermore, groups of people living in the United States may not be able to follow the traditional funeral rituals of their home countries because they lack the necessary resources and community support. However, some general cultural differences in funeral rituals can be seen in the following examples.

According to Purnell and Paulanka;[14] funeral rituals by the Amish are carried out in the deceased person's home. The church community takes care of the arrangements for visitors, relieving the grieving family of these tasks. In some Amish communities, a wakelike "sitting up" takes place in which family members are supported by friends throughout the night. The funeral itself is simple, with burial in an unadorned wooden coffin, often made by the local Amish carpenter. Children are encouraged to see death as a transition to a better life. Although the Amish clearly feel the pain of their loss, they often may not express this grief openly.

Muslim death rituals are based on their belief that death is the result of God's will. Death is foreordained. For Muslims (and for members of many other religious groups), life in this world is seen as a preparation for eternal life. At death, the deceased's bed is turned to face the Holy City of Mecca, and verses of hope and acceptance are read from the

Qur'an. The dead body is washed three times by a Muslim of the same sex as the deceased and then it is wrapped in white material and buried as soon as possible, usually in a brick or cement-lined grave facing Mecca. Prayers are offered for the dead at the cemetery, at the mosque, or at the home. Unless the deceased is a husband or close relative, women usually do not attend the burial. Cremation is not practiced among Muslims.

In Judaism, death is seen as part of the life cycle.[14] Traditional Jews believe in an afterlife in which a person's soul continues to flourish. In this afterlife, people are judged by their actions in life. People who have lived righteous lives are likely to be rewarded in the next world. Judaism does not have a form of last rites; any Jew may ask for God's forgiveness.

At traditional Jewish funerals, the body is rarely embalmed, unless there are unusual circumstances causing burial to be delayed. Burial routinely takes place within a short time after death. Cosmetic restoration is used minimally, if at all. The body is wrapped in a shroud and placed in an unadorned wooden casket. Traditionally, flowers are not displayed at the funeral or at the cemetery. The funeral service is directed at honoring the deceased, while praising God and encouraging people to reaffirm their faith. Traditionally, a 7-day period of immediate mourning *(shiva)* takes place after the burial. After this period there are established mourning periods. For example, mourning for a relative typically lasts 30 days; for a parent, 1 year.[14]

Embalming

Embalming is the process of using formaldehyde-based fluids to replace the blood components. Embalming helps preserve the body and return it to a natural look. Embalming permits friends and family members to view the body without being subjected to the odors associated with tissue decomposition. Embalming is often an optional procedure, except when death results from specific communicable diseases or when body *disposition* (disposal) is delayed.

Calling hours

Sometimes called a *wake,* this is an established time when friends and family members can gather in a room to share their emotions and common experiences about the deceased. Generally in the same room, the body will be in a casket, with the lid open or closed. Open caskets assist some people to confirm that death truly did occur. Some families prefer not to have any calling hours, sometimes called *visiting hours.*

Funeral service

Funeral services vary according to religious preference and the emotional needs of the survivors. Although some

services are held in a church, most funeral services today take place in a funeral home, where a special room might serve as a chapel. Some services are held at the graveside. Families may also choose to have a simple *memorial service* within a few days after the funeral. (Completing the Personal Assessment on page 489 will help you think about what kind of funeral arrangements you would prefer for yourself. As the Star Box on page 484 illustrates, some people choose some highly unusual ways to honor the memory of their loved ones.)

Disposition of the Body

Bodies are disposed of in one of four ways. *Ground burial* is the most common method. About 75 percent of all bodies are placed in ground burial. The casket is almost always placed in a metal or concrete vault before being buried. The vault serves to further protect the body (a need only of the survivors) and to prevent collapse of ground because of the decaying of caskets. Use of a vault is required by most cemeteries.

A second type of disposition is *entombment.* Entombment refers to nonground burial, most often in structures

Epitaphs in the Sky

Two interesting (and to some people, amusing) postmortem options have become available to those who want to connect with the cosmos. The first is the naming of distant celestial stars for people who have died. For a designated fee, ranging from about $100 to $500, a person, or his or her loved ones, can purchase the rights to name a star. The extent to which this naming is a legally binding arrangement between the payee and the "owner" of the star is subject to debate. However, this process seems to give some measure of comfort to the living.

The second new adventure in postmortem arrangements is the rocketing of ashes into outer space. For a fee approaching $5,000, Celestis, Inc., of Houston, Texas, will launch a cremated person's remains into orbit. However, only a small portion of the person's ashes—enough to fill a lipstick-size vial—will make the voyage. The ashes will be sent with about 100 other vials in a single launch. The Celestis company (www.celestis.com or 1-800-ORBIT-11) believes that these ash vials will orbit the Earth for 18 months to 10 years, when they will vaporize on reentry into the atmosphere.

Would you consider one of these two unusual options for yourself or a family member?

---

called **mausoleums.** A mausoleum has a series of shelves where caskets can be sealed in vaultlike areas called *niches.* Entombment can also occur in the basements of buildings, especially in old, large churches. The bodies of famous church leaders are sometimes entombed in vaultlike spaces called **crypts.**

Cremation is a third type of body disposition. In the United States, 29 percent of all bodies are cremated.[12] This practice is increasing. Generally both the body and casket (or cardboard cremation box) are incinerated so that only the bone ash from the body remains. The body of an average adult produces about 5–7 pounds of bone ash. These ashes can then be placed in containers called urns, and then buried, entombed, or scattered, if permitted by state law. The cost of cremation ($500–$850) is much less than ground burial. Some families choose to cremate after having full funeral services.[13]

A fourth method of body disposition is *anatomical donation.* Separate organs (such as corneal tissue, kidneys, or the heart) can be donated to a medical school, research facility, or organ donor network. Certain states permit people to indicate on their driver's licenses that they wish to donate their organs. However, family consent (by next of kin) is also required at the time of death for organ or tissue donation to occur. Recently, hospitals have been required by federal law to inform the family of a deceased person about organ donation at the time of his or her death. The need for donor organs is far greater than the current supply. For some, the decision to donate body tissue and organs is rewarding and comforting. Organ donors understand that their small sacrifice can help give life or improve the quality of life for another person. In this sense, their death can mean life for others. To become an organ donor, you must fill out a uniform organ donor card like the one in Changing for the Better on page 485.

Some people choose to donate their entire body to medical science. Often this is done through prior arrange-

Estimated Funeral Costs

Cemetery lot	$400–$1,200
Opening and closing of grave	$300–$800
Vault	$350–$1,000
Mausoleum space	$1,500–$5,000
Casket	$2,000–$10,000
Honorarium for minister	$75–$100
Organist and vocalists	$50–$75 each
Flowers over casket	$100+
Grave marker	$500–$1,500+
Hair styling/cosmetology	$250
Embalming	$200
Refrigeration	$85 per day

ments with medical schools. Bodies still require embalming. After they are studied, the remains are often cremated and returned to the family, if requested.

Costs

The full funeral services offered by a funeral home costs upward of $4,000 with other expenses added to this price. Casket prices vary significantly, with the average cost between

---

Key Terms

mausoleum (moz oh **lee** um) an above-ground structure, which frequently resembles a small stone house, into which caskets can be placed for disposition

crypts burial locations generally underneath churches

Planning an Organ Donation

I've thought about organ donation for a long time, and now I'm ready. What steps do I need to take to do this?

This is one of the most compassionate, responsible acts a person can do. Here are the simple steps that are involved:

1. You must complete a uniform donor card (Figure 17–2 see below). Obtain a card from a physician, a local hospital, or the nearest regional transplant or organ bank.
2. Print or type your name on the card.
3. Indicate which organs you wish to donate. You may also indicate your desire to donate all organs and tissues.
4. Sign your name in the presence of two witnesses, preferably your next of kin.
5. Fill in any additional information (for example, date of birth, city and state in which the card is completed, and date the card is signed).
6. Tell others about your decision to donate. Some donor cards have detachable portions to give to your family.
7. Always carry your card with you.
8. If you have any questions, you can call the United Network for Organ Sharing (UNOS) at 1-888-TXINFO1, or visit this organization's Web site at www.unos.org.

Uniform Donor Card

Of _____
(print or type name of donor)

In the hope that I may help others, I hereby make this anatomical gift, if medically acceptable, to take effect upon my death. The words and marks below indicate my wishes.
I give: ☐ any needed organs or parts
☐ only the following organs or parts

_____
specify the organ(s), tissue(s), or part(s)
for the purposes of transplantation, therapy, medical research or education:
☐ my body for anatomical study if needed.
Limitations or special wishes, if any: _____

National Kidney Foundation

Please detach and give this portion of the card to your family.

This is to inform you that, should the occasion ever arise, I would like to be an organ and tissue donor. Please see that my wishes are carried out by informing the attending medical personnel that I have indicated my wishes to become a donor. Thank you.

_____
Signature   Date
For further information write or call:
National Kidney Foundation
1522 K Street NW Suite 825 Washington, D.C. 20005-1213
www.kidney.org
(800)-622-9010

$1,500 and $2,500. If the family chooses an especially fancy casket, then the costs could spiral up to $10,000 or more. Costs that extend beyond these expenses include (should one choose them) those shown in the Star Box on page 484. When all the expenses associated with a typical funeral are added up, the average cost is between $5,500 and $7,000.

Regardless of the rituals you select for the handling of your body (or the body of someone in your care), most educators are encouraging people to prearrange their plans. Before you die, you can save your survivors a lot of misery by putting your wishes in writing. *Funeral prearrangements* relieve the survivors of many of the details that must be handled at the time of your death. You can gather much of the information for your obituary notice and your wishes for the disposition of your body. Prearrangements can be made with a funeral director, family member, or attorney. Many individuals also prepay the costs of their funeral. By making arrangements in advance of need, you can enhance your own peace of mind. Currently about 30–40 percent of funerals are preplanned or prepaid or both. Interestingly, in the 1960s, nearly all funerals were planned by relatives at the time of a person's death.

Personal Preparation for Death

This chapter is designed to help you to develop a new framework about death and form your own personal perspective on death and dying. Remember that the ultimate goal of death education is a positive one—to help you best use and enjoy your life. Becoming aware of the reality of your own mortality is a step in the right direction. Reading about the process of dying, grief resolution, and the rituals surrounding death can also help you accept that someday you too will die.

There are some additional ways in which you can prepare for the reality of your own death. Preparing a will, purchasing a life insurance policy, making funeral prearrangements, preparing a living will, and considering an anatomical or organ donation are measures that help you prepare for your own death (see Changing for the Better above). At the appropriate time, you might also wish to talk with family and friends about your own death. You may discover that an upbeat, positive discussion about death can help relieve some of your apprehensions and those of others around you.

Another suggestion to help you emotionally prepare for your death is to prepare your *obituary notice* or **eulogy.** Include all the things you would like to have said about you and your life. Now compare your obituary notice and eulogy with the current direction your life seems to be taking. Are you doing the kinds of activities for which you want to be known? If so, great! If not, perhaps you will want to consider why your current direction does not reflect how you would like to be remembered. Should you make some changes to restructure your life's agenda in a more personally meaningful fashion?

Another suggestion to help make you aware of your own eventual death is to write your own **epitaph.** Before doing this, you might want to visit a cemetery. Reading the epitaphs of others may help you develop yours.

Further awareness of your own death might come from attempting to answer these questions: (1) If I had only one day to live, how would I spend it? (2) What one accomplishment would I like to achieve before I die? (3) Once I am dead, what two or three things will people miss most about me? By answering these questions and accomplishing a few of the tasks suggested in this section, you will have a good start on accepting your own death and understanding the value of life itself.

Key Terms

eulogy a composition or speech that praises someone; often delivered at a funeral or memorial service

epitaph an inscription on a grave marker or monument

SUMMARY

- Death is determined primarily by clinical and legal factors.
- Euthanasia can be undertaken with either direct or indirect measures.
- The most current advance health care directives are the living will and the durable power of attorney for health care. Both documents permit critically ill people (especially those who cannot communicate) to die with dignity.
- Denial, anger, bargaining, depression, and acceptance are the five classic psychological stages that dying people commonly experience, according to Kübler-Ross.
- Hospice care provides an alternative approach to dying for terminally ill people and their families.
- The expression of grief is a common experience that can be expected when a friend or relative dies. The grief process can vary in intensity and duration.

- Death in our society is associated with a number of rituals to help survivors cope with the loss of a loved one and to ensure proper disposal of the body.
- In the past, most people died at home, whereas now the majority of people die in hospitals, nursing homes, and assisted-living facilities.
- The shortage of organ donations is the biggest problem facing people who need a transplant to save their lives.
- Hospice care is an alternative end-of-life health care option for terminally ill patients and their families.
- We dispose of bodies in four ways: ground burial, entombment, cremation, or anatomical donation.

REVIEW QUESTIONS

1. How does the experience of dying today differ from that in the early 1900s?
2. Identify and explain the clinical and legal determinants of death and indicate who establishes each of them.
3. Explain the difference between direct and indirect euthanasia.
4. How does a living will differ from a durable power of attorney for health-care document? Why are these advance health care directives becoming increasingly popular?
5. Identify the five psychological stages that dying people tend to experience. Explain each stage.

6. Identify and explain the four strategies that form the basis of hospice care. What are the advantages of hospice care for the patient and the family?
7. Explain what is meant by the term grief. Identify and explain the sensations and emotions most people have when they experience grief. When does the grieving process end?
8. What purposes do the rituals of death serve? What are the significant components of the full funeral service?
9. What are the four ways in which bodies are disposed?
10. What activities can we undertake to become better aware of our own mortality?

ENDNOTES

1. Leming MR, Dickinson GE: *Understanding Dying, Death, and Bereavement* (5th ed.). New York: Harcourt, 2001.
2. Kastenbaum RJ: *Death, Society, and Human Experience* (6th ed.). Boston: Allyn and Bacon, 1998.
3. www.pbs.org/wgbh/pages/frontline/kevorkian/law, The law on assisted suicide, December 16, 1999.
4. Partnership for Caring. Advance Directives, www.partnershipforcaring.org, accessed Sept 24, 2001.

5. Partnership for Caring: Personal correspondence, Sept 20, 2001.
6. Kübler-Ross E: *On Death and Dying,* reprint ed. New York: Collier Books, 1997.
7. Moody RA: *The Last Laugh: A New Philosophy of Near-Death Experiences, Apparitions, and the Paranormal,* Charlottsville, VA: Hampton Roads Publishing Co., 1999.
8. Ring K: *Life at Death: A Scientific Investigation of the Near-Death Experience.* New York: Coward, McCann & Geoghegan, 1980.
9. DeSpelder LA, Strickland AL: *The Last Dance: Encountering Death and Dying* (5th ed.). Mountain View, CA: Mayfield, 1999.
10. National Hospice and Palliative Care Organization: NHPCO *Facts and Figures,* www.mhpco.org, Sept 26, 2001.
11. Lindemann E: Symptomology and management of acute grief. In Fulton et al., Eds. *Death and Dying: Challenge and Change.* Boston: Addison-Wesley, 1978.
12. Cremation Association of North America (CANA). *2000 Data and Projections to the Year 2025,* Aug 29, 2001, pp. 1–4.
13. Bowman J (Licensed Funeral Director): Personal correspondence, Sept 25, 2001.
14. Purnell, LD, Paulanka BJ. *Transcultural Health Care: A Culturally Competent Approach.* Philadelphia: F. A. Davis, 1998.

As We Go to Press . . .

Over 100 legally deceased people are currently suspended in tanks of liquid nitrogen in the United States with thousands more making plans to join them. The legendary baseball Hall of Famer Ted Williams brought more spotlight to this alternative way of disposing of one's body, freezing it. Cryonics involves embalming the body with a glycerin-based solution, cooling it under dry ice until it reaches minus 40°F, and then gradually lowering the body into a pool of liquid nitrogen until the body reaches minus 320°F. All cell movement ceases at this temperature. The cost for this process and storage ranges from $28,000 to $120,000 per person. The first patient to be frozen was in 1967.

Why would you want to freeze your body when you die? Some believe that the body can be thawed and the cause of death be reversed. Sound like a science fiction movie? Proponents of cryonics predict that diseases such as cancer will have cures sometime in the future and so the deceased can be unfrozen and treated for whatever killed him or her in the first place. However, patients who are legally brain dead are not accepted for this procedure. Also, you can opt to freeze only your head (or your brain), presumably critical for revival. Freezing a severed head is less costly, around $40,000, and takes less effort to freeze and revive. In addition, it is though that when future people develop the technology to bring you back to life, they will also have the technology to generate a new body for you based on your DNA. While it is rumored that Walt Disney was frozen, this has not been substantiated. However, a few well-known scientists have also been put into cryonic suspension. Dr. Eric Drexler, known as the father of nanotechnology, and Dr. Marvin Minsky, the founder of artificial intelligence research in the United States, are also frozen. Is this an option you would consider for your future?

personal assessment

Planning your funeral

In line with this chapter's positive theme of the value of personal death awareness, here is a funeral service assessment that we frequently give to our health classes. This inventory can help you assess your reactions and thoughts about the funeral arrangements you would prefer for yourself.

After answering each of the following questions, you might wish to discuss your responses with a friend or close relative.

1. Have you ever considered how you would like your body to be handled after your death?

    _____ Yes _____ No

2. Have you already made funeral prearrangements for yourself?

    _____ Yes _____ No

3. Have you considered a specific funeral home or mortuary to handle your arrangements?

    _____ Yes _____ No

4. If you were to die today, which of the following would you prefer?

    _____ Embalming _____ Ground burial

    _____ Cremation _____ Entombment

    _____ Donation to medical science

5. If you prefer to be cremated, what do you want done with your ashes?

    _____ Buried _____ Entombed

    _____ Scattered

    _____ Other; please specify _____

6. If your funeral plans involve a casket, which of the following ones do you prefer?

    _____ Plywood (cloth covered)

    _____ Hardwood (oak, cherry, mahogany, maple, etc.)

    _____ Steel (sealer or nonsealer type)

    _____ Stainless steel

    _____ Copper or bronze

    _____ Other; please specify _____

7. How important is a funeral service for you?

    _____ Very important

    _____ Somewhat important

    _____ Somewhat unimportant

    _____ Very unimportant

    _____ No opinion

8. What kind of funeral service do you want for yourself?

    _____ No service at all

    _____ Visitation (calling hours) the day before the funeral service; funeral held at church or funeral home

    _____ Graveside service only (no visitation)

    _____ Memorial service (after body disposition)

    _____ Other; please specify _____

9. How many people do you want to attend your funeral service or memorial service?

    _____ I do not want a funeral or memorial service

    _____ 1–10 people

    _____ 11–25 people

    _____ 26–50 people

    _____ Over 51 people

    _____ I do not care how many people attend

10. What format would you prefer at your funeral service or memorial service? Select any of the following that you would like.

	Yes	No
Religious music	_____	_____
Nonreligious music	_____	_____
Clergy present	_____	_____
Flower arrangements	_____	_____
Family member eulogy	_____	_____
Eulogy by friend(s)	_____	_____
Open casket	_____	_____
Religious format	_____	_____

Other; please specify _____

11. Using today's prices, how much would you expect to pay for your total funeral arrangements, including cemetery expenses (if applicable)?

    _____ Less than $4,500

    _____ Between $4,501 and $6,000

    _____ Between $6,001 and $7,500

    _____ Between $7,501 and $9,000

    _____ Above $9,000

To Carry This Further . . .

Which items had you not thought about before? Were you surprised at the arrangements you selected? Will you share your responses with anyone else? If so, whom?

Glossary

A

abortion induced premature termination of a pregnancy

absorption passage of nutrients or alcohol through the walls of the stomach or intestinal tract into the bloodstream

abuse any use of a legal or illegal drug that is detrimental to health

acquired immunity (AI) significant component of the immune system associated with the formation of antibodies and specialized blood cells that are capable of destroying pathogens

acupuncture insertion of fine needles into the body to alter electroenergy fields and cure disease

acute alcohol intoxication potentially fatal elevation of the blood alcohol concentration, often resulting from rapid consumption of large amounts of alcohol

acute rhinitis the common cold; the sudden onset of nasal inflammation

adaptive thermogenesis physiological response of the body to adjust its metabolic rate to the presence or absence of calories

additive effect the combined (but not exaggerated) effect produced by the concurrent use of two or more drugs

aerobic energy production body's production of energy when the respiratory and circulatory systems are able to process and transport a sufficient amount of oxygen to muscle cells

agent causal pathogen of a particular disease

air pollution refers to a wide variety of substances found in the atmosphere that can have adverse effects on human health, crop productivity, and natural communities

air toxics a class of 188 toxic air pollutants identified by the U.S. Environmental Protection Agency as known or suspected causes of cancer or other serious health effects

alarm stage the first stage of the stress response involving physiological, involuntary changes which are controlled by the hormonal and nervous system; the fight or flight response is activated in this stage

alcoholism primary chronic disease with genetic, psychosocial, and environmental factors influencing its development and manifestations

allopathy system of medical practice in which specific remedies (often pharmaceutical agents) are used to produce effects different from those produced by a disease or injury

alveoli thin, saclike terminal ends of the airways; the sites at which gases are exchanged between the blood and inhaled air

Alzheimer's disease gradual development of memory loss, confusion, and loss of reasoning; will eventually lead to total intellectual incapacitation, brain degeneration, and death

amino acids chief components of protein; synthesized by the body or obtained from dietary sources

amotivational syndrome behavioral pattern characterized by widespread apathy toward productive activities

anabolic steroids drugs that function like testosterone to produce increases in weight, strength, endurance, and aggressiveness

anaerobic energy production body's production of energy when needed amounts of oxygen are not readily available

anal intercourse a sexual act in which the erect penis is inserted into the rectum of a partner

androgyny the blending of both masculine and feminine characteristics

angina pectoris chest pain that results from impaired blood supply to the heart muscle

anorexia nervosa an eating disorder in which the individual weighs less than 85% of their expected weight, and has an intense fear of gaining weight; in females, menstruation ceases for at least 3 consecutive months. People with anorexia perceive themselves as overweight, even though they are underweight

anovulatory not ovulating

antagonistic effect effect produced when one drug nullifies (reduces, offsets) the effects of a second drug

antibodies chemical compounds produced by the immune system to destroy antigens and their toxins

arrhythmias irregularities of the heart's normal rhythm or beating pattern

artificially acquired immunity (AAI) type of acquired immunity resulting from the body's response to pathogens introduced into the body through immunizations

asbestos a term used to refer to a class of minerals that have a fibrous crystal structure

asphyxiation death resulting from lack of oxygen to the brain

atherosclerosis the buildup of plaque on the inner walls of arteries

attention deficit hyperactivity disorder (ADHD) inability to concentrate well on a specified task; often accompanied by above-normal physical movement; also called *hyperactivity*

autoimmune immune response against the cells of a person's own body

axon portion of a neuron that conducts electrical impulses to the dendrites of adjacent neurons; neurons typically have one axon

ayurveda traditional Indian medicine based on herbal remedies

B

balanced diet diet featuring food selections from each of the five food groups

ballistic stretching a "bouncing" form of stretching in which a muscle group is lengthened repetitively to produce multiple quick, forceful stretches

basic needs deficiency needs that are viewed as essential and fundamental, including physiological safety, belonging, and love and esteem needs

benign noncancerous; tumors that do not spread

beta blockers drugs that prevent overactivity of the heart, which results in angina pectoris

beta endorphins mood-enhancing, pain-reducing, opiate-like chemicals produced within a smoker's body in response to the presence of nicotine

bias and hate crimes criminal acts directed at a person or group solely because of a specific characteristic, such as race, religion, ethnic background, or other difference

binge eating disorder an eating disorder formerly referred to as compulsive over-eating disorder; binge eaters use food in the same way to cope as bulimics do, but do not engage in compensatory purging behavior

biological air pollutants living organisms or substances produced by living organisms that cause disease or allergic reactions, including bacteria, molds, mildew, viruses, dust mites, plant pollen, and animal dander, urine or feces

biological sexuality male and female aspects of sexuality

biological water pollutants disease-causing organisms that are found in water

biopsychological model a model that addresses how biological, psychological, and social factors interact and affect psychological health

bipolar disorder a mood disorder characterized by alternating episodes of depression and mania

birth control all of the procedures that can prevent the birth of a child

bisexual choosing members of both genders as one's sexual preference

blackout temporary state of amnesia experienced by a drinker; an inability to remember events that occur during a period of alcohol use

blood alcohol concentration (BAC) percentage of alcohol in a measured quantity of blood

BOD POD body composition system used to measure body fat through air displacement

body image our subjective perception of how our body appears

body mass index (BMI) numerical expression of body weight based on height and weight

bolus theory a theory of nicotine addiction based on the bolus (ball) of nicotine delivered to the brain with each inhalation of cigarette smoke

brand name specific name assigned to a patented drug or product by its manufacturer

bulimia nervosa an eating disorder in which individuals engage in episodes of binging, consuming unusually large amounts of food and feeling out of control, and engaging in some form of compensatory purging behavior to eliminate the food

C

calcium channel blockers drugs that prevent arterial spasms; used in the long-term management of angina pectoris

calendar method form of periodic abstinence in which the variable lengths of a woman's menstrual cycle are used to calculate her fertile period

calipers device to measure the thickness of a skinfold from which percent body fat can be calculated

calories units of heat (energy); specifically, 1 calorie equals the heat required to raise 1 kilogram of water 1° C

carbohydrates chemical compounds comprised of sugar or saccharide units; the body's primary source of energy

carbon monoxide a gaseous by-product of the incomplete combustion of natural gas, kerosene, heating oil, wood, coal, gasoline, and tobacco

carcinogens environmental agents that stimulate the development of cancerous changes within cells

cardiac muscle specialized muscle tissue that forms the middle (muscular) layer of the heart wall

cardiorespiratory endurance ability of the body to process and transport oxygen required by muscle cells so that these cells can continue to contract

cardiovascular pertaining to the heart (cardio) and blood vessels (vascular)

carjacking a crime that involves a thief's attempt to steal a car while the owner is behind the wheel; carjackings are usually random and unpredictable and often involve handguns

catabolism metabolic process of breaking down tissue for the purpose of converting it to energy

cerebrovascular occlusion blockage to arteries supplying blood to the cerebral cortex of the brain; resulting in a stroke

cervical cap small, thimble-shaped contraceptive device designed to fit over the cervix

cesarean delivery surgical removal of a fetus through the abdominal wall

chemical name name used to describe the molecular structure of a drug

chemoprevention the safe and effective use of dietary supplements in the prevention of illness and disease

child maltreatment the act or failure to act by a parent or caregiver, which results in abuse or neglect of a child or which places the child in imminent risk of serious harm

chiropractic manipulation of the vertebral column to relieve pressure and cure illness

chlamydia the most prevalent sexually transmitted disease; caused by a nongono-coccal bacterium

cholesterol a primary form of fat found in the blood; lipid material manufactured within the body, as well as derived through dietary sources

chronic bronchitis persistent inflammation and infection of the smaller airways within the lungs

chronic fatigue syndrome (CFS) illness that causes severe exhaustion, fatigue, aches, and depression; mostly affects women in their thirties and forties

chronic stress a high level of physio-logical arousal for an extended period of time; it can also occur when an individual is not able to immediately react to a real or perceived threat

cilia small, hairlike structures that extend from cells that line the air passage

circadian rhythms The internal, biological clock that helps coordinate physiological processes to the 24-hour light/dark cycle

clinical depression a psychological disorder in which individuals experience a lack of motivation, decreased energy level, fatigue, social withdrawal, sleep disturbance, disturbance in appetite, diminished sex drive, feelings of worthlessness, and despair

codependence unhealthy relationship in which one person is addicted to alcohol or another drug and a person close to him or her is "addicted" to the alcoholic or drug user

cohabitation sharing of a residence by two unrelated, unmarried people; living together

coitus penile-vaginal intercourse

coitus interruptus (withdrawal) a contraceptive practice in which the erect penis is removed from the vagina before ejaculation

cold turkey immediate, total discontinuation of use of tobacco or other addictive substances

collateral circulation ability of nearby blood vessels to enlarge and carry additional blood around a blocked blood vessel

colonoscopy examination of the entire length of the colon, using a flexible fiberoptic scope to inspect the structure's lining

compliance willingness to follow the directions provided by another person

condom latex shield designed to cover the erect penis and retain semen on ejaculation

congestive heart failure inability of the heart to pump out all the blood that returns to it; can lead to dangerous fluid accumulation in veins, lungs, and kidneys

consumer fraud marketing of unreliable and ineffective services, products, or information under the guise of curing disease or improving health; quackery

contraception any procedure that prevents fertilization

contraceptive patch contraceptive skin patch containing estrogen and progestin; replaced each week for a three-week period

contraceptive ring thin, polymer contraceptive device containing estrogen and progestin; placed deep within the vagina for a three-week period

contraindications factors that make the use of a drug inappropriate or dangerous for a particular person

coronary arteries vessels that supply oxygenated blood and nutrients to heart muscle

coronary artery bypass surgery surgical procedure designed to improve blood flow to the heart by providing a new route for blood around points of blockage

corpus luteum cellular remnant of the graafian follicle after the release of an ovum

cross-tolerance transfer of tolerance from one drug to another within the same general category

cruciferous vegetables vegetables that have flowers with four leaves in the pattern of a cross

CT scan computed tomography scan; an x-ray procedure that is designed to visualize structures within the body that would not normally be seen through conventional x-ray procedures

cunnilingus oral stimulation of the vulva or clitoris

D

dehydration abnormal depletion of fluids from the body; severe dehydration can lead to death

dendrite portion of a neuron that receives electrical stimuli from adjacent neurons; neurons typically have several such branches or extensions

dependence general term that reflects the need to keep consuming a drug for psychological or physical reasons, or both

desertification a process that converts lands that historically supported grasslands, shrub lands, or dry forest to nonproductive desert

designated driver a person who abstains from or carefully limits alcohol use to drive others safely

desirable weight weight range deemed appropriate for people of a specific gender, age, and frame size

diaphragm soft rubber vaginal cup designed to cover the cervix

diastolic pressure blood pressure against blood vessel walls when the heart relaxes

dilation gradual expansion of an opening or passageway

dilation and curettage (D & C) surgical procedure in which the cervical canal is dilated to allow the uterine wall to be scraped

distillation the process of heating an alcohol solution and collecting its vapors into a more concentrated solution

distress stress that diminishes the quality of life; commonly associated with disease, illness, and maladaptation

drug synergism enhancement of a drug's effect as a result of the presence of additional drugs within the system

duration length of time one needs to exercise at the target heart rate to produce the training effect

E

ectopic pregnancy a pregnancy wherein the fertilized ovum implants at a site other than the uterus, typically in the fallopian tube

embolism potentially fatal situation in which a circulating blood clot lodges itself in a smaller vessel

emotional intelligence the ability to understand others and act wisely in human relations and measure how well you know your emotions, manage your emotions, motivate yourself, recognize emotions in others, and handle relationships

empower the ability to make choices and take responsibility for oneself

enabling in this case, the inadvertent support that some people provide to alcohol or drug abusers

enucleated egg an ovum with the nucleus removed

environment the physical conditions (temperature, humidity, light, presence of substances) and other living organisms that exist around your body

environmental tobacco smoke tobacco smoke that is diluted and stays within a common source of air

enzymes organic substances that control the rate of physiological reactions but are not themselves altered in the process

erection the engorgement of erectile tissue with blood; characteristic of the penis, clitoris, nipple, labia minora, and scrotum

ergogenic aids supplements that are taken to improve athletic performance

erotic dreams dreams whose content elicits a sexual response

estrogen ovarian hormone that initiates the development of the uterine wall

eustress stress that enhances the quality of life

exercise a subcategory of physical activity; it is planned, structured, repetitive, and purposive in the sense that an improvement or maintenance of physical fitness is an objective (Casperson, et al., 1985)

excitement stage initial arousal stage of the sexual response pattern

exhaustion stage the point at which the physical and psychological resources used to deal with stress have been consumed

F

false labor conditions that tend to resemble the start of true labor; may include irregular uterine contractions, pressure, and discomfort in the lower abdomen

FDA Schedule 1 list comprising drugs that hold a high potential for abuse but have no medical use

fecal coliform bacteria a category of bacteria that live within the intestines of warm-blooded animals. The presence of these bacteria is used as an indicator that water has been contaminated by feces

femininity behavioral expressions traditionally observed in females

fermentation chemical process whereby plant products are converted into alcohol by the action of yeast on carbohydrates

fertility ability to reproduce

fetal alcohol syndrome characteristic birth defects noted in the children of some women who consume alcohol during their pregnancies

fiber plant material that cannot be digested; found in cereal, fruits, and vegetables

fight-or-flight response the physiological response reaction to a stressor that prepares the body for confrontation or avoidance

flaccid nonerect; the state of erectile tissue when vasocongestion is not occurring

flexibility ability of joints to function through an intended range of motion

follicle-stimulating hormone (FSH) gonadotropic hormone required for initial development of ova (in the female) and sperm (in the male)

food additives chemical compounds that are intentionally or unintentionally added to our food supply that change some property of the food such as color or texture

food allergy a reaction in which the immune system attacks an otherwise harmless food or ingredient; allergic reactions can range from mildly unpleasant to life-threatening

food intolerance an adverse reaction to a specific food that does not involve the immune system; usually caused by an enzyme deficiency

foreplay activities, often involving touching and caressing, that prepare individuals for sexual intercourse

frequency number of times per week one should exercise to achieve a training effect

functional foods foods capable of contributing to the improvement/ prevention of specific health problems

G

gait pattern of walking

gaseous phase portion of tobacco smoke containing carbon monoxide and many other physiologically active gaseous compounds

gateway drugs easily obtained legal or illegal drugs (alcohol, tobacco, marijuana) whose use may precede the use of less common illegal drugs

gender general term reflecting a biological basis of sexuality; the male gender or the female gender

gender adoption lengthy process of learning the behaviors that are traditional for one's gender

gender identification achievement of a personally satisfying interpretation of one's masculinity or feminity

gender identity recognition of one's gender

gender preference emotional and intellectual acceptance of one's gender

general adaptation syndrome (GAS) sequenced physiological response to the presence of a stressor; the alarm, resistance, and exhaustion stages of the stress response

generalized anxiety disorder (GAD) an anxiety disorder that involves experiencing intense and nonspecific anxiety for at least six months, in which the intensity and frequency of worry is excessive and out of proportion to the situation

genetic counseling medical counseling regarding the transmission and management of inherited conditions

genetic predisposition inherited tendency to develop a disease process if necessary environmental factors exist

gonads male or female sex glands; testes produce sperm and ovaries produce eggs

green space areas of land that are dominated by domesticated or natural vegetation, including rural farmland, city lawns and parks, and nature preserves

greenhouse gases a category of gases in the atmosphere that allow solar radiation to pass through the atmosphere to the Earth, but then trap the heat that is radiated from the Earth back toward space; greenhouse gases include water vapor, carbon dioxide, methane, nitrous oxide, and tropospheric ozone

H

hallucinogens psychoactive drugs capable of producing hallucinations (distortions of reality)

health claims statements attesting to a food's contribution to the improvement/ prevention of specific health problems

health promotion movement in which knowledge, practices, and values are transmitted to people for their use in lengthening their lives, reducing the incidence of illness, and feeling better

healthy body weight body weight within a weight range appropriate for a person with an acceptable waist-to-hip ratio

herbalism an ancient form of healing in which herbal preparations are used to treat illness and disease

high-density lipoprotein (HDL) the type of lipoprotein that transports cholesterol from the bloodstream to the liver where it is eventually removed from the body; high levels of HDL are related to a reduction in heart disease

high-risk health behavior a behavioral pattern associated with a high risk of developing a chronic disease

holistic health broadest view of the composition of health; views health in terms of its physical, emotional, social, intellectual, spiritual, and occupational makeup

homeopathy the use of minute doses of herbs or minerals to stimulate healing

homicide the intentional killing of one person by another

hormone replacement therapy (HRT) medically administered estrogen and progestin to replace hormones lost at menopause

host negligence a legal term that reflects the failure of a host to provide reasonable care and safety for people visiting the host's residence or business

hot flashes temporary feelings of warmth experienced by women during and after menopause; caused by blood vessel dilation

human cloning the replication of a human being

human papillomavirus (HPV) sexually transmitted viruses, some of which are capable of causing precancerous changes in the cervix; causative agent for genital warts

hypercellular obesity form of obesity seen in individuals who possess an abnormally large number of fat cells

hyperglycemia elevated blood glucose levels; an important indicator of diabetes mellitus

hyperparathyroidism condition reflecting the overactive production of parathyroid hormone by the parathyroid glands

hypertonic saline solution salt solution with a concentration higher than that found in human fluids

hypoxia oxygen deprivation at the cellular level

I

immune system system of biochemical and cellular elements that protect the body from invading pathogens and foreign materials

immunizations laboratory-prepared pathogens that are introduced into the body for the purpose of stimulating the body's immune system

incest marriage or coitus (sexual intercourse) between closely related individuals

incubation stage time required for a pathogen to multiply significantly enough for signs and symptoms to appear

indoor air quality characteristics of air within homes, workplaces, and public buildings, including the presence and amount of oxygen, water vapor, and a wide range of substances that can have adverse effects on your health

infatuation a relatively temporary, intensely romantic attraction to another person

infertility inability of a male to impregnate or of a female to become pregnant

inhalants psychoactive drugs that enter the body through inhalation

inhibitions inner controls that prevent a person's engaging in certain types of behavior

insulin pancreatic hormone required by the body for the effective metabolism of glucose (blood sugar)

intensity level of effort one puts into an activity

interstitial cell stimulating hormone (ICSH) a gonadotropic hormone of the male required for the production of testosterone

intimacy any close, mutual verbal or nonverbal behavior within a relationship

intimate partner violence violence committed against a person by her or his current or former spouse, boyfriend, or girlfriend

intrauterine device (IUD) small plastic medicated or unmedicated device that when inserted in the uterus prevents continued pregnancy

ionizing radiation electromagnetic radiation that is capable of breaking chemical bonds, such as x-rays and gamma rays

isokinetic exercises muscular strength-training exercises that use machines to provide variable resistances throughout the full range of motion

isometric exercises muscular strength-training exercises that use a resistance so great that the resistance object cannot be moved

isotonic resistance exercises muscular strength-training exercises in which traditional barbells and dumbbells are used to provide variable resistances throughout the full range of motion

L

learned helplessness a theory of motivation explaining how individuals can learn to feel powerless, trapped, or defeated

learned optimism an attribution style, comprised of permanence, pervasiveness, and personalization; how people explain both positive and negative events in their lives, accounting for success and failure

lightening movement of fetus deeper into the pelvic cavity before the onset of the birth process

low-density lipoprotein (LDL) the type of lipoprotein that transports the largest amount of cholesterol in the bloodstream; high levels of LDL are related to heart disease

lumpectomy a surgical treatment for breast cancer in which a minimal amount of breast tissue is removed

luteinizing hormone (LH) female gonadotropic hormone required for fullest development and release of ova; ovulating hormone

Lyme disease systemic bacterial infection transmitted by deer ticks

M

mainstream smoke the smoke inhaled and then exhaled by a smoker

mania an extremely excitable state characterized by excessive energy, racing thoughts, impulsive and/or reckless behavior, irritability, and being prone to distraction

masculinity behavioral expressions traditionally observed in males

masturbation self-stimulation of the genitals

maximum contaminant level the highest concentration of a contaminant that is allowed in drinking water, as established and regulated by the U.S. Environmental Protection Agency

medical abortion an abortion caused by the use of prescribed drugs

medical power of attorney for health care a legal document that designates who will make health care decisions for people unable to do so for themselves

menarche time of a female's first menstrual cycle

menopause decline and eventual cessation of hormone production by the reproductive system

menstrual phase phase of the menstrual cycle during which the broken-down lining of the uterus (endometrium) is discharged from the body

metabolite breakdown product of a drug

metaneeds secondary concerns, such as spirituality, creativity, curiosity, beauty, philosophy, and justice, that can be addressed only after the basic needs are met

metastasis spread of cancerous cells from their site of origin to other areas of the body

misuse inappropriate use of legal drugs intended to be medications

monogamous paired relationship with one partner

mononuclear leukocytes large white blood cells that have only one nucleus

monounsaturated fats fats made of compounds in which one hydrogen-bonding position remains to be filled; semisolid at room temperature; derived primarily from peanut and olive oils

morbidity illness or disease

mortality death

MRI scan magnetic resonance imaging; an imaging procedure that uses a giant magnet to generate an image of body tissue

mucus clear, sticky material produced by specialized cells within the mucous membranes of the body; mucus traps much of the suspended particulate matter from tobacco smoke

multiorgasmic capacity potential to have several orgasms within a single period of sexual arousal

murmur an atypical heart sound that suggests a backwashing of blood into a chamber of the heart from which it has just left

muscular endurance the aspect of muscular fitness that deals with ability of a muscle or muscle group to repeatedly contract over a long period of time

muscular strength the aspect of physical fitness that deals with ability to contract skeletal muscles to a maximal level

myocardial infarction heart attack; the death of heart muscle as a result of a blockage in one of the coronary arteries

N

narcolepsy sleep-related disorder in which a person has a recurrent, overwhelming, and uncontrollable desire to sleep

narcotics psychoactive drugs derived from the oriental poppy plant; narcotics relieve pain and induce sleep

naturally acquired immunity (NAI) type of acquired immunity resulting from the body's response to naturally occurring pathogens

nature the innate factors that genetically determine personality traits

naturopathy a system of treatment that avoids drugs and surgery and emphasizes the use of natural agents to correct underlying imbalances

neuron nerve cell; the structural unit of the nervous system

nocturnal emission ejaculation that occurs during sleep; "wet dream"

nomogram graphic means of finding an unknown value

non-insulin-dependent (type 2) diabetes mellitus form of diabetes generally seen for the first time in people 35 years of age and older; adult-onset diabetes

nonionizing radiation electromagnetic radiation that cannot break chemical bonds, but may excite electrons (ultraviolet radiation) or heat biological materials (infrared, radio frequency, and microwave radiation)

nonoxynol 9 a spermicide commonly used with contraceptive devices

nontraditional-age students administrative term used by colleges and universities for students who, for whatever reason, are pursuing undergraduate work at an age other than that associated with traditional college years (18–24)

norepinephrine adrenaline-like neurotransmitter produced within the nervous system

nurture the effect that the environment, people, and external factors have on personality

nutrients elements in foods that are required for the growth, repair, and regulation of body processes

O

obesity condition in which a person's body weight is 20% above desirable weight

obsessive-compulsive disorder an anxiety disorder characterized by obsessions—intrusive thoughts, images, or impulses causing a great deal of distress—and compulsions—repetitive behaviors aimed at reducing anxiety or stress that is associated with the obsessive thoughts

oncogenes genes that are believed to activate the development of cancer

oral contraceptive pill taken orally, composed of synthetic female hormones that prevent ovulation or implantation; "the pill"

orgasmic platform expanded outer third of the vagina that during the plateau phase of the sexual response grips the penis

orgasmic stage third stage of the sexual response pattern; the stage during which neuromuscular tension is released

orthodontics dental specialty that focuses on the proper alignment of the teeth

osteoarthritis arthritis that develops with age; largely caused by weight-bearing and deterioration of joints

osteopathy system of medical practice that combines allopathic principles with specific attention to postural mechanics of the body

osteoporosis the loss of calcium from the bone caused by the inability of the body to use dietary calcium; seen primarily in postmenopausal women

outercourse sexual activity that does not involve intercourse

overload principle principle whereby a person gradually increases the resistance load that must be moved or lifted

overweight condition in which body weight is 1%–19% above desirable weight

ovolactovegetarian diet diet that excludes the use of all meat but does allow the consumption of eggs and dairy products

ovulation the release of a mature egg from the ovary

oxidation in this case, the process that removes alcohol from the bloodstream

oxygen debt physical state that occurs when the body can no longer process and transport sufficient amounts of oxygen for continued muscle contraction

P

panic disorder an anxiety disorder characterized by panic attacks, in which individuals experience severe physical symptoms; these episodes can seemingly occur "out of the blue" or because of some trigger, and can last for a few minutes or for hours

pap test a cancer screening procedure in which cells are removed from the cervix and examined for precancerous changes

particulate phase portion of tobacco smoke composed of small suspended particles

passively acquired immunity (PAI) temporary immunity achieved by providing extrinsic antibodies to a person exposed to a particular pathogen

pathogen disease-causing agent

pelvic inflammatory disease (PID) acute or chronic infections of the peritoneum or lining of the abdominopelvic cavity; associated with a variety of symptoms and a potential cause of sterility

perfectionism a tendency to expect perfection in everything one does, with little tolerance for mistakes

periodic abstinence birth control methods that rely on a couple's avoidance of intercourse during the ovulatory phase of a woman's menstrual cycle; also called *fertility awareness* or *natural family planning*

periodontal disease destruction of soft tissue and bone that surround the teeth

peripheral artery disease (PAD) damage resulting from restricted blood flow to the extremities, especially the legs and feet

permanence one of three dimensions of an individual's attribution style, related to whether certain events are perceived as temporary or long-lasting

peritonitis inflammation of the peritoneum or lining of the abdominopelvic cavity

personalization another dimension of attribution style, related to whether an individual takes things personally or is more balanced in accepting responsibility for positive and negative events

pervasiveness another dimension of an individual's attribution style, related to whether events are perceived as specific to a situation or generalized

pesco-vegetarian diet a vegetarian diet that includes fish, dairy products, and eggs, along with plant foods

phenylpropanolamine (PPA) active chemical compound once found in most over-the-counter diet products

physical activity any bodily movement produced by skeletal muscles that results in energy expenditure (Casperson, et al., 1985)

physical fitness a set of attributes that people have or achieve that relates to the ability to perform physical activity (Casperson, et al., 1985)

placebo medications that contain no active ingredients

platonic close association between two people that does not include a sexual relationship

positive caloric balance caloric intake greater than caloric expenditure

post-abortion syndrome long-term negative psychological effects of abortion

postpartum period of time after the birth of a baby during which the uterus returns to its prepregnancy size

potentiated effect phenomenon whereby the use of one drug intensifies the effect of a second drug

preventive or prospective medicine physician-centered medical care in which areas of risk for chronic illnesses are identified so that they might be lowered

primary care health provider the physician who sees a patient on a regular basis, particularly for preventative health care

problem drinking alcohol use pattern in which a drinker's behavior creates personal difficulties or difficulties for other people

Prochaska's stages of change the six predictable stages—precontemplation, contemplation, preparation, action, maintenance, and termination—people go through in establishing new habits and patterns of behavior

procrastination a tendency to put off completing tasks until some later time, sometimes resulting in increased stress

procreation reproduction

prophylactic mastectomy elective (voluntary) removal of the breast or breasts to prevent the development of breast cancer

prophylactic oophorectomy surgical removal of the ovaries to prevent cancer in women at high risk of the disease

prostaglandins chemical substances that stimulate smooth muscle contractions

prostate-specific antigen (PSA) test a blood test used to identify prostate-specific antigen, an early indicator that the immune system has recognized and mounted a defense against prostate cancer

prosthodontics dental specialty that focuses on the construction and fitting of artificial appliances to replace missing teeth

proteins compounds composed of chains of amino acids; primary components of muscle and connective tissue

protooncogenes normal genes that hold the potential of becoming cancer-causing oncogenes

psychoactive drugs any substance capable of altering feelings, moods, or perceptions

psychological health a broadly based concept pertaining to cognitive functioning in conjunction with the way people express their emotions, cope with stress, adversity, and success, and adapt to changes in themselves and their environment

psychosocial sexuality masculine and feminine aspects of sexuality

puberty achievement of reproductive ability

pulmonary emphysema irreversible disease process of the lungs in which the alveoli are destroyed

pulmonary hypertension a serious form of high blood pressure that affects lung vessels

purging using vomiting, laxatives, diuretics, enemas, or other medications, or such means as excessive exercise to eliminate food

R

radio frequency radiation electromagnetic radiation with frequency in the range of 3 kilohertz to 300 megahertz, emitted by cell phones, radios, communications transmitters, and other electronic devices

radon a naturally occurring radioactive gas that is emitted during the decay of uranium in soil, rock, and water

reflexology massage applied to specific areas of the feet to treat illness and disease in other areas of the body

refractory errors abnormal patterns of light wave transmission through the structures of the eye

refractory phase that portion of the male's resolution stage during which sexual arousal cannot occur

regulatory genes genes within the cell that control cellular replication and specialization, DNA repair, and tumor suppression

relaxation response physiological state of opposition to the fight-or-flight response of the general adaptation syndrome

resistance stage the second stage of a response to a stressor, during which the body attempts to reestablish its equilibrium or internal balance

resolution stage fourth stage of the sexual response pattern; the return of the body to a preexcitement state

retinal hemorrhage uncontrolled bleeding from arteries within the eye's retina

rheumatic heart disease chronic damage to the heart (especially heart valves) resulting from a streptococcal infection within the heart; a complication associated with rheumatic fever

risk factor a biomedical index or behavioral pattern associated with chronic illness

S

salt sensitive descriptive of people whose bodies overreact to the presence of sodium by retaining fluid and thus increasing blood pressure

satiety state in which there is no longer a desire to eat; fullness

saturated fats dietary fats that influence the formation of cholesterol

schizophrenia one of the most severe mental disorders, characterized by profound distortions in one's thought processes, emotions, perceptions and behavior; symptoms may include hallucinations, delusions, disorganized thinking, and/or maintaining a rigid posture and not moving for hours

sclerotic changes thickening or hardening of tissues

self-actualization the highest level of psychological health at which one reaches his or her highest potential and values truth, beauty, goodness, spirituality, love, humor, and ingenuity

self-care movement trend toward individuals taking increased responsibility for prevention or management of certain health conditions

self-concept an individual's internal picture of him or herself; the way one sees oneself

self-esteem an individual's sense of pride, self-respect, value, and worth

self-fulfilling prophecy the tendency to inadvertently make something more likely to happen as a result of your own expectations and attitudes

semen secretion containing sperm and nutrients discharged from the male urethra at ejaculation

set point a genetically programmed range of body weight beyond which a person finds it difficult to gain or lose additional weight

sex flush reddish skin response that results from increasing sexual arousal

sex reassignment operation surgical procedure designed to remove the external genitalia and replace them with genitalia appropriate to the opposite gender

sexual fantasies fantasies with sexual themes; sexual daydreams or imaginary events

sexuality the quality of being sexual; can be viewed from many biological and psychosocial perspectives

sexually transmitted diseases (STDs) infectious diseases that are spread primarily through intimate sexual contact

shock profound collapse of many vital body functions; evident during acute alcohol intoxication and other serious health emergencies

sidestream smoke the smoke that comes from the burning end of a cigarette, pipe, or cigar

smegma cellular discharge that can accumulate beneath the clitoral hood and the foreskin of an uncircumcised penis

social phobia a phobia characterized by feelings of extreme dread and embarrassment in situations in which public speaking or social interaction is involved

sodomy generally refers to anal or oral sex; a legal term whose definition varies according to state law

solid waste pollutants that are in solid form, including non-hazardous household trash, industrial wastes, mining wastes, and sewage sludge from wastewater treatment plants

spermatogenesis process of sperm production

spermicides chemicals capable of killing sperm

stalking a crime involving an assailant's planned efforts to pursue an intended victim

static stretching the slow lengthening of a muscle group to an extended level of stretch followed by holding the extended position for 10–30 seconds

stem cells premature cells that have the potential to turn into any kind of cells

sterilization generally permanent birth control techniques that surgically disrupt the normal passage of ova or sperm

stimulants psychoactive drugs that stimulate the function of the central nervous system

stress the physiological and psychological state of disruption caused by the presence of an unanticipated, disruptive, or stimulating event

stress response the physiological and psychological responses to positive or negative events that are disruptive, unexpected, or stimulating

stressors factors or events, real or imagined, that elicit a state of stress

sudden cardiac death immediate death resulting from a sudden change in the rhythm of the heart

synapse location at which an electrical impulse from one neuron is transmitted to an adjacent neuron

synergistic drug effect heightened, exaggerated effect produced by the concurrent use of two or more drugs

systolic pressure blood pressure against blood vessel walls when the heart contracts

T

tar particulate phase of tobacco smoke with nicotine and water removed

target heart rate (THR) number of times per minute that the heart must contract to produce a training effect

test anxiety a form of performance anxiety that generates extreme feelings of distress in exam situations

therapeutic cloning the use of certain human replication techniques to reproduce body tissues and cells

thermic effect of food (TEF) refers to the amount of energy our bodies require for the digestion, absorption, and transportation of food

thorax the chest; portion of the torso above the diaphragm and within the rib cage

titration determining a particular level of a drug within the body

tolerance an acquired reaction to a drug; continued intake of the same dose has diminished results

toxic shock syndrome (TSS) potentially fatal condition resulting from the proliferation of certain bacteria in the vagina, whose toxins enter the blood circulation

trace elements minerals whose presence in the body occurs in very small amounts; micronutrient elements

transcervical balloon tuboplasty the use of inflatable balloon catheters to open blocked fallopian tubes; a procedure used for some women with fertility problems

transient ischemic attack (TIA) temporary spasm of a cerebral artery that produces symptoms similar to those of a minor stroke; often a forewarning of a true cerebrovascular accident

trimester three-month period of time; human pregnancies encompass three trimesters

tropospheric ozone ozone is comprised of three oxygen atoms that are bound into a single molecule; tropospheric ozone refers to this substance as it occurs in the lower layer of the atmosphere, close to the ground

tumor mass of cells; may be cancerous (malignant) or noncancerous (benign)

U

unintentional injuries injuries that occur without anyone's intending that harm be done

urethra passageway through which urine leaves the urinary bladder

urethritis infection of the urethra

V

vasectomy surgical procedure in which the vasa deferentia are cut to prevent the passage of sperm from the testicles; the most common form of male sterilization

vegan vegetarian diet vegetarian diet that excludes the use of all animal products, including eggs and dairy products

virulent capable of causing disease

vitamins organic compounds that facilitate the action of enzymes

volatile organic compounds a wide variety of chemicals that contain carbon and readily evaporate into the air

W

wellness the promotion and achievement of optimal health, including physical, emotional, social, intellectual, spiritual, and occupational well-being

withdrawal illness uncomfortable, perhaps toxic response of the body as it attempts to maintain homeostasis in the absence of a drug; also called *abstinence syndrome*

Y

Yerkes-Dodson law a bell-shaped curve demonstrating that there is an optimal level of stress for peak performance. This law states that too little and too much stress are not helpful, while a moderate level of stress is positive and beneficial

Z

zero tolerance laws laws that severely restrict the right to drive for underage drinkers who have been convicted of driving under the influence of *any* alcohol

zoonosis the transmission of diseases from animals to humans

Credits

Chapter Two: p. 53 (Personal Assessment), Modified from Study Guide and Personal Exploration for *Psychology Applied to Modern Life: Adjustment in the 80s,* by Wayne Weitan. Copyright © 1983 by Wadsworth, Inc. Reprinted by permission of Brook/Cole Publishing, Pacific Grove, CA 93950.

Chapter Three: p. 77 (Personal Assessment), Modified from Holmes TH, Rahe RH: The social adjustment rating scale, *Journal of Psychosomatic Research* 11:213–218, 1967; p. 78 (Personal Assessment), Adapted with the permission of The Free Press, a Division of Simon and Schuster Adult Publishing Group, from *Never Good Enough: Freeing Yourself From the Chains of Perfectionism* by Monica Ramirez Basco, Ph.D. Copyright©1999 by Monica Ramirez Basco. All rights reserved.

Chapter Four: p. 80 (Figure 4-1), Data from *The Wirthlin Report,* Harris Interactive Inc. All rights reserved; p. 92 (Star Box),© 2005 American Academy of Orthopaedic Surgeons. Reprinted with permission from *Your Orthopaedic Connection,* the patient education Web site of the American Academy of Orthopaedic Surgeons, located at http:// orthoinfo.aaos.org; p. 96 (Table 4.2), Prentice, WE: *Fitness for College and Life.* ed 5; New York, 1997, McGraw Hill; pp. 99–100 (Personal Assessment), Data from the National Fitness Foundation.

Chapter Five: p. 103 (Table 5.1), From Dietary Guidelines for Americans 2005, United States Department of Health and Human Services; p. 110 (Table 5.2), From Dietary Guidelines for Americans 2005, United States Department of Health and Human Services; pp. 116–117 (Table 5.4), Data from Nutrition Action Newsletter, March 2005; pp. 121–122 (Figure 5-3), Data from US Food and Drug Administration and Wardlow G, Insel P: *Perspectives in Nutrition,* ed 3, St. Louis, 1986, Mosby.; p. 131 (Changing for the Better), Duyff, RL. *American Dietetic Association Complete Food and Nutrition Guide,* 2nd ed., © John Wiley & Sons. This material is used by permission of John Wiley and Sons, Inc.; p. 137 (Personal Assessment), From *Nutrition for a healthy life,* Courtesy of March Leeds.

Chapter Six: pp. 142–143 (Table 6.1), Adapted from *Clinical Guidelines on the Identification, Evaluation, and Treatment of Overweight and Obesity in Adults: The Evidence Report,* National Institutes of Health; p. 144 (Star Box), Data from C. Everett Koop Foundation, American Diabetes Association; p. 153(Table 6.4), Adapted from Guthrie H: *Introductory Nutrition,* ed 7, St. Louis, 1989, Mosby-Year Book, pp. 226–227; p. 154 (Figure 6-4), Opinion Research Institute for *Simply Lite Foods*; pp. 156–157 (Table 6.5), Adapted from Guthrie H: *Introductory Nutrition,* ed 7, St. Louis, 1989, Mosby; p. 159 (Table 6.7), USA Today. Copyright 2002. Reprinted with permission.

Chapter Seven: pp. 180 (Table 7.1), Modified from Muncie Star © 1987. Reprinted with permission; p. 193 (Personal Assessment), US Department of Education, A parent's guide to prevention.

Chapter Eight: p. 197 (Figure 8-1), Data from Core Institute: *2003 Statistics on alcohol and other drug use on American campuses,* Center for Alcohol and Other Drug Studies, Student Health Programs, Southern Illinois University at Carbondale, 2003; p. 200 (Figure 8-2), Data from Core Institute: 2003 *Statistics on alcohol and other drug use on American campuses,* Center for Alcohol and Other Drug Studies, Student Health Programs, Southern Illinois University at Carbondale, 2003; p. 202 (Figure 8-3), Feldman, *Understanding Psychology,* 5e, 2002, McGraw-Hill; p. 204 (Figure 8-4), From Wardlaw G: *Perspectives in Nutrition,* ed 3, St. Louis, Mosby; p. 207 (Changing for the Better), Modified from brochure of the Indiana Alcohol Countermeasure Program; p. 217 (Personal Assessment), From *Are You Troubled by Someone's Drinking?,* 1980, by Al-Anon Family Group Headquarters, Inc. Reprinted by permission of Al-Anon Family Group Headquarters, Inc.

Chapter Nine: p. 219 (Table 9.1), Data from *MMWR* 2004, 52(53): 1277–1280; p. 220 (Table 9.2), Data from *MMWR* 1999, 48(45): 1034–1039 and *MMWR* 2000, 49(SS-2): 1–60; p. 229 (Table 9.3) Adapted from Mulcahy S., *The Toxicology of Cigarette Smoke and Environmental Tobacco Smoke, A Review of Cigarette Smoke and Its Toxicological Effects*; p. 242 (Table 9.5), USA Today. Copyright 2001. Reprinted with permission; p. 247 (Personal Assessment), Reproduced with permission of the American Cancer Society.

Chapter Ten: p. 249 (Figure 10-1) Data from American Heart Association, *Heart Disease and Stroke Statistics—2005 Update,* 2005; p. 250 (Table 10.1) Data from American Heart Association, *Heart Disease and Stroke Statistics—2005 Update,* 2005; p. 256 (Figure 10-3) Reproduced with permission, © 1988, American Heart Association: Heart Facts; p. 259 (Figure 10-4) 1990 *Heart Facts,* art by Donald O'Connor; p. 267 (Personal Assessment) From Howard E: *Health Risks,* Tucson, 1985, Body Press.

Chapter Eleven: p. 272 (Figure 11-1), Data from National Cancer Institute: Horizons of cancer research, NIH Pub. No. 89-3011 © 1989; pp. 278, 284 (Changing for the Better), American Cancer Society; p. 279 (Table 11.2), American Cancer Society; p. 288 (Changing for the Better), Courtesy of the American Academy of Dermatology; p. 301 (Personal Assessment), American Cancer Society.

Chapter Twelve: p. 313 (Table 12.2) Courtesy of United States Department of Health and Human Services, Centers for Disease Control and Prevention; **p. 315 (Table 12.3)**, Courtesy of the National Institute of Allergy and Infectious Diseases; **p. 335 (Personal Assessment)**, Centers for Disease Control and Prevention, Atlanta.

Chapter Thirteen: p. 365 (Personal Assessment), Modified from USA Today.

Chapter Fourteen: p. 369 (Table 14.1), Adapted from Hatcher et al., *Contraceptive Technology*. 17th rev. ed., 1998, Ardent Media, Inc; **p. 395 (Personal Assessment)**, From Haas K, Haas A: *Understanding Sexuality*, 3rd ed., St. Louis, 1993, Mosby.

Chapter Fifteen: p. 402 (Changing for the Better), Pell, AR: *Making the Most of Medicare*, DCI Publishing, 1990, in *insynch*, Erie, PA Spring 1994, Erie Insurance.

Chapter Sixteen: p. 425 (Figure 16-1), Courtesy of the National Committee to Prevent Child Abuse, Chicago, IL; **p. 433 (Changing for the Better)**, From the American College Health Association; **p. 436 (Figure 16-2)**, National Safety Council; **p. 438 (Changing for the Better)**, Adapted from Pynoos J, Cohen E: *Creative ideas for a safe and livable home*, Washington DC, American Association of Retired Persons 1992, and Van Tassel D: *Home safe home*, St. Louis, 1996, GenCare Health Systems.

Chapter Seventeen: p. 457 (Figure 17-2), Environmental Protection Agency.

Chapter Eighteen: p. 485 (Changing for the Better), The National Kidney Foundation Uniform Donor Card is reprinted with permission from the National Kidney Foundation, Inc. Copyright 2000, New York, NY.

Photo Credits

Chapter 1 Page 8: Ryan McVay/PhotoDisc/Getty Images; p. 13: Digital Vision; p. 14: Don Farrall/PhotoDisc/Getty Images

Chapter 2 p. 35: Buccina Studios/Getty Images; p. 40: Mel Curtis/PhotoDisc/Getty Images

Chapter 3 p. 64: The McGraw-Hill Companies, Inc./Andrew Resek, photographer; p. 65: © K. Solveig/zefa/Corbis; p. 69: Ryan McVay/PhotoDisc/Getty Images; p. 81: Ryan McVay/PhotoDisc/Getty Images

Chapter 4 p. 84: Ryan McVay/PhotoDisc/Getty Images; p. 89: Ryan McVay/PhotoDisc/Getty Images; p. 90: Ryan McVay/PhotoDisc/Getty Images; p. 92: (top) www.asicsamerica.com, (left & right) Courtesy Stewart Halperin; p. 99: Courtesy Stewart Halperin; p. 100: Courtesy Stewart Halperin

Chapter 5 p. 111: Ryan McVay/PhotoDisc/Getty Images; p. 112: PhotoDisc/Getty Images; p. 120, © Royalty-Free/Corbis; p. 128: Ryan McVay/PhotoDisc/Getty Images

Chapter 6 p. 141: Suza Scalora/PhotoDisc/Getty Images; p. 145: © Custom Medical Stock Photo; p. 151: Ryan McVay/PhotoDisc/Getty Images

Chapter 7 p. 176: Image100/Corbis; p. 181: PhotoDisc/Getty Images; p. 183: Jack Star/PhotoLink/PhotoDisc/Getty Images; p. 187: © The Cover Story/Corbis

Chapter 8 p. 198: Jim Arbogast/PhotoDisc/Getty Images; p. 205: (top) George Steinmetz, (bottom) Courtesy Mothers Against Drunk Driving

Chapter 9 p. 224: Jack Star/PhotoLink/PhotoDisc/Getty Images; p. 232: Courtesy Wayne Jackson; p. 236: ©Photick/Superstock

Chapter 10 p. 250: Karl Weatherley/PhotoDisc/Getty Images; p. 254: Ryan McVay/PhotoDisc/Getty Images; p. 261: Keith Brofsky/PhotoDisc/Getty Images

Chapter 11 p. 276: © Kevin Laubacher/Getty Images/Taxi; p. 287: From Thibodeau G., Patton, K. *Anatomy and Physiology*, 3/e, St. Louis, 1996. Mosby

Chapter 12 p. 312: Janis Christie/PhotoDisc/Getty Images; p. 327: © Phototake; p. 328: © Custom Medical Stock Photo

Chapter 13 p. 340: Digital Vision/Getty Images; p. 358: Digital Vision/Getty Images; p. 359: Buccina Studios/PhotoDisc/Getty Images

Chapter 14 p. 371: Courtesy Stewart Halperin; p. 373: (left) Linsley Photographics, (right) Courtesy Stewart Halperin; p. 376: (left & right) © Laura J. Edwards, (bottom) Courtesy of Duramed Pharmaceuticals, Inc.; p. 377: Courtesy of Alza Corp.; p. 380: Courtesy Organon USA

Chapter 15 p. 401: Ryan McVay/PhotoDisc/Getty Images; p. 404: Anthony Saint James/PhotoDisc/Getty Images

Chapter 16 p. 432: Ryan McVay/PhotoDisc/Getty Images; p. 435: Ryan McVay/PhotoDisc/Getty Images; p. 437: Ryan McVay/PhotoDisc/Getty Images

Chapter 17 p. 451: Nick Koudis/PhotoDisc/Getty Images; p. 456: Kent Knudson/PhotoDisc/Getty Images; p. 463: Digital Vision/Getty Images; p. 464: Tomi/PhotoLink/PhotoDisc/Getty Images

Chapter 18 p. 478: © John Freilich/Corbis Sygma

Index

CNS. *See* central nervous system
CO. *See* carbon monoxide
cocaine, 181–183
    effects on body, 182*f*
    injecting, *183*
codependence, 210
coenzymes, 106
coffeehouses, *181*
cognitive self-talk, 72–73
cohabitation, 357
coitus, 350
Colbert, Don, 145
COLD. *See* chronic obstructive lung disease
cold turkey, 188
colds. *See* common cold
college students
    cigarette smoking among, 220
    disabled, 12
    minority, 11–12
    non-traditional age undergraduate, 11
    procrastination among, 66
    traditional-age undergraduate, 10–11
    working, 63*f*
colonoscopy, 285
colorectal cancer
    early detection of, 285
    prevention of, 285
    risk factors for, 285
    treatment of, 285–286
coming out, 355
Commercial Closet Association, 336
common cold, 312–314
    hand-washing and, *312*
    influenza *v.*, 315*t*
communication
    assertive, 35
    conflict resolution through, 359
    intergenerational, 11
    nonverbal, 34–35
    with patients, 399
    in relationships, 36
    style, 50
    verbal, 34
community environment, 453–460
community health promotion, 7
community of faith, 48
compatibility assessment, 365
complementary, alternative, integrative care
    practitioners, 403–405
    selecting, 406
complete protein, 105
compliance, 6
    defined, 398

comprehensive health assessment, 21–30
compulsion, 176, 223
computed tomography (CT), 144, 263
conditioning, 89
condoms, 372
    defined, 373
    effectiveness of, 375, *375*
    female, *373*
    male, *373*
conflict resolution, through
    communication, 359
conflict-management, enhancing skills for,
    35–36
congenital heart disease, 263
congenital rubella syndrome (CSR), 263
congestive heart failure, 264
consultation, 402
consumer advocacy groups, 399, 400*t*
consumer fraud, 416–417
contact inhibition, 271
contraception. *See also* birth control
    birth control *v.*, 367–368
    defined, 367
    effectiveness of, 368
    emergency, 380–381
    methods of, 368
contraceptive patch, 380
contraceptive ring, *380*
    defined, 379
contraceptive sponge, 376
contraindications, 379
Cookie Monster, 134
cooldown, 89
COPD. *See* chronic obstructive pulmonary
    disease
coping strategies, 68
cord blood stem cells, 310
coronary arteries, 250
coronary artery bypass surgery, 259
coronary artery disease, 258
coronary heart disease, 258–260
coronary repair
    alcohol and, 260
    angioplasty, 259
    artificial hearts, 260
    aspirin and, 259–260
    coronary artery bypass surgery, 259
    heart transplant, 260
corpus luteum, 346
cosmetic surgery, 139
court shoes, 92
Cowper's glands, 342
CPR. *See* cardiopulmonary resuscitation

crabs. *See* pubic lice
crack, 183–184
crank, 181
creatine, risks/benefits of, 93
creative expression, 48–49
creativity, 48–49
cremation, 484
crimes
    alcohol-related social problems and,
      206–207
    bias/hate, 427–428
    violent, 423, 426
criticism, accepting, 36
Crohn's disease, 291
cross-tolerance, 179
cross-training, 94
    shoes, 92
cruciferous vegetables, 111
cryonics, 487
crypts, 484
crystal, 181
crystal meth, 181–182
CSR. *See* congenital rubella syndrome
CT. *See* computed tomography
cultural factors, obesity and, 148
cunnilingus, 352
curette, 383
curiosity, 48
CVD. *See* cardiovascular disease
cystitis, 331

D

daily planner, keeping, 66
date rape, 430–431
    avoiding, 433
    depressants, 184
    drugs, 431
D&C. *See* dilation and suction curettage
D&E. *See* dilation and evacuation
de Varona, Donna, 176
death. *See also* dying
    accidental, 476
    brain, 474
    from cardiovascular disease, 249*f*
    causes of, 5, 10, 13
    cellular, 474
    of children, 479
    clinical determinants of, 473
    coping with causes of, 476–477
    cultural differences about, 483
    definitions of, 474–474
    by murder, 477
    near experiences of, 478

grain group foods, guidelines for eating, 112–114

GRAS. *See* generally recognized as safe

Greeks Advocating Mature Management of Alcohol (GAMMA), 208–209

green space, 459

"Greenhouse Effect," 462

greenhouse gases, 462

grief, 480–482

groin pull, 96

ground burials, 483

guided imagery, 71

gun violence, 426–427

H

H5N1, 322

HAART. *See* highly active antiretroviral therapy

haemophilus influenzae type B, 311

Hallelujah Diet (Malkmus), 145

hallucinations, 46, 186

hallucinogens, 184–185

hamstring pull, 96

hand-washing
  common cold and, *312*
  how to, 314

hantavirus pulmonary syndrome, 319

hashish, 186

HBV. *See* type B hepatitis

HCV. *See* type C hepatitis

HDLs. *See* high-density lipoproteins

health
  in 21st century, 10
  claims, 119
  composition of, 17–18
  concerns, 9–10
  consumer skills assessment, 421
  definition of, 4–6, 17–18
  educators, 400
  multiple dimensions of, 14–18
  role of, 17–18
  taking charge of, 409

health care
  access to, 414
  costs, 410–411
  quackery, 416–417

health care facilities, 409–410
  patients' rights in, 410*t*

health care providers, 401
  complementary, alternative, integrative care, 403–405
  consulting, 401–403
  patient communication and, 399

health information, 397–400
  on Internet, 3
  labels and, 398
  sources of, 397–400

health insurance, 411
  selecting, 412

health maintenance organizations (HMOs), 6, 413

health promotion, 6–7, 18

health reference publications, 399

health-related products, 414–415

healthy body weight, 143–144

Healthy People 2000, 8, 228

Healthy People 2010, 8, 18, 228

heart, 250–251, 251*f*
  artificial, 260
  exercise and, *250*
  stimulation, 251
  transplant, 260
  tumors of, 264

Heart and Stroke Statistical Update (2004), 249

heart attack. *See also* sudden cardiac death
  emergency response to, 258
  signs of, 257
  taking action for, 257

heart disease. *See also* congestive heart failure; coronary heart disease; rheumatic heart disease
  aerobic exercise and, 253
  children and, 251
  congenital, 263
  race and, 252
  risk assessment, 267–268
  women and, 253

heart rate, determining, 87

height-weight tables, 142–143

hemorrhage, 262*f*

hepatitis
  type A, 320
  type B, 310, 320–321
  type C, 321
  type D, 321

herbalism, 405

heredity, 50

heroin, 188

herpes simplex
  infection, 328*f*
  prevalence of, 328
  prevention of, 329
  talking about, 329

heterosexuality, 354
  bisexuality and, 355

hierarchy of needs, 46–47

high blood pressure, 254

high-density lipoproteins (HDLs), 106, 256–257
  classifications of, 258
  defined, 256
  nicotine and, 232

highly active antiretroviral therapy (HAART), 324

high-protein/low-carbohydrate diets, 155

high-risk health behavior, 18
  defined, 5

Hippocrates, 405

HIV
  diagnosis of, 323–324
  prenatal testing for, 19
  preventing, 325
  signs/symptoms of, 323
  spectrum of, 324*t*
  spread of, 322–323
  treatment of, 324–325
  women and, 323
  world statistics on, 323*f*

HMOs. *See* Health maintenance organizations

Hodgkin's disease, 286

holistic health, 14

home
  accident prevention in, 437–438
  care, 408

homeopathy, 404–405

homesickness, 61
  combating, 63

homicide, 423. *See also* murder

homosexuality, 336, 354. *See also* gays; lesbian

HONC. *See* Hooked on Nicotine Checklist

Hooked on Nicotine Checklist (HONC), 221

hormonal factors, obesity and, 147

hormone replacement therapy (HRT), 85, 275
  defined, 347

hospice, 409–410
  care, 480, *480*
  for terminal illness, 479–480

hospitals, 409
  wiring of, 419

host, 306

host negligence, 208

hot flashes, 347

HPV. *See* human papillomavirus

HRT. *See* hormone replacement therapy

human papillomavirus (HPV), 327, 327*f*

human papillomavirus infections, 280
humor, psychological health and, 36
humoral immunity, 307
hunger-satisfying products, 157
Hurricane Katrina, 76
hydrostatic weighing, 145–146
hymen, 344
hyperglycemia, 293
hypertension, 55, 260. *See also* high blood
    pressure
    analgesics and, 265
    children with, 248
    prevalence of, 260
    prevention/treatment of, 261
    as silent process, 248, 261
    women and, 265
hypertonic saline solution, 383
hypnosis, 71–72
hypothalamus, 147–148
hypothyroidism, 147
hypoxia, 230, 235
hysterectomy, 381

I

IBD. *See* inflammatory bowel disease
ice, 181
ICSH. *See* interstitial cell-stimulating
    hormone (ICSH)
ICSI. *See* intracytoplasmic sperm
    injection
identity forming, 12
identity theft, 441
    defined, 433
    reducing risk for, 434
illness. *See also* terminal illness
    foodborne, 124
    tobacco use and, 230–235
    withdrawal, 179
immune response, 308–310, 309*f*
immune system
    arming of, 308
    defined, 307
    divisions of, 307–308
immunity, 308–309
immunizations, 310–312
    for adults, 313*t*
    of children, 312
in vitro, 295
in vitro fertilization and embryo transfer
    (IVF-ET), 391
inactivity, obesity and, 150
incomplete protein, 105
incubation stage, 306

independence, 48
    in young adulthood, 12
independent practice associations
    (IPAs), 413
indirect (passive) euthanasia, 477
indirect transmission, 306
indoor air quality, 446
infatuation, 356
infection
    chain of, 304–306, 305*f*
    pelvic, 304
    stages of, 306–307
infectious disease. *See also* infection
    aging and, 311
    antimicrobial cleaning products and, 308
    causes/management of, 312–325
    living with, 317
    in older adults, 311
    pathogen and, 305*t*
    transmission, 304–307
infertility, 235, 390
    coping with, 391–392
    help for, 391
inflammatory bowel disease (IBD), 291
influenza, 314–315
    common cold *v.*, 315*t*
inhalants, 188–189
injectable contraceptives, 379
injuries
    during exercise, 95, 96*t*
    intentional, 423
    unintentional, 434
inner self, 48
Insel, Thomas, 50
Institute of Medicine, 7–8
insulin, 294
    defined, 292
intellectual dimension of health, 15–16, 18
intensity, 87
intentional injuries, 423
intercourse, 352–353
intergenerational communication, 11
Internet. *See also* Web sites
    addiction to, 49
    as health information source, 3, 396–399
    pornography, 432
    stress and, 54–55
interstitial cell-stimulating hormone
    (ICSH), 340
intimacy
    defined, 356
    nurturing in young adulthood, 13–14
intimate partner violence (IPV), 424–425

intracytoplasmic sperm injection (ICSI), 391
intrauterine device (IUD), 377
intrinsic resources, 17
involuntary regurgitation, 203
involuntary smoking, 237–239, 238, 239
ionizing radiation, 459–460
IPAs. *See* independent practice associations
IPV. *See* intimate partner violence
irradiation of food, 125
isokinetic exercises, 88
    defined, 83
isokinetic machines, 33
isometric exercises, 82
isotonic resistance exercises, 88
    defined, 82
It's Not about the Bike: My Journey Back to
    Life (Armstrong), 82
IVF-ET. *See* in vitro fertilization and
    embryo transfer

J

Jenny Craig, 155
Johnson, Magic, 303
Jones, Max, 437
Jordan, Michael, 176
"juice," 94
junk food, in schools, 134

K

Kennedy, John F., 86
Kennedy, Joseph P., 86
Kennedy, Rosemary, 86
ketamine, 185
ketosis, 155
Kevorkian, Jack, 478, *478*
Kirkpatrick, Jean, 213
"kissing disease," 318
Klu Klux Klan, 428
Kübler-Ross, Elisabeth, 474

L

labels
    "black box," 52
    children and, 122
    food, 115, 121*f*–122*f*, 122
    on OTC drugs, 416*f*
    as source of health information, 398
labia minora, 343
lactase deficiency, 130
lactose intolerance, 130
lactovegetarian diet, 130
The Lance Armstrong Performance Program:
    Seven Weeks to the Perfect Ride
    (Armstrong)

nitrate, 451
nitroglycerine, 258
NK. *See* natural killer
nocturnal emission, 337
noise, 452–453
nomogram
    for BMI, 144*f*
    defined, 142
nonconformity, 48
nonionizing radiation, 451–452
    cell phones and, 450–451
    defined, 450
nonspecific urethritis (NSU), 326
non-traditional students, 11
nonverbal communication, 34–35, *35*
Norcross, John, 9
norepinephrine, 226
No-Tobacco Day, 226
NRA. *See* National Rifle Association
NSU. *See* nonspecific urethritis
nurse professionals, 407
nurture, 40
nutraceuticals, 119
Nutri Sure Losers, 155
nutrient-dense foods, 108
nutrients, 102
nutrition, 69
    on food labels, 121*f*–122*f*
    international concerns for, 131
    older adults and, 130–131

O

oat bran, 108
obesity, 55
    in African Americans, 148
    in Asian Americans, 148
    as cardiovascular risk factor, 255
    in Caucasians, 148
    causes of, 146
    in children, 134, 150, 170
    cultural factors and, 148
    curbing, 150
    defined, 141
    diabetes mellitus and, 294
    dietary practices and, 148–149
    environmental factors and, 148–149
    genetic factors and, 146–147
    health risks of, 144
    hormonal factors and, 147
    inactivity and, 150
    metabolic factors and, 147–148
    morbid, 141
    physiological factors and, 147

psychological factors and, 149
    rates of, 140
    sleep and, 170
    societal factors and, 148
    surgeries, 180–182
obsessive-compulsive disorder (OCD), 45
occupational dimension of health, 16, 18
OCD. *See* obsessive-compulsive disorder
Office of Dietary Supplements, 42
oil group, guidelines for eating, 114
older adults
    home accident prevention for, 438
    infectious diseases in, 311
    maltreatment of, 426
    nutrition and, 130–131
oncogenes
    defined, 271
    formation of, 271
    HER-2, 280
opportunistic infections, 322
optimism, 37–38, 50
    compared to pessimism, 37
    learned, 37
optometrists, 407
oral cancer, detection of, 237
oral contraceptives, *377*
    defined, 377
    for men, 378
    negative side effects of, 378
    pill, 377
    tobacco use and, 236
oral-genital stimulation, 352
organ donation, 485
organic foods, 118, *120*, 145
orgasmic platform, 344
orgasmic stage, 347
orlistat, 160
Orser, Brian, 86
orthodontics, 406
osteoarthritis, 85
osteopathy, 403
osteoporosis, 85
OTC drugs, 157, 415
    labels on, 416*f*
OTC. *See* over the counter
outercourse, 368
ovarian cancer
    early detection of, 282
    prevention of, 282
    treatment of, 282–283
ovariectomy, 381
ovaries, 344
over the counter (OTC), 122

Overeaters Anonymous, 167
overeating, 149
overload principle, 82
overweight
    as cardiovascular risk factor, 255
    defined, 141
ovolactovegetarian diet
    defined, 128
    food pyramid for, 129
ovulation, 346
oxidation, 201
OxyContin, 188
oxygen debt, 81
ozone, 455–456
    depletion, 463
    nonattainment of, by U.S. county, 457*f*

P

PAD. *See* peripheral artery disease
Paget's disease, 277
PAHs. *See* polycyclic aromatic hydrocarbons
PAI. *See* passively acquired immunity
pancreatic cancer, 286
pandemic, 321–322
    defined, 304
panic disorder, 45
Pap test
    defined, 280
    meaning of results, 281*t*
parenting skills, young adults and, 14
Parents Against Drugs, 188
partial-birth abortion, 384
    U.S. Supreme Court and, 383
particulate phase, 228
parties, drinking and, 207–208
Partnership for a Drug-Free America, 188
passive immunity, 308
passive smoking, 237–239
passively acquired immunity (PAI), 308
patellofemoral knee pain, 96
pathogen
    defined, 304
    infectious disease and, 305*t*
patients' rights, 410*t*
peak smokers, 225
pelvic infection, 304
pelvic inflammatory disease (PID), 326, 372
penis, 343
perfectionism, 34, 67–68
    alleviating stress of, 68
    assessment of, 78
    defined, 67
    responding to, 67

periodic abstinence, 370–372, 370f

periodontal disease, 237

peripheral artery disease (PAD), 264

peritonitis, 327

permanence, 37

permanent language, 37

persistence, 49

personal environment, 445–453

personal space, 35

personalities, 39

personalization, 38

perspiration, 107

pervasiveness, 37

pesco-vegetarian diet, 130

pessimism, 33, 38

    compared to optimism, 37

    self-esteem and, 38

phagocytic leukocytes, 381

phencylidine (PCP), 185–186

phenfen, 159

phenlpropanolamine (PPA), 157

phish, 54–55

phlebitis, 264

PHT. *See* postmenopausal hormone

    replacement therapy

physical activity

    calories expended during, 153t

    defined, 80

    preferences, 80f

physical dimension of health,

    14–15, 18

physical fitness

    activity level and, 91

    assessing level of, 99–100

    of children, 94–95

    components of, 80–84

    defined, 80

    dreaming and, 95

    questions about, 90–95

    sleep and, 95

physician assisted suicide, 477–478

physicians, *401*

    choosing, 402

    training of, 403

Physicians' Desk Reference, 414

physiological factors, obesity and, 147

phytochemicals, 107

PID. *See* pelvic inflammatory disease

pipe smoking, 222–223

placebo pills, 378

placenta

    defined, 203

    delivery of, 389–390

Planned Parenthood Federation of

    America, 366

plasma nicotine, 226

plateau stage, 347

platelet adhesiveness, 232

platonic, 357

PMR. *See* progressive muscle relaxation

PMS. *See* premenstrual syndrome

pneumococcal infection, 311

pneumonia, 318

polio, 311

pollution

    from computers, 460

    land, 458–459

    water, 446–458, 464

polycyclic aromatic hydrocarbons (PAHs), 454

polyps, 285

polysaccharides, 103

polyvinyl chloride (PVC), 451

population explosion, 461–462

population, growth of, 461f

portal of entry, 306

portal of exit, 306

portion control, 155

positive caloric balance, 140

post-abortion syndrome, 384

postmenopausal hormone replacement

    therapy (PHT), 253

postmortem arrangements

    in outer space, 484

    star naming, 484

postpartum, 390

posttraumatic stress disorder, 76, 431

potentiated effect, 189

PPA. *See* phenlpropanolamine

PPOs. *See* preferred provider organizations

precontemplation stage, of change, 9

preferred provider organizations (PPOs), 413

pregnancy, 385–388

    drinking and, 203–205

    ectopic (tubal), 235

    gonorrhea and, 328

    signs of, 387

    tobacco smoke and, *236*

    weight gain/loss and, 17

premenstrual syndrome (PMS), 346

preparation stage, of change, 9

prepuce, 343

prescription drugs, 414

    development of new, 414–415

present situation, focusing on, 36

prevention, 402

preventive medicine, 4–6

primary health care providers, 402

private hospitals, 409

proactive approach to life, 38–40

probiotics, 123

    defined, 119

problem drinking, 208–212

Prochaska, James, 9

Prochaska's Stages of Change, 9

procrastination, 66–67

    among college students, 66

    defined, 66

    self-esteem and, 67

procreation, 352

prodromal stage, 306

professional journals, as health information

    source, 3

progressive muscle relaxation (PMR), 71

proof, 200

prophylactic mastectomy, 276

prophylactic oophorectomy, 282

prospective medicine, 4–6

prostate cancer

    early detection of, 283

    prevention of, 283

    risk factors for, 283

    treatment of, 283

prostate gland, 342

prostate-specific antigen (PSA), 283

prosthodontics, 406

prostitution, 432

protein-rich food, guidelines for eating, 112

proteins, 105

proto-oncogenes, 271

PSA. *See* prostate-specific antigen

pseudodoephedrine, restrictions on, 192

psilocybin, 185

psychoactive drugs, 175

    categories of, 180t

    defined, 178

    effects of on CNS, 175f

psychological disorders, 40

    ADD, 45–46

    anxiety, 44–45

    bipolar, 43–44

    mood, 40–43

    schizophrenia, 46

psychological factors, obesity and, 149

psychological health, 32–33

    challenges to, 40–46

    characteristics of, 33

    defined, 32

    enhancing, 34–35

    enhancing through humor, 36